INTEGRATIVE MEDICINE

A New Approach to Medical Diagnosis & Treatment

Jun Liu, M.D.

Copyright © 2007, 2008, 2009, 2010 by Jun Liu, M.D.

All rights reserved. This book, or any parts thereof, may not be used, reproduced or transmitted in any manner or by any means, electronic or mechanical, including photocopy, recording, or any information storage and retrieval system, without written permission.

Request for permission to make copies of any part of the work should be mailed to:

Jun Liu, M.D.
P.O. Box 1852
Dacula, GA 30019
info@mdliu.com
www.MDLIU.com

Notice: The author and the publisher of this book have made every effort to ensure that the information contained herein is accurate and compatible with the standards generally accepted at the time of publication. Nevertheless, it is difficult to ensure that all the information given is entirely accurate for all circumstances. This book is not intended as a substitute for the medical advice of a trained health professional. All matters regarding your health require medical supervision from your physician. Any application of the contents of this book is at the reader's discretion and sole risk. The author and publisher disclaim any liability, loss, or damage incurred as a consequence, directly or indirectly, of the use and application of any of the contents of this book.

ISBN: 978-0-578-02824-8

Printed in the United States of America

DEDICATION

To my wonderful and loving wife Ying, who is full of courage, enthusiasm, and intelligence.

To my children, Grace and Rachael, who bring joy and comfort to my life.

To my mother who encouraged me to obtain the best education possible.

To my father who always believed in me.

ACKNOWLEDGEMENTS

I gratefully acknowledge the thoughtful comments of Dr. John P. Heilman.

TABLE OF CONTENTS

INTRODUCTION 9

PART ONE: THE BASICS OF TRADITIONAL CHINESE MEDICINE 11

CHAPTER 1: ETIOLOGY OF DISEASE 13
- *1. The Six Exogenous Pathogenic Factors* 13
- *2. Pestilential Factors* 14
- *3. Seven Emotions* 14
- *4. Diet, Nutrition and Life Style* 15
- *5. Overstrain* 16
- *6. Traumatic Injuries* 16
- *7. Parasitosis* 16
- *8. Phlegm Retention and Blood Stasis* 16
- *9. Five Endogenous Pathogenetic Factors* 16
- *10. Weak Constitution* 17

CHAPTER 2: THE BASIC PHYSIOLOGY AND PATHOGENESIS OF DISEASE 18
- *1. Eight Principles/Parameters* 18
  - 1) Exterior and Interior 18
  - 2) Cold and Heat 19
  - 3) Deficiency and Excess 20
  - 4) Yin and Yang 21
- *2. The Five Phases/Elements* 23
  - 1) Generating 24
  - 2) Controlling/Restricting 25
  - 3) Overacting 25
  - 4) Insulting 25
- *3. The Three Humors: Qi, Blood, and Phlegm/Fluid* 26
  - 1) Qi 26
  - 2) Blood 28
  - 3) Phlegm and Fluid 30
- *4. The Ten Organ Systems* 33
  - A. Physiology and Pathology of the Ten Organ Systems 33
    - 1) Heart and Small Intestine 33
    - 2) Liver and Gallbladder 37
    - 3) Spleen and Stomach 42
    - 4) Lung and large Intestine 46
    - 5) Kidney and Bladder 50
  - B. The Relationship between Different Visceral Organs 53
  - C. Complicated Organ Dysfunctions 54
- *5. The Three Pathogens (Wind, Fire and Dampness) Playing both Internal and External Roles* 56
  - 1) Wind 56
  - 2) Dampness 57
  - 3) Fire 58
- *6. Six Stages (Syndromes of the Six Channels)* 60
- *7. Four Divisions/Levels of Febrile Diseases: Wei (defensive), Qi, Ying (nutritive) and Xue (blood)* 70
  - 1) Wei (Defensive) Level Syndrome 70
  - 2) Qi Level Syndrome 71
  - 3) Ying (Nutritive) Level Syndrome 71
  - 4) Xue (Blood) Level Syndrome 72

CHAPTER 3: DIAGNOSTIC METHODS OF DISORDERS 73
- *1. Inspection* 73
  - 1) Observation of the Spirit 73
  - 2) Observation of Complexion 73
  - 3) Observation of Body Structure, Posture and Movement 74

       4) Observation of the Tongue ... 74
   2. Auscultation and Olfaction ... 77
       1) Listening ... 77
       2) Smelling ... 77
   3. Interrogation ... 78
   4. Palpation ... 78
       1) Body Palpation ... 78
       2) Pulse Feeling ... 79

CHAPTER 4: THERAPEUTICS ... 81
   1. Therapeutic Principles ... 81
   2. Therapeutic Methods ... 82

PART TWO: MEDICAL DIAGNOSIS AND TREATMENT ... 85

CHAPTER 1: DISORDERS OF THE RESPIRATORY SYSTEM ... 87
   1. Acute Upper Respiratory Tract Infections (URIs, or Common Cold) ... 87
   2. Acute Bronchitis (Acute Tracheobronchitis) ... 91
   3. Chronic Bronchitis ... 94
   4. Obstructive Pulmonary Emphysema (Emphysema) ... 99
   5. Bronchial Asthma (Asthma) ... 102
   6. Bronchiectasis ... 109
   7. Chronic Respiratory Failure ... 112
   8. Acute Respiratory Distress Syndrome (ARDS) ... 116
   9. Pneumonia ... 119
   10. Lung Abscess ... 123
   11. Pulmonary Tuberculosis (TB) ... 126
   12. Primary Bronchogenic Carcinoma (Lung Cancer) ... 130
   13. Pleural Effusion ... 134
   14. Cough ... 136
   15. Influenza ... 142

CHAPTER 2: DISORDERS OF THE CARDIOVASCULAR SYSTEM ... 149
   1. Chronic Heart Failure ... 149
   2. Cardiac Arrhythmia ... 153
   3. Sudden Cardiac Arrest (Sudden Cardiac Death, SCA) ... 159
   4. High Blood Pressure (Hypertension) ... 162
   5. Atherosclerosis ... 166
   6. Coronary Atherosclerotic Heart Disease (Ischemic Heart Disease) ... 168
   7. Rheumatic Valvular Heart Disease ... 178
   8. Infective Endocarditis ... 182
   9. Cardiomyopathy ... 186
   10. Viral Myocarditis ... 189
   11. Acute Pericarditis ... 193
   12. Constrictive Pericarditis ... 197
   13. Chronic Cor Pulmonale (Pulmonary Heart Disease) ... 198

CHAPTER 3: DISORDERS OF THE GASTROINTESTINAL SYSTEM ... 203
   1. Chronic Gastritis ... 203
   2. Peptic Ulcer ... 207
   3. Upper Gastrointestinal Bleeding (UGIB) ... 211
   4. Ulcerative Colitis (UC) ... 213
   5. Crohn's Disease (CD) ... 217
   6. Gastric Carcinoma ... 221
   7. Carcinoma of Esophagus ... 225
   8. Carcinoma of the Large Intestine (Colon Cancer, Colorectal Carcinoma) ... 228

9. Primary Carcinoma of the Liver	*232*
10. Hepatic Cirrhosis	*235*
11. Hepatic Encephalopathy/Hepatic Coma	*239*
12. Viral Hepatitis	*242*
13. Cholecystitis	*247*
14. Acute Pancreatitis	*251*
15. Chronic Pancreatitis	*254*
CHAPTER 4: DISORDERS OF THE KIDNEY AND URINARY TRACT	259
1. Acute Glomerulonephritis (AGN)	*259*
2. Rapidly Progressive Glomerulonephritis (RPGN)	*264*
3. Chronic Glomerulonephritis (CGN)	*266*
4. Latent Glomerulonephritis (LGN)	*270*
5. Nephrotic Syndrome (NS)	*273*
6. Acute Tubulointerstitial Nephritis (Acute Interstitial Nephritis, AIN)	*277*
7. Chronic Tubulointerstitial Nephritis (Chronic Interstitial Nephritis, CTIN or CIN)	*281*
8. Diabetic Nephropathy (DN)	*285*
9. Lupus Nephritis (LN)	*288*
10. Urinary Tract Infection (UTI)	*291*
11. Urinary Stone Disease (Urolithiasis)	*295*
12. Acute Renal Failure (ARF)	*298*
13. Chronic Renal Failure (CRF)	*302*
CHAPTER 5: HEMATOLOGY	308
1. Anemia	*308*
2. Leukemia	*317*
3. Lymphoma	*325*
4. Allergic Purpura (Henoch-Schönlein Purpura)	*330*
5. Idiopathic Thrombocytopenia Purpura (ITP)	*333*
6. Leukopenia	*336*
7. Disseminated Intravascular Coagulation (DIC)	*339*
CHAPTER 6: ENDOCRINOLOGY AND METABOLISM	344
1. Diabetes Insipidus (DI)	*344*
2. Hyperthyroidism (Thyrotoxicosis)	*346*
3. Hypothyroidism and Myxedema	*350*
4. Subacute Thyroiditis	*353*
5. Hashimoto's Thyroiditis (Chronic Lymphocytic Thyroiditis)	*355*
6. Pheochromocytoma	*357*
7. Cushing's Syndrome (Hypercortisolism)	*360*
8. Addison's Disease (Chronic Adrenocortical Hypofunction)	*363*
9. Diabetes Mellitus (DM)	*366*
10. Hyperlipoproteinemia	*372*
11. Obesity	*376*
12. Gout	*380*
CHAPTER 7: DISORDERS OF CONNECTIVE TISSUE AND JOINTS	384
1. Rheumatoid Arthritis (RA)	*384*
2. Systemic Lupus Erythematosus (SLE)	*388*
3. Sjögren's Syndrome	*394*
4. Osteoarthritis	*396*
CHAPTER 8: NEUROLOGICAL DISORDERS	401
1. Trigeminal Neuralgia (tic douloureux)	*401*
2. Bell's Palsy (Idiopathic Facial Palsy)	*405*
3. Acute Idiopathic Polyneuropathy (AIDP, Guillain-Barré Syndrome)	*408*
4. Transient Ischemic Attacks (TIA)	*411*

5. Stroke (thrombotic Infarct, embolic Infarct and Hemorrhage)	*413*
6. Parkinson's Disease (Paralysis Agitans)	*419*
7. Epilepsy	*422*
8. Vascular Dementia (Multi-Infarct Dementia or Atherosclerotic Dementia)	*426*
9. Alzheimer's Disease (AD)	*429*
10. Myasthenia Gravis (MG)	*435*
CHAPTER 9: PSYCHIATRIC DISORDERS	440
1. Insomnia/Dyssomnias	*440*
2. Mood Disorders (Depression and Mania)	*442*
3. Schizophrenia	*447*
4. Autism	*449*
5. Impotence/Erectile Dysfunction	*451*
6. Frigidity and Disorders of Sexual Desire	*452*
7. Premature Ejaculation	*453*
CHAPTER 10: ENVIRONMENTAL HAZARDS AND POISONING	456
1. Acute Carbon Monoxide Poisoning	*456*
2. Barbiturates Poisoning	*459*
3. Alcohol (Ethanol) Poisoning	*461*
4. Heat Disorders (Heat Syncope, Heat Cramps, Heat Exhaustion and Heat Stroke)	*464*
CHAPTER 11: OTHER DISEASES	467
1. Headache	*467*
2. Chest Pain	*470*
3. Abdominal Pain	*473*
4. Lumbar Pain	*475*
5. Vertigo/Dizziness	*477*
6. Diarrhea	*480*
7. Constipation	*482*
8. Vomiting	*485*
9. Edema	*487*
10. Jaundice	*491*
11. Spermatorrhea (Nocturnal Emission and Spontaneous Emission)	*494*
12. Perspiration (Hidrosis)	*496*
13. Acquired Immune Deficiency Syndrome (AIDS)	*498*
14. Epistaxis	*503*
15. Gingival Hemorrhage	*505*
16. Hemoptysis	*505*
17. Hematemesis	*507*
18. Hematochezia	*508*
19. Hematuria	*508*
APPENDIX I: PREPARATION OF DECOCTION AND PRESCRIPTIONS	**511**
APPENDIX II: COMMONLY USED HERBS AND DOSAGE	**518**
APPENDIX III: COMMONLY USED HERBAL PRESCRIPTIONS/FORMULA	**558**
INDEX	**655**

INTRODUCTION

Conventional western medicine leads medical innovation, scientific research and the advancement of medical technology. However, conventional medicine often sees the patient as a collection of parts rather than a whole individual. It shows insufficient concern for overall feelings of patients during the 3-10min doctor's office/hospital visit, and it is often criticized for paying too much attention to laboratory tests, and for its relying too much on high-tech equipment or chemical manipulation. Practitioners of conventional medicine have been widely criticized for over-prescribing drugs. There is a growing displeasure of chemical drug treatments that sometimes appear to be worse than the disease itself. 225,000 patients die each year in the US from iatrogenic causes (direct result of treatments by physicians), including 7000 deaths from medication errors in hospitals and 106,000 deaths from adverse effects of medications. A recent study by CDC (Centers for Disease Control and Prevention) estimated that the number of healthcare-associated infections (HAIs) was approximately 1.7 million in 2002 and estimated deaths associated with HAIs alone in U.S. hospitals were 98,987.

Traditional Chinese Medicine (TCM) is attractive to many people because it searches for the primary cause of a disease and treats it accordingly; it promotes disease prevention and sets prevention of diseases as the priority; it makes an overall analysis of a disease and treats the whole person; it promotes good health and well-being, and it provides more personalized approach to patient concerns. In addition, Traditional Chinese medicine has thousands of years of history, but only those herbs, prescriptions, techniques that were proved to be effective have remained in use. National Center for Complementary and Alternative Medicine (NCCAM), which is a center within the National Institutes of Health, defines TCM as a "whole medical system", and describes it as involving "complete systems of theory and practice that have evolved independently from or parallel to allopathic (conventional) medicine."

Every medicine is effective for some but not all conditions; and many factors, e.g., body, heredity, mind, thoughts, beliefs, emotions, stress, spirit, nutrition, exercise, family issues, society, religion, culture, environment, nature, etc, have a great impact on both health and disease; therefore, an integrated medicine is needed to address the issue. Integrative medicine emphasizes the combination of both conventional and alternative approaches to address the biological, psychological, social and spiritual aspects of health and illness. It is a state-of-the-art modern medical care drawn from the very best conventional and alternative/complementary medicine evidence-based strategies. It focuses on the whole person; it addresses all dimensions of an individual's life and considers all factors that affect health and disease. Whenever possible, it favors the use of natural, low-tech, low-cost and less invasive interventions. It facilitates the human capacity for optimal health and healing. Integrative medicine emphasizes the importance of partnership between the practitioner and the patient and collaboration among practitioners.

In the United States, the practice of TCM has risen dramatically in recent years. NCCAM stated that more than one-third of American adults reported using some form of CAM (complementary and alternative medicine) and that visits to CAM providers each year exceed those to primary care physicians. The Food and Drug Administration (FDA) has also seen an increase in the number of CAM products imported into the Unites States. However, the barrier between conventional western medicine and TCM is still big. Most well-trained physicians in TCM, especially in the United States, lack the knowledge of western medicine, while many well-trained doctors in western medicine don't know anything about TCM at all. The world is flat now; many patients and health-conscious people have ways to access TCM and would like to apply it to their daily life; many healthcare practitioners would like to expand their practice to include TCM or would like to know enough to assess what their patients are taking. However, because of its complicated, mysterious and abstruse concepts, theories and philosophies, TCM is difficult for the west to understand, let alone to practice.

The book *INTEGRATIVE MEDICINE: A New Approach to Medical Diagnosis & Treatment* is a well designed and easy to read book. Its TCM part sources mainly from the classic Chinese medicine texts, including both ancient literature and modern books, and from the author's rich experience and training. It explains TCM in such a professional way that it makes complex and abstract TCM a concrete, real and easily understandable medical science and practice for western readers. In part two, it presents the readers with a brief but thorough understanding of various common clinical disorders; it demonstrates the readers how these diseases are diagnosed and treated by western medicine, and how they are differentiated and treated by TCM; it guides the readers through the process of evaluating symptoms and then accurately prescribing herbs or herbal formula; it offers the readers lots of modifications of herbal formulas that will further enhance the clinical results. In addition, this book offers readers a variety of strategies, treatment principles, detailed prescriptions of Chinese herbs and herbal formula for coping with common clinical diseases, and it offers doctors very workable and practical tools to easily apply TCM to their daily medical practice. The integration of the conventional and Chinese medicines in this book builds a bridge between the two subjects with ease.

PART ONE

THE BASICS OF TRADITIONAL CHINESE MEDICINE

Chapter 1: Etiology of Disease

1. The Six Exogenous Pathogenic Factors

The six pathogenic factors are also known as six climatic causes or six pernicious influences of disease. Wind (spring), Cold (winter), Summer Heat (summer), Dampness (long summer), Dryness (autumn) and Fire (summer) are not only six different climatic conditions of nature, but also exogenous pathogenic causes of disease. Abnormal changes of the six climatic conditions that surpass the body's adaptability, or compromised body's resistance to pathogenic factors, or both, can leave the body vulnerable to pathogens and, under such circumstances, the six climatic conditions become external causes of disease.

1) <u>Wind</u>: Wind is the most common cause of various diseases. Wind is yang pathogen and tends to rise and disperse outward. It usually affects upper and exterior parts of the body. Wind moves indefinitely, fluctuates or vacillates variably, and changes rapidly. Wind often invades the body with other pathogens. Wind can be divided into wind-warm, wind-cold, wind-heat, wind-dryness, wind-dampness and wind-fire, depending on different seasons and weathers. Wind can also attack channels (also known as meridians) and viscera and cause "wind-stroke syndrome". Wind plays both internal and external roles, so it can also be divided into internal pathogenic wind and external pathogenic wind. External pathogenic wind invades the pulmonary systems through mouth and nose; it invades the channels and viscera through the skin. Internal pathogenic wind is mainly caused by inappropriate emotion, diet, life style, extreme heat, hyperactivity of liver yang and blood deficiency.

2) <u>Cold</u>: Cold is yin pathogen and attacks yang qi. The main characteristic of cold is that it is stagnant, stiff and stringent, and it causes spasm. Cold induces varieties of pain syndromes. It causes febrile diseases and "syncope due to pathogenic cold" when it affects the body's exterior organs or interior organs respectively. Cold is differentiated as external cold syndromes and internal cold syndromes.

3) <u>Summer Heat</u>: Summer heat is yang pathogen. It can cause heat stroke, heat exhaustion, heat cramps and heat syncope. Heat rises and disperses, and it depletes qi and body fluids. Because heat stroke occurs in person undergoing strenuous exertion in a thermally stressful environment, it is also called "yang summer heat syndrome". "Yin summer heat syndrome" is due to a person's inactivity in

summer. Summer heat is often intermingled with dampness, thus summer heat and syndrome of dampness are often treated together.

4) <u>Dampness</u>: Dampness is yin pathogen and attacks yang. It is heavy, turbid and sticky. Dampness syndrome is due to extreme exposure to moisture, e.g. wet weather, drenched clothes or moist dwelling. Dampness is differentiated as external dampness syndromes and internal dampness syndromes. If dampness combines with wind, cold or heat, it is called wind-dampness, cold-dampness or damp-heat respectively. Dampness plays both internal and external roles. It plays an external role because it is one of the six exogenous pathogenic factors of disease; it also plays an internal role because it closely related to the pathological changes of the spleen and stomach.

5) <u>Dryness</u>: Dryness relates to autumn and is a residue of pathogenic fire. It is a yang pathogen. Dryness represents symptoms that are aggravated by dry climates. Dryness depletes body fluids and adversely affects lung. It is differentiated as external dryness and internal dryness. External dryness is further divided into warm-dryness (usually occurs in early autumn) and cold-dryness (usually occurs in late autumn).

6) <u>Fire</u>: Fire is caused by excess of yang. The difference between fire and summer heat is that fire is usually generated from inside human body. Fire is the extreme condition of heat and it inflames upward. Fire depletes body fluid. It also impairs channels and blood circulation. Fire manifests many common heat syndromes in an aggravating degree, and it tends to demonstrate ruddy complexion, red swollen tongue with yellow coating, toothache, fever sore (herpes simplex of the lips), sore throat, and dark colored and even blood tinged urine. Other five climatic causes of disease, i.e., wind, cold, summer heat, dampness and dryness, can transform into fire syndromes. Fire plays both internal and external roles. It plays an external role because it is one of the six exogenous pathogenic factors of disease; it also plays an internal role because it can be generated in the process of disorders. Fire can be divided into excess fire and deficiency fire.

2. Pestilential Factors

Pestilential factors are more pernicious, dangerous and fiercer in pathogenicity than other pathogenic factors. Pestilential diseases are epidemic and even pan-epidemic, with rapid drastic changes as seen in small pox, plague, cholera, pestilence, bird flu, AIDS, SARS, etc.

3. Seven Emotions

The seven emotions are joy, anger, melancholy, pensiveness, grief, fear and fright. They are physiological reflections of the human mental state and are induced by various environmental stimulations.

Under normal conditions these physiological phenomena do not cause disease; however, extreme and constant emotions can induce acute and long-standing changes, resulting in psychiatric disorders and other diseases. Therefore the seven emotions are endogenous pathogenic causes of disease.

1) <u>Joy</u> means too much celebrating. Excessive joy can damage the heart and causes qi to flow slowly. It is associated with insomnia, muddled thought, inappropriate laugh or tears, hysteria, and insanity.
2) <u>Anger</u> causes qi to flow inappropriately upward. The excess of anger can impair the liver and causes hypertension, headache, tinnitus, dizziness, blurred vision, confusion, red face, and hematemesis.
3) <u>Melancholy</u> abnormally affects the lung and is associated with depression, shortness of breath, asthma, allergies, cold, etc.
4) <u>Pensiveness</u> causes qi to stagnate and weakens the spleen. It is associated with symptoms of low appetite, edema, fatigue, and digestive disorders.
5) <u>Grief</u> causes qi to eradicate and impairs the lung. It causes cold, asthma, allergies, etc.
6) <u>Fear</u> causes qi to flow inappropriately downward and impairs the kidney. It is associated with pains in the lower back and joints, bed wetting, urinary incontinence, abnormal libido, etc.
7) <u>Fright</u> makes qi flow disorderly and abnormally affects the heart and kidney. It is associated with symptoms of palpitations, shortness of breath, insomnia, urinary incontinence, night sweats, dizziness, etc.

4. Diet, Nutrition and Life Style

Hippocrates, the father of western medicine, once said: "let your food be your medicine and your medicine be your food". What you eat, who you are. Choose high quality diet, e.g., low sodium, low fat, high fiber food, whole grains, tofu, organic vegetable and white meat, for your body and let it become your lifestyle.

Uncontrolled binge eating, eating too less (because of intense fear of becoming fat and disturbance of body image), anorexia, eating contaminated food, or being too picky about food can cause dysfunction of the spleen and stomach. Overeating damages the digestive and absorptive functions, and can induce gastrointestinal diseases, dampness accumulation and phlegm formation. Hunger causes malnutrition and leads to an insufficient supply of qi and blood, which causes general body weakness. Contaminated, poisonous, or stale food can cause vomiting, nausea, diarrhea and parasitosis. Cold food impairs spleen qi and stomach qi and causes stomachache and diarrhea. Spicy food can cause constipation and hemorrhoids. Partiality to a particular food may bring on disease due to insufficient nutrients. For example, long-term intake of polished white rice may cause beriberi.

5. Overstrain

Overstrain is excessive fatigue or excessive leisure. It includes over exertion (mental overwork, physical overwork, and excessive physical exercise), excessive sexual activity, drug indulgence, alcoholic, and longtime lack of exercise, physical exertion or work. Over exertion causes deficiency or depletion of qi, blood, yin, and kidney essence. Lack of physical exertion causes stagnation of qi and blood circulation, and weakens spleen and stomach function.

6. Traumatic Injuries

Traumatic injuries include gun shot, sword or knife cut, fall, beat, heavy load, burn, scald, cold, electric shock, radiation, drowning, insect bit, animal attack, food or drug poisoning, contusions and sprains. Traumatic injuries cause not only injuries, but also dysfunction of the viscera.

7. Parasitosis

Many parasitoses are due to contaminated food and drinking water. They include Amebiasis, Giardiasis, Toxoplasmosis, Tapeworm infection, Nematode infection (roundworm), Angiostrongyliasis, Ascariasis and Enterobiasis (pinworm), etc.

8. Phlegm Retention and Blood Stasis

Retention of phlegm and fluid is mainly due to impaired function of the lung, spleen and kidney. The difference between phlegm and fluid is that phlegm is thick and sticky while fluid is thin and clear. Phlegm exists in everywhere and can cause various symptoms. Fluid stays in cavities and porous tissues.

Blood stasis is the result of qi stagnation, qi deficiency, yin-blood deficiency, yang-qi insufficiency, internal cold, and internal heat and injury. It is usually associated with pricking pain, tumor, ecchymosis or petechia, hemorrhage, dry skin, purple lips and tongue.

9. Five Endogenous Pathogenetic Factors

The five endogenous pathogenic factors include internal wind, internal cold, internal dampness, internal dryness and internal heat (fire). Although they are the results of abnormal function of the viscera, the five endogenous pathogens cause many clinical syndromes.

1) <u>Internal wind</u> is mainly caused by excessive liver yang, excessive phlegm fire, or yin deficiency. It induces dizziness, syncope, convulsion, numbness and opisthotonus.

2) <u>Internal cold</u> is mainly caused by qi and yang deficiency. Cold syndrome of insufficiency type, e.g., vague abdomen pain, diarrhea, weak pulse and cold extremities, is caused by heart yang insufficiency, lung qi deficiency, spleen yang insufficiency, and kidney yang insufficiency.

3) <u>Internal dampness</u> is mainly caused by dysfunction of spleen qi. Over ingestion of fatty, sweet and greasy food, and raw fruit, or invasion of the body by exogenous dampness, induce abnormal function of spleen qi and cause epigastric distention, oppressed chest feeling, stuffiness, anorexia, nausea, vomiting, scanty urine, loose stools, and edema in the face and extremities.

4) <u>Internal dryness</u> is caused by phlegm and blood deletion after febrile diseases, or by excessive sweating, vomiting and purgation, or by taking too much warm and hot drugs. It is often associated with dry skin, parched lips, dry eyes, dry and hot nostrils, thirst, hunger, dry throat, dysphagia, constipation, flaccidity syndrome, phthisic cough, and convulsive seizure.

5) <u>Internal heat (fire)</u> is divided into Internal Heat (fire) of Excess Type and Internal Heat (fire) of Deficiency Type. Internal heat (fire) of excess type is mainly caused by excessive function of the five internal organs. It is associated with vexation, insomnia, congestion of conjunctivae, bitter taste in the mouth, dizziness, headache, abdominal pain, constipation, hematemesis, sore throat, hemoptysis, yellowish sputum, dark urine, seminal emission, and stranguria. Internal heat (fire) of deficiency type is mainly caused by yin-blood deficiency and is associated with hectic fever, night sweats, flushed cheeks, tinnitus, vexation, and insomnia.

10. Weak Constitution

Constitution depends on parents' general health at conception and mother's health in pregnancy, and it is largely fixed at that time. Some factors can adversely affect a person's constitution, e.g., old age of the mother during conception, smoking or using alcohol and drugs during pregnancy. Weak constitution has compromised resistance to pathogenic factors and is therefore vulnerable to diseases.

Although a person's basic constitution is largely determined at conception and during the mother's pregnancy, those with weak constitution can develop a healthier one by a balanced lifestyle, avoidance of overstrains and over exertion, adequate rest, proper diet and nutrition, and appropriate physical exercises.

Chapter 2: The Basic Physiology and Pathogenesis of Disease

1. Eight Principles/Parameters

The Eight Principles, also known as Eight Parameters, are the foundation of diagnosis and treatment. They are Exterior and Interior, Cold and Heat, Deficiency and Excess, Yin and Yang. Exterior and interior relate to the depth of a disease, cold and heat relate to the nature of a disease, deficiency and excess relate to the opposing force in the struggle between the anti-pathogenic factors and pathogenic factors, and yin and yang relate to the categories of the disease. All the exterior syndromes, heat syndromes and excess syndromes fall into the category of yang, while all the interior syndromes, cold syndromes and deficiency syndromes fall into the category of yin. The eight principles are not isolated; they are related to each other. For example, exterior and interior stages could demonstrate exterior-heat syndrome, exterior-cold syndrome, interior-heat syndrome or interior-cold symptom, and there is a difference between deficiency and excess in both the exterior and interior. Under certain circumstances, one principle can develop into another principle. Yin and yang are not only the foundation and chief principle of the eight principles; they are also the definition of a specific symptom.

1) Exterior and Interior

Exterior and interior indicate the depth of penetration of a disease. They also indicate the difference in degree of a disease. Exterior stage usually stays superficially and is not very serious. It is located in the skin or channels, and is contracted from exposure to one or several of the six climatic causes or exogenous pathogenic factors. Exterior stage represents an initial stage of acute disease or skin disorders. On the contrary, interior stage usually penetrates deeply in the body and is more serious. It is located in the visceral organs.

(1) <u>Exterior Syndrome</u>: Aversion to cold, fever, headache, sweating or absence of sweats, thin and white tongue coating, and floating pulse.

(a) Exterior-Cold Syndrome: Serious aversion to cold, light fever, headache, body pain, with or without sweats, pale tongue with thin and white coating, tense and floating or slow and floating pulse.

(b) Exterior-Heat Syndrome: Slight aversion to cold, high fever, sore throat, red tongue with thin, white and dry coating, rapid and floating pulse.

The Differential Points between Exterior-Cold, Exterior-Warm, Interior-Cold and Interior-Heat Syndromes

	Clinical Manifestations	Tongue	Pulse
Exterior-Cold	Serious aversion to cold, Light fever, chill, with or without sweat,	Pale tongue, thin white coating	Slow and floating or tense and floating
Exterior-Heat	Little aversion to cold, High fever, wind intolerance, may have sweat	Red tongue, thin yellow coating	Floating and rapid
Interior-Cold	Absence of thirst, desire for hot drinks, clear profuse urine or diarrhea, chill, cold limbs	Pale tongue, white coating	Deep and slow
Interior-Heat	Thirst, desire for cold drink, dark scanty urine or constipation, irritability, restlessness, flushed face, red eyes	Red tongue, yellow coating	Rapid

(2) Interior Syndrome: Interior syndrome is located in the visceral organs and is the general name for visceral organ disorders. As long as a syndrome is not diagnosed as an exterior one, it is interior syndrome. Specific interior syndromes will be introduced in the ten organ systems and the three humors.

(3) Half Exterior and Half Interior Syndrome: This is a special syndrome. The pathogens have left the exterior but have not invaded the interior yet. In other words, the pathogens invade an area that is between the interior and the exterior. Clinical manifestations include alternate attack of cold and heat, feeling of stuffiness and fullness in the chest, bitter taste in the mouth, dry throat, vexation, vomiting, and thready pulse.

2) Cold and Heat

Cold and heat are two different characteristics of a disease. Cold stage is caused by exposure to cold or by deficiency of yang qi. Heat stage is usually caused by exposure to heat or by insufficiency of yin fluid that generates internal deficiency heat (fire). Cold and heat can transform into each other.

(1) Cold Syndrome: Absence of fever, pale complexion, cold extremities, absence of thirst, desire

for warm drinks, clear urine, diarrhea, pale tongue with white coating, and slow pulse.

(2) <u>Heat Syndrome</u>: Fever, red complexion, thirst, desire for cold drinks, fidgety, dark and even blood tinged urine, constipation, red tongue with yellow and dry coating, and rapid pulse.

3) Deficiency and Excess

Deficiency stage indicates qi insufficiency or impaired qi, impaired immunity or weak immune response. Excess indicates accumulation or retention of pathological conditions.

(1) <u>Excess Syndrome</u>: Fidgety, restlessness of the extremities, sonorous voice, sensation of distention and pain in the chest and abdomen that is aggravated by pressure, constipation, aged looking tongue with thick greasy coating, full and forceful pulse.

(2) <u>Deficiency Syndrome</u>: Listlessness, fatigue, weakness in the body and extremities, feeble voice, shortness of breath, cold intolerance, distending sensation and pain in the chest and abdomen that are alleviated by pressure, chubby and tender tongue with scanty coating, weak and thready pulse.

The Differential Points between Excess and Deficiency

	Clinical Manifestations	**Tongue**	**Pulse**
Deficiency	Listless, weak extremities, feeble voice, pain alleviated by touch	Chubby and tender tongue, scanty coating	Weak
Excess	Fidgety, restless extremities, loud voice, pain aggravated by touch	Aged tongue, thick coating	Strong

The Differential Points between Excess Cold, Excess Heat, Deficiency Cold and Deficiency Heat

	Excess Syndromes		Deficiency Syndromes	
	Excess Cold	*Excess Heat*	*Deficiency Cold*	*Deficiency Heat*
Pathogenesis	Exposure to cold	Exposure to heat	Deficiency of yang qi	Insufficiency of yin fluid
Clinical findings	Pale or dark green complexion, pale or green purple tongue with white or grey, thick and greasy coating, slow, taut and forceful pulse, absence of fidg-	Crimson complexion, crimson red aged tongue with yellow and dry coating, full, rapid and forceful pulse, excitedness, restlessness or delirium, high	Pale complexion, pale, chubby and tender tongue with scanty white coating, deep, slow and weak pulse, listlessness, aversion to cold, cold extremities,	Red malar, bright red chubby and tender tongue with scanty coating, weak, rapid and thready pulse, vexation, hectic fever, night sweats, dry mouth

	ety, extremely cold extremities, abdominal pain that is alleviated by heat, joints pain that is aggravated by cold, absence of thirst, clear urine.	fever, thirst, desire for cold drinks, abdominal pain that is aggravated by touch, constipation, dark urine, yellow sputum.	abdominal pain that is alleviated by touch, diarrhea, frequent urination, spontaneous perspiration, clear sputum, or vomit clear water.	and throat, sensation of heat in the palms and soles, or constipation, or blood tinged sputum.
Treatment	Warm and clear cold	Resolve heat	Warm yang qi	Nourish yin and resolve heat

4) Yin and Yang

In Chinese philosophy the yin and yang are generalized descriptions of the antitheses or mutual correlations in human perceptions of phenomena in the natural world. Yin and yang combine to create a unity of opposites in the theory of the Taiji. Yin and yang describe two primal opposing but complementary principles or cosmic forces and are found in all non-static objects and processes in the universe. This seemingly paradoxical concept is the cornerstone of most branches of Chinese philosophy, as well as traditional Chinese medicine.

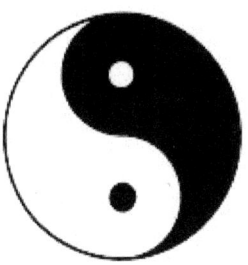

Yin and yang represent two opposite aspects of all phenomena. The nature of yin and yang is relative. Yin and yang theory indicates that everything in the universe can be divided into two opposite but complementary aspects of yin and yang, i.e., there are two aspects of yin and yang within either yin or yang. For example, day is yang and evening is yin, but the morning is yang within yang, and the afternoon is yin within yang; the evening before midnight is yin within yin, and the evening after midnight is yang within yin. Both yin and yang are prerequisite to each other for their existence; neither yin nor yang can exist without its opposite aspect. Although the two opposite aspects of yin and yang are relatively balanced, they do not remain static, but are constantly movable and changing. Under certain conditions, yin and yang can transform into each other. Yang stage indicates heat symptom, excess symptom and external influences, while yin stage indicates internal influences, cold and deficiency. Yin and yang are two dynamically interdependent parts of a whole.

(1) Yin and Yang Are Two Opposite Aspects of All Phenomena

The theory of yin and yang indicates that everything in the universe has two opposite aspects that are mutually restricted and interacted. For example, hot and cold, front and back, light and dark, sun and moon etc.

Two opposite Aspects of Yin and Yang

Yin	Yang
Rest	Activity
Cold	Hot
Descending	Ascending
Interior	Exterior
Inward	Outward
Dark	Light
Hypo-activity	Hyperactivity
Depression	Excitement
Weak	Strong
Light	Heavy
Introvert	Extrovert
Receptive	Aggressive
Winter	Summer
Moon	Sun
Earth	Heaven
Front	Back
Zang organs	Fu organs
Deficiency	Excess
Timid	Bold
Female	Male
Water	Fire
Form	Function
Matter	Energy

(2) Yin and Yang Are Interdependent

Neither yin nor yang exists as a single entity; they rely on and constantly interact with each other for their existence. If there were no yin, there would be no yang; if there were no yang, there would be no yin. Yang is born from yin, yin is born from yang. For example, day contrasts with night, excess contrasts with deficiency. One cannot exist without the other.

(3) Yin and Yang Mutually Consume and Increase Each Other

Yin and yang do not exist in a static condition; they are in a state of constant motion and change. They mutually consume and increase each other. Decreased yin leads to increased yang, or vise versa. For example, the transition from winter to spring and summer is the process of decreasing yin and increasing yang; whereas the transition from summer to autumn and winter is the process of decreasing yang and increasing yin.

(4) Yin and Yang Mutually Transform into Each Other

Under certain circumstances and at certain stage of development, yin and yang can transform into each other. For example, water (yin) can be transformed into cloud (yang); cloud (yang) can be transformed into rain (yin). A patient with high fever (yang syndrome) sweats profusely and then demonstrates pale complexion, cold extremities and feeble pulse (yin syndrome) is another example of yang transforms into yin.

(5) Yin and Yang Maintain A Relative Balance

Although yin and yang are in a state of constant change, motion, transformation and development, they maintain in a relatively balanced condition. If one changes, the other will always attempt to compensate and adjust. If the relative balance is interfered, pathological changes may occur.

2. The Five Phases/Elements

The Five Phases, also known as Five Elements, is a philosophy that correlates every aspect of human life and nature with an underlying cosmic cycle influencing life in the cosmos. The Five Elements are analogized and abstractly summarized entities of five substances represented by Metal, Water, Wood, Fire and Earth. These elements are in constant movement and change, and are interdependent and mutually restrained. The Five Phases theory is used to interpret the relationship between the different phenomena in the universe and the changes of mutual interactions of the five elements. In traditional Chinese medicine, the Five Phases theory is used to explain the correlation of the physiology and pathology of visceral organs with nature. It serves as one of the major diagnostic and treatment protocols and may be used to help make a diagnosis when there are conflicting signs and symptoms.

Typical Categories of the Five Elements

	Wood	**Fire**	**Earth**	**Metal**	**Water**
Planet	Jupiter	Mars	Saturn	Venus	Mercury
Seasons	Spring	Summer	Late summer	Autumn	Winter
Weather	Wind	Hot	Humid	Dry	Cold
Biochemical Process	Birth	Growth	Transformation	Harvest	Storage
Colors	Green	Red	Yellow	White	Black
Tastes	Sour	Bitter	Sweet	Pungent	Salty
Zang Organs	Liver	Heart	Spleen	Lung	Kidney
Fu Organs	Gallbladder	Small intes-	Stomach	Large intes-	Urinary blad-

		tine		tine	der
Tissues	Tendons	Vessels	Muscles	Skin, hair	Bone
Pulse	Taut	Full	Slow	Floating	Deep
The Five Sense Organs	Eye	Tongue	Mouth	Nose	Ear, genitals, and anus
Direction	East	South	Center	West	North
Emotions	Anger	Joy	Pensiveness/worry	Sadness/grief	Fear
Mental Quality	Sensitivity	Creativity	Clarity	Intuition	Spontaneity
Martial Arts	Crushing	Pounding	Crossing	Splitting	Drilling
The Five-note Scale	jue (mi) 角	zhi (so) 徵	gong (do) 宮	shang (re) 商	yu (la) 羽
Chinese Astrology	Jia 甲 Yi 乙	Bing 丙 Ding 丁	Wu 戊 Ji 己	Geng 庚 Xin 辛	Ren 壬 Gui 癸

The five elements are related through four cycles: sheng (generating, also called mother-son relationship), ke (controlling or restricting), cheng (overacting), and wu (insulting).

1) Generating

This cycle describes the interaction of the five elements where one element promotes the growth and development of the next one. For example, water generates or provides the generative force for wood (water makes plants and wood grow), wood generates fire (wood can catch fire), fire generates earth (burned substances become ashes that can be regarded as earth), earth generates metal (metals are mined underground), metal generates water (metal can be melted into a liquid form, which is a property of water). Each element in this cycle has two characteristics: generating and being generated. Generating element in this cycle is also called mother, generated element is also called son. Each element is the mother of the element following it, and a son of the one preceding it. Wood is the mother of fire,

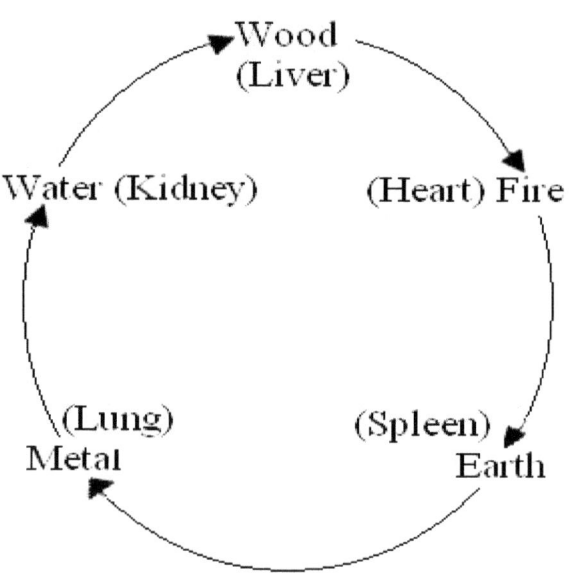

whereas fire is the son of wood, etc. On the other hand, as wood is generated by water, wood is the mother of fire and the child of water.

2) Controlling/Restricting

This cycle describes the relationship where one element restricts, controls, suppresses or inhibits another element. Wood controls earth (plants or woods deplete earth as they extract nutrients from it), metal controls wood (a metal axe can split wood), fire controls metal (fire can melt metal), water controls fire (water quenches fire), and earth controls water (the banks of water control water flow). Each element in this cycle

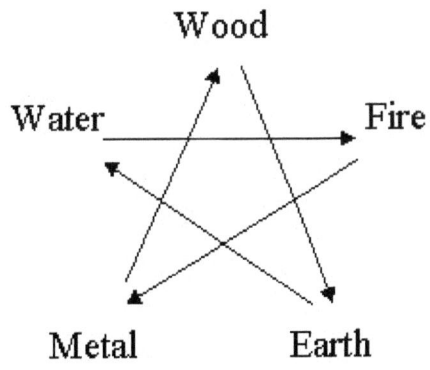

has two characteristics: controlling and being controlled. Each element controls the element following it, and is controlled by the one preceding it. For example, wood controls earth and it is controlled by metal.

3) Overacting

This cycle is an imbalance within the controlling cycle where the controlling element is too strong or the controlled element is too weak. Under the circumstances, the controlling element provides too much control over the controlled element and weakens the controlled element. For example water put out fire, earth soaks up water and so on.

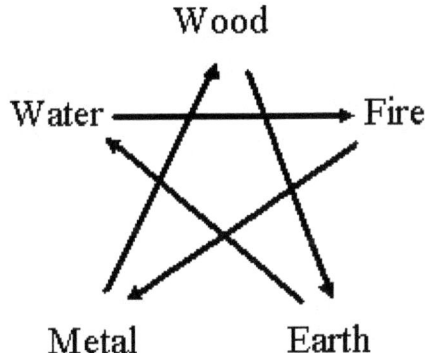

4) Insulting

This cycle is also an imbalance within the controlling cycle where the controlled element is too strong or the controlling element is too weak. Under the circumstances, the controlled element insults or returns the controlling force that is generated by the controlling element. For example, if fire is too fierce or there is not enough water, the fire can not be extinguished but rather

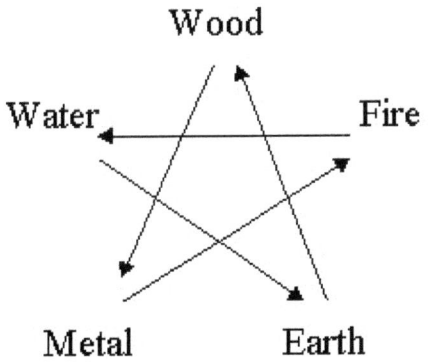

the water is vaporized. If there is flood, water may destroy the dam (earth) that prevents flood.

3. The Three Humors: Qi, Blood, and Phlegm/Fluid

Qi, blood and phlegm/fluid is the foundation of physiological and pathological activities of the body. They are also the products of physiological processes of the body.

1) Qi

Qi is a fundamental concept of traditional Chinese culture. Qi is believed to be part of every living thing that exists, as a kind of "life force", "vital force" or "spiritual energy". Theories of traditional Chinese medicine state that the body has natural patterns of qi that circulate in channels (also called meridians). Symptoms of various illnesses are often believed to be resulted from disrupted, blocked, or unbalanced qi movement through the body's channels, as well as deficiencies or imbalances of qi (homeostatic imbalance) in the various Zang Fu organs. Traditional Chinese medicine often seeks to relieve these imbalances by adjusting the interrupted qi circulation in the body using a variety of therapeutic techniques.

Qi is divided into primordial qi (yuan qi, sometimes called primary qi), pectoral qi (zong qi), nutritive qi (ying qi, also known as nutrient qi), defensive qi (wei qi), and visceral qi (zang fu qi). Primordial qi is usually described as "innate" or "pre-natal" qi to distinguish it from acquired qi that a person may develop of their lifetime. It is derived from congenital essence, housed in the kidney, and distributed to the whole body through San Jiao (Triple Warmer) to activate functions of visceral organs. Pectoral qi is generated in the lung from the combination of fresh air and the essence of food and water. It is housed in the chest and regulates blood and qi circulation in the heart, blood vessels and lymphatics. It controls respiration via throat. Nutritive qi is generated from the essence of food and water in the stomach and spleen. It is yin qi. It circulates within channels and blood vessels, and nourishes visceral organs, extremities and skeleton. Like nutritive qi, defensive qi is also generated from the essence of food and water in the stomach and spleen. The difference is that defensive qi circulates within the skin and muscles but outside channels to nourish muscles and skin. It is yang qi. It protects the surface of body from invasion of exogenous pathogens. Visceral qi manifests the functions of visceral organs.

Qi diseases are caused by exogenous and endogenous pathogenic factors. Exogenous pathogenic factors include: wind-cold invasion, wind-heat flaring up, heat invasion of pericardium, and retention of dampness. Endogenous pathogenic factors include: overstrain, improper diet, anger, joy, grief, fear, emotional stress, fatigue, and anxiety. There is a close relationship between qi diseases and visceral organs. Qi originates from the kidney and spleen. It is controlled by lung to ascend, descend, exit or enter. Liver governs the normal qi flow, while heart controls blood circulation in the vessels. Therefore, diseases of visceral organs can directly or indirectly reflect different symptoms of pathological changes of qi.

Qi diseases can be divided into deficiency syndrome and excess syndrome, although they often manifest the types of changes of ascent, descent, exit and entry.

(1) <u>Qi Deficiency Syndrome</u>

Symptoms: Overstrain and malnutrition due to chronic diseases deplete primordial qi. Qi deficiency is associated with lassitude, weak voice, spontaneous perspiration, shortness of breath, dizziness, tinnitus, anorexia, clear urine, frequent micturition, weak extremities, proctoptosis, feeble and weak pulse or feeble and full pulse, and soft large tongue with thin coating.

Treatment principle: To reinforce qi, regulate qi flow, and effectively control qi circulation.

Treatment with herbs: Radix Ginseng (Ren Shen), Radix Codonopsitis Pilosulae (Dang Shen), Radix Astragali (Huang Qi), Radix Glycyrrhizae Uralensis (Gan Cao).

Treatment with formula: Si Jun Zi Decoction or Bu Zhong Yi Qi Decoction is used to reinforce spleen and stomach qi. Bu Fei Decoction is used to reinforce lung qi. Da Bu Yuan Decoction or Jin Gui Shen Qi Pill is used to reinforce kidney qi.

(2) <u>Qi Excess Syndrome</u>

Qi excess syndrome maybe divided into qi stagnation syndrome and adverse flow of qi syndrome. It is caused by phlegm fire, indigestion, damp heat, stagnation of qi, or improper treatment of diseases caused by exogenous pathogenic factors.

Symptoms: Stuffy sensation, distention and pain in the chest, hypochondriac region and abdomen. Pain does not have fixed location; it is often wandering and related with emotion. Qi excess syndrome also manifests indigestion, abundant phlegm, asthma, shortness of breath, constipation, nausea, vomiting, hiccup, and dysphagia. Female patients often complain of irregular menstruation and breast distention. The pulse is taut and slippery or rapid and forceful.

Treatment principle: To remove fire from the liver, regulate the spleen and lung function, suppress the adverse flow of qi, and expel cold and dissolve stagnation.

Treatment with herbs:

(a) <u>Treatment of qi stagnation with herbs</u>: Pericarpium Citri Reticulatae (Chen Pi), Radix Aucklandiae Lappae (Mu Xiang), Fructus Citri Sarcodactyli (Fo Shou), Fructus Citri Aurantii Immaturus (Zhi Shi), Fructus Amomi Kravanh (Bai Dou Kou), Fructus Amomi Villosi (Sha Ren), Cortex Magnoliae Officinalis (Hou Po), Semen Areca Catechu (Bing Lang), Rhizoma

Cyperi Rotundi (Xiang Fu), Pericarpium Citri Reticulatae Viride (Qing Pi), Fructus Meliae Toosendan (Chuan Lian Zi), Radix Bupleuri (Chai Hu), and Radix Curcumae (Yu Jin).

(b) <u>Treatment of adverse flow of qi with herbs</u>: Lignum Aquilariae Resinatum (Chen Xiang), Fructus Perillae (Su Zi), Inulae Flos (Xun Fu Hua), and Ochra Haematitum (Dai Zhe Shi).

Treatment with formula:

(a) <u>Treatment of qi stagnation with formula</u>: Zhi Shi Dao Zhi Pill, Shu Gan Powder, or Xiao Yao Powder.

(b) <u>Treatment of adverse flow of qi with formula</u>: Su Zi Jiang Qi Decoction, Ju Pi Zhu Ru Decoction, or Xuan Fu Dai Zhe Decoction.

2) Blood

Blood originates from water and food essence in the spleen and stomach. It is also closely related to the kidney. "The kidney is a water visceral organ, stores essence and transforms it into blood". The main function of blood is to nourish the body. Visual acuity, walking, hand movement, skin sensation, and functional coordination of visceral organs rely on blood nourishment.

The circulation of blood in the blood vessels is not only related to heart function, but also related to qi function. Blood belongs to yin category and its circulation relies on yang qi. Blood circulation follows qi movement. Qi stagnation leads to blood stasis and so does qi deficiency to blood exhaustion. "Blood circulates with qi, and qi is the commander of blood".

Generally, blood disorders are divided into blood deficiency, blood stasis, and bleeding. Although their etiology and pathology are different, they are related to each other.

(1) <u>Blood Deficiency</u>

Blood deficiency is mainly caused by excessive bleeding, hematopenia or impaired hematopoiesis due to impaired function of spleen and stomach, or impaired hematopoiesis due to blood stagnation. Disorders, such as hematemesis, epistaxis, postpartum hemorrhage, traumatic bleeding, deficient generation of blood from essence in the spleen and stomach, chronic diseases, malnutrition due to parasitic infection and depletion of nourishing qi, cause malnutrition of visceral organs and blood vessels, leading to blood deficiency syndromes.

Symptoms: Pale complexion, pale lips, pale tongue and nails, dizziness, numbness of the extremities, severe palpitation, insomnia, shortness of breath, lethargy, and weak and thready pulse.

Treatment principle: To enrich blood, or enrich both blood and qi. Better clinical results are shown with the combination of kidney nourishment.

Treatment with herbs: Radix Angelicae Sinensis (Dang Gui), Radix Paeoniae Alba (Bai Shao Yao), Radix Rehmanniae Praeparatae (Shu Di Huang), Radix Polygoni Multiflori (He Shou Wu), Arillus Longanae Euphoriae (Long Yan Rou), and Radix Salviae Miltiorrhizae (Dan Shen).

Treatment with formula: Ren Shen Yang Rong Decoction or Shi Quan Da Bu Decoction is applied to replenish qi and enrich blood. Si Wu Decoction or Dang Gui Bu Xue Decoction is used for blood deficiency in female patients. Deficiency of both essence and blood should be treated with herbs and substances to nourish kidney and replenish essence.

(2) Blood Stasis

Blood stasis can be the result of blood flowing out of blood vessels but staying inside the body, or of obstruction of blood in the blood vessels by pathogenic factors, phlegm fire, damp heat or cold. Pathogenic mechanism includes: a) invasion of pathogenic factors, b) obstruction of blood flow in blood vessels, c) improper treatment of bleeding, which leaves residual blood stay inside the body, d) postpartum complications, e) channels or vessels injury, f) impaired qi or blood function.

Symptoms: Blood stasis can affect various areas of the body with symptoms such as prickling pain at a fixed part of the body where blood stagnation stays, feeling of stuffiness, tightness, distention and fullness, dyspnea with smothery sensation, black eyelids, dry and peeled lips or skin, purple skin spots or streaks, ecchimosis, petechiae, dark tongue, thready and uneven pulse.

Treatment principle: To invigorate blood and dissolve stagnation.

Treatment with herbs: Rhizoma Ligustici Chuanxiong (Chuan Xiong), Radix Angelicae Sinensis (Dang Gui), Gummi Olibanum (Ru Xiang), Myrrha (Mo Yao), Rhizoma Corydalis (Yan Hu Suo), Radix Salviae Miltiorrhizae (Dan Shen), Semen Pruni Persicae (Tao Ren), Flos Carthami Tinctorii (Hong Hua), Excrementum Trogopteri seu Pteromydis (Wu Ling Zhi), Radix Paeoniae Rubra (Chi Shao), Rhizoma Sparganii Stoloniferi (San Leng), and Rhizoma Curcumae Ezhu (E Zhu).

Treatment with formula: Accumulation of blood stasis is treated with Tao Ren Cheng Qi Decoction or Di Dang Decoction to promote blood circulation in order to remove blood stagnation. Obstruction of blood stasis is treated with Xue Fu Zhu Yu Decoction to promote qi and circulation to remove blood stagnation. Blood stasis due to internal cold is treated with Wen Jing Decoction to warm channels and promote blood circulation. Blood stasis due to weakened body resistance is treated with Bu Yang Huan Wu Decoction to strengthen body resistance and eliminate blood stagnation.

(3) Bleeding

Bleeding is defined as blood flows out of blood vessels. Generally, bleeding is caused by fire or by qi deficiency. Specifically, bleeding is caused by the followings: impairment of vessels by wind, fire, dryness and heat; uncontrolled eating of pungent, fatty and sweet food; alcoholic, disturbance of seven emotions, kidney yin depletion, impaired vessels by fire deficiency due to chronic diseases; sexual indulgence, and physical injury. Bleeding is classified by its location or organ, for example, pulmonary bleeding, gastric bleeding, hematochezia, hematuria, epistaxis, metrorrhagia, and metrostaxis.

Symptoms: Clinical symptoms of bleeding are different.

Treatment with herbs: Herba seu Radix Cirsii Japonici (Da Ji), Herba Cephalanoploris (Xiao Ji), Radix Sanguisorbae Officinalis (Di Yu), Herba Agrimoniae Pilosae (Xian He Cao), Rhizoma Bletillae Striatae (Bai Ji), Radix Notoginseng (San Qi), and Pollen Typhae (Pu Huang).

Treatment with formula: Bleeding due to fire flaming-up in the liver and gallbladder should be treated with Long Dan Xie Gan Decoction. Bleeding due to blood heat should be treated with Xi Jiao Di Huang Decoction. Bleeding due to stomach fire flaming-up should be treated with Jin Gui Xie Xin Decoction. Hemoptysis due to fire hyperactivity caused by yin deficiency should be treated with Sha Shen Mai Men Dong Decoction. Hematochezia should be treated with Huai Hua Powder. Hematuria due to heat in the lower visceral organs should be treated with Xiao Ji Decoction. Bleeding due to failure of the spleen to govern blood or failure of qi to astringe blood should be treated with Gui Pi Decoction or Bu Zhong Yi Qi Decoction.

3) Phlegm and Fluid

Phlegm is thick, fluid is thin and water is thinner. Accumulated water becomes fluid retention; whereas coagulated fluid becomes phlegm. The main function of phlegm and fluid is to nourish visceral organs, muscles, skin and appendages, channels and pulse. They generate or replenish bone marrow, cerebrospinal fluid, sinus fluid, blood and joint fluid. The metabolism of phlegm and fluid is regulated with lung, spleen, kidney and bladder. Through these organs, essence of water and food is transformed into fluid or blood to nourish the body. Essence of water and food is also transformed into sweat, qi or urine to excrete from the body.

(1) Fluid Deficiency

Fluid deficiency if caused by high fever, perspiration, bleeding, vomiting, purgation, diarrhea and polyuria.

Symptoms: The primary characteristic of fluid deficiency is dryness associated with dry skin and lips, dry throat, constipation, dry tongue or red tongue with little or no coating, and oliguria. The pulse is rapid and thready.

Treatment principle: To reproduce fluid and nourish yin.

Treatment with herbs: Radix Ophiopogonis Japonici (Mai Dong), Herba Dendrobii (Shi Hu), Rhizoma Polygonati Odorati (Yu Zhu), Radix Glehniae (Bei Sha Shen), Fructus Pruni Mume (Wu Mei), Rhizoma Phragmitis Communis (Lu Gen), Radix Rehmanniae (Di Huang), Radix Scrophulariae Ningpoensis (Xuan Shen), Carapax et Plastrum Testudinis (Gui Ban), Radix Polygoni Multiflori (He Shou Wu), and Radix Paeoniae Alba (Bai Shao Yao).

Treatment with formula: Zeng Ye Decoction or Wu Zhi Decoction.

(2) <u>Phlegm or Fluid Retention</u>

Water accumulates and causes fluid retention. Retained fluid coagulates and causes phlegm. Etiology of phlegm includes:

(a) Impaired function of visceral organs. Under the circumstances, essence of water and food meets yin cold and forms fluid retention; essence of water and food meets fire and forms phlegm.

(b) Spleen insufficiency, middle warmer yang failure, impaired transformation, transportation and distribution of essence of water and food. Then fluid is retained and phlegm formed.

(c) Heat due to yin deficiency and fire due to liver qi stagnation. Heat and fire then make fluid form phlegm.

(d) Heat and dryness due to lung invasion of wind-cold. Then fluid forms phlegm in the lung.

Phlegm invades the central nervous system and causes coma and epilepsy. Phlegm invades the lung and causes cough with abundant sputum. Phlegm stagnates in the middle warmer and causes loud borborygmi (rumbling sounds in the bowel or stomach "growling") and diarrhea. Phlegm invades muscle and bone and causes scrofula and subcutaneous nodules.

Fluid retention usually affects the chest, abdomen and extremities; it is closely related to the spleen and stomach. When phlegm affects the whole body, it is closely related with visceral organ diseases.

Symptoms

(a) Fluid Retention Syndrome: Clinical symptoms of fluid retention syndrome depend on where fluid retains.

- Fluid or phlegm retention in the intestine and stomach is associated with epigastric fullness and rigidity, no desire to drink water, vomiting clear fluid, salivation, loud bowel sound, white tongue coating, taut and slippery pulse.
- Retention of fluid in the chest and hypochondrium is associated with hypochondriac pain induced and aggravated by cough and expectoration, difficulty in turning over in bed, fever with sweats, white or greasy tongue coating, and taut pulse.
- Fluid retention in the extremities is associated with heaviness sensation of the limbs, pain, edema, white or yellowish tongue coating, floating and scattered pulse. Patients may also manifest retching, fever and thirst.
- Retention in hypochondrium and epigastrium is associated with asthma, cough, dyspnea, shortness of breath, slight edema in the body, salivation, and inability to lie flat. Tongue has white coating. Pulse is taut and thready.

(b) Phlegm Retention Syndrome: Phlegm retention is associated with cough, abundant sputum (sputum could be white and thin or yellowish and sticky), nausea, vomiting, diarrhea, palpitation, dizziness, madness, skin numbness, painful and swollen joints, subcutaneous nodules or abscess, white slippery or thick tongue coating, and slippery pulse.

Treatment principle: To warm yang and dissolve water, or strengthen spleen and dissolve dampness.

Treatment with herbs: Sclerotium Poriae Cocos (Fu Ling), Sclerotium Polypori Umbellati (Zhu Ling), Rhizoma Alismatis Orientalis (Ze Xie), Semen Plantaginis (Che Qian Zi), Exocarpium Benincasae Hispidae (Dong Gua Pi), Rhizoma Atractylodis Macrocephalae (Bai Zhu), and Cortex Cinnamomi Cassiae (Rou Gui).

Treatment with formula:

(a) Fluid Retention Syndrome: For fluid or phlegm retention in the intestine and stomach, use Ling Gui Zhu Gan Decoction; for fluid retention in the chest and hypochondriac region, use Shi Zao Decoction; for fluid retention in the extremities, use Xiao Qing Long Decoction; for fluid retention in hypochondrium and epigastrium, use Ting Li Da Zao Xie Fei Decoction.

(b) Phlegm Syndrome: For common cold with cough and sputum due to wind phlegm, use Xing Su Powder; for phlegm dampness invading the lung with cough, abundant white and thin sputum, use San Zi Yang Qin Decoction; for lung accumulation of phlegm heat with sticky and yellow sputum, use Qing Jin Hua Tan Decoction; for mental confusion caused by phlegm with sudden coma, accumulated saliva and sputum, use Xi Xian Powder, for subcutaneous nodules and scrofula under the neck, use Xiao He Powder; for interaction between phlegm and qi (phlegm causes stagnation of qi and, vice versa, stagnated qi causes accumulation of phlegm) with asthma, cough, shortness of breath and obstruction of the epigastrium, use Su Zi Jiang Qi Decoction.

4. The Ten Organ Systems

Despite the fact that the terminology of visceral organs in Traditional Chinese Medicine (TCM) is identical with that of anatomy of human body, the visceral organs in TCM are not simply anatomical substances, but more broadly represent the physiological function, pathological changes, and mutual relationships of every organ of certain systems of the human body. They are not defined to their anatomical structures. So the concept and meaning of visceral organs in TCM is different from that of conventional western medicine.

The visceral organs in TCM consist of Zang Viscera and Fu Viscera, i.e., five zang organs and six fu organs. The Five Zang Viscera are the heart (including the pericardium), lung, spleen, liver, and kidney. The Six Fu Viscera are the gallbladder, stomach, large intestine, small intestine, urinary bladder and San Jiao (also called Triple Warmer or Triple Burner). San Jiao mostly represents function rather than a specific organ, and it consists of Shang Jiao, Zhong Jiao and Xiao Jiao. Zhong Jiao (Middle Warmer) is located at gastral cavity; above that is Shang Jiao (Upper Warmer), below that is Xiao Jiao (Lower Warmer). Upper Warmer includes the heart, lung and pericardium; Middle Warmer includes the spleen, stomach and gallbladder; and Lower Warmer includes the liver, kidney, colon, intestine and urinary bladder.

Zang organs and fu organs are classified by the different features of their functions. The five zang organs mainly manufacture and store essence, i.e., qi, blood, and body fluid. The six fu organs mainly receive and digest food, absorb nutrient substances, and transmit and excrete wastes.

A. Physiology and Pathology of the Ten Organ Systems

1) Heart and Small Intestine

(1) Physiology of the Heart

The heart with pericardium as its external membrane is located in the chest, and it is functionally related to small intestine through channel connections. Heart is interior and yin, small intestine is exterior and yang. The heart is the most important visceral organ.

   (a) It controls mentality that includes spirit, emotion, sensation, mind and thinking.

(b) It governs blood and blood vessels. Its activity is reflected in the face and pulse.

(c) It governs fluid and sweat.

(d) Tongue is the orifice of the heart.

(2) Physiology of the Small Intestine

The physiology and pathology of small intestine along with gallbladder, stomach, large intestine and urinary bladder in TCM are similar to those of western medicine, and will not be discussed in details in this book.

The small intestine is the length of bowel that extends from the pylorus to the cecum. Its channels connect to the heart. It is a yang organ relatively to the heart. The primary functions of the small intestine are receiving and transforming ingested food and fluid, and separating "the pure" from "the impure".

(3) Pathology of the Heart

I. <u>Deficiency of Heart Yang and Heart Qi</u>

Pathogenesis: Heart yang deficiency is caused by heart qi deficiency or overtaxed mentality due to restless anxiety, irritability, hysteria, mania, exhausting mental activity and other psychotic disorders.

Symptoms: Main symptoms are palpitation, shortness of breath and spontaneous perspiration.

(a) Deficiency of heart qi: Pale complexion, pale tongue with white coating, feeble and thready pulse. Under certain circumstances, pulse may be slow with irregular interval or with regular interval but with retarded onset.

(b) Deficiency of heart yang: Cold intolerance, cold extremities, palpitation, asthma, chest pain, pale complexion, feeble and thready pulse. In serious conditions, patients may manifest confusion, spontaneous perspiration, dark purple extremities, lips and face.

Treatment principle: To replenish heart qi, nourish heart yang and tranquilize the mind.

Treatment with herbs:

(a) <u>Herbs to replenish heart qi</u>: Radix Ginseng (Ren Shen), Radix Codonopsitis Pilosulae (Dang Shen), Radix Astragali (Huang Qi), and Radix Glycyrrhizae Uralensis (Gan Cao).

(b) <u>Herbs to nourish heart yang</u>: Ramulus Cinnamomi Cassiae (Gui Zhi) and Radix Aconiti Lateralis Praeparatae (Fu Zi).

(c) <u>Herbs to tranquilize the mind</u>: Semen Ziziphi Spinosae (Suan Zao Ren), Semen Biotae Orientalis (Bai Zi Ren), Radix Polygalae Tenuifoliae (Yuan Zhi), Cortex Albizziae Julibrissin (He Huan Pi), Ganoderma (Ling Zhi), and Concha Ostreae (Mu Li).

Treatment with formula: Sheng Mai Powder, Yang Xin Decoction, Zhi Gan Cao Decoction, or Shen Fu Decoction.

II. Deficiency of Heart Yin and Heart Blood

Pathogenesis: Excessive mental activity causes blood insufficiency and yin essence deficiency. Under the circumstances, yin fails to keep yang well, resulting in heart yang floating.

Symptoms: Main symptoms are palpitation, shortness of breath, amnesia, insomnia and multi-dreams.

Deficiency of heart blood also demonstrates pale complexion, pale tongue, feeble and thready pulse.

Deficiency of heart yin also demonstrates vexation, restlessness, anxiety, suspicion, vague chest pain, pink tongue with scanty coating, dry and red tongue tip, thready pulse, rosy cheeks, warm palms and soles, nocturnal seminal emission and night sweats.

Treatment principle: To replenish heart yin, nourish heart blood and tranquilize the mind.

Treatment with herbs: Radix Salviae Miltiorrhizae (Dan Shen), Radix Angelicae Sinensis (Dang Gui), Radix Paeoniae Alba (Bai Shao Yao), Gelatinum Corii Asini (E Jiao), Radix Ophiopogonis Japonici (Mai Dong), Radix Rehmanniae Recens (Sheng Di Huang), Fructus Zizyphi Jujubae (Da Zao), Radix Polygalae Tenuifoliae (Yuan Zhi), and Semen Biotae Orientalis (Bai Zi Ren).

Treatment with formula: Tian Wang Bu Xin Pill, Zhu Sha An Shen Pill, or Gui Pi Decoction.

III. Heart Blood Stasis

Pathogenesis: Fatigue and anxiety affect the heart so adversely that heart qi can not consolidate, resulting in heart qi stagnation. Heart qi stagnation itself or together with chronic arthralgia or rheumatism (is defined as pain or numbness caused by cold, damp, etc by TCM), or so called heart diseases by western medicine, lead to heart blood stasis and circulatory system disorder.

Symptoms: Pricking chest pain (may radiate to hypochondriac region, shoulder or the back), palpitation, dark red tongue with purple petechiae and scanty coating, purple face, purple lips and nails, and irregular pulse.

Treatment principle: To promote blood circulation and resolve blood stasis.

Treatment with herbs: Rhizoma Ligustici Chuanxiong (Chuan Xiong), Radix Curcumae (Yu Jin), Radix Salviae Miltiorrhizae (Dan Shen), Semen Pruni Persicae (Tao Ren), Flos Carthami Tinctorii (Hong Hua), Excrementum Trogopteri seu Pteromydis (Wu Ling Zhi), Radix Paeoniae Rubra (Chi Shao), Bulbus Allii Macrostemonis (Xie Bai), Radix Angelicae Sinensis (Dang Gui), Pollen Typhae (Pu Huang), Fructus Trichosanthis (Gua Lou), and Ramulus Cinnamomi Cassiae (Gui Zhi).

Treatment with formula: Shi Xiao Powder or Xue Fu Zhu Yu Decoction.

IV. Mental Disorders Caused by Phlegm

Pathogenesis: 1) Anxiety, stress and other excessive mental activities cause qi stagnation that in turn leads to fluid accumulation and phlegm. 2) Impaired function of the spleen in transportation of fluid and nutrient causes damp retention. Chronic retention of dampness and phlegm causes damp-heat (fire) accumulation. Both phlegm and damp-heat affect mental status and, in serious cases, disturb pericardium and cause irritability or coma.

Symptoms: Palpitation, dysphoria, insomnia, insanity, clouded consciousness, delirium, dementia, mania, flushed face, craving for cold drinks, hematemesis, epistaxis, hot dark tea-colored urine, hematuria, dysuria, red parched tongue with yellow coating, slippery and rapid pulse.

Treatment principle: To resolve phlegm, induce resuscitation and relieve heat (fire).

Treatment with herbs:

(a) Herbs to resolve phlegm: Rhizoma Pinelliae Ternatae (Ban Xia), Rhizoma Arisaematis (Tian Nan Xing), Pericarpium Citri Reticulatae (Chen Pi), and Radix Polygalae Tenuifoliae (Yuan Zhi).

(b) Herbs to relieve phlegm-heat (fire): Bulbus Fritillariae Cirrhosae (Bei Mu), Concretio Silicea Bambusae (Tian Zhu Huang), Succus Bambosae (Zhu Li), and Rhizoma Arisaematis (Tian Nan Xing).

(c) Herbs to induce resuscitation: Moschus (She Xiang), Borneolum Syntheticum (Bing Pian), Styrax (Su He Xiang), Rhizoma Acori Tatarinowii (Shi Chang Pu), and Radix Curcumae (Yu Jin).

Treatment with formula: Huang Lian Wen Dan Decoction, Wen Dan Decoction, Dao Tan Decoction, Su He Xiang Pill, Xiao Xian Xiong Decoction, Niu Huang Qing Xin Pill, or Meng Shi Gun Tan Pill.

V. Invasion of the Small Intestine by Heart Heat (Fire)

Pathogenesis: The channels of small intestine are connected to the heart. The small intestine and the heart are related to each other, i.e. the small intestine is an exterior organ relative to the heart and the heart is an interior organ relative to the small intestine. Therefore, heart heat (fire) could cause the small intestine disorders when it invades the small intestine.

Symptoms: Vexation, aphthae, red tongue or red tongue tip with yellow coating, lingual ulcer, sore throat, deafness, thirsty, dark tea-colored urine, dysuria, difficult micturition, urethra pain and "feel hot inside urethra", slippery and rapid pulse.

Treatment principle: To eliminate excessive heat (fire).

Treatment with herbs: Folium Phyllostachydis Henonis (Zhu Ye), Rhizoma Coptidis (Huang Lian), Plumula Nelumbinis Nuciferae (Lian Zi Xin), Fructus Gardeniae Jasminoidis (Zhi Zi), and Caulis Akebiae (Mu Tong).

Treatment with Formula: Huang Lian Shang Qing Pill, Dao Chi Powder, or Liang Ge Powder.

VI. <u>Obstruction of Heart Yang due to Fluid Retention</u>

Symptoms: Palpitation, sensation of pressure in the chest, dizziness, nausea, vomiting, white greasy tongue coating, and slippery or deep and tense pulse.

Treatment principle: To warm yang and resolve fluid retention.

Treatment with Formula: Xiao Ban Xia Jia Fu Ling Decoction or Ling Gui Zhu Gan Decoction.

(4) Pathology of the Small Intestine

The small intestine disorders are mainly caused by improper diet.

I. <u>Cold Syndrome of the Small Intestine (Deficiency Type)</u>

Symptoms: Dull pain in the lower abdomen that is alleviated by massage, increased bowel sound, diarrhea, frequent and difficult urination, pale tongue with white and thin coating, thready and slow pulse.

Treatment principle: To warm and clear the small intestine.

Treatment with formula: Wu Zhu Yu Decoction.

II. <u>Heat Syndrome of the Small Intestine (Excess Type)</u>

Symptoms: Vexation, aphtha, sore throat, dysuria, difficult micturition, dark colored urine, abdominal distention that is slightly alleviated by passing flatus, red tongue with yellow coating, slippery and rapid pulse.

Treatment principle: To eliminate excess heat.

Treatment with formula: Dao Chi Powder or Liang Ge Powder.

III. <u>Qi Disorders of the Small Intestine</u>

Symptoms: Acute lower abdominal pain radiating to the testicle, the waist and the back, white tongue coating, and deep and taut or slippery and taut pulse.

Treatment principle: To promote qi circulation and resolve mass.

Treatment with formula: Tian Tai Wu Yao Powder.

2) Liver and Gallbladder

(1) Physiology of the Liver

(a) The liver regulates the smooth flow and proper direction of qi and blood throughout the body. It keeps qi, blood and temperament in balance.
  i. Disposition: deficient liver qi causes fear, whereas excessive liver qi causes anger. "The liver likes optimism and dislikes depression".
  ii. Digestion: liver regulates functions of the spleen and stomach. Stagnation of liver qi has an impact on the digestive function of the spleen and stomach.
(b) The liver stores blood, and regulates blood supply by the heart.
(c) The liver governs the ligaments, tendons and joints of the body. Its activities are reflected in the fingers and toes. If liver blood is deficient, blood can not nourish tendons.
(d) The eyes are the orifice of the liver. The function of the eyes relies on the nourishment of lover qi and blood. Eye malfunctions can reflect underlying liver disorders.

(2) Physiology of the Gallbladder

The gallbladder is located on the inferior aspect of the liver. Its channels connect to the liver. It is a yang organ relatively to the liver. The functions of the gallbladder include storage of the clean bile, concentration of bile, and release of bile. The gallbladder is a "clean visceral organ"; it only stores clean bile, which makes it different from other visceral organs. Resolute by nature, the gallbladder is in charge of making decisions.

(3) Pathology of the Liver

Sorrow, grief, melancholy, depression or other emotions cause liver qi stagnation, and chronic qi stagnation transforms itself into liver heat (fire) syndrome that in turn gives rise to liver yang hyperactivity. Liver yang hyperactivity brings about endogenous wind. Both wind and heat (fire) can then rise to vertex or invade channels and collaterals, and make blood rise with qi and fire, instead of circulating in the blood vessels.

  I. <u>Liver Qi Stagnation</u>

Pathogenesis: The liver regulates the smooth flow and proper direction of qi and blood throughout the body. Sorrow, grief, melancholy, depression or other emotions impair liver function and cause liver qi stagnation. The stagnant liver qi impedes blood circulation and causes blood stagnation. The stagnant liver qi can also invade stomach and spleen and impair their digestive functions.

Symptoms: Depression or mania, oppressive sensation in the chest, chest discomfort, wandering hypochondriac pain, inability to turn around because of pain; belching, regurgitation, anorexia, vomiting of yellow, green, bitter and watery fluid, lower quadrant abdominal pain, diarrhea, wandering abdominal distension or lumps that fluctuate in size and converge or diverge in an uncertain pattern;

white and thin tongue coating, and taut pulse. Female patients may demonstrate dysfunctional uterine bleeding, dysmenorrhea or breast distending pain during premenstrual phase of menstrual cycle.

Treatment principle: To soothe liver, regulate qi circulation and resolve lumps and masses.

Treatment with herbs: Pericarpium Citri Reticulatae Viride (Qing Pi), Fructus Citri Sarcodactyli (Fo Shou), Radix Aucklandiae Lappae (Mu Xiang), Rhizoma Cyperi Rotundi (Xiang Fu), Fructus Meliae Toosendan (Chuan Lian Zi), Radix Bupleuri (Chai Hu), Radix Curcumae (Yu Jin), and Caulis Perillae (Su Geng).

Treatment with formula: Chai Hu Shu Gan Powder or Xiao Yao Powder.

II. Liver Fire Flaming-Up

Pathogenesis: Chronic liver qi stagnation transforms itself into liver heat (fire) that in turn scurries with liver qi. Liver fire can also follow liver qi to rise and invade the vertex.

Symptoms: Headache (hot forehead with chopping or distending pain), dizziness, tinnitus, deafness, irritability, vexation, hypochondriac burning pain, hot red face, dry mouth with bitter taste, conjunctival congestion, hematemesis, epistaxis, vomiting bitter, yellow and watery fluid, difficult micturition, hot dark urine, red and smooth tongue with yellow or dry and greasy coating, taut and rapid pulse.

Treatment principle: To resolve liver heat (fire).

Treatment with herbs: Radix Gentianae (Long Dan Cao), Radix Scutellariae Baicalensis (Huang Qin), Fructus Gardeniae Jasminoidis (Zhi Zi), Folium Mori Alba (Sang Ye), Flos Chrysanthemi Morifolii (Ju Hua), Spica Prunellae Vulgaris (Xia Ku Cao), Semen Celosiae Argenteae (Qing Xiang Zi), and Semen Cassiae (Jue Ming Zi).

Treatment with formula: Long Dan Xie Gan Decoction.

III. Liver Yang Hyperactivity

Pathogenesis: Liver qi stagnation leads to excessive liver fire and sudden expansion of yang qi. Fire then scurries with qi and transversely invades channels and collaterals. Blood also ascends with qi all the way to the vertex.

Symptoms: Headache, dizziness, dysphoria, hot red face, red tongue, and thready, taut and rapid pulse.

Treatment principle: To calm the liver and suppress hyperactivity of liver yang.

Treatment with herbs: Rhizoma Gastrodiae Elatae (Tian Ma), Ramulus Uncariae cum Uncis (Gou Teng), Concha Haliotidis (Shi Jue Ming), and Flos Chrysanthemi Morifolii (Ju Hua).

Treatment with formula: Tian Ma Gou Teng Decoction.

IV. Liver Yin Deficiency

Pathogenesis: The liver is nourished by kidney yin. If kidney yin is deficient, the kidney can not produce blood from the essence, and as a result, there is not enough blood to nourish the liver. Failure of nourishing the liver by blood leads to liver yin deficiency and liver yang hyperactivity.

Symptoms: Tottering and distending headache, dizziness, tremor, blurred vision, nyctalopia (night blindness), scanty saliva, tinnitus, deafness, numbness, hypochondriac vague pain alleviated by massage, red and dry tongue with little coating, and thready, taut and rapid pulse.

Treatment principle: To nourish liver yin, replenish kidney and suppress liver yang.

Treatment with herbs: Fructus Lycii (Gou Qi Zi), Fructus Ligustri Lucidi (Nu Zhen Zi), Carapax et Plastrum Testudinis (Gui Ban), Carapax Trionycis (Bie Jia), Radix Polygoni Multiflori (He Shou Wu), Radix Rehmanniae Praeparatae (Shu Di Huang), and Fructus Corni Officinalis (Shan Zhu Yu).

Treatment with formula: Yi Guan Decoction or Da Bu Yin Pill.

V. <u>Internal Liver Wind</u>

Pathogenesis: Internal liver wind is caused by extreme deficiency of liver yin and kidney yin. Excessive liver yang, deficient liver blood and/or excessive liver fire develop to such an extent that they can result in interior liver wind.

Symptoms: Floating and throbbing headache, dizziness, numbness (a feeling as if ants are crawling on the extremities, face, lips or other parts of the body), tremor, convulsions, syncope, tetany, seizures (neck stiffness, or tonic-clonic seizures with rigid extremities or opisthotonus), dysphasia, deviated mouth and eyes, or hemiplegia and coma in worse case; red, deviated and quivering tongue with thin and yellow coating, and taut, rapid and forceful pulse.

Treatment principle: To calm the liver and stop the wind.

Treatment with herbs: Cornu Saigae Tataricae (Ling Yang Jiao), Buthus Martensi (Quan Xie), Scolopendra Subspinipes (Wu Gong), Bombyx Batryticatus (Bai Jiang Can), and Lumbricus (Di Long).

Treatment with formula: Zhen Gan Xi Feng Decoction.

VI. <u>Stagnation of cold in the Liver Channel</u>

Pathogenesis: Exterior pathogenic cold invades Jueyin channel and leads to dysfunction of liver qi and obstruction of channel qi.

Symptoms: Debility, timidity, distending sensation and pain in the lower quadrant abdomen, groin and testicles that is aggravated by cold and alleviated by heat; smooth and moist tongue with white coating, and deep, taut or slow pulse. The patient usually curls up.

Treatment principle: To warm the liver channel.

Treatment with herbs: Cortex Cinnamomi Cassiae (Rou Gui), Fructus Evodiae Rutaecarpae (Wu Zhu Yu), Fructus Feoniculi (Xiao Hui Xiang), Fructus Anisi Stellati (Ba Jiao Hui Xiang), and Radix Angelicae Sinensis (Dang Gui).

Treatment with formula: Nuan Gan Decoction.

VII. <u>Stagnation of Phlegm and Heat in the Liver and Gallbladder</u>

Pathogenesis: Dysfunction of the spleen and stomach retains fluid and forms phlegm, resulting in internal dampness. Chronic dampness turns into fire. Phlegm and fire invade the liver and gallbladder, and cause excess syndrome.

Symptoms: Yellow complexion and conjunctivae, hypochondriac pain, abdominal distension, oliguria, dark urine, fever, thirst, anorexia, nausea, vomiting of bitter and watery fluid, bitter taste in the mouth, red tongue with yellow and greasy coating, taut and rapid pulse.

Treatment principle: To resolve phlegm and clear away heat.

Treatment with herbs: Herba Artemisiae Scopariae (Yin Chen Hao), Sclerotium Poriae Cocos (Fu Ling), Sclerotium Polypori Umbellati (Zhu Ling), Rhizoma Alismatis Orientalis (Ze Xie), Semen Plantaginis (Che Qian Zi), Talcum (Hua Shi Fen), Fructus Gardeniae Jasminoidis (Zhi Zi), Radix Scutellariae Baicalensis (Huang Qin), Rhizoma Coptidis (Huang Lian), and Cortex Phellodendri (Huang Bai).

Treatment with formula: Yin Chen Hao Decoction, Long Dan Xie Gan Decoction, or Huang Lian Wen Dan Decoction.

(4) The Pathology of the Gallbladder

The gallbladder disorders mainly manifest hyperactive yang, excessive fire and phlegm syndrome (e.g. mental disturbance caused by phlegm fire)

I. <u>Deficiency Syndrome of the Gallbladder</u>

Symptoms: Dizziness, nausea, insomnia, blurred vision, timidity, thin and smooth tongue coating, taut and thready pulse.

Treatment principle: To calm the mind and spirit, and nourish the gallbladder and the stomach.

Treatment with formula: Suan Zao Ren Decoction.

II. <u>Excess Syndrome of the Gallbladder</u>

Symptoms: Dizziness, insomnia, sallow complexion, decreased hearing ability, vomiting bitter and watery fluid, bitter taste in the mouth, hypochondriac distending sensation and pain, fidgetiness, timidity, multi-dreams, alternate chill and fever, red tongue with yellow coating, and taut, rapid, full or slippery pulse.

Treatment principle: To clear away heat and resolve phlegm from the gallbladder.

Treatment with formula: Long Dan Xie Gan Decoction or Huang Lian Wen Dan Decoction. For jaundice, use Yin Chen Hao Decoction.

3) Spleen and Stomach

(1) Physiology of the Spleen

The spleen and stomach are the primary organs for digestion. "The spleen and stomach are the basis of the postnatal constitution", i.e. they are considered to be the root of postnatal qi, or the source of all qi produced by the body after birth.

(a) The spleen rules transformation and transportation of nutrients. First, the spleen, together with stomach, digests and absorbs food and drink and transports nutrients to the whole body. Second, the spleen regulates the metabolism of fluid and electrolyte and maintains them at a certain volume and concentration by absorbing fluid from organs and by transporting fluid to the kidney. The kidney then passes fluid to the bladder where the fluid is excreted from the body.

(b) The spleen controls blood and supplements qi. It controls blood circulation and keeps blood from circulating out of blood vessels.

(c) It governs muscles and extremities. The spleen transforms and transports nutrients to the body and nourishes muscles and extremities.

(d) The mouth is the orifice of the spleen and its activities are reflected in the lips.

(2) Physiology of the Stomach

The Stomach is located beneath the diaphragm. Its upper cardia part is connected to the esophagus through gastroesophageal junction and its lower antrum part ends at pylorus. The functions of the stomach include food storage and digestion. The stomach receives food and transforms it into chyme. The impure portion of food and fluid goes to the intestine for further digestion, while the nutrients are sent to the spleen for transportation and transformation. Its channels connect to the spleen. Relatively speaking, it is a yang organ.

(3) Pathology of Spleen

Factors, such as unhealthy diet, debilitated body, external pathogenic cold-dampness, lack of proper care after illness, anxiety and fatigue, affect the digestion and absorption of food and fluid, and impair the function of transportation and transformation of the spleen and stomach. Spleen channel disorders can be divided into deficiency syndrome, excess syndrome, cold syndrome and heat syndrome.

Treatment with formula: Li Zhong Decoction.

V. <u>Failure of the Spleen to Control Blood Circulation</u>

Pathogenesis: The spleen controls the blood and supplements qi. It controls blood circulation and keeps blood circulating within blood vessels. If spleen qi is deficient, the spleen can not control blood circulation, resulting in blood circulating out of blood vessels.

Symptoms: Failure of the spleen to control blood circulation manifests symptoms of spleen qi deficiency plus the followings: menorrhagia or dysfunctional uterine bleeding, melena or hematochezia, skin purpura (thrombocytopenia), pale complexion, lethargy, palpitation, shortness of breath, pale tongue, weak and thready pulse.

Treatment principle: To replenish qi, strengthen the spleen and promote blood to circulate in the vessels.

Treatment with herbs: Pollen Typhae (Pu Huang), Herba Agrimoniae Pilosae (Xian He Cao), and herbs that treat spleen qi deficiency.

Treatment with formula: Gui Pi Decoction.

(4) Pathology of the Stomach

The stomach disorders are mainly caused by improper diet.

I. <u>Cold Syndrome of the Stomach</u>

Symptoms: Distending sensation in the stomach, dull stomach pain that can be alleviated by warmth and massage, hiccup, vomiting of watery fluid, white and smooth tongue coating, and slow pulse.

Treatment principle: To warm the stomach and relieve cold.

Treatment with formula: Liang Fu Pill.

II. <u>Heat Syndrome of the Stomach</u>

Symptoms: Thirst with a desire for cold drinks, scanty saliva, hyperorexia, frequent vomiting, halitosis (mouth odor), swollen gum, gum pain, gum decay, gum bleeding, red tongue with yellow coating, slippery and rapid pulse.

Treatment principle: To resolve stomach heat.

Treatment with formula: Qing Wei Powder.

III. <u>Deficiency Syndrome of the Stomach</u>

Symptoms: Sensation of fullness in the stomach, dyspepsia, belching, loose stools, scanty tongue coating, soft and feeble pulse.

Treatment principle: To replenish qi and strengthen the spleen.

Treatment with formula: Xiao Jian Zhong Decoction.

IV. Excess Syndrome of the Stomach

Symptoms: Dyspepsia, sensation of distention and fullness in the stomach and abdomen, difficult defecation, halitosis (mouth odor), belching with decaying odor, vomiting, thin and yellow tongue coating, and slippery pulse.

Treatment principle: To promote digestion, evacuate food stagnation and normalize stomach function.

Treatment with formula: Xiang Su Powder or Bao He Pill.

4) Lung and large Intestine

(1) Physiology of the Lung

The lung is located in the chest and is connected upwards to trachea. It is the uppermost visceral organ and covers other visceral organs below in the body. The lung is related to the large intestine via channels. The lung is an interior organ relative to the large intestine; and vice versa the large intestine is an exterior organ.

(a) The lung controls respiration and governs qi (both natural air and pectoral qi). Respiratory air is internally and externally exchanged in the lung; natural air from the environment is drawn in and exchanged for waste air. The lung also forms pectoral qi (zong qi), which is the combination of essential qi transformed from water and food with the inhaled qi of the lung. Pectoral qi accumulates in the chest, and then flows up to the throat to control respiration. Pectoral qi along with blood also circulate throughout the body to nourish the tissues and organs and maintain the body's normal functional activities. If lung qi is deficient, deficiency syndrome with feeble respiration, uneven breathing, weak speech, lassitude, etc. will occur. The lung also dominates the function of dispersion and descent, which involves in the distribution of qi, blood, and body fluid to the zang-fu organs, the channel-collaterals, muscles, skin, and hair.

(b) The lung facilitates the circulation of fluid. The normal circulation of fluid in the body also relies on lung qi that facilitates other organs to balance the metabolism of fluid.

(c) The lung is in charge of the skin. Pectoral qi circulates with blood throughout the body and nourish the skin. Defensive qi, which is generated from the essence of food and water in the stomach and spleen, is transferred (facilitated by the lung) to muscles and skin and nourishes these tissues. The defensive qi also protects the surface of body from invasion of exogenous pathogens.

(d) The nose is the orifice of the lung. The nose is the gateway of respiration. Nasal breathing and smelling rely upon the functioning of lung qi. Since the nose is the opening of the lung, it will also be a passage for the invasion of external pathogenic factors that may attack the lung. The throat is also a gateway of respiration, and a vocal organ.

(2) Physiology of the Large Intestine

The upper part of the large intestine is connected with the small intestine through ileocecal junction and its lower part ends at anus. Its channels connect to the lung. Relatively it is a yang organ. The large intestine is a "transport organ"; it absorbs fluid, and transports, transforms and excretes waste.

(3) Pathology of the Lung

The lung is a tender respiratory organ and is prone to cold, heat, wind and other external pathogenic factors. Because the lung is connected to other visceral organs via channels, disorders of other organs often affect the lung.

I. <u>Lung Qi Deficiency</u>

Pathogenesis: It is mainly caused by overstrain, chronic illness or disorders of other visceral organs.

Symptoms: Cough, thin sputum, shortness of breath, asthma, low energy, lassitude, disinclination to talk, low voice, pale complexion, spontaneous perspiration, aversion to wind and cold, pale tongue with thin and white coating, and feeble pulse.

Treatment principle: To replenish and restore lung qi.

Treatment with herbs: Radix Ginseng (Ren Shen), Radix Codonopsitis Pilosulae (Dang Shen), and Radix Astragali (Huang Qi).

Treatment with formula: Bu Fei Decoction.

II. <u>Lung Yin Deficiency</u>

Pathogenesis: External pathogenic factors (e.g. wind-dryness), pulmonary tuberculosis, chronic cough and other chronic illness lead to lung yin deficiency that can transform into fire syndrome of deficiency type.

Symptoms: Dry cough, or cough with scanty sticky blood-streaked or blood-clotted sputum, belching, dry mouth and throat, hectic fever, night sweats, flushed cheeks in the afternoon, hot sensations in palms and soles, dyspnea, insomnia, red tongue with scanty coating, rapid and thready pulse.

Treatment principle: To nourish yin and moisten the lung.

Treatment with herbs: Radix Adenophorae (Nan Sha Shen), Radix Glehniae (Bei Sha Shen), Radix Ophiopogonis Japonici (Mai Dong), Tuber Asparagi Cochinchinensis (Tian Dong), Rhizoma Polygonati Odorati (Yu Zhu), Rhizoma Polygonati (Huang Jing), Bulbus Lilii (Bai He), Radix Rehmanniae

Recens (Sheng Di Huang), Folium Mori Alba (Sang Ye), and Folium Eriobotryae Japonicae (Pi Pa Ye).

Treatment with formula: Bai He Gu Jin Decoction or Yang Yin Qing Fei Decoction. Qing Zao Jiu Fei Decoction is the primary treatment of dryness syndrome of the lung.

III. <u>Heat Syndrome of the Lung</u>

Pathogenesis: External pathogenic factors (e.g. wind-heat), cold stagnation (it transforms into heat-syndrome), or accumulation of phlegm and heat, lead to heat congestion in the lung, resulting in dysfunction of the lung in purification and descent.

Symptoms: Fever, cough, yellow, sticky and stink sputum with pus or blood; asthma, dry nostrils, nostril flaring, epistaxis, thick nasal discharge, chest pain, thirst, sore throat, constipation, difficult micturition, dark urine, red tongue with dry and yellow coating, and rapid pulse.

Treatment principle: To eliminate heat from the lung, dissolve the sputum, and relieve cough and asthma.

Treatment with herbs: Radix Scutellariae Baicalensis (Huang Qin), Cortex Mori Alba Radicis (Sang Bai Pi), Rhizoma Phragmitis Communis (Lu Gen), Fructus Trichosanthis (Gua Lou), Bulbus Fritillariae Cirrhosae (Bei Mu), and Semen Descurainiae seu Lepidii (Ting Li Zi).

Treatment with formula: Sang Bai Pi Decoction, Wei Jing Decoction, or Ma Xing Shi Gan Decoction.

IV. <u>Wind-Cold Attacks the Lung</u>

Pathogenesis: External pathogenic wind-cold attacks the lung and obstructs lung qi, resulting in cold-fluid retention in the lung, which further impairs the function of lung in purification and descent.

Symptoms: Cough with abundant clear and thin sputum, stuffy nose, rhinorrhea, fever, aversion to cold, malaise, headache, muscle aches, cold extremities, thin and white tongue coating, floating and tense pulse.

Treatment principle: To disperse wind cold, warm the lung and resolve cold fluid retention.

Treatment with herbs: Rhizoma Zingiberis Officinalis (Gan Jiang), Herba cum Radice Asari (Xi Xin), Herba Ephedrae (Ma Huang), Rhizoma Pinelliae Ternatae (Ban Xia), and Semen Sinapis Albae (Bai Jie Zi).

Treatment with formula: San Ao Decoction or Xiao Qing Long Decoction.

V. <u>Phlegm Stagnation in the Lung</u>

Pathogenesis: Accumulation of fluid and phlegm obstructs lung qi, resulting in dysfunction of lung in purification and descent.

Symptoms: Cough, wheezing, asthma, thick and sticky sputum, distention and pain in the chest and hypochondriac region, increased pain and difficulty in breathing when lying down, yellow and greasy tongue coating, and slippery pulse.

Treatment principle: To resolve dampness and phlegm, and descend lung qi that abnormally rises.

Treatment with herbs: Rhizoma Pinelliae Ternatae (Ban Xia), Rhizoma Atractylodis (Cang Zhu), Cortex Magnoliae Officinalis (Hou Po), Sclerotium Poriae Cocos (Fu Ling), and Pericarpium Citri Reticulatae (Chen Pi).

Treatment with formula: Er Chen Decoction, San Zi Yang Qin Decoction, or Ting Li Da Zao Xie Fei Decoction.

(4) Pathology of the Large Intestine

   I. Cold Syndrome of the Large Intestine

Symptoms: Abdominal pain, increased bower sound, loose stools, clear urine, white and slippery tongue coating, and slow pulse.

Treatment principle: To disperse cold and resolve abdominal pain.

Treatment with formula: Wei Ling Decoction plus Liang Fu Pill.

   II. Heat Syndrome of the Large Intestine

Symptoms: Dry mouth, parched lips, constipation, foul feces, burning heat sensation and swelling pain in the anus, oliguria with dark urine, yellow and dry tongue coating, and rapid pulse. Dysentery due to damp-heat pathogen invasion is associated with fever, bloody diarrhea, tenesmus, left lower quadrant cramps, yellow and greasy tongue coating, rapid and slippery pulse.

Treatment principle: To induce laxation and purge heat. In dysentery, the treatment is to relieve fever and induce diuresis.

Treatment with formula: Liang Ge Power. Dysentery should be treated with Shao Yao Decoction or Bai Tou Weng Decoction.

   III. Deficiency Syndrome of the Large Intestine

Symptoms: Chronic diarrhea, dysentery, rectal prolapse, cold extremities, pale tongue with thin coating, rapid and thready pulse.

Treatment principle: To nourish the bowel and induce astringency.

Treatment with formula: Zhen Ren Yang Zang Decoction.

   IV. Excess Syndrome of the Large Intestine

Symptoms: Fever, vomiting, constipation, dyschezia (difficult defecation), abdominal pain that is aggravated by pressure, yellow tongue coating, deep and full pulse.

Treatment principle: To resolve heat and stagnation.

Treatment with formula: Cheng Qi Decoction (Da Cheng Qi Decoction, Xiao Cheng Qi Decoction, or Tiao Wei Cheng Qi Decoction).

5) Kidney and Bladder

(1) Physiology of the Kidney

The two kidneys are located on either side of the vertebral column retroperitoneally. TCM believes that the kidney is closely related with the development, ageing and reproduction of the body, and it is the origin of congenital constitution. The kidney is an internal organ of water and fire; it stores kidney yin, kidney yang, and congenital essence (an inherited constitution of life). The kidney houses the life gate fire (the foundation of yang qi and life, the vital activity power) of the body. Its channel connects to the bladder. The kidney and bladder are related to each other as interior and exterior organs.

(a) The kidney stores congenital essence and food essence, the root of reproduction and development of the body.

(b) The kidney regulates fluid metabolism of the body. Kidney yang regulates nutrimental composition of the fluid and maintains the proper volume and composition of the body's fluid. The kidney also transports surplus fluid to the bladder to eliminate from the body.

(c) The kidney governs the bone, produces bone marrow; its activities are reflected in the hair. TCM believes that the brain is composed of marrow (Sea of Marrow) and it depends on the kidney essence to develop.

(d) The orifice of the kidney is the ear, genitals and anus. Ear function relies on the nourishment of kidney qi. The kidney is the gate of stomach.

(2) Physiology of the Bladder

The urinary bladder is relatively a yang organ. Its channels connect to the kidney. It receives, stores and excretes fluid. Fluid is the source of urine, and qi circulation facilitates urine to excrete from the body.

(3) Pathology of the Kidney

The kidney disorders are caused by depletion of kidney qi due to over fatigue, excessive sexual activities and chronic illness. The kidney disorders are mainly deficiency syndromes. It is appropriate to reinforce the kidney but inappropriate to purge it.

I. <u>Kidney Yin Deficiency</u>

Pathogenesis: Over fatigue, alcohol indulgence, sex indulgence and chronic illness deplete kidney yin. Febrile diseases also cause kidney yin deficiency. Kidney yin deficiency develops until kidney yin can not balance kidney yang, leading to internal heat or fire, which results in water insufficiency and fire hyperactivity.

Symptoms: Dizziness, tinnitus, insomnia, amnesia, lassitude in the waist and legs, low-grade fever, seminal emission, dry mouth, red tongue with scanty coating, and thready pulse. Patients with fire hyperactivity also demonstrate red cheeks and lips, hectic fever, night sweats, vexation, nocturnal emission, dry mouth, dry and sore throat, hot sensation in palms and soles, dark yellow urine, constipation, thready and rapid pulse.

Treatment principle: To nourish kidney yin and relieve hyperactive fire.

Treatment with herbs: Radix Rehmanniae Praeparatae (Shu Di Huang), Radix Polygoni Multiflori (He Shou Wu), Rhizoma Polygonati (Huang Jing), Fructus Lycii (Gou Qi Zi), Fructus Ligustri Lucidi (Nu Zhen Zi), Carapax et Plastrum Testudinis (Gui Ban), and Fructus Corni Officinalis (Shan Zhu Yu).

Treatment with formula: Liu Wei Di Huang Pill, Zuo Gui Pill, or Zhi Bai Di Huang Pill.

II. <u>Kidney Yang Deficiency</u>

Pathogenesis: Kidney yang, i.e., the life gate fire, is the motive force of all functions. Chronic illness, inherited weakness, sex indulgence and deficiency of primordial qi attenuate the fire from the life gate, resulting in kidney yang deficiency.

Symptoms: Cold pain in the waist and legs, impotence, premature ejaculation, pale complexion, dizziness, tinnitus, aversion to cold, frequent micturition, oliguria, pale tongue with white coating, and deep, slow and feeble pulse.

Treatment principle: To warm and nourish kidney yang.

Treatment with herbs: Herba Cistanches (Rou Cong Rong), Radix Morindae officinalis (Ba Ji Tian), Herba Epimedii (Yin Yang Huo), Rhizoma Curculiginis Orchioidis (Xian Mao), Fructus Psoraleae Corylifoliae (Bu Gu Zhi), Semen Cuscutae Chinensis (Tu Si Zi), Semen Allii Tuberosi (Jiu Cai Zi), Radix Aconiti Lateralis Praeparatae (Fu Zi), Cortex Cinnamomi Cassiae (Rou Gui), and Aspongopus (Jiu Xiang Chong).

Treatment with formula: Jin Gui Shen Qi Pill or You Gui Pill.

III. <u>Edema due to Kidney Yang Deficiency</u>

Pathogenesis: Overstrain, congenital weakness and chronic illness lead to kidney yang deficiency, which fails to warm and transform fluid, resulting in pathogenic fluid overflow.

Symptoms: Edema throughout the body, pain and weakness in the waist and legs, cold extremities, feeling of distention in the abdomen, diarrhea, oliguria, palpitation, dyspnea, cough, abundant sputum, pale tongue, and deep, thready and slow pulse.

Treatment principle: To warm kidney yang and induce diuresis.

Treatment with herbs: herbs that treat kidney yang deficiency plus the following diuretics: Sclerotium Poriae Cocos (Fu Ling), Sclerotium Polypori Umbellati (Zhu Ling), Rhizoma Alismatis Orientalis (Ze Xie), Semen Plantaginis (Che Qian Zi), and Pericarpium Areca Catechu (Da Fu Pi).

Treatment with formula: Zhen Wu Decoction or Ji Sheng Shen Qi Pill.

IV. <u>Kidney Qi Deficiency</u>

Pathogenesis: Deficient kidney yang, overstrain, deficient primordial qi and malnutrition due to chronic illness lead to kidney qi deficiency, resulting in dysfunction of kidney in assimilating, storing and consolidating essence or qi.

Symptoms: Pale complexion, or edema in the face, weakness and soreness in the waist and lower back, shortness of breath, dyspnea worsened by exertion, hearing loss, frequent urination or even urinary incontinence, urinary dribbling after micturition or induced by cough, perspiration induced by cough, infertility, premature ejaculation, spermatorrhoea (involuntary emission), pale tongue with thin and white coating, thready and feeble pulse.

Treatment principle: To reinforce kidney qi.

Treatment with herbs: Fructus Schisandrae Chinensis (Wu Wei Zi), Semen Nelumbinis Nuciferae (Lian Zi), Semen Euryales Ferocis (Qian Shi), Fructus Corni Officinalis (Shan Zhu Yu), Fructus Rosae Laevigatae (Jin Ying Zi), Fructus Rubi Chingii (Fu Pen Zi), Radix Ginseng (Ren Shen), Lignum Aquilariae Resinatum (Chen Xiang), Radix Linderae Strychnifoliae (Wu Yao), and Rhizoma Dioscoreae (Shan Yao).

Treatment with formula: Da Bu Yuan Decoction to reinforce kidney qi, Ren Shen Hu Tao Decoction or Shen Ge Powder to assimilate kidney qi.

(4) Pathology of the Bladder

Bladder disorders are mainly manifested by impaired qi circulation, urine retention, difficult urination, frequent urination and urinary incontinence.

I. <u>Cold Syndrome of the Bladder (Deficiency Type)</u>

Symptoms: Frequent urination, urinary dribbling, enuresis, pale tongue with moist coating, deep and thready pulse.

Treatment principle: To strengthen and astringe the kidney qi.

Treatment with formula: Sang Piao Xiao Powder.

II. Heat Syndrome of the Bladder (Excess Type)

Symptoms: Scanty dark urine, cloudy urine, hematuria, difficult urination, dribbling urination, dysuria with a burning sensation, red tongue with yellow coating, and rapid pulse.

Treatment principle: To resolve damp-heat.

Treatment with formula: Ba Zheng Powder.

B. The Relationship between Different Visceral Organs

Although different visceral organs have different functions, they are not independent; they are interrelated with and interacted on each other. They share out the work and cooperate with each other. In studying the physiology and pathology of visceral organs, we must not only focus on different functions of organs, but also on their relationship to each other.

1) Heart and Kidney

The heart is located above kidney and relatively speaking, the heart is yang and the kidney is yin. By their very nature, heart yang descends and kidney yin ascends. Heart yang coordinates with kidney yin, thus heart yang is not hyperactive and the kidney is not hypoactive. If the coordination is broken, disorders occur.

2) Liver and Spleen

The liver stores blood, but the generation of blood depends on the spleen. The spleen rules transformation and transportation of nutrients, but the transformation and transportation depend on liver qi.

3) Kidney and Lung

The lung controls respiration, but it is assisted with the assimilation of kidney qi. Lung yin also needs the nourishment of kidney yin.

The lung facilitates the circulation of fluid and the kidney regulates fluid metabolism of the body, thus together they succeed in the normal metabolism of fluid.

4) Spleen and Lung

The spleen rules transformation and transportation of nutrients and is the origin of transformation of blood and qi. Lung qi is nourished by the essence qi of food and water from the spleen. The lung controls respiration and governs qi of the body, including the essence qi of food and water of the spleen. The transformation of dampness (the spleen) also needs to be regulated by lung qi.

   5) Heart and Lung

The heart governs the blood of the body and the lung governs qi of the body. The blood circulation depends on qi propelling and the qi circulation relies on blood as its carrier. Thus "qi is the general of the blood, and the blood is the mother of qi. If qi circulates, so does the blood; if qi is stagnated, so is the blood."

   6) Liver and Kidney

The liver stores blood and the kidney stores essence. Both blood and essence rely on the replenishment of the essence of food and water, and blood and essence can be transformed into each other. Liver yang relies on the nourishment of kidney yin that keeps liver yang from being hyperactive. Thus "the liver and kidney have the same origin."

C. Complicated Organ Dysfunctions

   1) Deficiency of Qi and Blood in the Heart and Spleen

Symptoms: Dyspnea, palpitation, insomnia, fatigue, lassitude, anorexia, amnesia, sallow complexion, irregular menstruation, pale tongue with white tongue coating, soft and feeble pulse.

Treatment: Gui Pi Decoction to replenish the heart and spleen.

   2) Impaired Coordination between Heart Yang and Kidney Yin

Symptoms: Vexation, insomnia, palpitation, amnesia, dizziness, tinnitus, lassitude in the waist and legs, nocturnal emission, hectic fever, night sweats, dry throat, polyuria, red tongue with scanty coating, thready and feeble pulse.

Treatment: Huang Lian E Jiao Decoction, Bu Xin Pill or Jiao Tai Pill to coordinate the heart and kidney.

   3) Liver Qi Attacks the Stomach

Symptoms: Vexation, irritation, sensation of oppression in the chest and stomach, wandering pain in the hypochondriac region, dyspepsia, belching, acid regurgitation, thin and yellow tongue coating, and taut pulse.

Treatment: Si Ni Powder plus Zuo Jin Pill to quench liver fire and regulate the stomach.

   4) Liver Fire Attacks the Lung

Symptoms: Cough, dizziness, irritability, dysphoria, conjunctival congestion, hematemesis, pricking pain in the chest and hypochondriac region, bitter taste in the mouth, red tongue with thin coating, taut and rapid pulse.

Treatment: Dai Ge Powder or Xie Bai Powder to relieve liver and lung heat.

5) Impaired Coordination between the Liver and Spleen

Symptoms: Anorexia, abdominal distention, bowel sound, diarrhea, white and greasy tongue coating, taut and slow pulse.

Treatment: Xiao Yao Powder to coordinate the liver and spleen.

6) Disturbance of the Liver and Gallbladder

Symptoms: Vexation, insomnia, nightmare, panic, shortness of breath, lassitude, blurred vision, bitter taste in the mouth, thin and white tongue coating, taut and thready pulse.

Treatment: Suan Zao Ren Decoction to nourish the liver, resolve gallbladder heat and tranquilize the mind. If it is accompanied with symptoms of phlegm and heat with greasy and yellow tongue coating, taut and slippery pulse, Huang Lian Wen Dan Decoction should be used.

7) Yin Deficiency in the Liver and Kidney

Symptoms: Dizziness, dry eyes, sore throat, dysphoria, dyschezia, seminal emission, night sweats, irregular menstruation, leukorrhea, sallow complexion, flushed cheeks, lassitude in the waist and knees, hot sensation in palms and soles, red tongue without coating, and thready pulse.

Treatment: Qi Ju Di Huang Pill to nourish yin and reduce fire.

8) Impaired Coordination between the Spleen and Stomach

Symptoms: Sensation of fullness and stuffiness in the stomach, dull abdominal pain, dyspepsia, belching, nausea, vomiting, diarrhea, thin and white tongue coating, and thready pulse.

Treatment: Ban Xia Xie Xin Decoction to nourish qi and coordinate the spleen and stomach.

9) Yang Deficiency in the Spleen and Kidney

Symptoms: Low energy, aversion to cold, disinclination to talk, cold extremities, spontaneous perspiration, diarrhea, lassitude in the waist and knees, pale tongue with thin and white coating, thready and deep pulse.

Treatment: Li Zhong Decoction plus Si Shen Pill to strengthen the spleen and warm the kidney.

10) Splenic Dampness Attacks the Lung

Symptoms: Cough, abundant sputum, sensation of constriction in the chest, shortness of breath, anorexia, little, white and greasy tongue coating, and slippery pulse.

Treatment: Er Chen Decoction or Ping Wei Powder to resolve dampness and phlegm.

11) Qi Deficiency in the Lung and Spleen

Symptoms: Cough, abundant sputum, anorexia, loose stools, lassitude, edema, abdominal distension, white tongue coating, soft and feeble pulse.

Treatment: Si Jun Zi Decoction to replenish the spleen, thus strengthening both spleen and lung qi.

12) Deficiency of Qi and Yin in the Lung and Kidney

Symptoms: Cough worsened at night, shortness of breath and dyspnea worsened by exertion, tectic fever, lassitude in the waist and legs, night sweats, seminal emission, red tongue with little coating, thready and rapid pulse.

Treatment: Sheng Mai Powder to nourish yin and the lung.

13) Kidney Yang Deficiency Affects the Heart

Symptoms: Cough, palpitation, restlessness, shortness of breath and dyspnea aggravated by recumbency, edema, sensation of distention and fullness in the chest and abdomen, cyanotic fingers and lips, cold extremities, pale tongue with thin coating, feeble and rapid pulse.

Treatment: Zhen Wu Decoction to warm yang and resolve fluid retention.

5. The Three Pathogens (Wind, Fire and Dampness) Playing both Internal and External Roles

1) Wind

External pathogenic wind invades the pulmonary systems through mouth and nose; it invades the channels and viscera through the skin. Internal pathogenic wind is mainly caused by inappropriate emotion, inappropriate diet, inappropriate life style, extreme heat, hyperactivity of liver yang, and blood deficiency.

(1) External Pathogenic Wind Syndrome

  (a) <u>Wind-Cold Syndrome</u>:

    Symptoms: Severe headache, stuffy nose, fever, absence of sweats, aversion to cold, white and thin tongue coating, tense and floating pulse.

    Treatment: Cong Chi Decoction or Jing Fang Bai Du Powder to expel wind and disperse cold.

  (b) <u>Wind-Heat Syndrome</u>:

    Symptoms: Sore throat, rhinorrhea, tonsillitis, conjunctival congestion and pain, photophobia, distending sensation in the head, fever without aversion to cold, little sweats, aversion to wind, cough, yellow sputum, flushed face, and facial swelling pain. Hemoptysis, yellow urine, rapid and full pulse may also be demonstrated.

Treatment: Sang Ju Decoction or Yin Qiao Powder to expel wind and resolve heat.

(c) <u>Wind-Dampness Syndrome</u>:

Symptoms: Headache, wandering pain in the joints, eczema, chickenpox, increase bowel sound, abdominal pain, and watery diarrhea.

Treatment: Qiang Huo Sheng Shi Decoction to dispel wind and reduce dampness. Huo Xiang Zheng Qi Powder for gastrointestinal syndromes.

(2) Internal Pathogenic Wind Syndrome

(a) <u>Wind Syndrome due to extreme heat</u>:

Symptoms: Fever, tic, stiff neck, opisthotonus, and upward deviation of the eyes.

Treatment: Tian Ma Gou Teng Decoction. An Gong Niu Huang Pill, Zhi Bao Pill or Zi Xue Pellet can be added according to condition.

(b) <u>Wind Syndrome due to liver yang hyperactivity</u>:

Symptoms: Vertigo, shaking extremities, coma, hemiplegia, or hemiparesis, and deviation of the eyes and mouth.

Treatment: Da Ding Feng Pill.

(c) <u>Wind Syndrome due to blood deficiency</u>:

Symptoms: Vertigo, dizziness, numbness or paresthesias of the limbs, shaking extremities, and muscle spasm.

Treatment: Modified Fu Mai Decoction.

2) Dampness

Dampness plays both internal and external roles. It plays an external role because it is one of the six exogenous pathogenic factors or climatic causes of disorders; dampness also plays an internal role because it closely related to the pathological changes of the spleen and stomach.

(1) External Pathogenic Dampness Syndrome

It is related to the climate and environment. It invades the skin, joints, muscle and the viscera. It often attacks the lower extremities first. Symptoms include sensation of heaviness in the extremities, body lassitude, joints pain in fixed locations, articular stiffness, white and slightly greasy tongue coating, soft and slow pulse.

(a) <u>Cold-Dampness</u>

Symptoms: Body pain, severe joints pain worsened by movement, absence of sweats, loose stools, edema of extremities, white and greasy tongue coating, soft and slow pulse.

Treatment: Juan Bi Decoction.

(b) <u>Damp-Heat</u>

Symptoms: Vexation, fever, thirst, spontaneous perspiration, articular pain, swollen joints, sensation of fullness in the chest, jaundice, dark urine, yellow and greasy tongue coating, soft and rapid pulse.

Treatment: Bai Hu Jia Cang Zhu Decoction. For syndrome with jaundice, use Yin Chen Wu Ling Powder; for syndrome with swollen joints, use Bai Hu Jia Gui Zhi Decoction.

(c) <u>Summer Dampness</u>

Symptoms: Anorexia, vomiting, diarrhea, fever, sweating, sensation of fullness and tightness in the chest and abdomen, white and smooth tongue coating, soft and feeble pulse.

Treatment: Huo Xiang Zheng Qi Powder.

(2) Internal Pathogenic Dampness Syndrome

It mainly caused by improper diet that impairs the functions of the spleen and stomach.

Symptoms: Headache, lassitude, sensation of heaviness in the extremities, sensation of fullness and tightness in the chest and stomach, stomatitis, insipidness or greasy taste in the mouth, anorexia, belching, diarrhea, thick and greasy tongue coat, soft and feeble pulse.

Treatment: Wei Ling Decoction to regulate the spleen and resolve dampness. The internal damp-heat syndromes (caused by the combination of dampness and heat) can, depending on situations, be treated in the reference to the treatment of fire syndromes, with the addition of herbs or formula to remove dampness.

3) Fire

Fire plays both internal and external roles. It plays an external role because it is one of the six exogenous pathogenic factors or climatic causes of disorders; fire also plays an internal role because it can be generated in the process of disorders. Fire can be divided into excess fire and deficiency fire. Generally, fire caused by external pathogens belongs to excess fire; whereas fire generated by internal causes belongs to deficiency fire.

(1) Excess Fire

It is caused by pathogenic fire directly or by other exogenous pathogenic factors, e.g. cold, dampness, etc. Excess fire usually demonstrates acute pattern and short course. Symptoms include high fever, flushed face, flushed ears, thirst, vexation, desire for cold drinks, mania, delirium, scanty dark urine, constipation, parched lips. Tongue coating is yellow, dry or has prickles. Pulse is rapid and full.

(a) <u>Excess Fire in the Heart</u>

Symptoms: Flushed face and ears, dysphoria, a sensation of heat or burning in the soles and palms, dry mouth, parched lips, necrosis of the tongue, delirium, coma, hematemesis, epistaxis, and abnormal laughing.

Treatment: Xie Xin Decoction.

(b) <u>Excess Fire in the Liver and Gallbladder</u>

Symptoms: Hypochondriac pain, insomnia, multi-dreams, dizziness, conjunctivitis, decreased hearing acuity, bitter taste in the mouth, myasthenia, stranguria (strangury), cloudy urine or hematuria.

Treatment: Long Dan Xie Gan Decoction.

(c) <u>Excess Fire in the Lung</u>

Symptoms: Dyspnea, nares flaring, cough, thick sputum, extreme thirst, desire for drinks, constipation, hard stools, epistaxis, and hemoptysis.

Treatment: Qian Jin Wei Jing Decoction or Sang Bai Pi Decoction.

(d) <u>Excess Fire in the Stomach</u>

Symptoms: Extreme thirst, acute and painful gingival inflammation and necrosis, often with bleeding and halitosis (necrotizing ulcerative gingivitis); vomiting, gastric acid regurgitation, hyper-metabolism, and increased appetite.

Treatment: Qing Wei Powder.

(e) <u>Excess Fire in the Large Intestine</u>

Symptoms: Constipation, or watery diarrhea, burning sensation in the anus.

Treatment: Da Cheng Qi Decoction.

(f) <u>Excess Fire in the Small Intestine</u>

Symptoms: Lower abdominal pain, stranguria, cloudy urine or hematuria.

Treatment: Dao Chi Powder.

(g) <u>Excess Fire in the Spleen</u>

Symptoms: Dry mouth and dry lips, extreme thirst, hyper-metabolism, increased appetite.

Treatment: Xie Huang Powder.

(h) <u>Excess Fire in the Urinary Bladder</u>

Symptoms: Abdominal pain, urinary retention, post-void dribbling, hematuria, enuresis (bed-wetting), and cloudy urine.

Treatment: Ba Zheng Powder.

(i) <u>Impaired Mental Activity due to Excess Fire</u>

Symptoms: Coma, delirium, and clonic convulsion.

Treatment: An Gong Niu Huang Pill or Zhi Bao Pill.

(2) Deficiency Fire

Deficiency fire is a product of pathological changes of the visceral organs. Depression, overstrain, sex indulgence, chronic diseases or malnutrition lead to the depletion of yin fluid and deficiency of essence and blood. Deficiency fire usually demonstrates chronic pattern and long course. Symptoms include hectic fever, night sweats, flushed cheeks in the afternoon, vexation, insomnia, tinnitus, amnesia, dry mouth, dry throat, dry cough, or scanty sputum tinged with blood, aching and sore waist, seminal emission, red smooth tongue with little tongue coating, rapid and thready pulse.

(a) <u>Deficiency Fire of the Kidney</u>

Symptoms: Dizziness, tinnitus, insomnia, amnesia, red cheeks and lips, hectic fever, night sweats, vexation, nocturnal emission, painful and dry mouth and throat, hot palms and soles, dark yellow urine, constipation, thready and rapid pulse.

Treatment: Zhi Bai Di Huang Pill or Qing Gu Powder.

(b) <u>Deficiency Fire of the Spleen and Stomach</u>

Symptoms: Gastric discomfort, gastric acid regurgitation, dry mouth, hunger without desire for drinks and food, and hard stools.

Treatment: Yi Wei Decoction.

6. Six Stages (Syndromes of the Six Channels)

The theory about the syndromes of the six channels, known as Six Stages, is a diagnosis and treatment system created by Zhang Zhongjing (an eminent Chinese physician of Eastern Han Dynasty and author of Treatise on Cold-Induced and Miscellaneous Diseases) who analyzed and differentiated febrile diseases on the basis of Huangdi's Canon of Medicine theory. He inherited the names of the six channels from Huangdi's Canon of Medicine (Huang Di Nei Jing, also known as The Yellow Emperor's Internal Classic, which was written during the Spring and Autumn Period and Warring States Period in ancient China) and divided febrile diseases into six different stages or types of manifestations: Tai Yang Syndrome, Shao Yang Syndrome, Yang Ming Syndrome, Tai Yin Syndrome,

Shao Yin Syndrome, and Jue Yin Syndrome. We need to understand the basics of channels and collaterals in traditional Chinese medicine before we can understand these syndromes.

1) Physiology of the Channels and Collaterals

Huangdi's Canon of Medicine divided "jing luo", the Chinese term for channels and collaterals (also known as meridians), into two categories: jing mai (channels) and luo mai (collaterals). Channels mean "pathways" and their locations are usually more interior than those of collaterals. They pass vertically through the spaces between the deep muscles. Collaterals mean "networks" and are the transverse branches of the deep vertical channels. They pass horizontally through the superficial parts of the body. Branches from the collaterals are called "sun luo" or sun collaterals, which are tiny collaterals. Both channels and collaterals mean link or connection, and they are closely bound together to form channels and collaterals.

Channels and collaterals are mainly composed of 12 regular channels, 8 extraordinary channels and 15 collaterals.

- <u>12 Regular Channels</u>: The 12 Regular Channels, also known as 12 Principal Channels or 12 Primary Channels, are Arm Tai Yang Small Intestine Channel, Arm Shao Yang Triple Warmer Channel, Arm Yang Ming Large Intestine Channel, Arm Tai Yin Lung Channel, Arm Shao Yin Heart Channel, Arm Jue Yin Pericardium Channel; Leg Tai Yang Bladder Channel, Leg Shao Yang Gallbladder Channel, Leg Yang Ming Stomach Channel, Leg Tai Yin Spleen Channel, Leg Shao Yin Kidney Channel, and Leg Jue Yin Liver Channel.

- <u>8 Extraordinary Channels</u>: The 8 Extraordinary Channels, also known as 8 Extra Channels or 8 Unusual Channels, are Yang Wei Channel, Yin Wei Channel, Yang Qiao Channel, Yin Qiao Channel, Chong Channel, Ren Channel, Du Channel, and Dai Channel

- <u>15 Collaterals</u>: The 12 Regular Channels plus Ren Channel and Du Channel of the 8 Extraordinary Channels are called "14 Channels". Each of the 14 channels has its collateral. The 15 Collaterals consist of 14 collaterals corresponding to the 14 Channels and the Great Collateral (Da Luo or Da Bao, also called Great Luo) of the spleen.

(1) Distribution of the 12 Regular Channels

The distribution of 12 regular channels is symmetrical. Every channel has one on the left of the body and another identical one on the right. Actually, the 12 regular channels are named according to their corresponding organs, limb positions, and yin and yang properties.

How 12 Regular Channels are named

Limb Positions	Yin and Yang	Organs
Arm	Yang Ming Tai Yang Shao Yang Tai Yin Shao Yin Jue Yin	Large Intestine Small Intestine Triple Warmer Lung Heart Pericardium
Leg	Yang Ming Tai Yang Shao Yang Tai Yin Shao Yin Jue Yin	Stomach Bladder Gallbladder Spleen Kidney Liver

The followings are the distribution of 12 regular channels:

(a) <u>Arm Tai Yang Small Intestine Channel</u>

It starts from the tip of the little finger and crosses the wrist. It runs upwards along the posterior side of the forearm and the back of shoulder until it reaches a point at the bottom of the neck where it splits into two branches. The first branch runs internally through the heart and stomach to reach the small intestine. The second branch runs upwards across the neck and cheek externally until it reaches a point where it splits again into two branches. The first branch runs across the cheek until it reaches the outer corner of the eye and then enters the ear. The second branch moves upward to the inner corner of the eye where it connects with the bladder channel.

(b) <u>Arm Shao Yang Triple Warmer Channel</u>

It begins at the tip of the ring finger and goes along the back of the hand, wrist, forearm and upper arm, until it reaches a point at the shoulder region where it splits into two branches. The first branch runs internally into the chest and passes through the pericardium and diaphragm, uniting the upper, middle and lower warmer (triple warmer). The second branch runs externally upward along the side of the neck, circles the back of ear and finally ends at the outer end of the eyebrow where it connects with the gallbladder channel.

(c) <u>Arm Yang Ming Large Intestine Channel</u>

It starts from the tip of the index finger and runs between the thumb and the index finger. It then runs upward along the lateral side of the forearm and the anterior side of the upper arm, until it reaches the highest point of the shoulder. From there, it splits into two branches. The first branch goes internally towards the lungs, diaphragm and large intestine. The second branch runs externally upwards and passes the neck and cheek until it reaches the point where it splits again into two branches. One branch then curves externally around the upper lip and crosses to the opposite side of the nose. The other branch goes internally to the lower teeth and gums.

(d) <u>Arm Tai Yin Lung Channel</u>

It originates in the middle portion of the body, and runs downward and connects with the large intestine. It then turns upward and passes through the diaphragm to connect with the lungs. It comes out at the axilla and runs downward the medial aspect of the upper arm where it crosses the elbow crease. It continues until it passes above the major artery of the wrist and ends at the tip of the thumb. Another branch emerges from the back of the wrist and ends at the radial side of the tip of the index finger to connect with the large intestine channel.

(e) <u>Arm Shao Yin Heart Channel</u>

It starts from the heart, and splits into three branches. The first branch goes downwards and ends at the small intestine. The second runs upwards, goes along the throat and ends at the eyes. The third branch goes toward the axilla and emerges under the arm. It then runs downward along the inner side of the upper arm, elbow, forearm, wrist and palm and ends at the inside tip of the little finger where it connects with the small intestine channel.

(f) <u>Arm Jue Yin Pericardium Channel</u>

It starts from the pericardium and splits into two branches. One branch runs downwards and passes through the diaphragm to connect with the triple warmer. The other branch goes toward the axilla and it emerges from the chest before it reaches the axilla. From the medial side of the upper arm, it runs downward between the lung and heart channels, until it reaches the elbow crease. It then runs down the forearm and enters the palm where it splits into two branches. The first branch runs downward and ends at the tip of the middle finger. The second branch runs downward and connects with the triple warmer meridian at the end of the ring finger.

(g) <u>Leg Tai Yang Bladder Channel</u>

It starts at the inner side of the eye, goes across the forehead and reaches the top of the head where it branches into the brain. The main channel then goes across the back of the head and neck and splits into two branches. The first branch runs downward, paralleling to the spine. At the bottom of the spine, it branches into the bladder. The second branch runs downward on the outside of the first branch and parallels to the first branch. It continues downward until it reaches the buttocks from where the first and second branches run across the back of thigh along different pathways until they join at the back of the knee. This channel continues along the back of the lower leg, circles behind the outer ankle, runs along the outside of the foot and ends at the lateral side of the small toe tip, where it connects with the kidney channel.

(h) <u>Leg Shao Yang Gallbladder Channel</u>

It starts from the outer corner of the eye and splits into two branches. One branch runs externally and weaves back and forth at the lateral side of the head. After curving behind the ear, it reaches the top of the shoulder and crosses the lateral side of the trunk until it ends up at the side of the hip. The other branch runs internally downward and passes the cheek, the neck and chest to connect with the gall bladder. It continues moving downwards all the way to the lower abdomen and joins with the first branch at the hip. The hip branch then runs toward the lateral side of the thigh and lower leg. After crossing the ankle, it goes over the foot to reach to the tip of the fourth toe. One small branch leaves the channel at the foot and ends at the big toe to connect with the liver channel.

(i) <u>Leg Yang Ming Stomach Channel</u>

It starts from one side of the nose, passes through the inner corner of the eye and emerges from the lower part of the eye. It then goes downwards, enters the upper gum, and curves around the corner of the lips and lower jaw. It then turns upwards and passes in front of the ear until it reaches the corner of the forehead where it splits into internal and external branches. The internal branch emerges from the lower jaw and runs downwards until it reaches the stomach. The external branch crosses the neck, chest, abdomen and groin, and it goes further downward along the front side of the thigh, the lower leg and the top of the foot. It ends at the lateral side of the tip of the second toe. One more branch emerges from the top of the foot and ends at the big toe to connect with the spleen channel.

(j) <u>Leg Tai Yin Spleen Channel</u>

It starts from the big toe and runs upward along the inside of the foot, the ankle, the leg and the thigh until it reaches the upper abdomen where it splits into internal and external branches. The internal branch connects with the spleen and continues upward to reach the heart channel. The external branch continues running upward along the chest until it reaches the throat and the root of the tongue.

(k) <u>Leg Shao Yin Kidney Channel</u>

It starts from the inferior side of the small toe and crosses the middle of the sole and the arch of the foot. It then circles behind the inner ankle and runs upward along the inner side of the leg and the thigh until it enters the trunk near the base of the backbone. After connecting with the kidney, one branch emerges at the pubic bone. It runs externally upward over the abdomen and the chest until it reaches the inner side of clavicle. The second branch emerges from the kidney and runs internally upwards and passes through the liver, diaphragm, lungs and throat. It ends at the root of the tongue. One small branch splits from the second branch at the lung and connects with the heart and the pericardium.

(l) Leg Jue Yin Liver Channel

It starts from the top of the big toe, goes along the top of the foot, and passes before the inner ankle. It goes upwards along the inner side of the leg and the thigh until it reaches the pubic region. It circulates around the external genitalia and then continues to go upward along the abdomen and the lower chest to connect with the liver and gallbladder. Here it splits into two branches. The first branch runs upwards along the throat, connects with the eyes and emerges from the forehead to reach the vertex of the head. The second branch passes through the diaphragm to reach the lung where it connects with the lung channel and completes the cycle of the twelve regular channels. One small branch originates internally from the eye and moves downwards to the cheek where it curves around the inner surface of the lips.

(2) Physiological Function of the Channels and Collaterals

(a) Facilitate Qi and Blood Circulation

Channels and collaterals are the pathway of qi and blood movement in the body. They connect with organs, tissues, extremities or even skin, and transport and distribute qi and blood to them. As a result, organs and tissues are nourished; joints are facilitated; normal metabolic activities are maintained.

Flow chart of qi and blood through channels and collaterals:

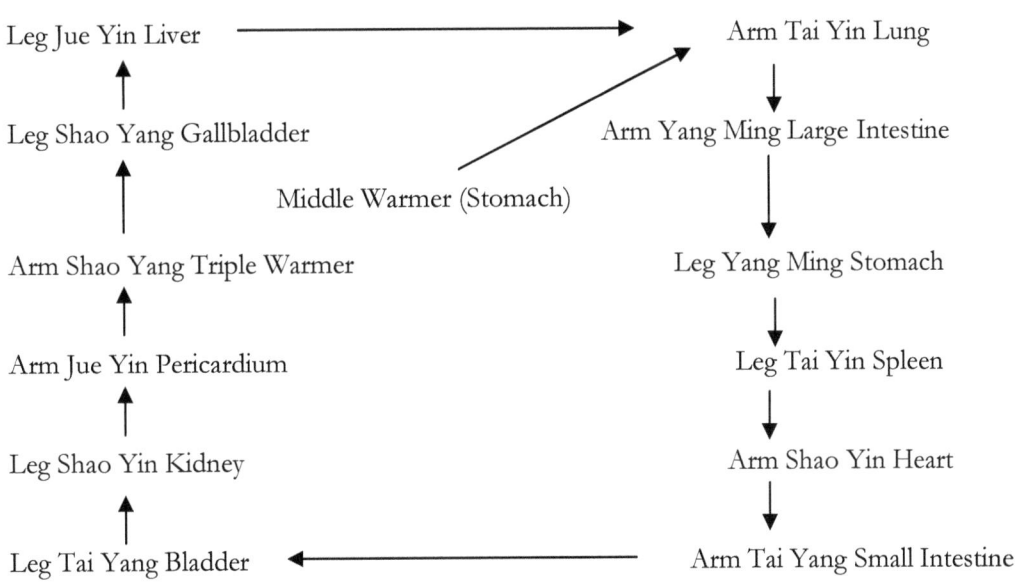

(b) <u>Display Defensive Function of Nutritive Qi and Defensive Qi</u>

Channels and collaterals are essential in supporting the flow of nutritive qi and defensive qi. Nutritive qi is yin qi and circulates in channels and nurtures visceral organs, extremities and skeleton. Day or night, it circulates continuously in the channels. Defensive qi is yang qi and circulates outside channels, and nourishes muscles and skin. It protects the surface of body from invasion of exogenous pathogenic factors. Defensive qi circulates outside yang channels during the day or during exercise; it circulates outside yin channels in the evening or during rest. The fact that yang channels bring defensive qi circulates in the surface of the body during the day means that it is difficult for exogenous pathogenic factors to invade the body during daytime or when the body is active. Yin channels bring the defensive qi to the interior organs to warm them at night or when the body is inactive. This may explain why people in sleeping are more vulnerable to the attack of exogenous pathogenic factors.

(c) <u>Connect Organs and Tissues</u>

Channels and collaterals work like a communication network between organs and tissues. Yang channels belong to Fu organs; their collaterals connect to Zang organs. Yin channels belong to Zang organs; their collaterals connect to Fu organs. As a result, yin and yang are regulated; organs and tissues are connected.

(d) <u>Make Clinical Diagnosis According to Reflected Symptoms</u>

Because channels and collaterals are the networks connecting organs and tissues, and they have unique distributions with unique beginnings and ends, clinical diagnosis can be made according to the symptoms reflected by the channels. For example, frontal headache or lower toothache is a Leg Yang Ming Channel type; headache of the temporal region or ear pain is Leg Shao Yang Channel type; occipital headache and nape pain is Leg Tai Yang Channel type; vertex headache is Leg Jue Yin Channel type.

(e) <u>Guide Herbal Prescriptions and Acupuncture Therapy</u>

The theory of channels and collaterals is important in guiding herbal treatment and acupuncture therapy. Acupuncture therapy replenishes, balances, and moves qi through acupuncture points on the channels and collaterals to resume normal organ functions. Moreover, different herbs belong to different channels and collaterals. These channel guiding properties of herbs help doctors to individually tailor herbal treatment plans for specific channels and their corresponding organs.

2) Pathology of the Channels and Collaterals

(1) Channels and Collaterals Are the Pathways through which Disorders Develop

Exogenous pathogenic factors invade the body from the exterior to the interior, from the outside to the inside along channels and collaterals. They affect skin and hair first, and then Sun collaterals, then collaterals, then channels and finally visceral organs. In this way exogenous pathogenic factors transform and progress along the channels and collaterals, and develop diseases. Because visceral organs are connected by channels and collaterals, impairment of one organ can affect other organs.

(2) Channels and Collaterals Reflect Disorders of Internal Visceral Organs

Disorders of internal visceral organs can show pathological changes at certain locations along the channels and collaterals with which these organs are connected. Namely, disorders inside the body can reflect to the surface, and disorders of one organ can affect other organs via channels and collaterals. For example, liver disorders can manifest lower chest pain because the liver channel passes through the lower chest region. The corresponding channels and acupuncture points usually demonstrate certain changes, e.g., painful feelings when these affected points are pressed.

In conclusion, the system of 12 channels and collaterals is the process through which the human body grows; is the explanation of how disease continues and develops; is the place where disease occurs; is the methods by which the body is treated; is the concept where philosophy begins; is the goal where successful outcome should be achieved.

The followings are the **SIX STAGES OF CHANNEL SYNDROMES** and their differentiation:

I. <u>Tai Yang Syndrome</u>

The Tai Yang Syndrome is the initial stage of diseases caused by exogenous pathogenic factors and uncoordinated Ying and Wei (nutritive level and defensive level). At this stage, cold and wind attack the skin of the body and cause a channel syndrome, which includes wind stroke syndrome and exogenous febrile syndrome. If the channel syndrome is not resolved, it will cause Fu organ syndrome, which includes water retention syndrome and blood retention syndrome. Tai Yang syndrome is mainly an exterior syndrome and manifests aversion to cold, fever, headache and floating pulse.

(a) Wind Stroke Syndrome

Wind stroke syndrome is an exterior and deficiency channel syndrome.

Symptoms: Fever, aversion to cold, sweating, headache, slow and floating pulse.

Treatment: Gui Zhi Decoction.

(b) Exogenous Febrile Syndrome

Exogenous febrile syndrome is an exterior and excess channel syndrome.

Symptoms: Fever, aversion to cold, no sweating, headache, stiffness in the neck and back, tense and floating pulse.

Treatment: Ma Huang Decoction.

(c) Water Retention Syndrome

Water retention syndrome is a Fu organ syndrome.

Symptoms: Fever, aversion to wind, difficult urination, extreme thirst, vomiting immediately after drinking, and floating pulse.

Treatment: Wu Ling Powder.

(d) Blood Retention Syndrome

Blood retention syndrome is a Fu organ syndrome.

Symptoms: Fever, aversion to wind, sensation of stiffness and fullness in the lower abdomen, urinary incontinence (enuresis), delirium, deep and thready pulse.

Treatment: Tao He Cheng Qi Decoction.

II. Shao Yang Syndrome

The Shao Yang Syndrome is caused by pathogens that have left Tai Yang (the exterior) but have not yet invaded Yang Ming (the interior). Pathogens could spread from exterior to interior or from interior to exterior, or come from channels and then stay between the exterior and interior. Shao yang syndrome is mainly a half exterior and half interior syndrome.

Symptoms: Bitter taste in the mouth, dry throat, dizziness, alternate attack of cold and fever, feeling of fullness in the chest and hypochondriac region, vexation, anorexia, vomiting, and taut pulse.

Treatment: Xiao Chai Hu Decoction.

Modifications: For headache, perspiration combined with the above symptoms (combination of Tai Yang and Shao Yang), use Chai Hu Gui Zhi Decoction; for constipation, or diarrhea, sensation of fullness and stiffness in the abdomen, combined with the above symptoms (combination of Yang Ming and Shao Yang), use Da Chai Hu Decoction.

III. Yang Ming Syndrome

The Yang Ming Syndrome is mainly an interior syndrome and is caused by external cold and wind, which invade from the exterior to interior and transform into heat. The heat accumulates in the stomach and intestine. The difference between channel syndrome and Fu organ syndrome is that channel syndrome does not have dry stools in the intestine while Fu organ syndrome does.

(a) Channel Syndrome

Symptoms: High fever, profuse perspiration, not aversion to cold but aversion to heat, extreme thirst, full and rapid pulse, yellow and dry tongue coating.

Treatment: Bai Hu Decoction

(b) Fu Organ Syndrome

Symptoms: Constipation, hectic fever, delirium, abdominal fullness sensation, aversion to heat, sweating, deep and forceful pulse.

Treatment: Cheng Qi Decoction (Da Cheng Qi Decoction, Xiao Cheng Qi Decoction, or Tiao Wei Cheng Qi Decoction).

IV. <u>Tai Yin Syndrome</u>

The Tai Yin Syndrome is mainly an interior, deficiency and cold syndrome. It is an early stage of yin channel syndrome. It is caused by cold pathogens that invade from the exterior to interior and damage the spleen and stomach, resulting in deficiency of spleen yang and impaired transformation and transportation of nutrients.

Symptoms: Sensation of fullness and pain in the abdomen, vomiting, diarrhea, anorexia, absence of fever, and slow pulse.

Treatment: Li Zhong Decoction or Fu Zi Li Zhong Decoction.

V. <u>Shao Yin Syndrome</u>

The Shao Yin Syndrome is mainly a deficiency and cold syndrome of the whole body and is the late and serous stage of a disease. It is caused by deeply invaded pathogens that impair the heart and kidney, resulting in deficiency of yin, yang, qi and blood.

(a) Cold Syndrome of Deficiency Type:

Symptoms: Aversion to cold, rolling up the body, cold extremities, somnolence, lethargy, diarrhea with undigested food, clear urine, feeble and thready pulse.

Treatment: Si Ni Decoction.

(b) Heat Syndrome of Deficiency Type:

Symptoms: Vexation, insomnia, dry mouth and throat, red tongue with scanty coating, thready and rapid pulse.

Treatment: Huang Lian E Jiao Decoction.

(c) Edema Type:

Symptoms: Dizziness, palpitation, shivering, edema, difficult urination, heavy and painful sensation in the extremities, and abdominal pain.

Treatment: Zhen Wu Decoction.

VI. Jue Yin Syndrome

The Jue Yin Syndrome is the last stage of yin channel syndromes. Pathogens invade the interior and seriously damage yin, yang, qi, blood and visceral organs, resulting in complicated and most serious condition with alternate attacks of cold and fever.

(a) Cold Type

Symptoms: Extremely cold extremities, aversion to cold, scanty tongue coating, retching, headache, and thready and extremely weak pulse.

Treatment: Dang Gui Si Ni Decoction supplemented with Fructus Evodiae Rutaecarpae (Wu Zhu Yu) and Rhizoma Zingiberis Recens (Sheng Jiang).

(b) Heat Type

Symptoms: Extremely cold extremities, vexation, thirsty, dark colored urine, yellow tongue coating, dysentery, rapid and slippery pulse.

Treatment: Bai Tou Weng Decoction.

(c) Simultaneously Occurred Cold and Heat Type

Symptoms: Vexation, vomiting after eating, or even vomiting roundworm (ascarid).

Treatment: Wu Mei Decoction or Wu Mei Pill.

7. Four Divisions/Levels of Febrile Diseases: Wei (defensive), Qi, Ying (nutritive) and Xue (blood)

Wei, Qi, Ying and Xue theory is the guiding principle for an overall analysis of febrile diseases, and is the classification method of all exogenous febrile diseases including infectious diseases. This theory is gradually formed and developed through clinical practice, observation, verification and experience on the basis of the six channels syndrome theory. It inherits the names of Wei (defensive), Qi, Ying (nutritive), Xue (blood) from Huangdi's Canon of Medicine to represent the four different divisions or levels of febrile disease development in order to illustrate the depth, the severity and the development of febrile diseases. Generally speaking, febrile diseases develop from the exterior to the interior, from the shallow to the deep, from the mild to the serious in the sequence of Wei, Qi, Ying and Xue levels (Wei → Qi → Ying → Xue). However, there are exceptions.

1) Wei (Defensive) Level Syndrome

Wei level syndrome is mainly the first stage of febrile disease. Warm pathogens attack the upper warmer or skin, and impair the lung function of purifying and descending.

Symptoms: Severe fever, little aversion to cold and wind, cough, sore throat, thirst, absence of sweats or little sweats, headache, thin and yellow tongue coating, red tongue tip or edge, floating and rapid pulse.

Treatment: Yin Qiao Power or Sang Ju Decoction.

2) Qi Level Syndrome

Warm pathogens invade qi system in Yang Ming, affecting the lung, diaphragm, stomach, intestine and gallbladder.

(1) Heat Accumulation in the Lung

Symptoms: Fever, chest pain, cough, thirsty, sweating, yellow tongue coating, and rapid pulse.

Treatment: Ma Xing Shi Gan Decoction.

(2) Heat Accumulation in the Stomach

Symptoms: High fever, profuse sweats, thirst, fidgety, yellow and dry tongue coating, and full pulse.

Treatment: Bai Hu Decoction or Bai Hu Jia Ren Shen Decoction.

(3) Heat Accumulation in the Intestine

Symptoms: Constipation, abdominal distension and pain, abdominal aversion to touch, sweating in the hands and feet, fidgety, delirium, red tongue with yellow and dry coating, and deep, rapid and forceful pulse.

Treatment: Da Cheng Qi Decoction, Xiao Cheng Qi Decoction, or Tiao Wei Cheng Qi Decoction.

3) Ying (Nutritive) Level Syndrome

Ying level syndrome is the serious stage of febrile diseases. Warm pathogens invade the interior (they have passed the Qi Level, have entered Ying Level, and nearly reach the Xue level) and transform into heat, resulting in impaired ying and mental activities. This syndrome is located in the heart and pericardium.

(1) Warm Pathogens Invade Ying Division/Level

Symptoms: Fever or high fever, fidgety, insomnia, delirium, dry throat, thirst, without desire to drink, skin rashes, red tongue with no coating, thready and rapid pulse.

Treatment: Qing Ying Decoction.

(2) Warm Pathogens Invade the Heart and Pericardium

Symptoms: High fever, slow response, delirium, even coma, or manic disorder, red tongue, and rapid pulse.

Treatment: An Gong Niu Huang Pill, Zi Xue Pellet, or Zhi Bao Pill.

4) Xue (Blood) Level Syndrome

Xue level syndrome is the life threatening stage of febrile diseases. Warm pathogens invade blood systems, resulting in heat accumulation, yin fluid depletion and internal wind stirring-up. This syndrome is located in the liver and the kidney.

(1) Heat Invades the Blood

Symptoms: Hematemesis, epistaxis, hematochezia, skin rashes, fever, vexation, insomnia, red tongue, and rapid pulse.

Treatment: Xi Jiao Di Huang Decoction.

(2) Heat Stirs Up Internal Wind

Symptoms: High fever, coma, stare, tight or closed mandibular joints, stiff nape, clonic convulsion of the extremities, or even opisthotonus, red and dry tongue with yellow coating, thready and rapid pulse.

Treatment: Ling Jiao Gou Teng Decoction or San Jia Fu Mai Decoction.

(3) Heat Depletes Yin

Symptoms: Hot body, flushed face, hot sensations in palms and soles, dry mouth, tremors of the extremities, purple tongue, and weak, thready and rapid pulse.

Treatment: Qing Hao Bie Jia Decoction.

Chapter 3: Diagnostic Methods of Disorders

The diagnostic procedure in TCM includes examination, diagnosis and treatment. There are four diagnostic methods: inspection (looking), auscultation (listening) and olfaction (smelling), interrogation (asking), and palpation (touching). Through the four diagnostic methods, the physicians obtain all the information about patients and make diagnoses in accordance with the theories of the channels and collaterals, the eight principles, the four levels of febrile diseases, the pathogenic changes of triple warmer and visceral organs, and the condition of wind, fire, phlegm and dampness.

1. Inspection

Inspection is a method to examine patients by observation of the outward manifestations, appearance, and the abnormal changes of spirit, color, tongue coating, secretion and excretion etc.

1) Observation of the Spirit

Observation of the spirit (shen), emotional state, consciousness, coordination, vigor of body movements, and keenness of response helps gain insight into the development of the disease, measure the strength or weakness of the disease, and judge the prognosis. Normal behavior, alertness, sparkled eyes, and cooperation indicate that the disease is usually mild. But spiritlessness, sluggish responses, dull eyes and confusion suggest that the disease might be serious.

2) Observation of Complexion

The color and luster of the facial region vary according to races. Generally speaking, a lustrous complexion with normal color indicates a good prognosis. Deep colored and withered complexion indicates a serious disease condition with a poor prognosis.

(1) Red Color: Red complexion indicates excess heat syndromes; malar flush indicates interior-heat of deficiency type caused by insufficiency of yin.

(2) White Color: Pale complexion indicates a yin excess with yang deficiency. Lusterless, pale and swollen complexion indicates a qi deficiency. Pale emaciated face indicates a blood deficiency. A

sudden pale complexion with cold sweats indicates febrile diseases caused by exogenous pathogenic wind-cold.

(3) Yellow Color: Yellowish, withered and lusterless complexion indicates qi deficiency of the spleen and stomach. Yellowish, chubby complexion indicates damp accumulation due to spleen dysfunction of transportation and transformation. Yellowish face, eyes, and skin indicates jaundice (bright orange yellow color indicates yang jaundice caused by pathogenic damp-heat; dark yellow color indicates yin jaundice due to pathogenic cold-damp).

(4) Purple-Green or Blue Color: Purple-green or bluish complexion indicates syndromes of cold, pain, and blood stasis or convulsion.

(5) Dark Gray or Black Color: Dark gray or black complexion indicates syndromes of kidney deficiency, cold, pain, humor accumulation and blood stasis.

3) Observation of Body Structure, Posture and Movement

Overweight indicates dampness, phlegm and splenic deficiency. Emaciation indicates yin and essence deficiency. Facing inside and huddling up indicates yin syndrome; whereas facing outside and stretching extremities indicates yang syndrome. Twitching of extremities indicates internal liver wind. Restlessness and agitation indicates yang heat; whereas listlessness and aversion to cold indicates yin cold. Numb and paralyzed limbs indicates stroke; whereas restricted movements of hands and feet with pain and swelling joints indicates rheumatism.

4) Observation of the Tongue

Observation of the tongue, also known as tongue diagnosis, is an important part of diagnostic methods. Changes of the tongue signs can objectively reflect the changes of the interior of the body, e.g. the deficiency or excess of visceral organs, the depth of external pathogenic invasion and the condition of phlegm and blood. The tongue can be divided into four parts: the tip, the middle, the root and the side. Different parts of the tongue correspond to different internal organs. The tip reflects the heart and lung; the middle part reflects the spleen and stomach; the sides of tongue reflect the liver and gallbladder; the root reflects the kidney. Tongue diagnosis includes tongue body observation and tongue coating (fur) observation. Tongue body refers to the tongue itself; tongue coating refers to the layer of "moss" on the tongue surface. A normal tongue is proper in size, soft in quality, free in motion, light red in color and has a thin layer of white coating that is neither dry nor overly moist.

(1) Tongue Body

(a) Appearance
- Big, Enlarged and Fat Tongue (Chubby Tongue): Chubby tongue indicates stagnation of phlegm, fluid or dampness. A pale and chubby tongue body with teeth marks on the margin indicates yang deficiency of the spleen and kidney, and/or qi deficiency. A deep red and chubby tongue (the mouth is full with the enlarged tongue) indicates excessive pathogenic heat in the heart and spleen.
- Thin and Small Tongue: A thin and small tongue indicates deficiency of phlegm, fluid and water. A thin and small tongue with pale color indicates deficiency of both qi and blood. A thin and dry tongue with deep red color indicates excess of pathogenic heat impairing phlegm, and hyperactivity of fire due to yin deficiency.
- Old Tongue: An old tongue texture that appears wrinkled and rough indicates excess of pathogenic factors.
- Tender Tongue: A tender tongue texture that appears smooth and delicate indicates deficiency of anti-pathogenic qi.
- Flaccid Tongue: A flaccid, soft or flabby tongue is weak and lacks strength and firmness. It usually indicates deficiency of qi and blood.
- Rigid Tongue: A stiff or rigid tongue is difficult to move and may cause speech abnormalities such as slurring or mumbled speech. It indicates invasion of exogenous pathogenic heat or obstruction of pathogenic phlegm in febrile diseases, depletion of body fluids, excess heat, or potential or impending Wind-Stroke.
- Cracked Tongue: Cracked tongue surface indicates excess of pathogenic heat and depletion of phlegm in febrile diseases. Crimson tongue with cracks indicates chronic diseases caused by hyperactivity of fire due to yin deficiency. A pale, chubby and tender tongue with cracks indicates deficiency of blood and qi. However, cracked tongue can be seen in normal people.
- Trembling Tongue: A trembling or quivering tongue with deep red color indicates external febrile disease or excess heat consuming yin. A pale and trembling tongue usually indicates a chronic deficiency of qi and blood. Medications may cause tongue tremor.
- Deviated Tongue: Deviated tongue indicates wind-stroke.

(b) Color
- Pale Tongue: Pale tongue indicates bleeding, blood deficiency, insufficiency of ying (nutritive) qi and blood, or deficiency of yang qi. Pale and atrophy tongue indicates great deficiency of qi and

blood.

- Red Tongue: Red tongue indicates heat syndromes, i.e., pathogenic heat invading Ying (nutritive) level, pathogenic heat impairing yin, blood getting thicker and more concentrated. Red tongue with yellow coating indicates Interior, Excess and Heat. Red tongue with scanty coating indicates hyperactivity of fire due to yin deficiency.
- Crimson Tongue: Crimson tongue is deep red or dark red in color and indicates excessive heat and invasion of pathogenic heat in Ying (nutritive) and Xue (blood) levels. It also indicates hyperactivity of fire due to yin deficiency in chronic diseases.
- Purple Tongue: A purple tongue is purplish dark in color or a tongue with purplish plaques and spots (petechiae or ecchymosis). It indicates blood stasis.

(2) Tongue Coating

(a) Appearance

- Thinness and Thickness: Thinness and thickness of tongue coating reflects the depth of pathogenic qi. Thin tongue coating indicates exterior syndromes; whereas thick coating indicates interior syndromes and serious diseases.
- Moistness and Dryness: Moistness and dryness of tongue coating reflects the body fluid condition. Slippery tongue coating indicates pathogenic damp syndromes. Dry tongue coating indicates exogenous pathogenic heat impairing phlegm in febrile diseases, or deficiency of phlegm and fluid in internal syndromes.
- Stickiness and Greasiness: Sticky, greasy, smooth and thick coating indicates hyperactive endogenous pathogenic phlegm and dampness or food accumulation. Thick but not smooth, and tofu-debris like coating indicates damp-heat in the stomach and intestine. A curdled tongue coating is the outcome of ascent of turbid qi due to food accumulation in the stomach. It is also seen in disease caused by phlegm-dampness.
- Peeling: Peeling of tongue coating is mostly due to insufficiency of qi and yin.
- No Coating: Smooth or shiny tongue without coating is mostly seen in chronic diseases or serious diseases due to severely damaged anti-pathogenic qi. Appearance or disappearance of the tongue coating reflects changes of disease conditions.

(b) Color

- White Coating: White tongue coating indicates exterior and/or cold syndromes. White and thin coating is seen in exterior-cold syndromes, whereas a white and thick coating is seen in interior-cold syndromes. Red tongue with white thin coating indicates exterior-heat syndromes. White and slippery tongue coating indicates cold-damp and phlegm syndromes. White, dry, cracked and powder-like coating indicates hyperactivity of internal pathogenic heat and impairment of phlegm and fluid. It is usually seen in serious infectious diseases.

- <u>Yellow Coating</u>: Yellow tongue coating indicates interior and heat syndromes. The deeper the yellow color, the more severe the heat. A slightly yellow and thin coating is seen in exterior-heat syndrome. Thick, dry and yellow coating indicates injured phlegm due to pathogenic heat accumulation in the stomach. Thick, greasy and yellow coating indicates damp-heat in the stomach and spleen or accumulation of pathogenic heat in the stomach and intestine.

- <u>Gray and Black Coating</u>: Gray and black tongue coating indicates serious diseases. Pale tongue with black and slippery coating indicates serious yang qi deficiency and interior cold-damp and fluid accumulation. Bright red tongue with black and dry coating indicates consumption of body fluid due to excessive heat or yin deficient fire. Black and dry coating with thorns or spikes on the tongue surface indicates depletion of body fluid and yin due to extreme heat. It is a dangerous stage of disease.

2. Auscultation and Olfaction

Auscultation (listening) is a diagnostic method to listen to the patient's speech, respiration and sound changes. Olfaction (smelling) is a method to smell abnormal odors of patient's body, breath, excretions and secretions.

1) Listening

Loud and sonorous voice indicates excess and heat syndromes, whereas weak and low voice indicates deficiency and cold syndromes. Forceful breathing with a coarse voice indicates excess and heat syndromes, often seen in exterior-cold or exterior-heat syndromes. Feeble breathing with shortness of breath usually indicates qi deficiency in the lung or the kidney. Loud and coarse coughing usually indicates excess syndromes. A weak cough indicates deficiency syndromes. A dry hacking, unproductive cough with little sticky yellow sputum indicates heat and dryness in the lung.

2) Smelling

Foul odor usually indicates excess-heat syndromes while fishy odor indicates deficiency-cold syndromes. For example, foul breath indicates pathogenic heat in the stomach. Sour breath indicates food retention in the stomach. Thick and foul sputum indicates heat in the lung while thin, clear and odorless sputum indicates cold in the lung.

3. Interrogation

Interrogation (asking) is a diagnostic method to ask a patient or the patient's relatives about the disease condition, including patient's immediate complaint, the onset and duration of diseases, relevant medical and family history, and previous treatments. The following "Ten Questions Song" is an outline to guild physicians about interrogation during medical practice.

> **Ten Questions Song**
> First ask hot and cold, second ask sweat,
> Third ask head and body, fourth ask stools and urine,
> Fifth ask food and drink, sixth ask chest and abdomen,
> Seventh ask hearing, eighth ask thirst and sleep,
> Ninth ask old disease, tenth ask cause.
> Taking medicines according to what changes appear.
> For women especially, ask menses, discharges and child bearing.
> For children, ask experience of measles and chicken pox.

As in the West, it is always the best to combine interrogation with other diagnostic methods.

4. Palpation

Palpation (touching) includes body palpation and pulse feeling. Pulse feeling is one of the most important aspects of diagnostic methods in TCM.

1) Body Palpation

Body palpation is a method of diagnosis using the hand to touch, feel and press certain areas of the body to judge the location, nature and state of an illness.

(1) <u>Chest and Abdomen</u>: Pain in this area, which is alleviated by pressure or massage, indicates deficiency syndromes; pain that is aggravated by pressure indicates excess syndromes. A mass in this area, which gathers and scatters irregularly, indicates qi stagnation; otherwise it is blood stagnation.

(2) <u>Extremities and Skin</u>: Yang deficiency syndromes manifest cold limbs, no fever and aversion to cold; heat syndromes manifest hot hands, feet and skin. Interior-heat due to yin deficiency manifests sensation of heat in the palms and soles.

(3) <u>Acupuncture Points</u>: Acupuncture points are given areas of the body where the organ's qi to meet; abnormal sensations in these points reflect dysfunction of the visceral organs.

2) Pulse Feeling

According to TCM, pathological changes of the body can be reflected by the pulse. Pulse feeling helps in judging the location and nature of a disease and in generating treatment plans.

The location of pulse feeling consist of three divisions: cun, guan, and chi along the radial artery in the wrist. To feel the pulse correctly, place the patient's hand comfortably on a cushion with the palm facing upward. The hand should be at the same level with the heart. First, the practitioner should put their middle finger on the guan division, then the index and ring fingers should naturally fall on the cun and chi divisions. An even finger force should be applied on the three regions to get a general picture of the depth, speed, rhythm, strength, and form of the pulse. Through comparisons of the three regions, the practitioner can gain a correct impression of the pulse as a whole. A normal pulse is smooth, even and forceful with regular rhythm and with the frequency of 4-5 beats per breath. However, the pulse may vary due to age, sex, body constitution, emotional state, and climatic changes.

Abnormal pulses commonly seen in the clinic

Pulse	Characteristics	Clinical Significance
Floating pulse (fu mai)	Pulse appears on light finger pressure but becomes weak on heavy finger pressure	Exterior syndromes
Deep pulse (chen mai)	Pulse is not clear with light finger pressure but is clear with heavy finger pressure	Interior syndromes
Slow pulse (chi mai)	Pulse frequency is less than 4 beats per breath (less than 60/min)	Cold syndromes
Rapid pulse (shu mai)	Pulse frequency is less than 5 beats per breath (less than 90/min)	Heat syndromes
Full pulse (hong mai)	Pulse is broad, large and forceful. It beats like dashing waves that ebb and flow	Excessive heat
Thready pulse (xi mai)	Pulse is as fine as a silk thread, but is very distinct and clear	Exhaustion of qi and blood
Slippery pulse (hua mai)	Pulse is smooth and flowing, like a pearl rolling on a plate	Excessive phlegm, excess heat and food retention. But it is also seen pregnant

		women and in healthy people with ample qi and blood
Rough pulse (se mai)	Pulse is uneven and rough, like scraping bamboo with a knife. It is opposite to rolling pulse.	Deficiency of blood and essence, stagnation of qi and blood
Taut pulse (xuan mai)	Pulse is taut, straight and long, like a music string	Disorders of liver, gall bladder, pain, or phlegm-humor
Excess pulse (shi mai)	Pulses of the three regions are forceful with either light or heavy touching and pressing	Excess syndrome, heat syndrome
Deficiency pulse (xu mai)	Pulses of the three regions are weak, forceless, empty with pressing	Deficiency of qi and blood. Seen in chronic diseases.
Weak pulse (ruo mai)	Pulse is weak, fine and deep. It appears with heavy deep pressing, otherwise disappears	Deficiency of yang
Tinny pulse (wei mai)	Scarcely perceptible pulse that is extremely fine, soft and vague	Depletion of yang, severe deficiency of qi and blood
Tense pulse (jin mai)	Pulse is tight and forceful, like a tightly stretched rope	Syndromes of cold, pain and retention of food
Hollow pulse (kou mai)	Pulse is floating, large, soft and empty inside, feeling like a scallion stalk	Massive loss of blood and yin essence
Hesitant pulse (cu mai)	Pulse is rapid with irregular intermittent beats	Excess heat, stagnation of qi and blood
Knot pulse (jie mai)	Pulse is slow and uneven with irregular intervals	Excessive yin, stagnation of qi and blood, cold phlegm
Intermittent pulse (dai mai)	Pulse is slow with regular intermittent intervals	Exhaustion of qi in zang organs, or emotion of fright and fear
Soft pulse (ru mai)	Pulse is soft, fine and floating, its tension is decreased. Scarcely perceptible with heavy pressing but appears with light pressing	Syndromes of qi deficiency or dampness
Long pulse (chang mai)	Pulse is long and straight, like feeling a long rod.	Sufficiency of qi
Short pulse (duan mai)	The length of pulse is short and seems not have the head and the tail	Insufficiency of qi
Leather pulse (ge mai)	Pulse is taut, hollow, floating, large and forceful, like feeling the skin of a drum	Chronic deficiency, blood deficiency, urine bleeding or seminal emission

Chapter 4: Therapeutics

Therapeutics consists of therapeutic principles and therapeutic methods. Therapeutic principles are the basis for guiding clinical practice. Therapeutic methods can be classified as internal treatment and external treatment. Internal treatment is a treatment method by using decoction, powder, pill, ointment, pellet, wine, tablet, granule, oral liquid and injection. External treatment includes sticking, plastering, topical application, compress, hot medicated compress, fumigation, infusing, washing, rubbing, steaming, powder applying, sneezing, blowing, inhaling, chiropractic, plugging, lying, pillow, full-filling, inducing, wearing, scrapping, cupping, massage and moxibustion. Only 8 commonly used therapies in the clinic are listed here.

1. Therapeutic Principles

The therapeutic principles of TCM include:
1) To make an overall analysis of a disease.
2) Prevention of diseases is the priority. Strengthen and maintain the body's resistance to pathogenic factors; diagnose and treat diseases as early as possible.
3) To treat the human body as an organic whole.
4) To strengthen the body resistance (for deficiency syndromes) and eliminate pathogenic factors (for excess syndromes with hyperactive pathogenic factors).
5) To differentiate Ben (primary or root cause) and Biao (secondary or branch cause) of a disease, and its insidious and acute conditions.
6) To treat acute and chronic diseases differently. If it is a chronic disorder, treat its primary cause first; if it is an acute disease, treat its secondary cause first, e.g., its symptoms first; if both primary and secondary causes are important, treat them simultaneously.
7) To pay special attention to climatic and seasonal conditions, geographic locations, environment, and personal conditions when formulating treatment plans.
8) To use routine treatment and treatment contrary to routine wisely. A routine treatment for a disease should be applied when clinical manifestations are identical to its nature, e.g. treat a cold syndrome by using drugs hot in nature; otherwise use treatment contrary to routine if its clinical

manifestations are not identical to its nature, e.g. a cold syndrome caused by flaming up of interior heat should be treated with drugs cold in nature.

9) To strengthen anti-pathogenic qi and eliminate pathogenic factors.
10) To use replenishing and eliminating methods for visceral organs wisely. Human body is an organic whole. Visceral organs are interrelated physiologically and pathologically. Disease of a given organ affects other organs. The replenishing and eliminating methods are given according to the principles defined by the five-element theory among visceral organs. These methods include: replenishing the mother-organ for deficiency syndrome and reducing the child-organ for excess syndrome; replenishing water to inhibit pathogenic yang and invigorating fire to eliminate pathogenic yin; purging the exterior fu organ to calm the interior zang organ, opening the interior zang organ to relieve the exterior fu organ, and clearing the interior zang organ to lubricate the exterior fu organ.
11) To pay attention to the transformation of a syndrome and implement treatment with a dynamic viewpoint, and to change recipes according to the changes of conditions of diseases. Because conditions of diseases change, it is important to have regular follow-up evaluations.
12) To differentiate cold and heat, true nature and false manifestation.
13) To combine treatment with healthy diet, healthy daily life, healthy mind and nursing care.
14) Above all, the primary therapeutic principle is to search for the primary cause of a disease and treat it accordingly, and prevention of diseases is the priority.

2. Therapeutic Methods

The therapeutic methods include:
1) <u>Diaphoretic Therapy</u>: A sweating method of dispersion and purgation to expel pathogens out of the body. Its function includes relieving exterior syndrome, subsiding fever and swelling, expelling wind and dampness, and promoting skin eruptions. It is applicable to the early stage of exterior syndromes of cold or heat, and the early stage of measles. Contraindications: severe loss of body fluids from vomiting and diarrhea, or deficiency of blood or yin.
2) <u>Emetic Therapy</u>: A method of removing pathogens or toxic substances from the body by vomiting. It is primarily used for treating accumulation of phlegm, indigestion with food accumulation in the stomach or food poisoning. Contraindication: pregnancy, postpartum, blood loss.
3) <u>Purgative Therapy</u>: A therapeutic method of purging stagnation of waste, excessive heat and pathogenic fluid, relieving constipation through the colon. It is applicable to constipation, reten-

tion of undigested food, stagnation of phlegm or blood, distention or parasitosis. Contraindication: menstruation, pregnancy, postpartum etc.

4) <u>Regulating/Harmonizing Therapy</u>: A therapeutic method of mediation or regulation to eliminate pathogens and at the same time to strengthen body resistance. It is applicable to Shao Yang syndromes, incoordination between liver and stomach, incoordination between liver and spleen, incoordination between stomach and intestine, incoordination between gallbladder and stomach, and irregular menstruation. Contraindication: clear external or internal conformation.

5) <u>Warming Therapy</u>: A therapeutic method of eliminating cold pathogens and invigorating yang qi. It is applicable to interior-cold syndromes such as vomiting, diarrhea, cold limbs, intolerance to cold and spasmodic pain. Contraindication: yin deficiency, blood deficiency, diarrhea with fever, blood tinged sputum or stool.

6) <u>Cooling/Clearing Therapy</u>: A therapeutic method of reducing fever, removing pathogenic heat, reserving body fluid, eliminating vexation and quenching thirst. It is applicable to disorders due to heat pathogenic factors such as interior-heat or exterior-heat syndromes. Contraindication: individuals with delicate health, cold extremities, loose stools, diarrhea and anemia.

7) <u>Nourishing/Tonifying Therapy</u>: A therapeutic method of replenishing and invigorating qi, blood, yin, yang or viscera of the human body. It is applicable to congenial and postnatal deficiency, and deficiency of qi, blood, yin, yang and body fluid due to chronic or serious illness. Contraindications: excess syndromes or stagnation of qi and blood.

8) <u>Resolving Therapy</u>: A therapeutic method of eliminating the tangible lumps formed by the accumulation and stagnation of qi, blood, phlegm, retained food and fluids. It is applicable to stagnation of qi, blood and phlegm, and retention of indigested food, including abdominal mass, subcutaneous nodules, scrofula, calculus, and sore and pyogenic infection of the skin. Contraindication: deficiency syndromes.

In short, the procedure of diagnosis and treatment of diseases in TCM follows five steps:
(1) To recognize the disease based on the information obtained with the four diagnostic methods.
(2) To identify the nature and location of a disease.
(3) To dig for the cause and the pathogenesis of a disease.
(4) To formulate treatment principles, plan and methods.
(5) To choose drugs and make a prescription.

PART TWO

MEDICAL DIAGNOSIS AND TREATMENT

Chapter 1: Disorders of the Respiratory System

1. Acute Upper Respiratory Tract Infections (URIs, or Common Cold)

Upper respiratory tract infections (URIs) represent the most common acute illness evaluated in the outpatient setting. URIs is a nonspecific term used to describe acute infections involving the nose, paranasal sinuses, pharynx, larynx, trachea, and bronchi. Common cold is the prototype. Although URIs may occur year round, in the United States, most URIs occurs during fall and winter. URIs includes rhinitis, sinusitis, nasopharyngitis, pharyngitis, epiglottitis, laryngitis, laryngotracheitis and tracheitis.

URIs involves direct invasion of the mucosa lining the upper airway. Most URIs is viral in origin. More than 200 different viruses are known to cause URIs; however, most common viruses are rhinoviruses, parainfluenza virus, coronaviruses, adenoviruses, or coxsackieviruses. Group A beta hemolytic streptococci (GABHS) cause 5% to 10% of cases of pharyngitis in adults. The virus can spread through droplets in the air, but it also spreads by hand-to-hand contact with someone who has URIs or by using shared objects. Incubation times before the appearance of symptoms vary among pathogens. Rhinoviruses and group A streptococci may incubate for 1-5 days; influenza and parainfluenza, for 1-4 days; and respiratory syncytial virus (RSV), for a week. Pertussis typically incubates 7-10 days or even as long as 21 days before causing symptoms. Diphtheria incubates for 1-10 days. The incubation period of Epstein-Barr virus (EBV) is 4-6 weeks. Most URIs resolve spontaneously in 3 to 10 days with symptomatic therapy alone. Acute bacterial sinusitis develops in 0.5% to 2% of cases of viral URIs.

Symptoms include runny or stuffy nose, itchy or sore throat, cough, congestion, slight body aches or a mild headache, sneezing, watery eyes, low-grade fever (up to 102 F), mild fatigue. The nasal discharge may become thicker and yellow or green in color as a common cold runs its course. Colds occasionally can lead to bacterial infections of the middle ear or sinuses. High fever, significantly swollen glands, severe sinus pain, and a cough that produces mucus, may indicate a complication or more serious illness.

How is URIs Diagnosed by Conventional Western Medicine?

Most common colds are diagnosed based on reported symptoms. However, cold symptoms may be similar to certain bacterial infections, allergies, and other medical conditions. Because viruses cause most URIs, the diagnostic role of laboratory tests and radiologic studies is limited.

How is URIs Treated by Conventional Western Medicine?

There is no cure for the common cold, but one can get relief from the cold symptoms by (1) resting in bed, (2) drinking plenty of fluids, (3) gargling with warm salt water or using throat sprays or cough syrups for a scratchy or sore throat, (4) using petroleum jelly for a raw nose, (5) taking aspirin or acetaminophen, Tylenol, for example, for headache or fever.

Several studies have linked aspirin use to the development of Reye's syndrome in children recovering from flu or chickenpox. The American Academy of Pediatrics recommends children and teenagers not be given aspirin or medicine containing aspirin when they have any viral illness such as the common cold. Adults shouldn't use decongestant drops or sprays for more than a few days and children shouldn't use decongestant drops or sprays at all. There's little evidence that they work in young children, and they may cause side effects. American College of Chest Physicians strongly discourages the use of cough syrups because they're not effective at treating the underlying cause of cough due to colds. Antibiotics should be used only if a rare bacterial complication, such as sinusitis or ear infections, has occurred.

What Causes URIs According to Traditional Chinese Medicine?

1) **Dysfunction of the Defensive Level (Wei Fen) and the Exterior**. Improper living habit, sudden change of climate or seasons, overstrain, emotional disturbance, and delicate constitution may result in failure of the defense system to protect the body against diseases, resulting in the invasion of the body by pathogenic factors.

2) **The Pathogenic Factors Attacking the Lung**: The lung and the defense system are the first organs to be affected by the invasion of pathogenic factors that impair the purifying and descending function of the lung and induce abnormal rising of lung qi.

3) **Disharmony between the Defense Systems and the Exterior**

How is URIs Differentiated and Treated by Traditional Chinese Medicine?

1) <u>Wind-Cold Attacking the Exterior</u>

Symptoms: Severe chill, mild fever, no sweating, headache, sore limbs, nasal stuffiness, running nose, muffled voice, sneezing, itching throat, cough, no thirst or preference to hot drink, moist tongue with thin and white coating, and floating or floating and tense pulse.

Therapeutic Principle: To relieve exterior syndrome with pungent and warm herbs.

Prescription: Modified Jing Fang Bai Du Powder composed of Semen Sojae Preparatum (Dan Dou Chi)10g, Folium Perillae Frutescentis (Su Ye) 10g, Herba Schizonepetae (Jing Jie) 10g, Radix Saposhnikoviae Divaricatae (Fang Feng) 10g, Radix Platycodi Grandiflori (Jie Geng) 6g, Rhizoma Cynanchi Stauntonii (Bai Qian) 10g, Radix Ligustici Chuanxiong (Chuan Xiong) 10g, Radix Glycyrrhizae Uralensis (Gan Cao) 6g, Semen Armeniacae Amarum(Xing Ren) 6g, Fructus Citri Aurantii (Zhi Ke) 9g, Rhizoma Zingiberis Recens (Sheng Jiang) 10g.

Modifications: For severe exterior-cold, add Herba Ephedrae (Ma Huang) 6g and Ramulus Cinnamomi Cassiae (Gui Zhi) 6g; for cough, profuse sputum, oppressive sensation in the chest, poor appetite, add Semen Raphani Sativi (Lai Fu Zi) 10g, Pericarpium Citri Reticulatae (Chen Pi) 6g, Rhizoma Pinelliae Ternatae (Ban Xia) 10g; for cold-wind combined with dampness, severe headache and general aching, fever, white greasy tongue coating, soft pulse, add Rhizoma et Radix Notopterygii (Qiang Huo) 10g and Radix Angelicae Pubescentis (Du Huo) 10g or modified Qiang Huo Sheng Shi Decoction.

2) <u>Wind-Heat Attacking the Exterior</u>

Symptoms: Severe fever, slight aversion to wind and cold, obstructed sweating, distending pain in the head, distending feelings in the eyes, stuffy nose, turbid nasal discharge, dry mouth, thirst with a desire to drink, cough, yellow and sticky sputum, dry and sore or red and swelling throat, red tongue tip, slight yellow and thin tongue coating, and floating and rapid pulse.

Therapeutic Principle: To relieve exterior syndrome with pungent and cool herbs.

Prescription: Modified Yin Qiao Powder or Cong Chi Jie Geng Decoction composed of Herba Schizonepetae (Jing Jie) 10g, Herba Menthae Haplocalycis (Bo He), Semen Sojae Preparatum (Dan Dou Chi) 10g, Flos Lonicerae (Jin Yin Hua) 10g, Fructus Forsythiae Suspensae (Lian Qiao) 10g, Radix Platycodi Grandiflori (Jie Geng) 6g, Radix Glycyrrhizae Uralensis (Gan Cao) 6g, Fried Fructus Arctii Lappae (Chao Niu Bang Zi) 10g and Rhizoma Phragmitis Communis (Lu Gen) 10g.

Modifications: For severe distending pain in the head, add Folium Mori Alba (Sang Ye) 10g and Flos Chrysanthemi Morifolii (Ju Hua) 10g; for cough with abundant sputum, add Pericarpium Trichosanthis (Gua Lou Pi) 15g, Bulbus Fritillariae Thunbergii (Zhe Bei Mu) 10g and Semen Armeniacae Amarum (Xing Ren) 10g; for severe sore, swelling and red throat, add Radix Isatidis seu Baphicacanthi (Ban Lan Gen) 10g, Fructificatio Lasiosphaerae seu Calvatiae (Ma Bo) 6g and Radix Scrophulariae Ningpoensis (Xuan Shen) 10g; for persistent severe fever, add Radix Puerariae (Ge Gen) 15g, Radix Bupleuri (Chai Hu) 10g and Gypsum Fibrosum (Shi Gao) 30g.

3) <u>Summer-heat and Dampness Impairing the Exterior</u>

Symptoms: Fever, slight aversion to cold, little sweating, heavy or sore limbs, dizziness, heavy and distending sensation in the head, cough, sticky sputum, turbid nasal discharge, restlessness, thirst without much desire to drink, sticky and greasy feeling of the mouth, feeling of oppression in the chest and hypochondriac region, acid regurgitation, scanty dark urine, thin, yellow and greasy tongue coating, and soft and rapid pulse.

Therapeutic Principle: To clear away summer-heat, resolve dampness and relieve exterior syndrome.

Prescription: Modified Xin Jia Xiang Ru Decoction composed of Herba Elsholtziae seu Moslae (Xiang Ru) 6g, Flos Lonicerae (Jin Yin Hua) 10g, Fresh Semen Dolichoris Lablab (Bian Dou) 10g, Fructus Forsythiae Suspensae (Lian Qiao) 10g, Fresh Folium Nelumbinis Nuciferae (He Ye) 10g, Cortex Magnoliae Officinalis (Hou Po) 8g, Rhizoma Phragmitis Communis (Lu Gen) 15g and Radix Glycyrrhizae Uralensis (Gan Cao) 6g.

Modifications: For predominant summer-heat, add Rhizoma Coptidis (Huang Lian) 5g, Radix Scutellariae Baicalensis (Huang Qin) 10g and Herba Artemisiae Apiaceae seu Annuae (Qing Hao) 6g; for dampness attacking the exterior and defensive division/level (Wei Fen), add Sojae Semen Germinatum Siccus (Da Dou Huang Juan) 10g, Herba Agastache seu Pogostemonis (Huo Xiang) 10g and Herba Eupatorii (Pi Lan) 10g; for predominant endogenous dampness, add Rhizoma Atractylodis (Cang Zhu) 10g, Fructus Amomi Cardamomi (Bai Kou Ren) 5g and Pericarpium Citri Reticulatae (Chen Pi) 9g; for predominant interior heat, scanty and dark urine, add Sclerotium Poriae Cocos Rubra (Chi Fu Ling) 15g or Liu Yi Powder.

4) <u>Qi Deficiency Common Cold</u>

Symptoms: Strong aversion to cold, fever, absence of sweat, lassitude, general aching, headache, nasal stuffiness, cough, white sputum, lassitude, shortness of breath, and being tired of words, repeated cold or susceptibility to cold, pale tongue with white coating, and floating and weak pulse.

Therapeutic Principle: To replenish qi and relieve exterior syndrome.

Prescription: Modified Shen Su Decoction.

Modifications: For spontaneous perspiration and susceptibility to exogenous wind pathogen, add Yu Ping Feng Powder; for yang deficiency with severe aversion to cold, mild fever, cold limbs, pale and chubby tongue, weak and deep pulse, add Radix Aconiti Lateralis Praeparatae (Fu Zi) 10g, Herba cum Radice Asari (Xi Xin) 5g and Ramulus Cinnamomi Cassiae (Gui Zhi) 10g.

5) <u>Yin Deficiency Common Cold</u>

Symptoms: Headache, fever, slight aversion to wind-cold, no sweating or mild sweating or night sweating, dizziness, vexation, thirst, dry throat, hot sensation in the palms and soles, non-productive cough with scanty sputum or blood tinged sputum, tender and red tongue with scanty coating, and thready and rapid pulse.

Therapeutic Principle: To nourish yin and relieve exterior syndrome.

Prescription: Modified Wei Rui Decoction.

Modifications: For severe exterior syndrome, add Herba Schizonepetae (Jing Jie) 10g and Radix Saposhnikoviae Divaricatae (Fang Feng) 10g; for cough, dry throat and difficult expectoration, add Fructus Arctii Lappae (Niu Bang Zi) 10g, Pericarpium Trichosanthis (Gua Lou Pi) 10g and Rhizoma Belamcandae Chinensis (She Gan) 10g; for distinct yin deficiency with dry throat and thirst, add Radix Adenophorae (Sha Shen) 10g and Radix Ophiopogonis Japonici (Mai Dong) 10g; for blood deficiency with pale complexion, pale lips and nails, add Radix Rehmanniae (Di Huang) 20g and Radix Angelicae Sinensis (Dang Gui 10g.

What Kinds of Chinese Patent Drugs are Available to Treat URIs?

1) Gan Mao Soft Capsule: 2-4 capsules each time, twice daily.
2) Chai Hu Oral Liquid: 10-20ml each time, thrice daily.

2. Acute Bronchitis (Acute Tracheobronchitis)

Acute bronchitis is an acute infectious disease of the trachea and bronchi characterized by cough and chest pain. Acute bronchitis is the inflammation of mucous membranes of the bronchial tubes. Bronchitis often follows a respiratory infection such as a cold. Smoking and exposure to smoke, allergy, air pollution and gastroesophageal reflux disease (GERD) are also risk factors for bronchitis. Influenza A and B viruses, parainfluenza viruses, respiratory syncytial virus, adenovirus, rhinovirus, and others are the infectious agents causing acute bronchitis in older children and adults.

Most cases of acute bronchitis disappear within a few days without lasting effects, although coughs may linger for weeks. Older adults, infants, smokers and people with chronic respiratory disorders or heart problems are at greatest risk of pneumonia.

Symptoms include cough that initially is nonproductive but later brings up yellowish-gray or green mucopurulent sputum, and substernal discomfort worsened by coughing are the main signs of bronchitis. Acute bronchitis is often accompanied by common signs and symptoms of an upper respiratory infection, including soreness and a feeling of constriction or burning in the chest, sore throat, chest congestion, sinus fullness, breathlessness, wheezing, slight fever and chills and overall malaise. Physical findings are minimal or absent. Rhonchi and wheezing may be evident.

How is Acute Bronchitis Diagnosed by Conventional Western Medicine?

Bronchitis is usually diagnosed solely on the history and physical examination of the patient. Many tests may be ordered to rule out other diseases, such as pneumonia or asthma. In addition, the following tests may be ordered to help confirm diagnosis: chest x-rays, blood tests, pulse oximetry, sputum cultures, and pulmonary function test (PFT).

How is Acute Bronchitis Treated by Conventional Western Medicine?

In many cases, antibiotic treatment is not necessary because the condition usually results from a viral infection. Instead, the cornerstones of acute bronchitis treatment are supportive of the symptoms, and may include: (1) get plenty of rest, (2) drink extra liquids, (3) take a nonprescription cough medicine and analgesics, such as acetaminophen (for fever and discomfort), (4) cool mist humidifier in the room may be helpful.

Antihistamines should be avoided, in most cases, because they dry up the secretions and can make the cough worse. It's best not to suppress a cough that brings up mucus. However, if the cough is keeping the patient awake at night, use just enough cough medicine so that the patient can rest, but not enough to suppress the cough completely. If bacterial infection is suspected, or the patient has a chronic lunge disorder, or the patient smokes, antibiotics may be prescribed. An inhaler and other asthma medications may be recommended to reduce inflammation and open narrowed passages in the lungs if asthma is present.

What Causes Acute Bronchitis According to Traditional Chinese Medicine?

1) **Exogenous Pathogenic Factors**: Sudden change of climate or seasons can cause six exogenous pathogenic factors to invade the body and impair the purifying and descending function of the lung, resulting in accumulation and obstruction of lung qi, abnormal production of phlegm and impeded air flow in the respiratory tracts.

2) **Dysfunction of Zang-fu organs**: Dysfunction of zang-fu organs can lead to disturbance of the lung by endogenous pathogenic factors.

How is Acute Bronchitis Differentiated and Treated by Traditional Chinese Medicine?

1) <u>Wind-Cold Attacking the Lung</u>

Symptoms: Initial stage of cough, low and vague cough sound, itching throat, white and thin sputum, headache, nasal stuffiness, running nose, joints aching, aversion to cold, absence of sweat, white and thin tongue coating, and floating or floating and tense pulse.

Therapeutic Principle: To disperse wind, expel cold, release lung qi and stop cough.

Prescription: Modified San Ao Decoction and Zhi Sou Powder.

Modifications: For distending feeling in the chest, white and greasy tongue coating, add Rhizoma Pinelliae Ternatae (Ban Xia) 10g, Cortex Magnoliae Officinalis (Hou Po) 10g and Sclerotium Poriae Cocos (Fu Ling) 10g; for wind-cold attacking the exterior and lung-heat stagnated in the interior with cough, sore throat, hoarse sound, shortness of breath, thick sputum difficult to be expectorated, thirst, vexation or fever (Exterior cold and interior heat type or so called fire wrapped by cold type), add Ma Xing Shi Gan Decoction.

2) Wind-Heat Attacking the Lung

Symptoms: Newly occurred cough, coarse and loud or hoarse cough sound, yellow and thick sputum, difficult expectoration, sweating, fever, aversion to wind, headache, thirst, yellow nasal discharge, dry and sore throat, thin and yellow tongue coating, and floating and rapid or floating and slippery pulse.

Therapeutic Principle: To dispel wind, clear away heat, ventilate the lung and resolve phlegm.

Prescription: Modified Sang Ju Decoction.

Modifications: For aversion to wind, add Herba Schizonepetae (Jing Jie) 10g and Radix Saposhnikoviae Divaricatae (Fang Feng) 10g; for severe lung-heat, add Radix Scutellariae Baicalensis (Huang Qin) 10g, Gypsum Fibrosum (Shi Gao) 30g and Rhizoma Anemarrhenae (Zhi Mu) 10g; for epistaxis, add Rhizoma Imperatae Cylindricae (Bai Mao Gen) 20g and Nodus Nelumbinis Nuciferae Rhizomatis (Ou Jie) 10g; for sore throat, add Fructus Arctii Lappae (Niu Bang Zi) 10g, Rhizoma Belamcandae Chinensis (She Gan) 10g, Radix Isatidis seu Baphicacanthi (Ban Lan Gen) 10g and Fructificatio Lasiosphaerae seu Calvatiae (Ma Bo) 6g; for difficult expectoration, add Semen Benincasae Hispidae (Dong Gua Zi) 15g and Fructus Trichosanthis (Gua Lou) 15g.

3) Dry-Heat Attacking the Lung

Symptoms: Newly occurred cough, hoarse cough sound, non-productive cough or cough with scanty thick and sticky sputum that is difficult to be expectorated, chest pain induced by cough, dry nose, dry throat and dry mouth, aversion to wind, fever, red tongue tip, dry, yellow and thin tongue coating, and floating and rapid or slightly rapid pulse.

Therapeutic Principle: To dispel wind, moisten the lung, clear away lung heat and stop cough.

Prescription: Modified Sang Xing Decoction.

Modifications: For severe dry-heat, dry cough and hoarse sound, add Fructus Trichosanthis (Gua Lou) 15g and Radix Ophiopogonis Japonici (Mai Dong) 10g; for severe cough and itching throat, add

Radix Peucedani (Qian Hu) 10g, Periostracum Cicadae (Chan Tui) 10g, Radix Platycodi Grandiflori (Jie Geng) 6g and Radix Glycyrrhizae Uralensis (Gan Cao) 6g; for blood tinged sputum or epistaxis, add Rhizoma Imperatae Cylindricae (Bai Mao Gen) 20g and Nodus Nelumbinis Nuciferae Rhizomatis (Ou Jie) 10g; for sever fever, add Gypsum Fibrosum (Shi Gao) 30g and Rhizoma Anemarrhenae (Zhi Mu) 10g.

4) <u>Cool-Dryness Attacking the Lung</u>

Symptoms: Cough with little sputum or no sputum, dry nose, dry throat, headache, fever, absence of sweat, dry, thin and white tongue coating, and floating and tense pulse.

Therapeutic Principle: To dispel wind and cold, moisten the lung and stop cough.

Prescription: Modified Xing Su Powder.

Modifications: For severe aversion to cold and absence of sweat, add Herba Schizonepetae (Jing Jie) 10g and Radix Saposhnikoviae Divaricatae (Fang Feng) 10g; for distinct non-productive cough, add Radix Asteris Tatarici (Zi Wan) 10g and Radix Stemonae (Bai Bu) 10g.

What Kinds of Chinese Patent Drugs are Available to Treat Acute Bronchitis?

1) Zhi Sou Pill: 20 pills each time, thrice daily.
2) Ji Zhi Syrup: 20-30ml each time, 3-4 times per day.

3. Chronic Bronchitis

Chronic obstructive pulmonary disease (COPD) is the overall term for a group of chronic lung conditions characterized by the presence of airflow obstruction due to chronic bronchitis and emphysema, but it can also refer to damage caused by asthmatic bronchitis. It is a major smoking-related public health problem, which currently affects over 21 million Americans and ranks as the fourth leading cause of death worldwide.

Chronic bronchitis is characterized by inflammation and narrowing of the major and smaller bronchial tubes and increased bronchial mucus production, and is manifested by productive cough for 3 mouth or more in at least 2 consecutive years in the absence of any other disease that might account for this symptom. Although cigarette smoking is clearly the most important cause of chronic bronchitis, air pollution, airway infection, familial factors, allergy, age and other irritants have also been implicated. Complications of chronic bronchitis include respiratory infections, high blood pressure, heart problems, lung cancer and depression.

Symptoms include:

- Persistent and severe cough with copious and mucopurulent or purulent sputum production

- Increased mucus production
- Intermittent, mild to moderate shortness of breath, especially during physical activities
- Wheezing
- Chest tightness
- Hemoptysis occurs occasionally
- Frequent respiratory infections
- Right heart failure may be present
- Wheezes, rhonchi on physical examination
- Increased markings ("dirty lungs") on chest x-ray

How is Chronic Bronchitis Diagnosed by Conventional Western Medicine?

Chronic bronchitis is usually diagnosed on symptoms, a history of exposure to lung irritants (especially cigarette smoke) and physical examination. The following tests may be ordered to help confirm diagnosis: Pulmonary function tests, chest X-ray, arterial blood gas analysis, sputum examination and CT scan.

How is Chronic Bronchitis Treated by Conventional Western Medicine?

There's no cure for chronic bronchitis, but the following treatments can control symptoms, reduce the risk of complications and improve a patient's ability to lead an active life:

- Smoking cessation
- Bronchodilators
- Inhaled steroids, which are usually reserved for people with moderate or severe COPD
- Antibiotics help fight bacterial infections
- Emerging medications
- Oxygen therapy
- Pulmonary rehabilitation program
- Managing exacerbations

What Causes Chronic Bronchitis According to Traditional Chinese Medicine?

1) Six Exogenous Pathogenic Factors Invading the Lung
2) Deficiency of the Lung
3) Deficient Spleen Inducing Phlegm
4) Deficiency of the Kidney

How is Chronic Bronchitis Differentiated and Treated by Traditional Chinese Medicine?

1) Excess Syndrome (usually seen in acute stage of attack)

(1) <u>Wind-Cold Attacking the Lung</u>

Symptoms: Cough, dyspnea, distending feeling in the chest, profuse white sputum, fever or aversion to cold, absence of sweat and thirst, white, thin and slippery tongue coating, and floating and tense pulse.

Therapeutic Principle: To release lung qi, expel cold, resolve phlegm and stop cough.

Prescription: Modified San Ao Decoction.

Modifications: For retention of cold-phlegm in the lung, abundant sputum and distending feeling in the chest, add Rhizoma Pinelliae Ternatae (Ban Xia) 10g, Exocarpium Citri Rubrum (Ju Hong) 10g and Fructus Perillae (Su Zi) 10g; for persistent dyspnea, add Ramulus Cinnamomi Cassiae (Gui Zhi) and Hou Po Xing Zi Decoction.

(2) <u>Wind-Heat Attacking the Lung</u>

Symptoms: Severe and frequent cough, hoarse breathing or cough sound, yellow and sticky sputum that is difficult to be expectorated, distending feeling or dull pain in the chest, yellow nasal discharge, fever, sweating, thirst, constipation, dark urine, yellow or thin and white tongue coating, and floating or slippery and rapid pulse.

Therapeutic Principle: To clear away heat, relieve exterior syndrome, stop cough and resolve dyspnea.

Prescription: Modified Ma Xing Shi Gan Decoction.

Modifications: For severe lung-heat, add Radix Scutellariae Baicalensis (Huang Qin) 10g, Rhizoma Anemarrhenae (Zhi Mu) 10g and Herba cum Radice Houttuyniae Cordatae (Yu Xing Cao) 20g; for severe wind-heat syndrome, add Flos Lonicerae (Jin Yin Hua) 15g, Fructus Forsythiae Suspensae (Lian Qiao) 10g, Folium Mori Alba (Sang Ye) 10g and Flos Chrysanthemi Morifolii (Ju Hua) 10g; for abundant sputum and severe dyspnea, add Semen Descurainiae seu Lepidii (Ting Li Zi) 10g and Rhizoma Belamcandae Chinensis (She Gan) 10g; for yellow and sticky sputum, add Fructus Trichosanthis (Gua Lou) 15g, Bulbus Fritillariae Cirrhosae (Bei Mu) 10g and Pumex (Fu Hai Shi) 10g.

(3) <u>Turbid Phlegm Accumulated in the Lung</u>

Symptoms: Cough with muffled sound, abundant, white and sticky sputum, distending and suffocative sensation in the chest, poor appetite, sticky feeling of the mouth, absence of thirst, nausea and vomiting in severe cases, white, thick and greasy tongue coating, and slippery pulse.

Therapeutic Principle: To clear away dampness, resolve phlegm, lower qi and stop cough.

Prescription: Modified Er Chen Decoction and San Zi Yang Qin Decoction.

Modifications: For severe turbid phlegm and distending sensation in the chest, add Rhizoma Atractylodis (Cang Zu) 10g and Cortex Magnoliae Officinalis (Hou Po) 10g; for white sticky sputum with foam, aversion to cold and cold feeling in the back of the body, add Rhizoma Zingiberis Officinalis (Gan Jiang) 10g and Herba cum Radice Asari (Xi Xin) 5g; for deficiency of the spleen with severe dampness, poor appetite and spiritlessness, add Radix Codonopsitis Pilosulae (Dang Shen) 10g and Rhizoma Atractylodis Macrocephalae (Bai Zhu) 10g.

(4) Phlegm-Heat Accumulated in the Lung Type

Symptoms: Cough, panting, feverish and distending feeling in the chest, chest pain, profuse yellow, thick and sticky sputum, difficult expectoration or blood tinged sputum, thirst with desire to cold drinks, flushed face, dry throat, dark urine, constipation, yellow and greasy tongue coating, and slippery and rapid pulse.

Therapeutic Principle: To clear away heat, resolve phlegm, release lung qi and stop cough.

Prescription: Modified Sang Bai Pi Decoction.

Modifications: For fever, add Gypsum Fibrosum (Shi Gao) 30g and Rhizoma Anemarrhenae (Zhi Mu) 10g; for abundant and sticky sputum, add Concha Meretricis seu Cyclinae (Hai Ge Qiao) 12g or Dai Ge Powder; for panting, inability to lie flat, profuse sputum and constipation, add Semen Descurainiae seu Lepidii (Ting Li Zi) 10g, Radix et Rhizoma Rhei (Da Huang) 6g and Natrii Sulfas (Mang Xiao) 10g; for stinky sputum, add Herba cum Radice Houttuyniae Cordatae (Yu Xing Cao) 20g, Semen Coicis (Yi Yi Ren) 20g, Semen Benincasae Hispidae (Dong Gua Zi) 15g and Rhizoma Phragmitis Communis (Lu Gen) 20g.

(5) Phlegm-Cold Accumulated in the Lung Type

Symptoms: Cough, dyspnea, inability to lie down, abundant, clear, thin, white and foamy sputum that is worsened by cold air, edema, aversion to cold, cold limbs, mild fever, difficult urination, white and slippery or white and greasy tongue coating, and taut and tense pulse.

Therapeutic Principle: To warm the lung, resolve phlegm, relieve cold and stop cough.

Prescription: Modified Xiao Qing Long Decoction.

Modifications: For severe phlegm and mild cold, absence of exterior syndrome, severe dyspnea and cough, add Semen Descurainiae seu Lepidii (Ting Li Zi) 10g, Rhizoma Atractylodis Macrocephalae (Bai Zhu) 10g and Sclerotium Poriae Cocos (Fu Ling) 10g; for abundant, sticky and greasy sputum, distending sensation in the chest, belching and turbid tongue coating, add Semen Sinapis Albae (Bai Jie Zi) 10g and Semen Raphani Sativi (Lai Fu Zi) 10g.

2) Deficiency Syndrome (usually seen in stage of remission and stage of chronic procrastination)

(1) <u>Deficiency of Lung Qi</u>

Symptoms: Cough, shortness of breath, clear and thin sputum, liability to catching cold that is frequently induced by climate changes, lassitude, indolence of speaking, low voice, timidness, dim complexion, spontaneous sweating, aversion to wind, pale tongue with white coating, and thready and weak pulse.

Therapeutic Principle: To replenish lung qi, resolve phlegm and stop cough.

Prescription: Modified Bu Fei Decoction.

Modifications: For abundant and thin sputum, add Semen Sinapis Albae (Bai Jie Zi) 10g, Rhizoma Pinelliae Ternatae (Ban Xia) 10g and Flos Farfarae (Kuan Dong Hua) 10g; for kidney deficiency with inability to receive lung qi, frequent and severe shortness of breath, add Fructus Psoraleae Corylifoliae (Bu Gu Zhi) 10g, Fructus Corni Officinalis (Shan Zhu Yu) 10g and Placenta Hominis (Zi He Che) 3g.

(2) <u>Deficiency of Lung Qi and Spleen Qi</u>

Symptoms: Cough, shortness of breath, lassitude, weakness, profuse sputum that is easy to be expectorated, dim complexion, abdominal distension and diarrhea induced by intake of food or moving the bowels right after intake of food, white, thin and greasy or white and thin tongue coating, chubby tongue with teeth marks on lateral sides, and thready and weak pulse.

Therapeutic Principle: To replenish lung qi, invigorate the spleen, stop cough and resolve phlegm.

Prescription: Modified Yu Ping Feng Powder and Liu Jun Zi Decoction.

Modifications: For deficiency of lung qi with thin sputum, aversion to cold and cold limbs, add Rhizoma Zingiberis Officinalis (Gan Jiang) 10g and Herba cum Radice Asari (Xi Xin) 5g; for diarrhea, add Shen Ling Bai Zhu Powder; for frequent cough, abundant clear and thin sputum, add Ling Gui Zhu Gan Decoction.

(3) <u>Deficiency of Lung Yin and Kidney Yin</u>

Symptoms: Cough and dyspnea worsened by exertion, little sticky sputum difficult to be expectorated, dry mouth and dry throat, night sweating, hectic fever, flushed face, dysphoria, feverish sensation in the chest, palms and soles, sore lower back, tinnitus, red tongue with thin and yellow coating, and thready and rapid pulse.

Therapeutic Principle: To nourish yin, invigorate the kidney, moisten the lung and stop cough.

Prescription: Modified Sha Shen Mai Dong Decoction and Liu Wei Di Huang Pill.

Modifications: For severe cough and sticky sputum difficult to be expectorated, add Bulbus Fritillariae Cirrhosae (Bei Mu) 10g, Radix Stemonae (Bai Bu) 10g and Radix Asteris Tatarici (Zi Wan) 10g;

for shortness of breath, feverish sensation in the chest, palms and soles, flushed face and night sweating, add Fructus Schisandrae Chinensis (Wu Wei Zi) 6g, Cortex Lycii Radicis (Di Gu Pi) 10g and Radix Stellariae Dichotomae (Yin Chai Hu) 10g.

What Kinds of Chinese Patent Drugs are Available to Treat Chronic Bronchitis?

1) Qing Qi Hua Tan Pill: 6-9g each time, twice daily.
2) Ren Shen Bao Fei Pill: 1 pill each time, twice daily.

4. Obstructive Pulmonary Emphysema (Emphysema)

Emphysema is a progressive lung disease that results in shortness of breath and reduces the capacity for physical activity. The cause of emphysema is that inflammation destroys the fragile walls of the air sacs, causing them to lose their elasticity. As a result, the bronchioles collapse, and air becomes trapped in the air sacs, which overstretches them. In time, this overstretching may cause several air sacs to rupture, forming one larger air space.

Cigarette smoke is by far the most common cause of emphysema. In a small percentage of people, emphysema results from low levels of alpha-1-antitrypsin (AAt), which leads to progressive lung damage that eventually results in emphysema. Respiratory infections such as acute bronchitis, pneumonia and influenza are a leading complication of emphysema. Spontaneous pneumothorax occurs in a small fraction of patients with emphysema.

Symptoms and signs include:

- The main emphysema symptoms are progressive, constant and severe dyspnea and a reduced capacity for physical activity.
- Chronic, mild and nonproductive cough, although cough is uncommon with emphysema
- Loss of appetite and weight loss
- Fatigue
- Decreased markings in periphery on chest x-ray

How is Emphysema Diagnosed by Conventional Western Medicine?

Chronic bronchitis is usually diagnosed on symptoms, a history of exposure to lung irritants (especially cigarette smoke) and physical examination. The following tests may be ordered to help confirm diagnosis: Pulmonary function tests (PFTs), chest X-ray, arterial blood gas analysis, pulse oximetry, sputum examination and CT scan. Additionally, researchers are studying whether magnetic resonance imaging (MRI) could detect emphysema even before signs and symptoms appear.

How is Emphysema Treated by Conventional Western Medicine?

- Smoking cessation. The most important step in any treatment plan for smokers with emphysema is stopping smoking; it's the only way to stop the damage to the lungs from becoming worse
- Bronchodilators
- Inhaled steroids. They are usually reserved for people with moderate or severe COPD
- Broad-spectrum antibiotics help fight bacterial infections, but should be used with caution to avoid the serious and growing problem of antibiotic-resistant bacteria
- Oxygen therapy
- Protein therapy. Infusions of AAt may help slow lung damage in people with an inherited deficiency of the protein
- Inoculations against influenza and pneumonia. Experts recommend an influenza (flu) shot annually and a pneumonia shot every five years after age 65 for people who have emphysema or other forms of COPD
- Lung volume reduction surgery (LVRS)
- Lung transplantation
- Pulmonary rehabilitation program

What Causes Emphysema According to Traditional Chinese Medicine?

1) Dysfunction of Zang-Fu Organs

2) Invasion of Six Pathogenic Factors and other Pestilential Toxicity

How is Emphysema Differentiated and Treated by Traditional Chinese Medicine?

1) <u>Exterior-Cold and Internal Fluid Retention Syndrome</u>

Symptoms: Cough, dyspnea, inability to lie flat, abundant, clear and thin sputum, aversion to cold, fever, cold back, absence of sweat, thirst without much desire to drinks, or thirst with preference to hot drinks, dark and bluish complexion, white and slippery tongue coating, and taut and tense pulse.

Therapeutic Principle: To warm the lung, dispel cold, relieve exterior syndrome and resolve phlegm.

Prescription: Modified Xiao Qing Long Decoction.

Modifications: For phlegm-heat, dysphoria and dyspnea, add Gypsum Fibrosum (Shi Gao) 30g and Radix Scutellariae Baicalensis (Huang Qin) 10g; for edema, cough, dyspnea and inability to lie flat, add Semen Descurainiae seu Lepidii (Ting Li Zi) 10g and Radix Stephaniae Tetrandrae (Fang Ji) 10g.

2) <u>Retention of Phlegm-Heat in the Lung</u>

Symptoms: Cough, dyspnea, hoarse breathing sound, irritability, distending sensation in the chest, yellow or white, sticky and thick sputum that is difficult to be expectorated, fever, slight aversion to cold, little sweat, dark urine, constipation, thirst, red tongue with yellow or yellow and greasy coating, and rapid or slippery pulse.

Therapeutic Principle: To clear away lung heat, resolve phlegm, lower adverse flow of lung qi and arrest asthma.

Prescription: Modified Yue Bi Jia Ban Xia Decoction or Sang Bai Pi Decoction.

Modifications: For severe phlegm-heat, add Herba cum Radice Houttuyniae Cordatae (Yu Xing Cao) 20g and Concha Meretricis seu Cyclinae (Hai Ge Qiao) 12g; for wheezing sound in the throat, dyspnea and inability to lie flat, add Rhizoma Belamcandae Chinensis (She Gan) 10g and Semen Descurainiae seu Lepidii (Ting Li Zi) 10g; for consumption of body fluid by phlegm-heat, dry mouth and dry throat, add Radix Trichosanthis (Tian Hua Fen) 10g, Rhizoma Anemarrhenae (Zhi Mu) 10g and Rhizoma Phragmitis Communis (Lu Gen) 20g; for constipation, add Radix et Rhizoma Rhei (Da Huang) 6g and Natrii Sulfas (Mang Xiao) 10g.

3) <u>Accumulation of Turbid Phlegm in the Lung</u>

Symptoms: Cough, abundant, white, sticky and greasy sputum, dyspnea worsened by exertion, abdominal distension, lassitude, light pale tongue with thin and greasy or curdy and greasy coating, and slippery pulse.

Therapeutic Principle: To strengthen the spleen, resolve phlegm, lower qi and stop asthma.

Prescription: Modified San Zi Yang Qin Decoction and Er Chen Decoction.

Modifications: For profuse sputum, distending feeling in the chest and inability to lie flat, add Semen Descurainiae seu Lepidii (Ting Li Zi) 10g and Cortex Mori Alba Radicis (Sang Bai Pi) 12g; for phlegm-heat with sticky sputum difficult to be expectorated, add Radix Scutellariae Baicalensis (Huang Qin)10g and Fructus Trichosanthis (Gua Lou) 15g; for turbid phlegm with stasis, dark and bluish lips and nails, dim tongue with ecchymosis, add Semen Pruni Persicae (Tao Ren) 10g, Radix Salviae Miltiorrhizae (Dang Shen) 10g and Radix Paeoniae Rubra (Chi Shao) 10g.

4) <u>Deficiency of Lung Qi and Spleen Qi</u>

Symptoms: Chronic cough and dyspnea, shortness of breath, abundant, thin and white sputum, suffocative sensation in the chest and abdominal distension, lassitude, indolence of speaking, pale and lusterless complexion, poor appetite, loose stool, pale and white tongue coating and thready and weak pulse.

Therapeutic Principle: To nourish the lung, strengthen the spleen, replenish qi and stop asthma.

Prescription: Bu Fei Decoction and Si Jun Zi Decoction.

Modifications: For severe phlegm-dampness with abundant sputum, add Semen Sinapis Albae (Bai Jie Zi) 10g, Semen Raphani Sativi (Lai Fu Zi) 10g and Fructus Perillae (Su Zi) 10g; for aversion to cold, cold limbs, oliguria and edema of extremities, add Radix Aconiti Lateralis Praeparatae (Fu Zi) 10g, Rhizoma Zingiberis Officinalis (Gan Jiang) 10g and Rhizoma Alismatis Orientalis (Ze Xie) 10g.

5) <u>Deficiency of Both the Lung and the Kidney</u>

Symptoms: Rapid, short and shallow respiration, dyspnea worsened by exertion, low voice, shortness of breath, cough, white and foamy sputum, difficult expectoration, suffocative sensation in the chest, palpitation, cold limbs, sweating, pale or dark and purplish tongue, and deep, thready and weak or knot and intermittent pulse.

Therapeutic Principle: To nourish the lung, invigorate the kidney, lower qi and arrest asthma.

Prescription: Modified Ping Chuan Gu Ben Decoction and Bu Fei Decoction.

Modifications: For aversion to cold, clear, thin and foamy sputum, add Cortex Cinnamomi Cassiae (Rou Gui) 5g, Rhizoma Zingiberis Officinalis (Gan Jiang) 10g and Stalactitum (Zhong Ru Shi) 10g; for mild fever, red tongue with scanty coating, add Radix Ophiopogonis Japonici (Mai Dong) 12g and Rhizoma Polygonati Odorati (Yu Zhu) 12g; for cyanosis of the face, lips and fingers, add Radix Salviae Miltiorrhizae (Dan Shen) 10g, Radix Angelicae Sinensis (Dang Gui) 10g and Lignum Sappan (Su Mu) 10g; for panting prostration with sweating, cold limbs, palpitation, rapid respiration, dyspnea, irritability, feeble pulse that is about to disappear, inability to maintain recumbency with mouth opened and shoulders elevated, and flapping of alae nasi, emergency treatment with Shen Fu Decoction and Gecko (Ge Jie) Powder 7g or Hei Xi Pill should be given.

What Kinds of Chinese Patent Drugs are Available to Treat Emphysema?

1) Su Zi Jiang Qi Pill: 6g each time, twice daily.
2) Ge Jie Ding Chuan Capsule: 3 capsules each time, twice daily.

5. Bronchial Asthma (Asthma)

Asthma is a chronic, inflammatory disease in which the airways become sensitive to allergens (any substance that triggers an allergic reaction). The lining of the airways become swollen and inflamed, the muscles that surround the airways tighten, and cells in the lungs produce extra mucus further narrowing the airways. Approximately 20.5 million people in the US have been diagnosed with asthma; at least 6 million of them are children under the age of 18. Asthma accounts for millions of missed school days and workdays each year. It's also a common reason for emergency room visits and hospitalizations. Asthma is a chronic but treatable condition.

The exact cause of asthma is not completely known. It is probably due to a combination of genetic, environmental, infectious, and chemical factors. The following may trigger the asthma symptoms:

- Allergens, such as pollen, animal dander or mold
- Cockroaches and dust mites
- Air pollutants and irritants
- Smoke
- Strong odors or scented products or chemicals
- Respiratory infections, including the common cold
- Physical exertion, including exercise
- Strong emotions and stress
- Cold air
- Certain medications, including beta blockers, aspirin and other nonsteroidal anti-inflammatory drugs
- Sulfites, preservatives added to some perishable foods
- Gastroesophageal reflux disease (GERD), a condition in which stomach acids back up into the esophagus. GERD may trigger an asthma attack or make an attack worse.
- Sinusitis

Most asthma attacks are preceded by warning signs. Recognizing these warning signs and treating symptoms early can help prevent attacks or keep them from becoming worse. Symptoms of asthma may include:

- Constant, intermittent or night time cough
- Increased shortness of breath or wheezing
- Disturbed sleep caused by shortness of breath, coughing or wheezing
- Chest tightness or pain
- Fatigue
- Increased need to use bronchodilators
- Noisy breathing with whistling or wheezing sound in children
- A fall in peak flow rates as measured by a peak flow meter

How is Asthma Diagnosed by Conventional Western Medicine?

Diagnosing asthma can be difficult. To diagnose asthma and distinguish it from other lung disorders, physicians rely on a combination of medical history, physical examination, and laboratory tests, which may include spirometry, peak flow monitoring (PFM), chest x-rays, blood tests and allergy tests.

How is Asthma Treated by Conventional Western Medicine?

There are several types of medications available for treating asthma. Most people use a combination of long-term control medications and quick relief medications.

Long-term-control medications

- Inhaled corticosteroids
- Long-acting beta-2 agonists (LABAs), such as salmeterol (Serevent Diskus) and formoterol (Foradil)
- Leukotriene modifiers, which include montelukast (Singulair) and zafirlukast (Accolate)
- Cromolyn and nedocromil
- Theophylline

Quick-relief medications

- Short-acting beta-2 agonists, such as albuterol
- Ipratropium (Atrovent)
- Oral and intravenous corticosteroids for asthma attacks

Medications for allergy-induced asthma

- Immunotherapy
- Anti-IgE monoclonal antibodies, such as Xolair
- Treatment based on asthma severity for better control

What Causes Asthma According to Traditional Chinese Medicine?

1) Attack by Exterior Pathogenic Factors
2) Improper Diet
3) Deficiency of the Lung and the Kidney

How is Asthma Differentiated and Treated by Traditional Chinese Medicine?

1) Stage of Attack

(1) <u>Cold Type</u>

Symptoms: Dyspnea, wheezing sound in the throat, white and greasy sputum or thin and foamy sputum, sensation of chest tightness, dim or bluish complexion, absence of thirst or thirst with preference to hot drinks, fever, headache, aversion to cold, absence of sweat, cold extremities, white and greasy or white and slippery tongue coating, and floating and tense pulse.

Therapeutic Principle: To warm the lung, dispel cold, remove phlegm and relieve asthma.

Prescription: Modified She Gan Ma Huang Decoction.

Modifications: For severe dyspnea with abundant sputum and inability to lie flat, add Semen Descurainiae seu Lepidii (Ting Li Zi) 10g; for exterior-cold and internal fluid retention, add Xiao Qing Long Decoction combined with Fructus Perillae (Su Zi) 10g, Rhizoma Cynanchi Stauntonii (Bai Qian) 10g, Semen Armeniacae Amarum (Xing Ren) 10g and Pericarpium Citri Reticulatae (Ju Pi) 6g; for chronic asthma and deficiency of yang, frequent attack with severe wheezing, shortness of breath, clear and thin sputum, pale complexion, diaphoresis, cold limbs, pale and thin tongue coating, and deep and thready pulse, use Su Zi Jiang Qi Decoction supplemented with Radix Astragali (Huang Qi) 10g, Fructus Corni Officinalis (Shan Zhu Yu) 10g, Fructus Terminaliae Chebulae (He Zi) 10g and Lignum Aquilariae Resinatum (Chen Xiang) 1g; for severe deficiency of yang, add Radix Aconiti Lateralis Praeparatae (Fu Zi) 10g and Fructus Psoraleae Corylifoliae (Bu Gu Zhi) 10g.

(2) Heat Type

Symptoms: Dyspnea with hoarse voice, paroxysmal cough, wheezing sound in the throat, over inflated chest, irritability, sweating, flushed face, thirst with a desire to drink, bitter taste in the mouth, thick, yellow, greasy and sticky sputum that is difficult to be expectorated, no aversion to wind, red tongue with yellow and greasy coating, and slippery and rapid or slippery and taut pulse.

Therapeutic Principle: To clear away heat, ventilate the lung, resolve phlegm and relieve asthma.

Prescription: Modified Ding Chuan Decoction.

Modifications: For predominant heat in the lung and attack of the exterior by cold pathogen, add Gypsum Fibrosum (Shi Gao) 30g and Herba Ephedrae (Ma Huang) 10g; for severe exterior-cold syndrome, add Ramulus Cinnamomi Cassiae (Gui Zhi) 10g and Rhizoma Zingiberis Recens (Sheng Jiang) 10g; for severe dyspnea, wheezing and inability to lie flat due to stagnation of lung qi, add Semen Descurainiae seu Lepidii (Ting Li Zi) 10g and Lumbricus (Di Long) 10g; for dry and yellow tongue coating, add Radix et Rhizoma Rhei (Da Huang) 6g and Natrii Sulfas (Mang Xiao) 10g; for yellow, thick and sticky sputum, add Concha Meretricis seu Cyclinae Powder (Hai Ge Fen) 10g, Rhizoma Belamcandae Chinensis (She Gan) 10g, Rhizoma Anemarrhenae (Zhi Mu) 10g and Herba cum Radice Houttuyniae Cordatae (Yu Xing Cao) 20g.

(3) Wind Type

Symptoms: Sudden onset of asthma induced by certain factors, mental distress or certain odor, wheezing without sputum or with little sputum that is difficult to be expectorated, distending and suffocative sensation in the chest, absence of sputum or little amount of sputum that is difficult to be expectorated, dry throat, dry mouth, flushed face or sallow complexion, loose stool, red and dry tongue with little coating, taut and thready pulse.

Therapeutic Principle: To nourish the liver, dispel wind, regulate the lung and stop asthma.

Prescription: Modified Guo Min Decoction.

Modifications: For severe stagnation of liver qi, add Fructus Citri Aurantii Immaturus (Zhi Shi) 10g and Radix Paeoniae Rubra (Chi Shao) 12g; for paroxysmal heat-predominant wheezing with clear predisposing factors, add Bombyx Batryticatus (Jiang Can) 10g and Periostracum Cicadae (Chan Tui) 10g; for cold predominant wheezing, add Buthus Martensi (Quan Xie) 5g and Radix Ligustici Chuanxiong (Chuan Xiong) 10g; for severe asthma with wheezing and hoarse breathing sound, and distending sensation in the chest, add Herba Ephedrae (Ma Huang) 6g and Semen Descurainiae seu Lepidii (Ting Li Zi) 10g; for coexistence of exterior-cold and interior-heat (so called "cold wrapping fire syndrome"), add Herba Ephedrae (Ma Huang) 6g and Gypsum Fibrosum (Shi Gao) 30g.

(4) <u>Blood Stasis Type</u>

Symptoms: chronic and lingering asthma that attacks frequently, distending pain in the chest and hypochondriac region, cyanosis of nails, dim complexion, dry throat, bitter taste in the mouth, constipation, abdominal distention, or slight edema or abnormal menstruation, dark and purplish tongue or with ecchymosis, and deep and rough pulse.

Therapeutic Principle: To promote blood circulation, remove blood stasis, lower adverse qi and relieve asthma.

Prescription: Modified Xue Fu Zhu Yu Decoction.

Modifications: For insufficiency of liver blood, internal dampness stagnation induced by spleen deficiency and combination of turbid phlegm and blood stasis, use Dang Gui Shao Yao Powder supplemented with Caulis Perillae (Su Geng) 10g, Fructus Perillae (Su Zi) 10g, Semen Armeniacae Amarum (Xing Ren) 10g Lumbricus (Di Long) 10g and Herba Ephedrae (Ma Huang) 6g; for coexistence of excess-heat and blood stasis of Shao Yang and Yang Ming Channels, use Da Chai Hu Decoction and Modified Gui Zhi Fu Ling Pill.

Example prescription: Radix Angelicae Sinensis (Dong Gui) 10g, Radix Ligustici Chuanxiong (Chuan Xiong) 10g, Radix Paeoniae Rubra (Chi Shao) 10g, Sclerotium Poriae Cocos (Fu Ling) 12g, Radix Bupleuri (Chai Hu) 10g, Radix Scutellariae Baicalensis (Huang Qin) 10g, Fructus Citri Aurantii

(Zhi Ke) 10g, Rhizoma Pinelliae Ternatae (Ban Xia) 10g, Fructus Perillae (Xu Zi), Semen Armeniacae Amarum (Xing Ren) 10g and wine-fried Radix et Rhizoma Rhei (Da Huang) 4g.

(5) <u>Blockage of Phlegm in the Lung</u>

Symptoms: Dyspnea, feeling of oppression in the chest, wheezing sound in the throat, cough with abundant thick and white sputum aggravated in the early morning, nausea, sticky and greasy sensation in the mouth, thick and greasy tongue coating, and slippery pulse.

Therapeutic Principle: Remove phlegm, dredge aperture, lower adverse qi and stop asthma.

Prescription: Modified Er Chen Decoction and San Zi Yang Qin Decoction.

Modifications: For poor appetite, Charred Fructus Crataegi (Shan Zha Tan) 10g, stir-baked Massa Medicata Fermentata (Shen Qu) 12g, Fructus Germinatus Oryzae Sativae (Gu Ya) 12g and Fructus Hordei Germinatus (Mai Ya) 12; for predominant dampness, add Fructus Amomi Villosi (Sha Ren) 3g.

2) Stage of Remission

(1) <u>Deficiency of the Lung</u>

Symptoms: Dyspnea, shortness of breath, low voice, aversion to wind, spontaneous sweating, liability to catching cold that is frequently induced by climate changes, clear, white and thin sputum, frequent sneezing, nasal stuffiness, clear nasal discharge, pale and lusterless complexion, mild wheezing sound in the throat, pale tongue with thin and white coating, and thready and weak pulse or deficient and large pulse.

Therapeutic Principle: To reinforce the lung and consolidate the Wei-system.

Prescription: Modified Yu Ping Feng Powder.

Modifications: For severe aversion to wind and cold, add Radix Paeoniae Alba (Bai Shao Yao) 10g, Ramulus Cinnamomi Cassiae (Gui Zhi) 10g, Rhizoma Zingiberis Recens (Sheng Jiang) 10g and Fructus Ziziphi Jujubae (Da Zao) 20g; for deficiency of both qi and yin with irritable cough, little sticky sputum, dry mouth and throat, red tongue, use Sheng Mai Powder supplemented with Radix Glehniae (Bai Sha Shen) 10g, Rhizoma Polygonati Odorati (Yu Zhu) 12g, Bulbus Fritillariae Cirrhosae (Bei Mu) 10g and Herba Dendrobii (Shi Hu) 12g; for severe deficiency of yang, add Radix Aconiti Lateralis Praeparatae (Fu Zi) 12g; for dysfunction of both the lung and the spleen, poor appetite and diarrhea, use Bu Zhong Yi Qi Decoction.

Example prescription: Radix Astragali (Huang Qi) 12g, Radix Saposhnikoviae Divaricatae (Fang Feng) 8g, Rhizoma Atractylodis Macrocephalae (Bai Zhu) 6g, Radix Glycyrrhizae Uralensis (Gan Cao) 5g, Radix Codonopsitis Pilosulae (Dang Shen) 10g, Radix Ophiopogonis Japonici (Mai Dong)

10g, Fructus Schisandrae Chinensis (Wu Wei Zi) 10g and Cordyceps Sinensis (Dong Chong Xia Cao) 10g.

(2) <u>Deficiency of the Spleen</u>

Symptoms: Lassitude, shortness of breath, feeble voice, poor appetite, nausea, loose stool, frequent diarrhea induced by intake of greasy food, epigastric stuffiness, dim and lusterless complexion, abundant and sticky sputum, difficult expectoration, pale tongue with white and slippery or greasy coating, and thready and weak pulse.

Therapeutic Principle: To strengthen the spleen and resolve phlegm.

Prescription: Modified Liu Jun Zi Decoction.

Modifications: For spleen yang deficiency with cold limbs and loose stool, add Radix Aconiti Lateralis Praeparatae (Fu Zi) 12g and Rhizoma Zingiberis Officinalis (Gan Jiang) 10g; for abundant sputum and tachypnea, add San Zi Yang Qin Decoction.

Example prescription: Radix Codonopsitis Pilosulae (Dang Shen) 15g, Rhizoma Atractylodis Macrocephalae (Bai Zhu) 10g, Sclerotium Poriae Cocos (Fu Ling) 10g, Pericarpium Citri Reticulatae(Chen Pi), Rhizoma Pinelliae Ternatae (Ban Xia) 10g and Radix Glycyrrhizae Uralensis (Gan Cao) 6g.

(3) <u>Deficiency of the Kidney</u>

Symptoms: Shortness of breath and tachypnea worsened by exertion, spiritlessness, palpitation, lumbago (weakness of the waist and legs), tinnitus, liability to asthma attacks induced by overstrain; or aversion to cold, pale complexion, cold limbs, spontaneous sweating, pale, chubby and tender tongue with white coating, and deep and thready pulse (yang deficiency); or flushed cheeks, dysphoria, feverish sensation in the chest, palms and soles, night sweating, red tongue with little coating, and thready and rapid pulse (yin deficiency).

Therapeutic Principle: To invigorate the kidney to receive lung qi.

Prescription: Modified Jin Gui Shen Qi Pill or Qi Wei Du Qi Pill.

Modifications: For severe deficiency of yang, add Fructus Psoraleae Corylifoliae (Bu Gu Zhi) 10g, Herba Epimedii (Yin Yang Huo) 12g and sliced Cornu Cervi (Lu Jiao) 10g; for deficiency of the kidney with inability to accept lung qi, use Ge Jie Powder supplemented with Semen Juglandis (Hu Tao Ren) 20g, Fructus Schisandrae Chinensis (Wu Wei Zi) 5g and Placenta Hominis (Zi He Che) 2g.

Example prescription: Radix Rehmanniae Praeparatae (Shu Di Huang) 12g, Radix Rehmanniae (Di Huang) 12g, Fructus Corni Officinalis (Shan Zhu Yu) 10g, Sclerotium Poriae Cocos (Fu Ling) 12g, Radix Angelicae Sinensis (Dang Gui) 10g, Fructus Psoraleae Corylifoliae (Bu Gu Zhi) 10g, Fructus

Ligustri Lucidi (Nu Zhen Zi) 10g, Pericarpium Citri Reticulatae (Chen Pi) 10g, Fructus Schisandrae Chinensis (Wu Wei Zi) 8g and Fructus Perillae (Su Zi) 10g.

(4) <u>Wheezing Prostration</u>

Symptoms: Vomiting, diarrhea, muscle cramps, purple complexion, lassitude, irritability, cloudy mentality, greasy sweat, cold extremities, purple tongue with slippery and greasy coating, and faint pulse.

Therapeutic Principle: To restore yang from collapse, resolve phlegm and remove blood stasis.

Prescription: Modified Si Wei Hui Yang Decoction.

Modifications: For purplish face and tongue, add Semen Pruni Persicae (Tao Ren) 10g and Flos Carthami Tinctorii (Hong Hua) 10g; for cloudy mentality, add Rhizoma Acori Tatarinowii (Shi Chang Pu) 10g, Radix Curcumae (Yu Jin) 10g and Moschus (She Xiang) 0.06g; for deficiency of both yang-qi and body fluid, add Fructus Corni Officinalis (Shan Zhu Yu) 10g, Radix Ophiopogonis Japonici (Mai Dong) 12g and Fructus Schisandrae Chinensis (Wu Wei Zi) 5g.

What Kinds of Chinese Patent Drugs are Available to Treat Asthma?

1) Bu Shen Fang Chuan Tablet: 4-6 tablets each time, thrice daily.
2) Bai He Gu Jin Pill: 1 pill each time, twice daily.
3) He Che Da Zao Pill: 9g each time, twice daily.

6. Bronchiectasis

Bronchiectasis is a congenital or acquired lung disorder of the large bronchi characterized by permanent, abnormal dilation and destruction of bronchial walls. This impairs their ability to clear mucus from the lungs. Bronchiectasis may affect multiple areas of one or both lungs and may be caused by recurrent inflammation and infection of the airways due to the following:

- Cystic fibrosis, which causes about half of all cases of bronchiectasis
- Bacterial lung infection, such as chronic bronchitis, pneumonia, tuberculosis and lung abscess
- Fungal infections in people with asthma
- Abnormal lung defense mechanisms, such as humoral immunodefiency, alpha 1-antiprtease deficiency with cigarette smoking, mucociliary clearance disorders and rheumatic diseases
- Localized airway obstruction, such as foreign body, tumor and mucoid impaction
- Immunodeficiency states
  Signs and symptoms include:
- Chronic cough

- Production of copious amounts of yellow or green sputum
- Hemoptysis
- Shortness of breath
- Fatigue
- Recurring pneumonia
- Persistent crackles at the lung bases on physical examination
- Infrequent clubbing
- Roentgenographic abnormalities

Complications of bronchiectasis include cor pulmonale, amyloidosis and secondary abscesses at distant sites.

How is Bronchiectasis Diagnosed by Conventional Western Medicine?

To diagnose bronchiectasis, physicians rely on a combination of medical history, physical examination and imaging, which includes chest x-rays and CT scan. A diagnosis of bronchiectasis can be confirmed by a CT scan of the chest.

How is Bronchiectasis Treated by Conventional Western Medicine?

Treatment depends on the extent and severity of the condition and may include:

- Avoiding irritants such as smoke and dust
- Bronchodilator medications, if the condition is associated with asthma
- Antibiotics to treat or prevent lung infections
- Daily postural drainage of the affected part of the lung
- Bronchoscopy to evaluate hemoptysis, remove retained secretions and rule out obstructing airway lesions
- Surgical removal of the affected lung tissue

What Causes Bronchiectasis According to Traditional Chinese Medicine?

1) Attack by Exogenous Pathogenic Factors
2) Deficiency of Anti-pathogenic Qi or Deficiency of Both the Lung and the Spleen
3) Phlegm Stagnation Blending with Blood Stasis

How is Bronchiectasis Differentiated and Treated by Traditional Chinese Medicine?

1) <u>Retention of Phlegm-Heat in the Lung</u>

Symptoms: Recurrent cough, expectoration of foul purulent or blood-tinged sputum, or massive hemoptysis, fever in severe cases, distending pain in the chest, dry mouth with bitter taste, dark and red tongue with yellow and greasy coating, and slippery and rapid pulse.

Therapeutic Principle: To clear away heat, resolve phlegm, release hung qi and stop cough.

Prescription: Modified Qing Jin Hua Tan Decoction and Qian Jin Wei Jing Decoction.

Modifications: For foul, pyoid and yellow sputum, add Herba cum Radice Violae (Zi Hua Di Ding) 15g and Herba cum Radice Houttuyniae Cordatae (Yu Xing Cao) 20g; for abundant sputum, fullness sensation in the chest and constipation, add Semen Descurainiae seu Lepidii (Ting Li Zi) 10g, fresh Succus Bambosae (Zhu Li) 30g and Radix et Rhizoma Rhei (Da Huang) 6g; for hemoptysis, add Radix Sanguisorbae Officinalis (Di Yu) 12g and Radix Rubiae Cordifoliae (Qian Cao) 12g.

2) <u>Attack on the Lung by Liver Fire</u>

Symptoms: Paroxysmal cough, recurrent expectoration of little blood or blood-tinged sputum, or persistent massive hemoptysis, distending pain in the chest and hypochondriac region, irritability, dry mouth with bitter taste, constipation, red and dry tongue with yellow and thin coating, and taut and rapid pulse.

Therapeutic Principle: To clear away liver-fire, cool blood and stop hemoptysis.

Prescription: Modified Dai Ge Powder and Xie Bai Powder.

Modifications: For severe cough and copious amounts of sputum, add Fructus Trichosanthis (Gua Lou) 15g, Herba cum Radice Houttuyniae Cordatae (Yu Xing Cao) 20g, Succus Bambosae (Zhu Li) 30g, Flos Lonicerae (Jin Yin Hua) 15g, Semen Armeniacae Amarum (Xing Ren) 10g, Rhizoma Cynanchi Stauntonii (Bai Qian) 10g and Radix Peucedani (Qian Hu) 10g; for distending pain in the chest, add Radix Curcumae (Yu Jin) 10g, Luffae Fasciculus Vascularis (Si Gua Lou) 12g, Fructus Citri Aurantii (Zhi Ke) 10g and Flos Inulae (Xuan Fu Hua) 10g; for dry mouth and dry throat, add Radix Ophiopogonis Japonici (Mai Dong) 12g, Radix Trichosanthis (Tian Hua Fen) 12g and Radix Adenophorae (Sha Shen) 12g; for hemoptysis, add charred Radix et Rhizoma Rhei (Da Huang) 6g, Radix Sanguisorbae Officinalis (Di Yu) 12g, Radix Rubiae Cordifoliae (Qian Cao) 12g and fried Pollen Typhae (Pu Huang) 10g.

3) <u>Deficiency of Qi and Yin</u>

Symptoms: Chronic cough, emaciation, little sputum or non-productive cough, cough with low sound, sputum tinged with bright red blood, dry mouth and throat, feverish sensation in the chest, palms and soles, red tongue with little moisture, and thready and rapid pulse.

Therapeutic Principle: To replenish yin, nourish the lung, resolve phlegm and stop hemoptysis.

Prescription: Modified Bai He Gu Jin Decoction.

Modifications: For severe deficiency heat, Cortex Lycii Radicis (Di Gu Pi) 12g, Radix Stellariae Dichotomae (Yin Chai Hu) 10g, Rhizoma Picrorrhizae (Hu Huang Lian) 10g and Radix Cynanchi Atrati (Bai Wei) 10g; for night sweating, add Fructus Tritici Aestivi Levis (Fu Xiao Mai) 20g and Fructus Pruni Mume (Wu Mei) 20g; for hemoptysis, add Cortex Moutan Radicis (Mu Dan Pi) 10g, Fructus Gardeniae Jasminoidis (Zhi Zi) 10g, Gelatinum Corii Asini (E Jiao) 10g and Nodus Nelumbinis Nuciferae Rhizomatis (Ou Jie) 12g; for massive hemoptysis and drenching sweat, use Du Shen Decoction.

4) <u>Deficiency of Lung Qi and Spleen Qi</u>

Symptoms: Lusterless complexion, shortness of breath, indolence of speaking, poor appetite, spiritlessness, lassitude, feeling of oppression in the chest, cough with little or blood-tinged sputum, pale tongue with white coating, and deep and thready pulse.

Therapeutic Principle: To replenish the lung qi, invigorate the spleen, moisten the lung and relieve cough.

Prescription: Modified Bu Fei Decoction.

Modifications: For poor appetite, add Rhizoma Atractylodis Macrocephalae (Bai Zhu) 12g, Rhizoma Dioscoreae (Shan Yao) 20g and Sclerotium Poriae Cocos (Fu Ling) 12g; for persistent hemoptysis, add Radix Ampelopsis (Bai Lian) 10g; for persistent diaphoresis, add Fructus Corni Officinalis (Shan Zhu Yu) 10g and Concha Ostreae (Mu Li) 20g.

What Kinds of Chinese Patent Drugs are Available to Treat Bronchiectasis?

1) Xian Zhu Li Oral Liquid: 15-30ml each time, 2-3 times each day.
2) Tan Ke Jing: 6g each time, thrice daily.

7. Chronic Respiratory Failure

Respiratory failure may be acute or chronic. While acute respiratory failure is characterized by life-threatening derangements in arterial blood gases and acid-base status, the manifestations of chronic respiratory failure are less dramatic and may not be as readily apparent. The most etiology of chronic respiratory failure is COPD. Chronic respiratory failure develops over several days or longer, allowing time for renal compensation and an increase in bicarbonate concentration. Therefore, the pH usually is only slightly decreased. The clinical markers of chronic hypoxemia, such as polycythemia and cor pulmonale, suggest a long-standing disorder.

Respiratory failure can arise from an abnormality in any of the components of the respiratory system. Patients who have hypoperfusion secondary to cardiogenic, hypovolemic, or septic shock often present with respiratory failure. The mortality rate associated with respiratory failure varies according to the underlying etiology. Respiratory failure remains an important cause of morbidity and mortality in the United States. Symptoms and signs of respiratory failure are those of underlying disease combined with those of hypoxemia and hypercapnia.

<u>Signs of hypoxemia:</u> Dyspnea, cyanosis, restlessness, confusion, anxiety, delirium, tachypnea, tachycardia, hypertension, cardiac arrhythmias, and tremor.

<u>Signs of hypercapnia:</u> Dyspnea, headache, peripheral and conjunctival hyperemia, hypertension, tachycardia, tachypnea, impaired consciousness, papilledema, and asterixis.

How is Respiratory Failure Diagnosed by Conventional Western Medicine?

- Arterial blood gas analysis: confirmation of the diagnosis.
- Chest x-ray
- Full blood count
- Renal and hepatic function tests
- Serum creatine kinase and troponin I tests
- Thyroid function tests
- Echocardiography
- Pulmonary function tests
- ECG
- Right heart catheterization
- Pulmonary capillary wedge pressure

How is Respiratory Failure Treated by Conventional Western Medicine?

Treatment of the patient with chronic respiratory failure includes (1) specific therapy directed toward the underlying disease, (2) respiratory supportive care directed toward the maintenance of adequate gas exchange, and (3) general supportive care. Only a few guidelines are listed below:

- A patient with acute respiratory failure generally needs prompt admission to hospital. Most patients with chronic respiratory failure can be treated at home with oxygen as well as therapy for their underlying disease.
- Ensure an adequate airway.
- Correction of hypoxemia
- Beware the prolonged use of high concentration oxygen

- Correct the underlying cause and/or provide assisted ventilation for hypercapnia and respiratory acidosis
- Mechanical ventilation
- Appropriate management of the underlying disease
- General supportive care

What Causes Chronic Respiratory Failure According to Traditional Chinese Medicine?

1) Chronic Diseases and Overstrain

2) Attack by Exterior Pathogenic Factors

How is Chronic Respiratory Failure Differentiated and Treated by Traditional Chinese Medicine?

1) <u>Blockage of Turbid Phlegm in the Lung</u>

Symptoms: Tachypnea, wheezing sound in the throat, abundant thick and sticky sputum difficult to be expectorated, feeling of oppression in the chest, dark red or bluish complexion, dark and purplish lips and tongue, white or white and greasy tongue coating, and slippery and rapid pulse.

Therapeutic Principle: Resolve phlegm, lower qi, promote blood circulation and remove blood stasis.

Prescription: Modified Er Chen Decoction and San Zi Yang Qin Decoction.

Modifications: For severe retention of turbid phlegm, dyspnea and inability to maintain recumbency, add Fructus Gleditsiae Sinensis (Zao Jia) 5g and Semen Descurainiae seu Lepidii (Ting Li Zi) 10g; for dark and purplish lips and tongue, add Semen Pruni Persicae (Tao Ren) 10g, Flos Carthami Tinctorii (Hong Hua) 10g and Radix Paeoniae Rubra (Chi Shao) 12g.

Example Prescription: Pericarpium Citri Reticulatae (Chen Pi) 10g, Rhizoma Pinelliae Ternatae (Ban Xia) 10g, Sclerotium Poriae Cocos (Fu Ling) 12g, Radix Glycyrrhizae Uralensis (Gan Cao) 5g, Fructus Perillae (Su Zi) 10g, Semen Sinapis Albae (Bai Jie Zi) 6g, Semen Raphani Sativi (Lai Fu Zi) 10g, Cortex Magnoliae Officinalis (Hou Po) 8g and Semen Armeniacae Amarum (Xing Ren) 10g.

2) <u>Deficiency of Both Lung Qi and Kidney Qi</u>

Symptoms: Dyspnea with rapid, short and shallow respiration, panting with mouth opened and shoulders elevated, inability to lie down, shortness of breath, distending feeling in the chest, palpitation, cough with white and frothy sputum, difficult expectoration, cold limbs, diaphoresis, pale or dark and purplish tongue, white and slippery tongue coating, and deep, thready and weak or knot and intermittent pulse.

Therapeutic Principle: To nourish the lung, replenish the kidney to receive qi and arrest panting.

Prescription: Modified Bu Fei Decoction and Shen Ge Powder.

Modifications: For aversion to cold and cold limbs, add Cortex Cinnamomi Cassiae (Rou Gui) 5g and Herba cum Radice Asari (Xi Xin) 5g; for deficiency of qi and blood stasis, cyanosis of lips and face, add Radix Angelicae Sinensis (Dang Gui) 12g, Radix Salviae Miltiorrhizae (Dan Shen) 12g and Radix Paeoniae Rubra (Chi Shao) 12g; for consumption of yin, mild fever, red tongue with little coating, add Rhizoma Polygonati Odorati (Yu Zhu) 12g, Radix Ophiopogonis Japonici (Mai Dong) 12g, Rhizoma Anemarrhenae (Zhi Mu) 10g and Radix Rehmanniae (Di Huang) 20g.

Example Prescription: Radix Codonopsitis Pilosulae (Dang Shen) 10g, Radix Ophiopogonis Japonici (Mai Dong) 10g, Fructus Schisandrae Chinensis (Wu Wei Zi) 10g, Radix Astragali (Huang Qi) 12g, Fructus Psoraleae Corylifoliae (Bu Gu Zhi) 10g, Radix Rehmanniae Praeparatae (Shu Di Huang) 12g, Pericarpium Citri Reticulatae (Chen Pi) 10g, Radix Angelicae Sinensis (Dang Gui) 10g, Radix Asteris Tatarici (Zi Wan) 10g and Flos Farfarae (Kuan Dong Hua) 10g.

3) <u>Deficiency of Both Spleen Yang and Kidney Yang</u>

Symptoms: Cough, dyspnea, palpitation, inability to lie flat worsened by exertion, abdominal distension, edema, cold limbs, oliguria, cyanosis of face and lips, dark, purplish and chubby tongue with white and slippery coating, and deep and thready or knot and intermittent pulse.

Therapeutic Principle: To warm kidney yang, invigorate the spleen, resolve fluid retention and induce diuresis.

Prescription: Modified Zhen Wu Decoction and Wu Ling Powder.

Modifications: For blood stasis, add Flos Carthami Tinctorii (Hong Hua) 10g, Radix Paeoniae Rubra (Chi Shao) 12g, Herba Lycopi Lucidi (Ze Lan) 12g and Cortex Acanthopanacis Radicis (Wu Jia Pi) 10g; for severe edema, palpitation and severe dyspnea, add Lignum Aquilariae Resinatum (Chen Xiang) 1g and Semen Descurainiae seu Lepidii (Ting Li Zi) 10g.

Example Prescription: Radix Aconiti Lateralis Praeparatae (Fu Pian) 10g, Rhizoma Atractylodis Macrocephalae (Bai Zhu) 10g, Ramulus Cinnamomi Cassiae (Gui Zhi) 10g, Sclerotium Poriae Cocos (Fu Ling) 30g, Rhizoma Alismatis Orientalis (Ze Xie) 15g, Sclerotium Polypori Umbellati (Zhu Ling) 15g, Radix Codonopsitis Pilosulae (Dang Shen) 10g, Semen Descurainiae seu Lepidii (Ting Li Zi) 10g, Herba Leonuri Heterophylii (Yi Mu Cao) 15g and Rhizoma Zingiberis Recens (Sheng Jiang) 10g.

4) <u>Mental Confusion due to Phlegm</u>

Symptoms: Tachypnea, or wheezing sound due to excessive phlegm, cloudy conscience, irritability, delirium, apathy, drowsiness, coma, muscle cramps of the extremities, cyanosis of complexion, dark and purplish tongue with white and greasy coating, and rapid and thready and slippery pulse.

Therapeutic Principle: To remove phlegm, cause resuscitation, suppress wind and arrest convulsion.

Prescription: Di Tan Decoction and An Gong Niu Huang Pill, or Di Tan Decoction and Zhi Bao Pill.

Modifications: For severe internal phlegm-heat, fever, coma, delirium, add Rhizoma Acori Tatarinowii (Shi Chang Pu) 10g, Radix Curcumae (Yu Jin) 10g, Semen Descurainiae seu Lepidii (Ting Li Zi) 10g, Succus Bambosae (Zhu Li) 30g, Cortex Mori Alba Radicis (Sang Bai Pi) 10g and Concretio Silicea Bambusae (Tian Zhu Huang) 5g; for convulsion and spasm, add Ramulus Uncariae cum Uncis (Gou Teng) 12g, Buthus Martensi (Quan Xie) 5g and Cornu Saigae Tataricae (Ling Yang Jiao) 2g; for severe blood stasis, cyanosis of lips and nails, add Semen Pruni Persicae (Tao Ren) 10g, Flos Carthami Tinctorii (Hong Hua) 10g and Radix Salviae Miltiorrhizae (Dan Shen) 10g; for mucocutaneous hemorrhage, hemoptysis, hematemesis and hemafecia, add Cornu Bubali (Shui Niu Jiao) 10g, Radix Rehmanniae (Di Huang) 20g, Cortex Moutan Radicis (Mu Dan Pi) 10g, Radix et Rhizoma Rhei (Da Huang) 6g and Radix Lithospermi seu Macrotomiae (Zi Cao) 10g.

Example Prescription: Exocarpium Citri Rubrum (Ju Hong) 10g, Rhizoma Pinelliae Ternatae (Ban Xia) 10g, Sclerotium Poriae Cocos (Fu Ling) 12g, Rhizoma Arisaematis cum Bile (Dan Nan Xing) 8g, Rhizoma Acori Tatarinowii (Shi Chang Pu) 10g, Radix Curcumae (Yu Jin) 10g, Fructus Forsythiae Suspensae (Lian Qiao) 10g, Radix Salviae Miltiorrhizae (Dan Shen) 15g, Fructus Citri Aurantii Immaturus (Zhi Shi) 10g and Succus Bambosae 10g.

5) <u>Weakness of Yang on the Verge of Collapse</u>

Symptoms: Severe dyspnea with mouth opened and shoulders elevated, flaring of nares, pale complexion, drenching cold sweat, extreme cold limbs, irritability, dark and bluish complexion and tongue, and deep, thready and weak or tinny and extremely faint pulse.

Therapeutic Principle: To replenish qi, warm yang and restore yang from collapse.

Prescription: Du Shen Decoction and Shen Fu Decoction.

8. Acute Respiratory Distress Syndrome (ARDS)

Acute respiratory distress syndrome (ARDS) is a severe and often fatal condition following a systemic or pulmonary insult; it is characterized by respiratory distress, bilateral infiltrate, hypoxemia, non-compliant lungs and normal pulmonary capillary wedge pressure.

ARDS usually occurs in people who are already critically ill or who have sustained massive injuries. Risk factors for ARDS include sepsis, aspiration of gastric contents, shock, infection, lung contusions, trauma, toxic inhalation, near-drowning, drugs, DIC, oxygen toxicity, radiation and multiple blood transfusions, etc. ARDS begins with widespread lung inflammation that in turn damages the cells and the alveolar-capillary membranes, causing fluid to leak into the air sacs. The mortality rate associated with ARDS is extremely high, especially when it is accompanied by sepsis. The major cause of death in ARDS is nonpulmonary multiple organ system failure, often with sepsis.

Symptoms include:

- Rapid onset of severe shortness of breath, usually a few hours to a few days after the original disease or trauma
- Labored breathing and tachypnea
- Cough or fever in some cases
- Intercostal retractions and crackles on physical examination
- Abnormalities in chest radiograph
- Marked hypoxemia may occur
- Most ARDS demonstrate multiple organ failure

How is ARDS Diagnosed by Conventional Western Medicine?

ARDS is usually confirmed with a chest X-ray and an arterial blood gas analysis. In certain cases, other tests to rule out heart problems may be ordered.

How is ARDS Treated by Conventional Western Medicine?

Because no specific treatment for ARDS exists, the goal is to treat the underlying condition and to supply oxygen until the lungs start functioning normally. Managing fluids carefully is also crucial. Broad-spectrum antimicrobial treatment should be started promptly when infection is known or suspected.

At one time, many people with ARDS were given corticosteroids to reduce lung inflammation. It is now believed that the side effects of these drugs outweigh any temporary benefits. A number of new therapies are now under investigation, such as surfactant supplementation, monoclonal antibodies to TNF, and human recombinant interleukin-1 receptor antagonist, etc.

What Causes ARDS According to Traditional Chinese Medicine?

1) Invasion of Exogenous Pathogenic Factors
2) Injury and Blood Stasis
3) Internal Injury (Dysfunction of Zang-Fu Organs) and Chronic Diseases

How is ARDS Differentiated and Treated by Traditional Chinese Medicine?

1) <u>Toxic Heat Attacking the Lung</u>

Symptoms: Tachypnea, or labored breathing with mouth opened and shoulders elevated, inability to lie flat, severe fever, irritability, cyanosis of the face and lips, dark red tongue with thin and white or thin and yellow coating, and rapid and full pulse.

Therapeutic Principle: To clear away heat, remove toxic substance, release lung qi and lower the adverse lung qi.

Prescription: Modified Qing Wen Bai Du Decoction and Ma Xing Shi Gan Decoction.

Modifications: For dark and red tongue, add Xi Jiao Di Huang Decoction; for cyanosis, add Radix Salviae Miltiorrhizae (Dan Shen) 12g and Radix Ligustici Chuanxiong (Chuan Xiong) 10g; for constipation, add Radix et Rhizoma Rhei (Da Huang) 6g or use Da Chen Qi Decoction enema.

2) <u>Retention of Phlegm-Heat in the Lung</u>

Symptoms: Tachypnea, cough, abundant yellow, sticky and thick sputum, or blood-tinged sputum, dysphoria and feverish sensation in the chest, dry throat, thirst, dark urine, constipation, red tongue with yellow and sticky coating, and slippery and rapid pulse.

Therapeutic Principle: To clear away heat, resolve phlegm, release lung qi and relieve asthma.

Prescription: Modified Qing Jin Hua Tan Decoction.

Modifications: For dysphoria and feverish sensation, add Gypsum Fibrosum (Shi Gao) 30g and Rhizoma Anemarrhenae (Zhi Mu) 10g; for abundant sticky and thick sputum, add Concha Meretricis seu Cyclinae Powder (Hai Ge Fen) 12g and Rhizoma Arisaematis cum Bile (Dan Nan Xing) 3g; for thirst and dry throat, add Radix Trichosanthis (Tian Hua Fen) 12g and Rhizoma Phragmitis Communis (Lu Gen) 20g; for constipation, add Radix et Rhizoma Rhei (Da Huang) 6g, Cortex Magnoliae Officinalis (Hou Po) 10g, Fructus Citri Aurantii Immaturus (Zhi Shi) 10g and Natrii Sulfas (Mang Xiao) 10g.

3) <u>Deficiency of Qi and Yin</u>

Symptoms: Tachypnea, shortness of breath that is aggravated by exertion, little sputum or clear and thin sputum, low voice and indolence of speaking, spontaneous sweating, aversion to wind, weakness and lassitude, dysphoria with feverish sensation in the chest, dry mouth, red complexion, pale and red tongue with thin and white or little coating, and deep and thready or weak pulse.

Therapeutic Principle: To replenish qi and nourish yin.

Prescription: Modified Sheng Mai Powder and Bu Fei Decoction.

Modifications: For severe deficiency of lung yin, add Bulbus Lilii (Bai He) 20g, Radix Adenophorae (Sha Shen) 12g and Rhizoma Polygonati Odorati (Yu Zhu) 12g; for deficiency of qi with cold, add Radix Astragali (Huang Qi) 12g, Rhizoma Zingiberis Officinalis (Gan Jiang) 10g and Fructus Evodiae

Rutaecarpae (Wu Zhu Yu) 3g; for profuse sweating, Mastodi Ossis Fossilia (Long Gu) 20g and Concha Ostreae (Mu Li) 20g.

4) <u>Deficiency of Heart Yang and Kidney Yang</u>

Symptoms: Tachypnea with mouth opened and shoulders elevated, more expiration than inspiration, dyspnea worsened by exertion, spiritlessness and shortness of breath, sweating, cold limbs, cyanosis of the face and lips, pale tongue, and deep, thready and weak pulse.

Therapeutic Principle: To warm heart yang and kidney yang.

Prescription: Modified Shen Fu Decoction.

Modifications: For dyspnea worsened by exertion, add Lignum Aquilariae Resinatum 1g; for sweating and cold limbs, add Cortex Cinnamomi Cassiae (Rou Gui) 3g and Rhizoma Zingiberis Officinalis (Gan Jiang) 10g; for cyanosis of the face and lips, add Radix Paeoniae Rubra (Chi Shao) 10g, Radix Salviae Miltiorrhizae (Dan Shen) 10g and Radix Ligustici Chuanxiong (Chuan Xiong) 10g.

9. Pneumonia

Pneumonia is an inflammation of the lungs usually caused by infection with bacteria, viruses, fungi, other organisms or chemical irritants. Pneumonia attacks older adults, very young children and people with chronic illnesses or impaired immune systems, but it also can strike young, healthy people. Worldwide, it's a leading cause of death in children, many of them younger than a year old. Pneumonia can occur year round, but is usually seen in the winter and spring. There is an increased chance of developing pneumonia in a crowded area.

There are more than 50 types of pneumonia ranging in seriousness from mild to life-threatening. The main types of pneumonia include: (1) bacterial pneumonia. Streptococcus pneumoniae is the most common bacterium that causes bacterial pneumonia; (2) viral pneumonia; (3) mycoplasma pneumonia; and (4) other less common pneumonias, which may be caused by the inhaling of food, liquid, gases, dust, or by fungi. Pneumonia is sometimes classified according to where or how a person is exposed to the disease: (1) community-acquired pneumonia; (2) hospital-acquired (nosocomial) pneumonia; (3) aspiration pneumonia; (4) pneumonia caused by opportunistic organisms.

Pneumonia often mimics a cold or the flu. Its signs and symptoms can vary greatly, depending on the underlying conditions and the type of organism causing the infection. However, many cases of pneumonia develop suddenly, with chest pain, fever, chills, cough and shortness of breath. Common symptoms may include:

- Fever

- Chest or stomach pain
- Decrease in appetite
- Cough
- Chills
- Breathing fast or hard
- Vomiting
- Headache
- Not feeling well
- Fussiness
- Rales and rhonchi on physical examination

How is Pneumonia Diagnosed by Conventional Western Medicine? Diagnosis is usually made based on the season, a thorough history and physical examination, but may include the following tests to confirm the diagnosis: (1) chest x ray; (2) blood tests; (3) sputum culture; (4) pulse oximetry; and (5) CT scan.

How is Pneumonia Treated by Conventional Western Medicine?

- Treatment may include antibiotics for bacterial pneumonia. Antibiotics may also speed recovery from mycoplasma pneumonia and some special cases. There is no clearly effective treatment for viral pneumonia, which usually resolves on its own.
- Appropriate diet
- Increased fluid intake
- Cool mist humidifier in the room
- Acetaminophen (for fever and discomfort)
- Medication for cough
- Oxygen therapy
- Breathing treatments

What Causes Pneumonia According to Traditional Chinese Medicine?

1) Wind-Heat Attacking the Lung
2) Retention of Phlegm-Heat in the Lung
3) Toxic Heat Disturbing and Blocking the Mind
4) Exhaustion of Yin and Prostration of Yang

How is Pneumonia Differentiated and Treated by Traditional Chinese Medicine?

1) <u>Pathogenic Factors Attacking the Wei (Defensive) Level and the Lung</u>

Symptoms: On the early stage of attack, cough, difficult expectoration, white or yellow, thick and sticky sputum, severe fever, slight aversion to cold, no sweating or little sweating, slight thirst, headache, nasal stuffiness, red tongue tip and margin, thin and white or little yellow tongue coating, and floating and rapid pulse.

Therapeutic Principle: To dispel wind, clear away heat, release lung qi and stop cough.

Prescription: Modified San Ao Decoction or Sang Ju Decoction.

Modifications: For severe headache, add Flos Chrysanthemi Morifolii (Ju Hua) 12g and Fructus Viticis (Man Jing Zi) 10g; for cough with thick sputum, add Radix Scutellariae Baicalensis (Huang Qin) 10g and Herba cum Radice Houttuyniae Cordatae (Yu Xing Cao) 20g; for sore throat and hoarse voice, add Rhizoma Belamcandae Chinensis (She Gan) 10g and Periostracum Cicadae (Chan Tui) 10g; for severe fever, add Flos Lonicerae (Jin Yin Hua) 15g, Gypsum Fibrosum (Shi Gao) 30g and Rhizoma Anemarrhenae (Zhi Mu) 10g; for dry mouth and throat, add Radix Adenophorae (Sha Shen) 12g and Radix Trichosanthis (Tian Hua Fen) 12g.

2) <u>Retention of Phlegm-Heat in the Lung</u>

Symptoms: Cough with yellow and thick or rust-colored sputum, tachypnea, persistent high fever, distending pain in the chest and hypochondriac region that is aggravated by pressing, thirst, irritability, dark urine, constipation, red tongue with yellow coating, and full and rapid or slippery and rapid pulse.

Therapeutic Principle: To clear away heat, resolve phlegm, relieve distending pain and stop cough.

Prescription: Modified Ma Xing Shi Gan Decoction and Qian Jin Wei Jing Decoction.

Modifications: For severe phlegm-heat, add Radix Scutellariae Baicalensis (Huang Qin) 10g and Herba cum Radice Houttuyniae Cordatae (Yu Xing Cao) 20g and Fructus Trichosanthis (Gua Lou) 15g; for severe chest pain, add Radix Curcumae (Yu Jin) 10g and Rhizoma Corydalis (Yan Hu Suo) 10g; for blood-tinged sputum, add Rhizoma Imperatae Cylindricae (Bai Mao Gen) 20g and Cacumen Biotae Orientalis (Ce Bai Ye) 12g.

3) <u>Mental Dysfunction due to Toxic Heat</u>

Symptoms: Cough, tachypnea, rumbling wheezing sound due to sputum, irritability, coma, delirium, persistent high fever, extremely cold limbs in severe cases, red tongue with yellow and dry coating, and thready, slippery and rapid pulse.

Therapeutic Principle: To clear away heat, remove toxic substance, resolve phlegm and cause resuscitation.

Prescription: Modified Qing Ying Decoction.

Modifications: For irritability and delirium, add Zi Xue Pill; for cramps, add Buthus Martensi (Quan Xie) 5g, Ramulus Uncariae cum Uncis (Gou Teng) 12g and Lumbricus (Di Long) 12g; for constipation, add Da Huang Fen Granule.

4) <u>Exhaustion of Yin and Prostration of Yang</u>

Symptoms: Sudden drop from high fever, drenching sweat, extremely cold extremities, pale complexion, tachypnea, cyanosis of lips and nails, mental confusion, pale and bluish tongue, and extremely tinny pulse.

Therapeutic Principle: To replenish qi and nourish yin and restore yang from collapse.

Prescription: Modified Sheng Mai Powder and Si Ni Decoction.

Modifications: For exhaustion of yin, use modified Sheng Mai Powder supplemented with Radix Panacis Quinquefolii (Xi Yang Shen) 6g, Radix Ophiopogonis Japonici (Mai Dong) 12g, Fructus Schisandrae Chinensis (Wu Wei Zi) 5g, Fructus Corni Officinalis (Shan Zhu Yu) 10g, fried Mastodi Ossis Fossilia (Long Gu) 20g and fried Concha Ostreae (Mu Li) 20g; or use Sheng Mai Injection 40ml, once daily. For Prostration of yang, use modified Shen Fu Decoction supplemented with Radix Ginseng (Ren Shen) 6g, Radix Aconiti Lateralis Praeparatae (Fu Zi) 10g, Radix Ophiopogonis Japonici (Mai Dong) 12g, Fructus Schisandrae Chinensis (Wu Wei Zi) 5g, fried Mastodi Ossis Fossilia (Long Gu) 20g and fried Concha Ostreae (Mu Li) 20g; or use Shen Fu Injection 50ml, 2-3 times each day.

5) <u>Deficiency of Anti-Pathogenic Qi and Lingering Attack by Pathogenic Factors</u>

Symptoms: Non-productive cough or with little sputum, low cough sound, shortness of breath, spiritlessness, fever, feverish sensation in palms and soles, spontaneous sweating or night sweating, dysphoria and distending sensation in the chest, thirst with a desire to drink, vexation, insomnia, red tongue with yellow and thin coating, and thready and rapid pulse.

Therapeutic Principle: To replenish qi, nourish yin, moisten the lung and resolve phlegm.

Prescription: Modified Zhu Ye Shi Gao Decoction.

Modifications: For stronger nourishing yin and relieving deficient-heat function, add Radix Scrophulariae Ningpoensis (Xuan Shen) 12g, Radix Rehmanniae (Di Huang) 20g and Cortex Lycii Radicis (Di Gu Pi) 12g; for stronger relieving phlegm and cough function, add Semen Armeniacae Amarum (Xing Ren) 10g, Cortex Mori Alba Radicis (Sang Bai Pi) 12g and Pericarpium Trichosanthis (Gua Lou Pi) 10g.

What Kinds of Chinese Patent Drugs are Available to Treat Pneumonia?

1) Lian Hua Qing Wei Capsule: 4 capsules each time, thrice daily.
2) Fu Fang Yu Xing Cao Tablet: 4 tablets each time, thrice daily.
3) Shuang Huang Lian Fen Injection: 60mg/kg/day.
4) Chuan Hu Ning Dong Gan Fen Injection: 80-120mg each time intravenously, twice daily; or 40-80mg each time intramuscularly, once or twice daily.

10. Lung Abscess

A lung abscess is a pus-filled cavity in the lung surrounded by inflamed tissue. It is usually caused by aspiration of bacteria that normally live in the mouth or throat. Periodontal disease is often the source of the bacteria that cause a lung abscess. Infection occurs primarily when a person is unconscious or very drowsy because of sedation, anesthesia, alcohol or drug abuse, seizures, or a disease of the nervous system. A lung tumor in smokers older than age 40, aspiration of foreign objects, tracheal or nasogastric tubes, pneumonia caused by certain bacteria or fungi, poorly functioning immune system and septic pulmonary emboli may also lead to the formation of a lung abscess.

Eventually, most abscesses rupture into an airway, producing a lot of sputum that gets coughed up. A ruptured abscess leaves a cavity in the lung that is filled with fluid and air. When a large abscess ruptures into an airway, it may cause widespread pneumonia and acute respiratory distress syndrome (ARDS). Sometimes an abscess ruptures into the pleural space and cause empyema. If an abscess destroys a blood vessel wall, serious bleeding may result, sometimes leading to death.

The death rate for people with lung abscesses is about 5%. The rate is higher when the person is debilitated or has an impaired immune system, lung cancer, or a very large abscess.

The symptoms may start slowly or suddenly. Early symptoms resemble those of pneumonia: malaise, loss of appetite, sweating, fever, poor dental hygiene and weight loss. Cough with expectoration of foul smelling purulent sputum suggests anaerobic infection. The sputum may be streaked with blood. The person also may feel chest pain with breathing. Chest x-rays nearly always reveal a lung abscess. CT scan of the chest can confirm the presence of a lung abscess and possibly determine its cause. Cultures of sputum from the lungs may help identify the organism causing the abscess, but this test is not always useful.

How is Lung Abscess Diagnosed by Conventional Western Medicine?

Diagnosis is usually made based on a thorough history, physical examination, chest x ray and CT scan. Cultures of representative material from the lung, which can be obtained by transtracheal or transthoracic aspiration, bronchoscopy or thoracentesis, may identify the organism.

How is Lung Abscess Treated by Conventional Western Medicine?

- Prompt, complete healing of a lung abscess requires the administration of antibiotics
- Postural drainage may be used to help drain the abscess
- Bronchoscopy is performed to confirm the presence of an obstruction due to a tumor or a foreign object. Bronchoscopy may also be used to remove a foreign object or to help drain a lung abscess that does not respond to antibiotics
- Occasionally, an abscess requires drainage through a tube
- Infected lung tissue may have to be removed surgically

What Causes Lung Abscess According to Traditional Chinese Medicine?

1) Invasion of Exogenous Pathogenic Factors
2) Retention of Phlegm-Heat in the Lung

How is Lung Abscess Differentiated and Treated by Traditional Chinese Medicine?

1) <u>Early Stage of Abscess</u>

Symptoms: Fever, aversion to cold, cough, chest pain worsened by cough, white and sticky or sticky and purulent sputum whose amount increases gradually, distending feeling in the chest, dyspnea, dry mouth and nose, red tongue with thin and yellow or thin and white coating, and floating, rapid and slippery pulse.

Therapeutic Principle: To dispel wind, release lung qi, clear away heat and remove toxicant.

Prescription: Modified Yin Qiao Powder.

Modifications: For severe exterior syndrome, add Folium Mori Alba (Sang Ye) 10g and Semen Sojae Preparatum (Dan Dou Chi) 12g; for severe fever, add Radix Scutellariae Baicalensis (Huang Qin) 10g, Gypsum Fibrosum (Shi Gao) 30g and Herba cum Radice Houttuyniae Cordatae (Yu Xing Cao) 20g; for copious amount of sputum and severe cough, add Fructus Trichosanthis (Gua Lou) 15g, Bulbus Fritillariae Thunbergii (Bei Mu) 10g, Semen Armeniacae Amarum (Xing Ren) 10g, Semen Benincasae Hispidae (Dong Gua Zi) 12g and Folium Eriobotryae Japonicae (Pi Pa Ye) 12g; for headache, add Radix Angelicae Dahuricae (Bai Zhi) 10g and Flos Chrysanthemi Morifolii (Ju Hua) 12g; for chest pain and dyspnea, add Semen Pruni Persicae (Tao Ren) 10g, Radix Curcumae (Yu Jin) 10g and Pericarpium Trichosanthis (Gua Lou Pi) 10g.

2) <u>Forming Stage of Abscess</u>

Symptoms: Fever that is getting worse until it becomes persistent high fever; chill, sweating, irritability, cough, dyspnea, distending pain in the chest that is aggravated by turning over, yellow, greenish, turbid and foul-smelling sputum, dry mouth and throat, red tongue with yellow and greasy coating, and rapid and slippery pulse.

Therapeutic Principle: To clear away heat, remove toxic substance, resolve stasis and subside abscess.

Prescription: Modified Qian Jin Wei Jing Decoction.

Modifications: For persistent high fever, add Taraxaci Mongolici Herba cum Radice (Pu Gong Yin) 20g, Radix Scutellariae Baicalensis (Huang Qin) 10g, Fructus Gardeniae Jasminoidis (Zhi Zi) 10g, Rhizoma Coptidis (Huang Lian) 10g, Patriniae Herba cum Radice (Bai Jiang Cao) 10g, Herba cum Radice Houttuyniae Cordatae (Yu Xing Cao) 20g, Gypsum Fibrosum (Shi Gao) 30g, Rhizoma Anemarrhenae (Zhi Mu) 10g, Herba cum Radice Violae (Zi Hua Di Ding) 15g and Flos Lonicerae (Jin Yin Hua) 15g; for distending sensation in the chest, cough, labored breathing, copious amount of yellow, turbid and purulent sputum, and inability to lie flat, add Cortex Mori Alba Radicis (Sang Bai Pi) 12g, Fructus Trichosanthis (Gua Lou) 15g, Semen Descurainiae seu Lepidii (Ting Li Zi) 10g, Rhizoma Belamcandae Chinensis (She Gan) 10g and Concha Meretricis seu Cyclinae (Hai Ge Qiao) 12g; for severe chest pain, add Radix Curcumae (Yu Jin) 10g, Gummi Olibanum (Ru Xiang) 10g, Myrrha (Mo Yao) 10g and Radix Salviae Miltiorrhizae (Dan Shen) 12g; for constipation, add Radix et Rhizoma Rhei (Da Huang) 6g and Fructus Citri Aurantii Immaturus (Zhi Shi) 10g; for hemoptysis, add Cortex Moutan Radicis (Mu Dan Pi) 10g and Radix Notoginseng (San Qi) 10g; for turbid, foul-smelling purulent sputum, add Xi Huang Pill.

3) <u>Necrotizing and Rupturing Stage of Abscess</u>

Symptoms: Copious amount of thick, sticky, foul-smelling, purulent and blood-tinged sputum, distending pain in the chest that is aggravated by turning over, shortness of breath, inability to lie flat, flushed face, fever, diaphoresis, irritability, thirst with a desire to drink, red tongue with yellow and greasy coating, and rapid and slippery or rapid and excess pulse.

Therapeutic Principle: To resolve phlegm, discharge pus, clear away heat and remove toxic substance.

Prescription: Jia Wei Jie Geng Decoction.

Modifications: For small amount of purulent sputum difficult to be expectorated, add Spina Gleditsiae Sinensis (Zao Jiao Ci) 10g and fresh Succus Bambosae (Zhu Li) 30g (contraindication for copious amount of sputum), or add Fructus Forsythiae Suspensae (Lian Qiao) 10g, Herba cum Radice Houttuyniae Cordatae (Yu Xing Cao) 20g, Patriniae Herba cum Radice (Bai Jiang Cao) 12g and Radix Scutellariae Baicalensis (Huang Qin) 10g; for severe hemoptysis, add Cortex Moutan Radicis (Mu

Dan Pi) 10g, Radix Notoginseng (San Qi) 10g, Fructus Gardeniae Jasminoidis (Zhi Zi) 10g, Radix Rehmanniae (Di Huang) 20g, Pollen Typhae (Pu Huang) 10g, Nodus Nelumbinis Nuciferae Rhizomatis (Ou Jie) 12g, Rhizoma Imperatae Cylindricae (Bai Mao Gen) 20g and Cacumen Biotae Orientalis (Ce Bai Ye) 12g; for dyspnea, lassitude, inability to expectorate due to lack of energy, add Radix Astragali (Huang Qi) 12g; for constipation, add Radix et Rhizoma Rhei (Da Huang) 6g and Fructus Citri Aurantii Immaturus (Zhi Shi) 10g; for dry mouth and tongue, add Radix Scrophulariae Ningpoensis (Xuan Shen) 12g, Radix Adenophorae (Sha Shen) 12g, Radix Trichosanthis (Tian Hua Fen) 12g and Radix Ophiopogonis Japonici (Mai Dong) 12g.

4) <u>Stage of Remission</u>

Symptoms: Fever that is gradually faded, mild cough, less amount of foul-smelling, purulent and blood-tinged sputum that is becoming thinner, appetite and spirit that are getting better, vague pain in the chest, inability to lie flat, lassitude, shortness of breath, spontaneous sweating, night sweating, vexation, dry mouth and dry throat, lusterless complexion, weight loss, pale and red tongue with yellow and thin coating, and thready or thready, rapid and weak pulse.

Therapeutic Principle: To clear away heat, nourish yin, replenish qi and nourish the lung.

Prescription: Sha Shen Qing Fei Decoction and Zhu Ye Shi Gao Decoction.

Modifications: For poor appetite and diarrhea, add Rhizoma Atractylodis Macrocephalae (Bai Zhu) 10g, Rhizoma Dioscoreae (Shan Yao) 20g and Sclerotium Poriae Cocos (Fu Ling) 12g; for mild fever, add Cortex Lycii Radicis (Di Gu Pi) 12g, Herba Artemisiae Apiaceae seu Annuae (Qing Hao) 10g and Radix Cynanchi Atrati (Bai Wei) 10g; for recurrent and persistent foul-smelling purulent sputum, add Patriniae Herba cum Radice (Bai Jiang Cao) 12g, Herba cum Radice Houttuyniae Cordatae (Yu Xing Cao) 20g and Fructus Forsythiae Suspensae (Lian Qiao) 12g; for blood-tinged sputum, add Radix Ampelopsis (Bai Lian) 10g and Gelatinum Corii Asini (E Jiao) 10g; for severe deficiency of yin, add Rhizoma Polygonati Odorati (Yu Zhu) 12g.

11. Pulmonary Tuberculosis (TB)

Tuberculosis (TB) is a life-threatening infection that primarily affects the lungs, although other organs are sometimes involved. Every year, tuberculosis kills nearly 2 million people worldwide. The infection is common — about one-third of the human population is infected with TB, with one new infection occurring every second. Today, despite advances in treatment, TB is a global pandemic.

Tuberculosis spreads by airborne droplets from infected people when they cough, talk or sneeze. Left untreated, tuberculosis can be fatal. With proper care, however, most cases of tuberculosis can be treated, even those resistant to the drugs commonly used against the disease. There are three important ways to describe the stages of TB: (1) exposure, (2) TB infection, and (3) TB disease.

TB is caused by Mycobacterium tuberculosis (M. tuberculosis). Most people infected with M. tuberculosis never develop active TB. However, with the spread of HIV/AIDS, poverty, a lack of health services and the emergence of drug-resistant strains of the bacterium, TB organisms can overcome the body's defenses, multiply, and cause an active disease. TB affects all ages, races, income levels, and both genders. Those at higher risk include the following:

- People who live or work with others who have TB
- Medically underserved populations
- Homeless people
- People from other countries where TB is prevalent
- People in group settings, such as nursing homes
- People who abuse alcohol
- People who use intravenous drugs
- People with impaired immune systems
- The elderly
- Healthcare workers who come in contact with high-risk populations

In pulmonary tuberculosis, coughing is often the only indication of infection initially. The symptoms of TB may resemble other lung conditions or medical problems. Signs and symptoms of active pulmonary TB include:

- A cough lasting three or more weeks that may produce discolored or bloody sputum
- Unintended weight loss
- Fatigue
- Slight fever
- Night sweats
- Chills
- Loss of appetite
- Pain with breathing or coughing (pleurisy)
- Or blood in their sputum

How is Tuberculosis Diagnosed by Conventional Western Medicine?

Tuberculosis is diagnosed with a TB skin test, such as Mantoux test. A blood test called QuantiFERON-TB Gold (QFT) is not yet widely available. Additional tests to determine if a person has active TB include chest x-ray and culture tests.

How is Tuberculosis Treated by Conventional Western Medicine?

Treatment for active TB may include: (1) short-term hospitalization, (2) medications, such as isoniazid, rifampin, pyrazinamide, ethambutol, or streptomycin, may be prescribed for a period of time up to six months or more for the medication to be effective.

What Causes Pulmonary Tuberculosis According to Traditional Chinese Medicine?

1) Pestilential Toxicant Attacking the Lung
2) Deficiency of Anti-Pathogenic Qi

How is Pulmonary Tuberculosis Differentiated and Treated by Traditional Chinese Medicine?

1) Deficiency of Lung Yin

Symptoms: Non-productive cough, shortness of breath, scanty white and sticky or bright red blood stained sputum, vague distending pain in the chest, low-grade fever, afternoon feverish sensation in palms and soles, dry skin, mouth and throat, little night sweating, red tongue tip and margin, little tongue coating, and thready and rapid pulse.

Therapeutic Principle: To nourish yin and moisten the lung.

Prescription: Modified Yue Hua Pill.

Modifications: For severe deficiency of yin, add Bulbus Lilii (Bai He) 20g and Rhizoma Polygonati Odorati (Yu Zhu) 12g; cough with little sticky sputum, add Bulbus Fritillariae Cirrhosae (Bei Mu) 10g and Semen Armeniacae Amarum (Xing Ren) 10g; for blood-stained sputum, add Herba Agrimoniae Pilosae (Xian He Cao) 12g and Rhizoma Bletillae Striatae (Bai Ji) 10g; for low-grade fever, add Radix Stellariae Dichotomae (Yin Chai Hu) 10g, Cortex Lycii Radicis (Di Gu Pi) 12g and Herba Artemisiae Apiaceae seu Annuae (Qin Hao) 10g; for fatigue and poor appetite, add Radix Pseudostellariae Heterophyllae (Tai Zi Shen) 15g, Sclerotium Poriae Cocos (Fu Ling) 12g, Rhizoma Atractylodis Macrocephalae (Bai Zhu) 12g, Endothelium Corneum Gigeriae Galli (Ji Nei Jin) 10g and Fructus Germinatus Oryzae Sativae (Gu Ya) 12g.

2) Fire Hyperactivity due to Yin Deficiency

Symptoms: Cough and shortness of breath, little thick and sticky or yellow sputum, cough with bright red blood constantly, afternoon hectic fever, dysphoria and feverish sensation in the chest, palms and soles, flushed cheek, night sweating, vexation, insomnia, irritability, distending pain in the hypochondriac region, seminal emission or abnormal menstruation, weight loss, crimson and dry tongue with yellow or peeled tongue coating, and rapid and thready pulse.

Therapeutic Principle: To replenish yin and clear fire.

Prescription: Modified Bai He Gu Jin Decoction and Qin Jiao Bie Jia Powder.

Modifications: For cough with clear sputum, add Radix Asteris Tatarici (Zi Wan) 10g, Flos Farfarae (Kuan Dong Hua) 10g and Fructus Perillae (Su Zi) 10g; for cough with yellow and thick sputum, add Cortex Mori Alba Radicis (Sang Bai Pi) 12g, Rhizoma Anemarrhenae (Zhi Mu) 10g, Concha Meretricis seu Cyclinae Powder (Hai Ge Fen) 12g and Herba cum Radice Houttuyniae Cordatae (Yu Xing Cao) 20g; for severe hemoptysis, add Fructus Gardeniae Jasminoidis (Zhi Zi) 10g, Folium Callicarpae Formosanae (Zi Zhu) 12g, fried Radix et Rhizoma Rhei (Da Huang) 6g and fried Radix Sanguisorbae Officinalis (Di Yu) 10g; for severe fire hyperactivity, add Rhizoma Picrorrhizae (Hu Huang Lian) 10g, Radix Scutellariae Baicalensis (Huang Qin) 10g and Cortex Phellodendri (Huang Bai) 10g.

3) <u>Consumption of Qi and Yin</u>

Symptoms: Cough, fatigue, shortness of breath, low voice, abundant clear and white sputum, or cough with blood-stained sputum or bright red blood (sometimes), afternoon hectic fever, aversion to wind and cold, spontaneous sweating and night sweating, poor appetite, spiritlessness, diarrhea, pale and lusterless complexion, pale and silky tongue with teeth marks on the margins, thin tongue coating and thready, weak and rapid pulse.

Therapeutic Principle: To replenish qi and nourish yin.

Prescription: Modified Bao Zhen Decoction.

Modifications: For clear and thin sputum, add Radix Asteris Tatarici (Zi Wan) 10g, Flos Farfarae (Kuan Dong Hua) 10g and Fructus Perillae (Su Zi) 10g; for severe hemoptysis, add Ophicalcitum (Hua Rui Shi) 12g, Pollen Typhae (Pu Huang) 10g, Herba Agrimoniae Pilosae (Xian He Cao) 12g and Radix Notoginseng (San Qi) 10g; for poor appetite, abdominal distension and diarrhea, add Semen Dolichoris Lablab (Bai Bian Dou) 20g, Semen Coicis (Yi Yi Ren) 20g, Semen Nelumbinis Nuciferae (Lian Zi) 12g and Rhizoma Dioscoreae (Shan Yao) 20g; for severe consumption with night sweating, add Carapax Trionycis (Bie Jia) Concha Ostreae (Mu Li) 20g, Fructus Pruni Mume (Wu Mei) 20g and Cortex Lycii Radicis (Di Gu Pi) 10g.

4) <u>Deficiency of Yin and Yang</u>

Symptoms: Cough, dyspnea, shortness of breath worsened by exertion, white or dark colored blood-tinged sputum, hectic fever, spontaneous sweating, night sweating, coarse voice, aphonia, edema of the face and extremities, palpitation, cyanosis of lips, cold body and limbs, diarrhea, aphthous stomatitis, emaciation, seminal emission, impotence, little menses or amenorrhea, pale and vague purplish tongue with little moisture, and tinny, thready and rapid or deficiency, large and weak pulse.

Therapeutic Principle: To replenish yin and nourish yang.

Prescription: Modified Bu Tian Da Zao Pill.

Modifications: For kidney deficiency with shortness or breath, add Semen Juglandis (Hu Tao Ren) 20g, Cordyceps Sinensis (Dong Chong Xia Cao) 10g, Gecko (Ge Jie) 5g and Stalactitum (Zhong Ru Shi) 10g; for severe palpitation, add Fluoritum (Zi Shi Ying) 12g and Radix Salviae Miltiorrhizae (Dan Shen) 12g; for diarrhea and seminal emission, add Semen Myristicae Fragrantis (Rou Dou Kou) 10g and Fructus Psoraleae Corylifoliae (Bu Gu Zhi) 10g.

What Kinds of Chinese Patent Drugs are Available to Treat Pulmonary Tuberculosis?

1) Qiang Li Pi Pa Capsule: 2 capsules each time, thrice daily.
2) Ren Shen Ge Jie Pill: 1-2 pills each time, twice daily.

12. Primary Bronchogenic Carcinoma (Lung Cancer)

Lung cancer is the leading cause of cancer deaths in the United States, among both men and women. Smoking accounts for nearly 90 percent of lung cancer cases. Other leading causes of lung cancer include asbestos, radon, secondhand smoke and other industrial carcinogens. Sex, race and heredity may play a role in causing lung cancer.

Lung cancer is commonly divided into two types: small cell lung cancer and non-small cell lung cancer. Surgical removal usually isn't an option for small cell lung cancer; instead, it's best treated with chemotherapy and radiation. The five-year survival rate for small cell lung cancer is very low. Non-small cell lung cancer accounts for more than 75 percent of lung cancers. It often can be removed surgically. There are four major categories of non-small cell lung cancer: squamous cell carcinoma, adenocarcinoma, large cell carcinoma and bronchoaveolar carcinoma. Prevention is critical because lung cancer usually isn't discovered until it's at an advanced stage.

Lung cancer doesn't manifest signs or symptoms in its earliest stages; the most common warning sign is a cough. Be alert for:

- Worsening cough in a person who smokes
- Coughing up blood, even a small amount
- Chest pain
- Shortness of breath
- New onset of wheezing

- Recurrent pneumonia or bronchitis
- Hoarseness that lasts more than two weeks

Lung cancer also may cause fatigue, loss of appetite and weight loss.

How is Lung Cancer Diagnosed by Conventional Western Medicine?

A standard chest X-ray can reveal an abnormal mass or nodule in the lungs. And a CT scan may show very small lesions and whether cancer has spread to other areas. Biopsy confirms the diagnosis. The sample may be removed using one of the following techniques: sputum cytology bronchoscopy, mediastinoscopy, transthoracic needle biopsy, thoracentesis and video thoracoscopy.

How is Lung Cancer Treated by Conventional Western Medicine?

Treatments for lung cancer depend on the type and stage of cancer, as well as on the patient's overall health.

<u>Small cell lung cancer:</u> surgery usually isn't a treatment option. Instead, the most effective treatment is chemotherapy, either alone or in combination with radiation therapy.

<u>Non-small cell lung cancer:</u> surgery is usually the best treatment for early-stage non-small cell lung cancer. More advanced non-small cell lung cancers are generally treated with chemotherapy, radiation, or a combination of both chemotherapy and radiation. Some patients may have surgery after first being treated with chemotherapy and radiation. Experimental therapies may be recommended.

Some new treatments include Erlotinib (Erlotinib has been approved for use in treating recurrent non-small cell lung cancers and is being studied for use in other stages of the disease) and Bevacizumab (it is only used in certain cases because the drug can have potentially fatal side effects)

What Causes Lung Cancer According to Traditional Chinese Medicine?

1) Deficiency of Anti-Pathogenic Qi
2) Retention of Phlegm-Dampness and Blood Stasis in the Lung
3) Imbalance of Seven Emotions and Overstrain
4) Smoking, Dust and Drinking
5) Invasion of the Lung by Six Exogenous Pathogenic Factors

How is Lung Cancer Differentiated and Treated by Traditional Chinese Medicine?

1) <u>Stagnation of Qi and Blood Stasis</u>

Symptoms: Rough cough, difficult expectoration, distending or stabbing pain in the chest, cyanosis of the face and lips, constipation, dark and purple tongue with ecchymosis, and taut or rough pulse.

Therapeutic Principle: To promote the circulation of blood and qi, and remove blood stasis and qi stagnation.

Prescription: Modified Xue Fu Zhu Yu Decoction, or modified Tao Hong Si Wu Decoction and Wu Ling Powder.

Modifications: For severe chest pain, add Cortex Moutan Radicis (Mu Dan Pi) 10g, Rhizoma Cyperi Rotundi (Xiang Fu) 10 and Rhizoma Corydalis (Yan Hu Suo) 10g; for recurrent hemoptysis with dark and red blood, add Pollen Typhae (Pu Huang) 10g, Nodus Nelumbinis Nuciferae Rhizomatis (Ou Jie) 12g, Herba Agrimoniae Pilosae (Xian He Cao) 12, Radix Notoginseng (San Qi) 10g and Radix Rubiae Cordifoliae (Qian Cao) 12g; for anorexia, fatigue and shortness of breath, add Radix Astragali (Huang Qi) 12g, Radix Codonopsitis Pilosulae (Dang Shen) 6g and Rhizoma Atractylodis Macrocephalae (Bai Zhu) 10g; for dry mouth and aphthous stomatitis, add Radix Adenophorae (Sha Shen) 10g, Radix Trichosanthis (Tian Hua Fen) 12g, Radix Rehmanniae (Di Huang) 15g and Rhizoma Anemarrhenae (Zhi Mu) 10g.

2) Accumulation of Toxic Phlegm-Dampness

Symptoms: Cough with abundant sputum, distending pain in the chest and hypochondriac region, anorexia, diarrhea, fever, dark urine, dim tongue with ecchymosis, thick and greasy tongue coating, and slippery and rapid pulse.

Therapeutic Principle: To eliminate dampness, resolve phlegm, clear away heat and remove toxic substance.

Prescription: Modified Dao Tan Decoction and Ting Li Da Zao Xie Fei Decoction.

Modifications: For yellow, thick and sticky sputum difficult to be expectorated, add Concha Meretricis seu Cyclinae (Hai Ge Qiao) 12g, Herba cum Radice Houttuyniae Cordatae (Yu Xing Cao) 20g and Radix Scutellariae Baicalensis (Huang Qin) 10g; for severe chest pain with distinct sign of stasis, add Radix Curcumae (Yu Jin) 10g, Radix Ligustici Chuanxiong (Chuan Xiong) 10g and Rhizoma Corydalis (Yan Hu Suo) 10g; for spiritlessness and poor appetite, add Radix Panacis Quinquefolii (Xi Yang Shen) 5g, Rhizoma Atractylodis Macrocephalae (Bai Zhu) 10g and Endothelium Corneum Gigeriae Galli (J Nei Jin) 10g.

3) Yin Deficiency and Toxic Heat

Symptoms: Cough with little or no sputum, or blood-stained sputum, or persistent hemoptysis in severe cases, vexation, insomnia, feverish sensation in palms and soles, low-grade fever, night sweating, thirst, constipation, red tongue with thin and yellow coating, and thready and rapid or rapid and large pulse.

Therapeutic Principle: To nourish yin, clear away heat, remove toxic substance and diminish stagnation.

Prescription: Sha Shen Mai Dong Decoction and Wu Wei Xiao Du Decoction.

Modifications: For constipation, add Fructus Trichosanthis (Gua Lou) 15g, Radix et Rhizoma Rhei Praeparatae (Zhi Da Huang) 6g, Radix Rehmanniae (Di Huang) 10g and Semen Pruni (Yu Li Ren) 10g.

4) <u>Deficiency of Qi and Yin</u>

Symptoms: Cough with low voice, little or no sputum, or blood-tinged sputum, spiritlessness, lassitude, frequent palpitation, sweating, shortness of breath, dry mouth, fever or afternoon hectic fever, feverish sensation in palms and soles, anorexia, abdominal distension, constipation or diarrhea, red tongue with thin coating, or bulgy and tender tongue with teeth marks, and thready, rapid and weak pulse.

Therapeutic Principle: To replenish qi, nourish yin, resolve phlegm and diminish stagnation.

Prescription: Modified Sha Shen Mai Dong Decoction, Da Bu Yuan Decoction, Sheng Mai Powder, or Mai Wei Di Huang Pill.

Modifications: For concurrent blood stasis, add Extremitas Radicis Angelicae Sinensis (Dang Gui Wei) 10g, Radix Paeoniae Rubra (Chi Shao) 12g, Semen Pruni Persicae (Tao Ren) 10g, Flos Carthami Tinctorii (Hong Hua) 10g, Radix Curcumae (Yu Jin) 10g, Rhizoma Corydalis (Yan Hu Suo) 10g, Radix Salviae Miltiorrhizae (Dan Shen) 10g, Rhizoma Sparganii Stoloniferi (San Leng) 10g and Rhizoma Curcumae Ezhu (E Zhu) 10g.

5) <u>Deficiency of Yin and Yang</u>

Symptoms: Pale complexion, cough with little sputum, feeling of oppression in the chest, shortness of breath, dyspnea on exertion, sweating, tinnitus, lumbago and weak legs, aversion to cold, cold limbs, pale tongue with thin and white coating, and deep and thready pulse.

Therapeutic Principle: To invigorate the lung, nourish the kidney and regulate both yin and yang.

Prescription: Modified Sheng Mai Decoction and Er Xian Decoction.

Modifications: For dyspnea and inability to lie flat, add Stalactitum (Zhong Ru Shi) 10g and Fluoritum (Zi Shi Ying) 12g; for cough with abundant sputum, add Radix Asteris Tatarici (Zi Wan) 10g, Flos Farfarae (Kuan Dong Hua) 10g and roasted Bombyx Batryticatus (Bai Jiang Can) 10g; for weak voice and spontaneous sweating, add Radix Astragali (Huang Qi) 12g, Radix Glycyrrhizae Uralensis (Gan Cao) 5g and Rhizoma Atractylodis Macrocephalae (Bai Zhu) 12g; for dysphoria with feverish sensation in the chest, palms and soles, and distinct dry mouth, add Carapax et Plastrum Testudinis (Gui Ban) 20g, Rhizoma Polygonati (Huang Jing) 12g and Fructus Ligustri Lucidi (Nu Zhen Zi) 12g.

What Kinds of Chinese Patent Drugs are Available to Treat Lung Cancer?

1) Fu Fang Ban Mao Capsule: 3 capsules each time, twice daily.
2) Ai Di Injection: 50-100ml each time, once daily.

13. Pleural Effusion

Pleural effusion is an abnormal collection of fluid in the pleural space. It is an indicator of a pathologic process due to primary pulmonary diseases, diseases in another organ system or systemic disease. Pleural effusion affects 1.3 million individuals each year in the United States. Morbidity and mortality of pleural effusions are directly related to cause, stage of disease at the time of presentation, and biochemical findings in the pleural fluid. There are five major types of pleural effusion, including transudates, exudates, empyema, hemorrhagic pleural effusion and chylous or chyliform effusion.

Dyspnea, dry cough and pleuritic chest pain are the most common symptom associated with pleural effusion. Other symptoms may suggest the etiology of the pleural effusion. Physical findings, which do not usually manifest until pleural effusions exceed 300 mL, include the following:

- Decreased breath sounds
- Dullness to percussion
- Decreased tactile fremitus
- Diminution of breath sounds
- Pleural friction rub
- Egophony in large effusions
- Contralateral mediastinal shift and bulging of the intercostals spaces

How is Pleural Effusion Diagnosed by Conventional Western Medicine?

Diagnosis is based on symptoms, physical findings, radiographic evidence of pleural effusion and diagnostic findings on thoracentesis.

How is Pleural Effusion Treated by Conventional Western Medicine?

Transudative effusions are usually managed by treating the underlying medical disorder. The management of exudative effusions depends on the underlying etiology of the effusion. Drain complicated parapneumonic effusions and empyemas to avoid fibrosing pleuritis. Malignant effusions are usually drained to palliate symptoms and may require pleurodesis to prevent recurrence. Drain large pleural effusions if they are causing severe respiratory symptoms.

Surgical intervention is most often required for parapneumonic effusions that cannot be drained adequately by needle or small-bore catheters, and surgery might be required for diagnosis. Restrictions of fat intake might help in the management of chylous effusions, although management remains controversial.

What Causes Pleural Effusion According to Traditional Chinese Medicine?

1) Exterior Cold-Dampness

2) Improper Food and Drink

3) Overstrain and Sex Indulgence

How is Pleural Effusion Differentiated and Treated by Traditional Chinese Medicine?

1) <u>Pathogenic factors Attacking the chest and the Lung</u>

Symptoms: Distending and stabbing pain in the chest and hypochondriac region, which is aggravated by respiration and turning over; dyspnea, cough with little sputum, alternate attacks of chills and fever, or tidal fever, little sweat, or fever without aversion to cold, persistent sweating, suffocative and stiff feeling in the chest, non-productive vomiting, bitter taste in the mouth, dry throat, thin and white or yellow tongue coating, and taut and rapid pulse.

Therapeutic Principle: To reduce fever by mediation, regulate qi, remove phlegm and relieve stagnation.

Prescription: Modified Chai Zhi Ban Xia Decoction.

Modifications: For severe fever with sweat, dyspnea and hoarse cough sound, remove Radix Bupleuri (Chai Hu) and add Ma Xing Shi Gan Decoction; for severe pain in the chest and hypochondriac region, remove Semen Armeniacae Amarum (Xing Ren) and add Rhizoma Corydalis (Yan Hu Suo) 10g, Radix Curcumae (Yu Jin) 10g and Fasciculus Vascularis Luffae (Si Gua Luo) 12g; for suffocative and stiff sensation in the chest, bitter taste in the mouth and vexation, add Rhizoma Coptidis (Huang Lian) 10g; for cough with yellow and thick sputum, add Liang Ge Powder; for constipation, add Radix et Rhizoma Rhei (Da Huang) 6g.

2) <u>Accumulation of Phlegm in the Chest and Hypochondrium</u>

Symptoms: Chest and hypochondriac pain worsened by cough and expectoration (but in less degree compared with that in early stage of onset), severer dyspnea (compared to early stage of onset), cough, shortness of breath, inability to lie flat, fullness in the affected hypochondriac region, or thoracic bulge in severe cases, white and greasy tongue coating, and deep and taut or slippery taut pulse.

Therapeutic Principle: To purge heat from the lung and remove water retention.

Prescription: Modified Shi Zao Decoction.

Modifications: For weak constitution, use Kong Xian Pill; for extremely weak constitution, use Ting Li DA Zao Xie Fei Decoction; for lingering water retention, fullness in the chest and hypochondriac region, weak constitution and anorexia, add Ramulus Cinnamomi Cassiae (Gui Zhi) 10g, Rhizoma Atractylodis Macrocephalae (Bai Zhu) 10g and Radix Glycyrrhizae Uralensis (Gan Cao) 10g.

3) Blockage of Collaterals due to Qi Stagnation

Symptoms: Burning or stabbing chest pain, or distending feeling in the chest, dyspnea, lingering muffled cough sound worsened under cloudy weather, dark and thin tongue coating, and taut pulse.

Therapeutic Principle: To regulate qi and mediate collaterals.

Prescription: Modified Xiang Fu Xuan Fu Hua Decoction.

Modifications: For severe cough, add Semen Armeniacae Amarum (Xing Ren) 10g, Pericarpium Trichosanthis (Gua Lou Pi) 10g and Folium Eriobotryae Japonicae (Pi Pa Ya) 12g; for distending feeling in the chest and abundant sputum, add Fructus Trichosanthis (Gua Lou) 15g, Bulbus Fritillariae Thunbergii (Zhe Bei Mu) 10g and Pumex (Fu Hai Shi) 10g; for chronic chest pain, add Semen Pruni Persicae (Tao Ren) 10g, Flos Carthami Tinctorii (Hong Hua) 10g and Radix Rubiae Cordifoliae (Qian Cao) 12g; for persistent water retention, add Medulla Tetrapanacis Papyriferi (Tong Cao) 3g, Fructus Liquidambaris Taiwanianae (Lu Lu Tong) 10g and Exocarpium Benincasae Hispidae (Dong Gua Pi) 20g.

4) Interior-Heat due to Yin Deficiency

Symptoms: Being in chronic and lingering disease, frequent cough with little sticky sputum, distending pain in the cheat and hypochondriac region, vexation, flushed cheek, dry mouth and throat, feverish sensation in palms and soles, afternoon hectic fever, night sweating, emaciation, red tongue with little coating, and thready and rapid pulse.

Therapeutic Principle: To nourish yin and clear away heat.

Prescription: Modified Sha Shen Mai Dong Decoction.

Modifications: For severe hectic fever, add Radix Stellariae Dichotomae (Yin Chai Hu) 10g, Carapax Trionycis (Bie Jia) 20g and Rhizoma Picrorrhizae (Hu Huang Lian) 10g; for concurrent deficiency of qi, add Radix Panacis Quinquefolii (Xi Yang Shen) 5g and Radix Pseudostellariae Heterophyllae (Tai Zi Shen) 15g; for distinct distending feeling of the chest, add Radix Curcumae (Yu Jin) 10g and Pericarpium Trichosanthis (Gua Lou Pi) 10g.

14. Cough

Coughing is an important way to keep the throat and airways clear. However, excessive coughing may indicate an underlying disease or disorder. Some coughs are dry, while others are productive. Coughs can be either acute or chronic. Acute coughs usually begin suddenly. They are often due to a cold, flu or sinus infection. They usually go away after 2 to 3 weeks. Chronic coughs last longer than 2 to 3 weeks. Common causes of cough include:

- Recent upper airway infections such as the common cold and flu
- Allergies and asthma
- Lung infections such as pneumonia or acute bronchitis
- COPD (chronic bronchitis or emphysema)
- Sinusitis leading to postnasal drip
- Lung disease such as bronchiectasis, interstitial lung disease, or tumors
- Gastroesophageal reflux disease (GERD)
- Cigarette smoking
- Exposure to secondhand smoke
- Exposure to air pollutants
- ACE inhibitors

The following symptoms need immediate attention:

- Violent cough that begins suddenly
- Stridor, a high-pitched sound when inhaling
- Cough that produces blood
- Fever
- Thick, foul-smelling, yellowish-green sputum
- A history of heart disease or swelling in the legs
- A cough that worsens in recumbent position
- Exposure to someone with tuberculosis
- Unintentional weight loss or night sweats
- Cough longer than 10-14 days
- Cough in an infant less than 3 months old

Diagnostic tests that may be performed include:

- Bronchoscopy
- Lung scan
- Pulmonary function tests
- Sputum analysis

- Chest X-ray

How is Cough Treated by Conventional Western Medicine?

Although coughing can be a troubling symptom, it is usually the defensive response of the body. Here are some tips to help ease the cough:

- For a dry and tickling cough, try cough drops or hard candy.
- Use a vaporizer or take a steamy shower
- Drink plenty of fluids.
- Guaifensin or decongestants. They are available without a prescription. Some medical experts have recommended against using cough suppressants in many situations

What Causes Cough According to Traditional Chinese Medicine?

1) Six Exogenous Pathogenic Factors Invading the Lung
2) Hypofunction of the Lung
3) Dysfunction of the Spleen
4) Attack of the Lung by Hyperactive Liver-Fire
5) Insufficiency of the Kidney

How is Cough Differentiated and Treated by Traditional Chinese Medicine?

1) Exogenous Cough

(1) <u>Wind-Cold Type</u>

Symptoms: Low and vague cough sound, white and thin sputum, aversion to cold, headache, nasal stuffiness, running nose, absence of sweat, joints pain, white and thin tongue coating, and floating pulse.

Therapeutic Principle: To disperse wind, expel cold, ventilate lung qi and stop cough.

Prescription: Modified San Ao Decoction and Xing Su Powder.

Modifications: For concurrent exterior-cold and interior-heat (so called cough of fire wrapped by cold), manifesting cough, sore throat, dry mouth, thirst, thick sputum difficult to be expectorated, hoarse cough sound, severe fever, white and greasy or yellow tongue coating, and floating and rapid pulse, remove Rhizoma zingiberis officinalis and add Cortex Mori Alba Radicis (Sang Bai Pi) 12g, Fructus Arctii Lappae (Niu Bang Zi) 10g and Radix Scutellariae Baicalensis (Huang Qin) 10g, or use Ma Xing Shi Gan Decoction.

Example Prescription: Prepared Herba Ephedrae (Ma Huang) 5g, Semen Armeniacae Amarum (Xing Ren) 10g, Caulis Perillae (Su Geng) 10g, Radix Glycyrrhizae Uralensis (Gan Cao) 5g, Radix Platycodi Grandiflori (Jie Geng) 8g, Radix Peucedani (Qian Hu) 10g, Exocarpium Citri Grandis Rubrum (Hua Ju Hong) 10g, Rhizoma Pinelliae Ternatae (Ban Xia) 5g and Fructus Citri Aurantii (Zhi Ke) 10g.

(2) <u>Wind-Heat Type</u>

Symptoms: Coarse and loud cough sound, yellow and thick sputum, aversion to wind, fever, headache, sore throat, thirst and sweating, thin and yellow tongue coating, and floating and rapid pulse.

Therapeutic Principle: To dispel wind, clear away heat, ventilate the lung and resolve phlegm.

Prescription: Modified Sang Ju Decoction.

Modifications: For severe lung-heat, add Radix Scutellariae Baicalensis (Huang Qin) 10g and Gypsum Fibrosum (Shi Gao) 30g; for severe cough, add Fructus Arctii Lappae (Niu Bang Zi) 10g and Rhizoma Phragmitis Communis (Lu Gen) 15g; for epistaxis, add Nodus Nelumbinis Nuciferae Rhizomatis (Ou Jie) 12g and Rhizoma Imperatae Cylindricae (Bai Mao Gen) 15g; for sore throat, add Fructus Arctii Lappae (Niu Bang Zi) 10g, Fructificatio Lasiosphaerae seu Calvatiae (Ma Bo) 5g and Radix Isatidis seu Baphicacanthi (Ban Lan Gen) 12g; for difficult expectoration, add Semen Benincasae Hispidae (Dong Gua Zi) 12g and Fructus Trichosanthis (Gua Lou) 15g.

Example Prescription: Herba Schizonepetae (Jing Jie) 10g, Herba Menthae Haplocalycis (Bo He) 5g, Radix Platycodi Grandiflori (Jie Geng) 10g, Fructus Forsythiae Suspensae (Lian Qiao) 10g, Fructus Arctii Lappae (Niu Bang Zi) 10g, Radix Peucedani (Qian Hu) 10g, Bulbus Fritillariae Thunbergii (Zhe Bei Mu) 10g, Radix Glycyrrhizae Uralensis (Gan Cao) 5g, Folium Mori Alba (Sang Ye) 10g and Flos Chrysanthemi Morifolii (Ju Hua) 10g.

(3) <u>Dry-Heat Type</u>

Symptoms: Hoarse or splitting cough sound, dry cough with little sticking sputum difficult to be expectorated, aversion to wind, fever, dry nose and mouth, blood tinged sputum, or chest pain caused by cough, red tongue tip, thin and yellow and dry tongue coating, and slightly rapid pulse.

Therapeutic Principle: To dispel wind, clear away heat, moisten the dryness and stop cough.

Prescription: Modified Sang Xing Decoction

Modifications: For severe cough and itching throat, add Radix Peucedani (Qian Hu) 10g, Periostracum Cicadae (Chan Tui) 10g, Radix Platycodi Grandiflori (Jie Geng) 6g and Radix Glycyrrhizae Uralensis (Gan Cao) 6g; for chronic dry cough, red tongue with little moisture and emaciation, use modified Qing Zao Jiu Fei Decoction; for severe fever, add Gypsum Fibrosum (Shi Gao) 30g and Rhizoma Anemarrhenae (Zhi Mu) 10g.

Example Prescription: Folium Mori Alba (Sang Ye) 10g, Semen Armeniacae Amarum (Xing Ren) 10g, Radix Adenophorae (Sha Shen) 12g, Radix Peucedani (Qian Hu) 10g, Prepared Folium Eriobotryae Japonicae (Pi Pa Ye) 10g, Rhizoma Anemarrhenae (Zhi Mu) 10g, Bulbus Fritillariae Cirrhosae (Bei Mu) 10g, Radix Glycyrrhizae Uralensis (Gan Cao) 5g and Radix Asteris Tatarici (Zi Wan)10g.

2) Endogenous Cough

(1) <u>Retention of Phlegm-Dampness in the Lung Type</u>

Symptoms: Chronic cough, abundant white and sticky sputum easy to be expectorated, poor appetite, fatigue, weakness, diarrhea and chest distress, greasy and white tongue coating, and soft and slippery pulse.

Therapeutic Principle: To invigorate the spleen, dry dampness, resolve phlegm and relieve cough.

Prescription: Modified Er Chen Decoction.

Modifications: For abundant sputum and stuffy sensation in the chest, add Rhizoma Atractylodis (Cang Zhu) 10g, Cortex Magnoliae Officinalis (Hou Po) 10g, Semen Armeniacae Amarum (Xing Ren) 10g and Semen Coicis (Yi Yi Ren) 15g; for severe cough, add Herba Ephedrae (Ma Huang) 6g, Semen Armeniacae Amarum (Xing Ren) 10g, Fructus Perillae (Su Zi) 10g and Rhizoma Cynanchi Stauntonii (Bai Qian) 10g; for distinct deficiency of the spleen with fatigue, pale tongue and weak pulse, add Radix Codonopsitis Pilosulae (Dang Shen) 6g and Rhizoma Atractylodis Macrocephalae (Bai Zhu) 10g or use modified Liu Jun Zi Decoction; for cough with severe adverse qi, add San Zi Yang Qin Decoction.

Example Prescription: Pericarpium Citri Reticulatae (Chen Pi) 10g, Sclerotium Poriae Cocos (Fu Ling) 10g, Rhizoma Pinelliae Ternatae (Ban Xia) 10g, Radix Glycyrrhizae Uralensis (Gan Cao) 5g, Semen Armeniacae Amarum (Xing Ren) 10g, Cortex Magnoliae Officinalis (Hou Po) 6g, Semen Coicis (Yi Yi Ren)15g, Fructus Perillae (Su Zi)10g and Caulis Perillae (Su Geng) 10g.

(2) <u>Accumulation of Phlegm-Heat in the Lung Type</u>

Symptoms: Coarse cough sound, shortness of breath, yellow and sticky sputum, fever, thirst, distending pain in the chest and hypochondriac region, dry mouth with bitter taste, stinky sputum or blood in sputum, yellow and greasy tongue coating, and rapid and slippery or rapid and taut pulse.

Therapeutic Principle: To clear away heat, resolve phlegm, release lung qi and relieve cough.

Prescription: Modified Qing Jin Hua Tan Decoction.

Modifications: For yellow, thick and foul-smelling purulent sputum, add Herba cum Radice Houttuyniae Cordatae (Yu Xing Cao) 20g, Fructus Forsythiae Suspensae (Lian Qiao) 12g, Semen Benincasae Hispidae (Dong Gua Zi) 12g and Semen Coicis (Yi Yi Ren) 20g; for cough and stuffy sensation in the chest worsened by lying flat, add Semen Descurainiae seu Lepidii (Ting Li Zi) 10g; for dry mouth, thirst and red tongue, add Radix Adenophorae (Nan Sha Shen) 12g, Radix Trichosanthis (Tian Hua Fen) 12g and Dai Ge Powder.

Example Prescription: Fructus Trichosanthis (Gua Lou) 20g, Radix Scutellariae Baicalensis (Huang Qin) 10g, Rhizoma Anemarrhenae (Zhi Mu) 10g, Bulbus Fritillariae Cirrhosae (Bei Mu) 10g, Charred Fructus Gardeniae Jasminoidis (Zhi Zi) 10g, Rhizoma Pinelliae Ternatae (Ban Xia) 10g, Rhizoma Arisaematis cum Bile (Dan Nan Xing) 6g, Radix Platycodi Grandiflori (Jie Geng) 6g, Semen Descurainiae seu Lepidii (Ting Li Zi) 10g and Cortex Mori Alba Radicis (Sang Bai Pi) 10g.

(3) <u>Liver-Fire Attacking the Lung Type</u>

Symptoms: Paroxysmal irritable dry cough with pain in the chest and hypochondriac region, flushed face, conjunctival congestion, dry throat and mouth, symptoms changes with emotional activity, red tongue margin, yellow, thin and dry tongue coating, and rapid and taut pulse.

Therapeutic Principle: To clear away lung heat, sooth the liver, lower the adverse flow of qi and purge fire.

Prescription: Modified Xie Bai Powder and Dai Ge Powder.

Example Prescription: Cortex Mori Alba Radicis (Sang Bai Pi) 10g, Cortex Lycii Radicis (Di Gu Pi) 10g, Radix Scutellariae Baicalensis (Huang Qin) 10g, Fructus Trichosanthis (Gua Lou) 15g, Radix Stemonae (Bai Bu) 10g, Fructus Gardeniae Jasminoidis (Zhi Zi) 10g, Radix Glycyrrhizae Uralensis (Gan Cao) 5g and plus Dai Ge Powder (wrapped in cloth and decocted).

(4) <u>Lung-Deficiency Type</u>

Symptoms: Chronic non-productive cough, blood tinged sputum, afternoon hectic fever, vexation, insomnia, fatigue, lack of vitality, flushed cheeks, hot sensation in palms and soles, night sweating, red tongue with scanty coating, and thready and rapid pulse.

Therapeutic Principle: To nourish yin, moisten the lung, relieve cough and resolve phlegm.

Prescription: Modified Sha Shen Mai Dong Decoction.

Modifications: For severe cough, add Semen Armeniacae Amarum (Xing Ren) 10g and Bulbus Fritillariae Cirrhosae (Bei Mu) 10g; for hemoptysis, add Cacumen Biotae Orientalis (Ce Bai Ye) 12g, Herba Agrimoniae Pilosae (Xian He Cao) 12g, Nodus Nelumbinis Nuciferae Rhizomatis (Ou Jie) 12g, Rhizoma Bletillae Striatae (Bai Ji) 10g, Gelatinum Corii Asini (E Jiao) 10g and Radix Notoginseng (San Qi) 10g; for afternoon hectic fever and flushed cheek, add Radix Stellariae Dichotomae (Yin Chai Hu) 10g, Cortex Lycii Radicis (Di Gu Pi) 10g, Radix Scutellariae Baicalensis (Huang Qin) 10g and Radix Cynanchi Atrati (Bai Wei) 10g; for cough with yellow sputum, add Radix Scutellariae Baicalensis (Huang Qin) 10g, Rhizoma Anemarrhenae (Zhi Mu) 10g and Concha Meretricis seu Cyclinae (Hai Ge Qiao) 12g; for cough and asthma, add Radix Rehmanniae Praeparatae (Shu Di Huang) 20g, Fructus Corni Officinalis (Shan Zhu Yu) 10g, Fructus Schisandrae Chinensis (Wu Wei Zi) 5g, Radix Ginseng (Ren Shen)5g and Gecko (Ge Jie) 5g.

Example Prescription: Radix Adenophorae (Sha Shen) 12g, Radix Ophiopogonis Japonici (Mai Dong) 10g, Schisandrae Fructus (Wu Wei Zi) 6g, Semen Armeniacae Amarum (Xing Ren) 10g, prepared Folium Eriobotryae Japonicae (Pi Pa Ye) 10g, Bulbus Fritillariae Cirrhosae (Bei Mu) 10g, Radix Asteris Tatarici (Zi Wan) 10g and Radix Glycyrrhizae Uralensis (Gan Cao) 6g.

What Kinds of Chinese Patent Drugs are Available to Treat Cough?

1) Sang Ju Gan Mao Tablet: 4-8 tablets each time, twice or thrice daily.
2) She Dan Chuan Bei Oral Liquid: 1 vial each time, thrice daily.
3) Qing Qi Hua Tan Pill: 6-9g each time, thrice daily.
4) Xing Su Er Chen Pill: 6-9g each time, twice daily.
5) Fu Fang Gan Cao Tablet: 2-3 tablets each time, thrice daily.

15. Influenza

Influenza (or flu) is a highly contagious viral infection that attacks respiratory system. It is characterized by the abrupt onset of fever, muscle aches, sore throat, and a nonproductive cough. An estimated 5 to 20 percent of the population in the US contract influenza each year. As many as 36,000 Americans die each year of complications of influenza and more than 200,000 are hospitalized.

The flu viruses can spread through droplets in the air when someone with the infection coughs, sneezes or talks. But it also spreads by hand-to-hand contact with someone who has a cold and then transfers the viruses to the eyes, nose or mouth of another person. Influenza is caused by three types of viruses — influenza A, B and C. Type A is responsible for the deadly influenza pandemics that strike every 10 to 40 years. Type B can lead to smaller, more localized outbreaks that generally occur every three to 15 years. And either types A or B can cause the flu that circulates almost every winter. Type C is less common and causes only mild symptoms. Numerous influenza A subtypes exist. At least 15 flu subtypes affect birds, the most virulent of which is H5N1. Avian influenza virus is spread from infected poultry to humans. Influenza viruses continually mutate or change, which enables the viruses to evade the immune system. People are susceptible to influenza infection throughout their lives.

Initially, the flu may seem like a common cold, with a runny nose, sneezing and sore throat. Common signs and symptoms of the flu include:

- Fever over 101 F. Children with the flu tend to have higher fevers than adults have — often as high as 103 to 105 F
- Chills and sweats
- Headache
- Dry cough, often becoming severe
- Muscular aches and pains, especially in the back and limbs
- Fatigue and weakness
- Nasal congestion or clear nose
- Loss of appetite
- Diarrhea, nausea and vomiting. Although children may have these signs, diarrhea and vomiting are rare in adults
- Most people recover from influenza within a week, but may be left feeling exhausted for as long as three to four weeks

How is Influenza Diagnosed by Conventional Western Medicine?

- Abrupt onset with fever, chills, malaise, cough, coryza, and muscle aches
- Aching, fever and prostration out of proportion to catarrhal symptoms
- Leukopenia
- Cases usually in epidemic pattern, not sporadic

How is Influenza Treated by Conventional Western Medicine?

The goal of treatment for influenza is to help prevent or decrease the severity of symptoms. Treatment may include:

- Bed rest
- Plenty of fluids
- Medications to relieve aches and fever, such as acetaminophen (Tylenol). Aspirin should not be used.
- Medications used for congestion and nasal discharge
- Medications for cough may be prescribed after a thorough evaluation
- Antiviral medications, such as oseltamivir (Tamiflu) or zanamivir (Relenza)
- Antibiotics may be given if a secondary bacterial infection is suspected or diagnosed
- Influenza vaccine is recommended for specific groups of people

What Causes Influenza According to Traditional Chinese Medicine?

1) Affection by Pathogenic Wind and Pestilential Toxicity
2) Deficiency of Anti-Pathogenic Qi and Dysfunction of the Lung and Wei Division/Level

How is Influenza Differentiated and Treated by Traditional Chinese Medicine?

1) <u>Wind-Cold Type</u>

Symptoms: Nasal congestion, watery rhinorrhea, muffled voice, sneezing, itching throat, thin and white sputum, aversion to cold, headache, arthralgia, muscular aching, malaise, fever or absence of fever, absence of sweat, moisture tongue with thin and white coating, and floating or floating and tense pulse.

Concurrent Symptoms:

(1) Dampness: Fatigue, nausea, poor appetite, diarrhea, chest distress, absence of thirst, white greasy tongue coating, and slippery pulse.

(2) Sputum: Cough with profuse sputum, poor appetite, chest distress, white greasy tongue coating, and slippery pulse.

(3) Qi Stagnation: Hypochondriac pain and chest discomfort, and taut pulse.

(4) Interior-fire: Cough, dyspnea, yellow, thick and sticky sputum, dark urine, constipation, irritability, yellow tongue coating, and floating and rapid pulse.

Therapeutic Principle: To relieve the exterior syndrome with pungent and warm herbs, promote the dispersing function of the lung, and resolve the pathogenic cold.

Prescription: Modified Cong Chi Decoction or Jing Fang Bai Du Powder.

Modifications: For concurrent wind-heat and dampness, add Cortex Magnoliae Officinalis (Hou Po) 10g, Pericarpium Citri Reticulatae (Chen Pi) 9g, Rhizoma Atractylodis (Cang Zhu) 10g and Rhizoma Pinelliae Ternatae (Ban Xia)10g, or change to modified Qiang Huo Sheng Shi Decoction; for turbid phlegm, add Er Chen Decoction; for stagnation of qi, add Rhizoma Cyperi Rotundi (Xiang Fu) 10g and Caulis Perillae (Su Geng) 10g; for combination of exterior-cold with interior-fire, use Ma Xing Shi Gan Decoction.

Example Prescription: Semen Sojae Preparatum (Dan Dou Chi)10g, Folium Perillae Frutescentis (Su Ye) 10g, Herba Schizonepetae (Jing Jie) 10g, Radix Saposhnikoviae Divaricatae (Fang Feng) 10g, Radix Platycodi Grandiflori (Jie Geng) 6g, Rhizoma Cynanchi Stauntonii (Bai Qian) 10g, Radix Ligustici Chuanxiong (Chuan Xiong) 10g, Radix Glycyrrhizae Uralensis (Gan Cao) 6g, Semen Armeniacae Amarum(Xing Ren) 6g, Fructus Citri Aurantii (Zhi Ke) 9g, Rhizoma Zingiberis Recens (Sheng Jiang) 10g.

2) Wind-Heat Type

Symptoms: Slight aversion to cold, headache, cough, fever, thirst, sweat, nasal stuffiness, turbid nasal discharge, dry mouth, reddish swelling and sore throat, yellowish and sticky sputum, yellowish and thin tongue coating, and floating and rapid pulse.

Concurrent Symptoms:

(1) Severe Wind-Heat Type: Irritability, chill, headache, thirst, persistent high fever, dry nose and mouth, and red tongue with yellow coating.

(2) Dampness: Nausea, lassitude, heaviness feeling of the head, chest distress, dark urine, and yellow greasy tongue coating.

(3) Summer-Dampness: Thirst, sweat, persistent high-grade fever, limb heaviness, scanty and dark urine, yellow and greasy tongue coating, and soft and rapid pulse.

(4) Autumn-Dryness: Dry mouth, dry lips, dry nose, dry throat, thirst, non-productive cough, little sputum or no sputum, red and dry tongue, and slightly rapid pulse.

Therapeutic Principle: To relieve exterior syndrome with pungent and cool herbs, and dispel pathogenic factors from the lung.

Prescription: Modified Yin Qiao Powder.

Modifications: For headache, add Folium Mori Alba (Sang Ye) 10g and Flos Chrysanthemi Morifolii (Ju Hua) 12g; for cough with abundant sputum, add Semen Armeniacae Amarum (Xing Ren) 10g, Bulbus Fritillariae Cirrhosae (Bei Mu) 10g and Fructus Trichosanthis (Gua Lou) 15g; for red, swollen and sore throat, add Radix Isatidis seu Baphicacanthi (Ban Lan Gen) 12g, Fructificatio Lasiosphaerae seu Calvatiae (Ma Bo) 5g and Radix Scrophulariae Ningpoensis (Xuan Shen) 10g; for severe wind-heat type or epidemic exterior syndrome, add Radix Puerariae (Ge Gen) 15g, Radix Scutellariae Baicalensis (Huang Qin) 10g, Gypsum Fibrosum (Shi Gao) 30g, Rhizoma Anemarrhenae (Zhi Mu) 10g and Radix Trichosanthis (Tian Hua Fen) 12g; for dampness, add Herba Agastache seu Pogostemonis (Huo Xiang) 10g and Herba Eupatorii (Pei Lan) 10g; for summer-dampness, use modified Xin Jia Xiang Ru Decoction; for autumn-dryness, add Semen Armeniacae Amarum (Xing Ren) 10g and Pericarpium Trichosanthis (Gua Lou Pi) 10g, or use modified Sang Xing Decoction.

Example Prescription: Herba Schizonepetae (Jing Jie) 10g, Herba Menthae Haplocalycis (Bo He), Semen Sojae Preparatum (Dan Dou Chi) 10g, Flos Lonicerae (Jin Yin Hua) 10g, Fructus Forsythiae Suspensae (Lian Qiao) 10g, Radix Platycodi Grandiflori (Jie Geng) 6g, Radix Glycyrrhizae Uralensis (Gan Cao) 6g, Fried Fructus Arctii Lappae (Chao Niu Bang Zi) 10g, Rhizoma Phragmitis Communis

(Lu Gen), Bulbus Fritillariae Thunbergii (Zhe Bei Mu) 10g and Semen Armeniacae Amarum (Xing Ren) 10g.

3) <u>Qi Deficiency Type</u>

Symptoms: Aversion to cold, fever, headache, nasal stuffiness, cough with white sputum, lassitude, shortness of breath, indolence of speaking, lusterless complexion, sweating, abdominal pain, pale tongue with thin and white coating, and floating and weak pulse.

Therapeutic Principle: To replenish qi and relieve exterior syndrome

Prescription: Modified Shen Su Decoction.

Modifications: For severe deficiency of qi, add Radix Astragali (Huang Qi) 12g or use Bu Zhong Yi Chi Decoction supplemented with Folium Perillae Frutescentis (Su Ye) 10g; for spontaneous sweating and susceptibility to exogenous pathogenic factors, use Yu Ping Feng Powder.

Example Prescription: Perillae Frutescentis (Su Ye) 10g, Radix Codonopsitis Pilosulae (Dang Shen) 10g, Sclerotium Poriae Cocos (Fu Ling) 10g, Radix Glycyrrhizae Uralensis (Gan Cao) 6g, Radix Peucedani (Qian Hu) 10g, Radix Platycodi Grandiflori (Jie Geng) 6g, Fructus Citri Aurantii (Zhi Ke) 10g, Rhizoma Pinelliae Ternatae (Ban Xia) 10g, Pericarpium Citri Reticulatae (Chen Pi) 10g, Semen Armeniacae Amarum (Xing Ren) 10g and Radix Ligustici Chuanxiong (Chuan Xiong) 10g.

4) <u>Yang Deficiency Type</u>

Symptoms: Headache, light fever, severe aversion to cold, pale complexion, cold extremities, feeble voice, general aching, diarrhea, edema, fatigue, pale and bulgy tongue with white and thin coating, and deep and weak pulse.

Therapeutic Principle: To strengthen yang and relieve exterior syndrome.

Prescription: Modified Shen Fu Zai Zao Pill.

Modifications: For aversion to cold, absence of sweat and light deficiency of yang, use modified Ma Huang Fu Zi Xi Xing Decoction.

Example Prescription: Radix Aconiti Lateralis Praeparatae (Fu Pian) 6g, Ramulus Cinnamomi Cassiae (Gui Zhi)10g, Radix Codonopsitis Pilosulae (Dang Shen) 10g, Radix Astragali (Huang Qi) 15g, Rhizoma et Radix Notopterygii (Qiang Huo) 10g, Radix Saposhnikoviae Divaricatae (Fang Feng) 10g, Herba cum Radice Asari (Xi Xin) 3g, Radix Platycodi Grandiflori (Jie Geng) 6g, Radix Glycyrrhizae Uralensis (Gan Cao) 6g, Semen Armeniacae Amarum (Xing Ren) 10g and Radix Cynanchi Stauntonii (Bai Qian) 10g.

5) <u>Blood Deficiency Type</u>

Symptoms: Headache, fever, slight aversion to cold, absence of sweat, dim and lusterless complexion, pale lips and finger nails, palpitation, dizziness, postpartum bleeding or menorrhagia, hemafesia, pale tongue with white coating, and thready or floating and weak pulse.

Therapeutic Principle: To nourish blood and relieve exterior syndrome.

Prescription: Modified Cong Bai Qi Wei Decoction.

Modifications: For severe aversion to cold, add Folium Perillae Frutescentis (Su Ye) 10g and Herba Schizonepetae (Jing Jie) 10g, or use Si Wu Decoction supplemented with Herba Schizonepetae (Jing Jie) 10g and Radix Saposhnikoviae Divaricatae (Fang Feng) 10g; for severe fever, add Flos Lonicerae (Jin Yin Hua) 15g, Fructus Forsythiae Suspensae (Lian Qiao) 12g and Radix Scutellariae Baicalensis (Huang Qin) 10g, or use Chai Hu Si Wu Decoction; for persistent bleeding, add Gelatinum Corii Asini (E Jiao) 10g, Nodus Nelumbinis Nuciferae Rhizomatis (Ou Jie) 12g, Rhizoma Bletillae Striatae (Bai Ji) 10g and Radix Notoginseng (San Qi) 10g.

Example Prescription: Radix Angelicae Sinensis (Dang Gui) 10g, Radix Rehmanniae (Shu Di Huang) 10g, Radix Paeoniae Alba (Bai Shao Yao) 10g, Radix Ligustici Chuanxiong (Chuang Xiong) 10g, Herba Schizonepetae (Jing Jie) 10g, Radix Saposhnikoviae Divaricatae (Fang Feng) 10g, Radix Bupleuri (Chai Hu) 10g, Radix Glycyrrhizae Uralensis (Gan Cao) 6g, Semen Armeniacae Amarum (Xing Ren) 10g and Radix Puerariae (Ge Gen) 10g.

6) Yin Deficiency Type

Symptoms: Headache, fever, slight aversion to wind and cold, absence of sweat or little sweating or night sweating, dizziness, vexation, thirst, dry throat, hot sensation in palms and soles, non-productive cough, or little or blood tinged sputum, tender and red tongue with scanty coating, thready and rapid pulse.

Therapeutic Principle: To nourish yin and relieve exterior syndrome.

Prescription: Modified Jia Jian Wei Rui Decoction.

Modifications: For severe exterior syndrome, add Herba Schizonepetae (Jing Jie) 10g and Herba Menthae Haplocalycis (Bo He) 10g; for dry throat, cough and difficult expectoration, add Fructus Arctii Lappae (Niu Bang Zi) 10g and Pericarpium Trichosanthis (Gua Lou Pi) 10g; for severe vexation and thirst, add Radix Trichosanthis (Tian Hua Fen) 12g and Herba Lophatheri Gracilis (Dan Zhu Ye) 12g.

Example prescription: Rhizoma Polygonati Odorati (Yu Zhu) 15g, Radix Cynanchi Atrati (Bai Wei) 10g, Radix Ophiopogonis Japonici (Mai Dong) 10g, Radix Adenophorae (Nan Sha Shen) 15g, Radix Scrophulariae Ningpoensis (Xuan Shen) 12g, Radix Glycyrrhizae Uralensis (Gan Cao) 6g, Radix

Platycodi Grandiflori (Jie Geng) 6g, Semen Oroxyli (Mu Hu Die) 5g, fried Fructus Arctii Lappae (Niu Bang Zi) 10g, Rhizoma Phragmitis Communis (Lu Gen) 30g and Herba Schizonepetae (Jing Jie) 10g.

What Kinds of Chinese Patent Drugs are Available to Treat Influenza?

1) Ban Lan Gen Granule: 15g each time, thrice daily.
2) Xiao Chai Hu Granule: 10g each time, thrice daily.

Chapter 2: Disorders of the Cardiovascular System

1. Chronic Heart Failure

Heart failure, also known as congestive heart failure (CHF), is a condition in which the heart cannot pump enough oxygenated blood to meet the body's needs. It can affect the right side of the heart, the left side of the heart, or both sides. Any number of underlying heart conditions can lead to heart failure. Heart failure is a serious condition. About 5 million people in the United States have heart failure, and the number is growing. Each year, another 550,000 people are diagnosed for the first time. It contributes to or causes about 300,000 deaths each year.

Heart failure is caused by other diseases or conditions that damage or overwork the heart muscle. Over time, the heart can no longer keep up with even the normal demands placed on it. Medical problems that can cause heart failure include, but are not limited to, the following:

- Coronary artery disease and heart attack
- Hypertension
- Diabetes
- Cardiomyopathy
- Heart valve diseases
- Abnormal heartbeats or arrhythmias
- Congenital heart defects
- Treatments for cancer, such as radiation and certain chemotherapy drugs
- Thyroid disorders
- Alcohol abuse
- HIV/AIDS
- Cocaine and other illegal drug use
- Chronic lung disease
- Anemia
- Excessive bleeding

Medications can improve the signs and symptoms of chronic heart failure and lead to improved survival. Lifestyle changes, such as exercising, reducing salt intake, managing stress, treating depression, and losing weight, also can improve the quality of life. The following are the most common symptoms of heart failure:

- Swelling in the ankles, feet, legs, and sometimes the abdomen
- Fast breathing during rest or exercise
- Shortness of breath or labored breathing
- Wheezing while breathing
- Fatigue
- Limitation on physical activity
- Nausea
- Lack of appetite
- Weight gain
- Frequent urination
- Cough and congestion in the lungs

The severity of the condition and symptoms depends on how much of the heart's pumping capacity has been affected. The symptoms of heart failure may resemble other conditions or medical problems.

How is Heart Failure Diagnosed by Conventional Western Medicine?

There is not a specific test to determine if a person has heart failure. A clinical diagnosis of heart failure is usually made based on a detailed medical history, a physical exam, and several tests, including blood and urine testes, chest x-ray, electrocardiogram (ECG or EKG), echocardiogram (echo), nuclear heart scan, cardiac catheterization Coronary angiography, stress test and thyroid functions tests.

How is Heart Failure Treated by Conventional Western Medicine?

The goals of treatment are to treat the underlying cause of the heart failure, improve the symptoms and quality of life, stop the heart failure from getting worse and prolong the life span. The treatment for heart failure includes:

- Treat the underlying diseases or conditions
- Lifestyle changes
- Medicines, such as digoxin, diuretics, potassium supplements, ACE inhibitors and beta blockers
- Specialized care for those in the most advanced stage of heart failure

The best defense against heart failure is to prevent or control risk factors and aggressively manage any underlying conditions such as coronary artery disease, high blood pressure, high cholesterol, diabetes or obesity

What Causes Chronic Heart Failure According to Traditional Chinese Medicine?

1) Attack by Exogenous Pathogenic Factors
2) Improper Emotional Activity
3) Improper Food and Drink
4) Overstrain and Sex Indulgence

How is Chronic Heart Failure Differentiated and Treated by Traditional Chinese Medicine?

1) <u>Deficiency of Heart Qi and Lung Qi</u>

Symptoms: Palpitation, shortness of breath, lassitude worsened by exertion, spiritlessness, cough, pale complexion, pale tongue or with teeth marks on the margin, and deep and thready or deficiency pulse.

Therapeutic Principle: To nourish the heart and the lung.

Prescription: Modified Yang Xin Decoction and Bu Fei Decoction.

Modifications: For severe internal cold-phlegm, add Flos Farfarae (Kuan Dong Hua) 10g and Fructus Perillae (Su Zi) 10g; for severe deficiency of lung yin, add Radix Adenophorae (Sha Shen) 10g, Rhizoma Polygonati Odorati (Yu Zhu) 12g and Bulbus Lilii (Bai He) 15g.

2) <u>Deficiency of Qi and Yin</u>

Symptoms: Palpitation, shortness of breath, fatigue, sweating aggravated by exertion, spontaneous sweating or night sweating, dizziness, restlessness, dry mouth, flushed cheeks, red tongue with little coating, and thready, rapid and weak or knot and intermittent pulse.

Therapeutic Principle: To replenish qi and nourish yin.

Prescription: Modified Sheng Mai Powder.

Modifications: For severe deficiency of yin, add Radix Paeoniae Alba (Bai Shao Yao) 10g and Radix Angelicae Sinensis (Dang Gui) 12g; for distinct deficiency of qi, add Rhizoma Atractylodis Macrocephalae (Bai Zhu) 12g, Sclerotium Poriae Cocos (Fu Ling) 12g and Radix Glycyrrhizae Uralensis (Gan Cao) 6g.

3) <u>Deficiency of Heart Yang and Kidney Yang</u>

Symptoms: Palpitation, shortness of breath, lassitude, dyspnea worsened by exertion, cold body and limbs, oliguria, edema, abdominal distention, diarrhea, crimson complexion, red tongue with little coating, and thready, rapid and weak or knot and intermittent pulse.

Therapeutic Principle: To warm and nourish the heart and the kidney.

Prescription: Modified Gui Zhi Gan Cao Long Gu Mu Li Decoction and Jin Gui Shen Qi Pill.

Modifications: For severe edema, add Cortex Acanthopanacis Radicis (Wu Jia Pi) 10g; for severe deficiency of qi, add Radix Ginseng Rubra (Hong Shen) 6g and Radix Astragali (Huang Qi) 12g.

4) <u>Deficiency of Qi and Blood Stasis</u>

Symptoms: Palpitation, shortness of breath, distending pain in the chest and hypochondriac region, jugular venous distention in the neck, hypochondriac lump, edema of extremities, pale and bluish complexion, cyanosis of lips and nails, dark and purplish tongue with ecchymosis, and rough or knot and intermittent pulse.

Therapeutic Principle: To replenish qi and promote blood circulation.

Prescription: Modified Ren Shen Yang Rong Decoction and Tao Hong Si Wu Decoction.

Modifications: For severe chest pain, add Fructus Citri Aurantii (Zhi Ke) 10g, Lignum Dalbergiae Odoriferae (Jiang Xiang) 5g and Radix Curcumae (Yu Jin) 10g.

5) <u>Deficiency of Yang and Water Retention</u>

Symptoms: Palpitation, shortness of breath, inability to lie flat, frothy sputum, edema of face and extremities, aversion to cold, cold limbs, irritability, sweating, pale complexion, cyanosis of lips, oliguria, abdominal distention, or hydrothorax, or ascites, pale or pale and red tongue with white and slippery coating, and thready and rapid or knot and intermittent pulse.

Therapeutic Principle: To warm yang and induce diuresis.

Prescription: Modified Zhen Wu Decoction.

Modifications: For severe deficiency of qi, add Radix Codonopsitis Pilosulae (Dang Shen) 9g and Radix Astragali (Huang Qi) 12g; for severe edema, add Cortex Acanthopanacis Radicis (Wu Jia Pi) 10g and Sclerotium Poriae Cocos (Fu Ling) 12g.

6) <u>Blockage of Phlegm in the Lung</u>

Symptoms: Palpitation, dyspnea, cough with white or yellow, thick and sticky sputum, inability to lie flat, distending feeling in the chest and hypochondriac region, dizziness, oliguria, edema, or wheezing sound caused by sputum, or fever and thirst, white and greasy or yellow and greasy tongue coating, and taut and slippery or rapid and slippery pulse.

Therapeutic Principle: To purge heat from the lung and resolve phlegm.

Prescription: Modified Ting Li Da Zao Xie Fei Decoction.

Modifications: For severe cold-phlegm, add Rhizoma Zingiberis Officinalis (Gan Jiang) 10g and Herba cum Radice Asari (Xi Xing) 3g; for severe cough and dyspnea, add Semen Raphani Sativi (Lai

Fu Zi) 10g and Fructus Perillae (Su Zi) 10g; for phlegm-heat, use Qing Jin Hua Tan Decoction and Qian Jin Wei Jing Decoction.

What Kinds of Chinese Patent Drugs are Available to Treat Chronic Heart Failure?

1) Sheng Mai Injection: 20-60ml each time, 1-2 times daily.
2) Shen Fu Injection: 50ml each time, 1-2 times daily.

2. Cardiac Arrhythmia

An arrhythmia (also called dysrhythmia) is a problem with the speed or rhythm of the heartbeat. There are four main types of arrhythmia: premature (extra) beats, supraventricular arrhythmias, ventricular arrhythmias, and bradyarrhythmias. Premature beats that occur in the atria are called premature atrial contractions, or PACs. Premature beats that occur in the ventricles are called premature ventricular contractions, or PVCs. Supraventricular arrhythmias are tachycardias that start in the atria or the atrioventricular node. Types of supraventricular arrhythmias include atrial fibrillation (AF), atrial flutter, paroxysmal supraventricular tachycardia (PSVT), and Wolff-Parkinson-White (WPW) syndrome. Ventricular arrhythmias include ventricular tachycardia and ventricular fibrillation (v-fib). Bradyarrhythmias are arrhythmias in which the heart rate is slower than normal.

An arrhythmia can occur when the electrical signals that control the heartbeat are delayed or blocked. This can happen when the special nerve cells producing the electrical signal don't work properly or when the electrical signal doesn't travel normally through the heart. An arrhythmia also can occur when another part of the heart starts to produce electrical signals, adding to the signals from the special nerve cells and disrupting the normal heartbeat. Stress, smoking, heavy alcohol use, heavy exercise, use of certain drugs (such as cocaine or amphetamines), use of certain prescription or over-the-counter medicines, and too much caffeine or nicotine can lead to arrhythmia in some people. Any pre-existing structural heart condition can lead to arrhythmia development due to inadequate blood supply and damage or death of heart tissue.

Millions of Americans have arrhythmias. They are very common in older adults. About 2.2 million Americans have atrial fibrillation. Most arrhythmias are harmless, but some can be serious or even life threatening. When the heart rate is too slow, too fast, or irregular, the heart may not be able to pump enough blood to the body. Lack of blood flow can damage the brain, heart, and other organs.

Many arrhythmias cause no signs or symptoms. Signs and symptoms of arrhythmias may include:

- Palpitations
- A slow heartbeat

- An irregular heartbeat
- Feeling of pauses between heartbeats
- Anxiety
- Weakness
- Dizziness and light-headedness
- Fainting or nearly fainting
- Sweating
- Shortness of breath
- Chest pain

How is Cardiac Arrhythmia Diagnosed by Conventional Western Medicine?

Arrhythmias can be hard to diagnose, especially types that only cause symptoms every once in a while. Diagnosis of arrhythmias is made based on family and medical history, physical exam, and diagnostic tests and procedures, which may include ECG or EKG, chest x ray, echocardiogram, transesophageal echocardiography (TEE), stress test, electrophysiologic study (EPS), tilt table testing and coronary angiography.

How is Cardiac Arrhythmia Treated by Conventional Western Medicine?

Common arrhythmia treatments include lifestyle modifications, medicines, medical procedures and surgery. Treatment is needed when an arrhythmia causes serious symptoms, such as dizziness, chest pain, or fainting, or when it increases the chances of developing complications.

What Causes Cardiac Arrhythmia According to Traditional Chinese Medicine?

1) Attack by Exogenous Pathogenic Factors
2) Internal Injury by Seven Emotions
3) Improper Food and Drinks
4) Overstrain and Sex Indulgence
5) Chronic Diseases and Malnutrition

How is Cardiac Arrhythmia Differentiated and Treated by Traditional Chinese Medicine?

1) Tachyarrhythmias

(1) <u>Restless Mind and Timidity</u>

Symptoms: Palpitation, timidity, restlessness, insomnia, dreamful sleep, thin and white tongue coating, and rapid and deficiency or knot and intermittent pulse.

Therapeutic Principle: To calm the emotions, nourish the heart and tranquilize the mind.

Prescription: Modified An Shen Ding Zhi Pill.

Modifications: Add Semen Ziziphi Spinosae (Suan Zao Ren) 15g and Cortex Albizziae Julibrissin (He Huan Pi) 12g to nourish the heart and tranquilize the mind; for deficiency of heart qi, add Radix Glycyrrhizae Uralensis (Gan Cao) 6g and Radix Codonopsitis Pilosulae (Dang Shen) 9g.

(2) <u>Insufficiency of Qi and Blood</u>

Symptoms: Palpitation and shortness of breath worsened by exertion, dizziness, lassitude, lusterless complexion, pale tongue with white and thin coating, and thready and weak pulse.

Therapeutic Principle: To replenish blood, nourish the heart, supplement qi and tranquilize the mind.

Prescription: Modified Gui Pi Decoction.

Modifications: For deficiency of qi and blood that can not nourish the heart, use Zhi Gan Cao Decoction; for severe palpitation, add Mastodi Ossis Fossilia (Long Gu) 20g and Concha Ostreae (Mu Li) 20g.

(3) <u>Hyperactivity of Fire due to Yin Deficiency</u>

Symptoms: Palpitation, timidity, restlessness, insomnia, dizziness, feverish sensation in palms and soles, tinnitus, lumbago, red tongue with little coating, and thready and rapid pulse.

Therapeutic Principle: To replenish yin, clear fire, nourish the heart and tranquilize the mind.

Prescription: Modified Tian Wang Bu Xin Pill.

Modifications: For restlessness, dry throat and mouth, and bitter taste in the mouth, use Zhu Sha An Shen Pill; for palpitation and restlessness, add Mastodi Ossis Fossilia (Long Gu) 20g, Concha Ostreae (Mu Li) 20g and Margarita (Zhen Zhu) 0.5g; for vexation, irritability, bitter taste in the mouth and aphthous stomatitis, add Fructus Forsythiae Suspensae (Lian Qiao) 10g, Plumula Nelumbinis Nuciferae (Lian Zi Xin) 2g and Fructus Gardeniae Jasminoidis (Zhi Zi) 10g; for feverish sensation in the chest, palms and soles, nocturnal seminal emission and lumbago, add Zhi Bai Di Huang Pill.

(4) <u>Deficiency of Qi and Yin</u>

Symptoms: Palpitation, shortness of breath, dizziness, fatigue, distending pain in the chest, indolence of speaking, feverish sensation in the chest, palms and soles, insomnia, dreamful sleep, red tongue with little coating, and deficiency and rapid pulse.

Therapeutic Principle: To supplement qi, replenish yin, nourish the heart and tranquilize the mind.

Prescription: Modified Sheng Mai Powder.

Modifications: For deficiency of heart yin with vexation and insomnia, add Radix Rehmanniae (Di Huang) 15g, Fructus Forsythiae Suspensae (Lian Qiao) 10g and Plumula Nelumbinis Nuciferae (Lian

Zi Xin) 2g; for soreness in the lower back and knees, tinnitus and dizziness, add Radix Polygoni Multiflori (He Shou Wu) 15g, Fructus Lycii (Gou Qi Zi) 10g and Carapax et Plastrum Testudinis (Gui Ban) 20g; for concurrent blood stasis that blocks the heart, add Radix Salviae Miltiorrhizae (Dan Shen) 10g and Radix Notoginseng (San Qi) 10g.

(5) <u>Phlegm-Fire Disturbing the Heart</u>

Symptoms: Paroxysmal palpitation, feeling of oppression in the chest, restlessness, insomnia, dreamfulness, dry mouth with bitter taste, constipation, dark scanty urine, yellow and greasy tongue coating, and taut and slippery pulse.

Therapeutic Principle: To clear away heat, resolve phlegm and tranquilize the mind.

Prescription: Modified Huang Lian Wen Dan Decoction.

Modifications: For severe phlegm-fire, add Radix Scutellariae Baicalensis (Huang Qin) 10g and Fructus Gardeniae Jasminoidis (Zhi Zi) 10g; for constipation, add Fructus Trichosanthis (Gua Lou) 15g and Radix et Rhizoma Rhei (Da Huang) 6g; for palpitation, timidity and restlessness, add Concha Margaritiferae (Zhen Zhu Mu) 20g, Mastodi Dentis Fossilia (Long Chi) 20g and Concha Ostreae (Mu Li) 20g; for red tongue with little coating due to stagnated fire impairing yin, add Radix Rehmanniae (Di Huang) 15g, Radix Ophiopogonis Japonici (Mai Dong) 12g and Rhizoma Polygonati Odorati (Yu Zhu) 12g.

(6) <u>Blood Stasis Blocking the Heart</u>

Symptoms: Palpitation, restlessness, chest distress, intermittent stinging pain in the chest, or cyanosis of lips and nails, purple tongue with ecchymosis, and rough or knot and intermittent pulse.

Therapeutic Principle: To promote blood circulation, remove blood stasis, regulate qi and activate the collaterals.

Prescription: Modified Tao Ren Hong Hua Decoction.

Modifications: For aversion to cold and cold extremities, add Ramulus Cinnamomi Cassiae (Gui Zhi) 10g, Lignum Santali Albi (Tan Xiang) 2g and Lignum Dalbergiae Odoriferae (Jiang Xiang) 5g; for distending pain in the chest, turbid and greasy tongue coating, add Fructus Trichosanthis (Gua Lou) 15g, Bulbus Allii Macrostemonis (Xie Bai) 10g and Rhizoma Pinelliae Ternatae (Ban Xia) 10g; for severe chest pain, add Gummi Olibanum (Ru Xiang) 10g, Myrrha (Mo Yao) 10g and Excrementum Trogopteri seu Pteromydis (Wu Ling Zhi) 10g.

(7) <u>Insufficiency of Heart Yang</u>

Symptoms: Palpitation, restlessness, feeling of oppression in the chest, shortness of breath, pale complexion, cold limbs, pale tongue, and deficiency and weak or thready and rapid pulse.

Therapeutic Principle: To warm and replenish heart yang and tranquilize the mind.

Prescription: Modified Shen Fu Decoction and Gui Zhi Gan Cao Long Gu Mu Li Decoction.

Modifications: For cold limbs and edema of lower extremities, add Zhen Wu Decoction; for dizziness, nausea and vomiting, add Sclerotium Poriae Cocos (Fu Ling) 12g, Rhizoma Pinelliae Ternatae (Ban Xia) 10g and Pericarpium Citri Reticulatae (Chen Pi) 5g; for concurrent pronounced yin consumption, add Radix Ophiopogonis Japonici (Mai Dong) 10g, Rhizoma Polygonati Odorati (Yu Zhu) 10g and Fructus Schisandrae Chinensis (Wu Wei Zi) 5g.

2) Bradyarrhythmias

(1) Insufficiency of Heart Yang

Symptoms: Palpitation and shortness of breath worsened by exertion, or sudden syncope, sweating, lassitude, pale complexion, cold limbs, pale tongue with white coating, and deficiency and weak or deep, thready and rapid pulse.

Therapeutic Principle: To warm and replenish heart yang, and tranquilize the mind.

Prescription: Modified Ren Shen Si Ni Decoction and Gui Zhi Gan Cao Long Gu Mu Li Decoction.

Modifications: For blood stasis, add Radix Salviae Miltiorrhizae (Dan Shen) 10g, Radix Paeoniae Rubra (Chi Shao) 10g and Flos Carthami Tinctorii (Hong Hua) 10g; for edema, add Rhizoma Alismatis Orientalis (Ze Xie) 10g, Semen Plantaginis (Che Qian Zi) 10g and Herba Leonuri Heterophylii (Yi Mu Cao) 10g; for deficiency of qi, add Radix Astragali (Huang Qi) 12g.

(2) Deficiency of Heart Yang and Kidney Yang

Symptoms: Palpitation and shortness or breath worsened by exertion, pale complexion, cold limbs, weak and sore loins and knees, frequent or dribbling urination with clear urine, edema of lower extremities, pale and chubby tongue, and deep and slow pulse.

Therapeutic Principle: To warm and replenish the heart and the kidney, warm yang and induce diuresis.

Prescription: Modified Shen Fu Decoction and Zhen Wu Decoction.

Modifications: For blood stasis in the heart, add Radix Salviae Miltiorrhizae (Dan Shen) 10g, Flos Carthami Tinctorii (Hong Hua) 10g and Herba Leonuri Heterophylii (Yi Mu Cao) 12g; for deficiency of qi, add Radix Astragali (Huang Qi) 12g and Rhizoma Dioscoreae (Shan Yao) 15g; for deficiency of yang without edema, add You Gui Pill.

(3) Deficiency of Qi and Yin

Symptoms: Palpitation, shortness of breath, fatigue, insomnia, dreamful sleep, night sweating, spontaneous sweating, feverish sensation in the chest, palms and soles, slight red tongue with little moisture, and deficiency and weak or knot and intermittent pulse.

Therapeutic Principle: To supplement qi, replenish yin, nourish the heart and activate circulation.

Prescription: Modified Zhi Gan Cao Decoction.

Modifications: For pronounced deficiency of yin, add Tuber Asparagi Cochinchinensis (Tian Men Dong) 10g and Rhizoma Polygonati (Huang Jing) 12g; for concurrent phlegm-dampness, add Fructus Trichosanthis (Gua Lou) 15g, Rhizoma Pinelliae Ternatae (Ban Xia) 10g, Caulis Bambusae in Taeniam (Zhu Ru) 10g and Rhizoma Arisaematis cum Bile (Dan Nan Xing) 5g.

(4) <u>Blockage of Turbid Phlegm</u>

Symptoms: Palpitation, shortness of breath, distending and stuffy sensation in the chest, abundant sputum, poor appetite, abdominal distention, or nausea, white and greasy or slippery and greasy tongue coating, and taut and slippery pulse.

Therapeutic Principle: To regulate qi, resolve phlegm, tranquilize the mind and activate circulation.

Prescription: Modified Di Tan Decoction.

Modifications: For concurrent blood stasis, add Radix Salviae Miltiorrhizae (Dan Shen) 10g, Flos Carthami Tinctorii (Hong Hua) 10g and Hirudo seu Whitmania (Shui Zhi) 5g; for phlegm-heat, use Huang Lian Wen Dan Decoction.

(5) <u>Blood Stasis Blocking the Heart</u>

Symptoms: Palpitation, feeling of oppression in the chest, dyspnea, paroxysmal chest pain, or cold limbs, dark tongue with ecchymosis, and deficiency or knot and intermittent pulse.

Therapeutic Principle: To promote blood circulation, remove blood stasis, regulate qi and activate the collaterals.

Prescription: Modified Xue Fu Zhu Yu Decoction.

Modifications: For aversion to cold and cold limbs, add Radix Ginseng (Ren Shen) 6g, Radix Aconiti Lateralis Praeparatae (Fu Zi) 10g, Ramulus Cinnamomi Cassiae (Gui Zhi) 10g and Radix Glycyrrhizae Uralensis (Gan Cao) 6g; for pronounced qi stagnation, add Radix Curcumae (Yu Jin) 10g, Lignum Dalbergiae Odoriferae (Jiang Xiang) 5g and Fructus Citri Aurantii Immaturus (Zhi Shi) 10g; for pronounced chest pain, add Rhizoma Corydalis (Yan Hu Suo) 10g, Pollen Typhae (Pu Huang) 10g and Radix Notoginseng (San Qi) 10g.

(6) <u>Excessive Fluid Attacking the Heart</u>

Symptoms: Palpitation, feeling of oppression in the chest, dyspnea, thirst without a desire to drink, oliguria, edema, cold limbs, dizziness, nausea, vomiting, productive expectoration, pale tongue with white and slippery coating, and taut and slippery pulse.

Therapeutic Principle: To activate heart yang, promote qi circulation and induce diuresis.

Prescription: Modified Ling Gui Zhu Gan Decoction.

Modifications: For nausea and vomiting, add Rhizoma Pinelliae Ternatae (Ban Xia) 10g, Pericarpium Citri Reticulatae (Chen Pi) 6g and Rhizoma Zingiberis Recens (Sheng Jiang) 10g; for severe palpitation, dyspnea, inability to lie flat, oliguria and edema, use modified Zhen Wu Decoction.

What Kinds of Chinese Patent Drugs are Available to Treat Cardiac Arrhythmia?

1) Tachyarrhythmias

(1) Shen Song Yang Xin Capsule: 2-4 capsules each time, thrice daily.
(2) Tian Wang Bu Xin Bolus: 3g each time, thrice daily.
(3) Sheng Mai Injection: 40ml each time, once daily.
(4) Fu Fang Dan Shen Di Pill: 10 pills each time, thrice daily.

2) Bradyarrhythmias

(1) Xin Bao Pill: 5-10 pills each time, thrice daily.
(2) Xue Fu Zhu Yu Oral Liquid: 10ml each time, thrice daily.
(3) Shen Fu Injection: 40ml each time, once daily.
(4) Xiang Dan Injection: 30ml each time, once daily.

3. Sudden Cardiac Arrest (Sudden Cardiac Death, SCA)

Sudden cardiac arrest (SCA), also known as sudden cardiac death, is when the heart suddenly and unexpectedly stops beating. When this occurs, blood stops flowing to the brain and other vital organs. SCA usually causes death if not treated in minutes. SCA occurs when the heart develops an arrhythmia that causes it to stop beating.

SCA is not the same thing as a heart attack. A heart attack is a problem with blocked blood flow to a part of the heart muscle. In a heart attack, the heart usually does not suddenly stop beating. SCA, however, may happen during recovery from a heart attack. People with heart disease have a higher chance of having SCA. But most SCAs happen in people who appear healthy and have no known heart disease or other risk factors for SCA.

Most cases of sudden cardiac arrest (SCA) are due to ventricular fibrillation (v-fib). Other electrical problems that can cause SCA are extreme slowing of the rate of the heart's electrical signals or when heart muscle stops responding to the electrical signals. Several factors can cause the electrical problems that lead to SCA, including coronary artery disease (CAD), severe physical stress, inherited disorders and structural changes in the heart.

Each year, between 250,000 and 450,000 Americans have sudden cardiac arrest (SCA). Ninety-five percent of these people die within minutes. SCA occurs most often in adults in their mid-thirties to mid-forties. It affects men twice as often as women. The major risk factor for SCA is having coronary artery disease (CAD). The risk factors for SCA include:

- Smoking
- A family history of early cardiovascular
- High blood cholesterol
- Diabetes
- Increasing age
- High blood pressure
- Overweight and obesity
- A sedentary lifestyle
- A personal or family history of SCA
- Arrhythmias
- Birth defects of the heart or blood vessels, or an enlarged heart
- Heart failure
- Recreational drug abuse

Signs and symptoms include:

- Sudden collapse
- No heartbeat or pulse
- No breathing
- Loss of consciousness

Sometimes, other signs and symptoms precede sudden cardiac arrest. These may include fatigue, fainting, blackouts, racing heartbeat, dizziness, chest pain, shortness of breath, palpitations or vomiting. But sudden cardiac arrest often occurs with no warning.

How is SCA Diagnosed by Conventional Western Medicine?

Sudden cardiac arrest (SCA) happens without warning and requires immediate treatment. Rarely is there a chance to diagnose it with medical tests as it is happening. Instead, SCA is often diagnosed after it happens, by ruling out other causes of the patient's sudden collapse.

Several tests to help detect the risk factors for SCA include ECG or EKG, echocardiogram, stress echocardiogram, MUGA test or MRI heart scans, cardiac catheterization and electrophysiology study.

How is SCA Treated by Conventional Western Medicine?

Sudden cardiac arrest (SCA) requires immediate treatment with a defibrillator. To be effective, defibrillation must be provided within minutes of cardiac arrest. Cardiopulmonary resuscitation (CPR) should be given to a person having SCA until defibrillation can be provided. A person who survives SCA is usually admitted to the hospital for observation and treatment. If CAD is detected, angioplasty may be ordered to restore blood flow through blocked coronary arteries. Often, implantable cardioverter defibrillator (ICD) will be surgically placed under the skin. An ICD continuously monitors the heart for dangerous rhythms. If SCA or another dangerous rhythm is detected, the ICD immediately delivers an electric shock to restore a normal rhythm.

What Causes SCA According to Traditional Chinese Medicine?

1) Weak Constitution with Deficiency of Heart Yang
2) Deficiency of Anti-Pathogenic Qi due to Chronic Diseases
3) Attack by Exogenous Pathogenic Factors
4) Turbid Phlegm and Blood Stasis

How is SCA Differentiated and Treated by Traditional Chinese Medicine?

1) <u>Prostration of Both Qi and Yin</u>

Symptoms: Spiritlessness, lassitude, shortness of breath, extremely cold extremities, vexation, feeling of oppression in the chest, oliguria, pale or dark red tongue with little coating, and deficiency and rapid or tinny pulse.

Therapeutic Principle: To replenish qi and save yin.

Prescription: Modified Sheng Mai Powder.

Modifications: Rhizoma Polygonati (Huang Jing) 12g and Fructus Corni Officinalis (Shan Zhu Yu) 10g can be added to the above prescription; for concurrent blood stasis, add Radix Salviae Miltiorrhizae (Dan Shen) 10g, Flos Carthami Tinctorii (Hong Hua) 10g and Radix Angelicae Sinensis (Dang Gui) 10g.

2) <u>Mental Confusion due to Phlegm</u>

Symptoms: Delirium, dyspnea with hoarse voice, wheezing sound in the throat, dark red lips and nails, dim tongue with thick and greasy or white or yellow coating, and deep and excess pulse.

Therapeutic Principle: To remove phlegm, promote blood circulation and cause resuscitation.

Prescription: Modified Chang Pu Yu Jin Decoction.

3) <u>Sudden Collapse of Primordial Qi and Yang</u>

Symptoms: Delirium, or dementia, dysphasia, pale complexion, extremely cold extremities, pale and moistured tongue, and tinny, thready and extremely faint pulse.

Therapeutic Principle: To restore yang from collapse.

Prescription: Modified Du Shen Decoction or Si Wei Hui Yang Decoction.

What Kinds of Chinese Patent Drugs are Available to Treat SCA?

1) Shen Fu Injection: 30-100ml each time, once daily.
2) Sheng Mai Injection: 40-100ml each time, once daily.
3) Xing Nao Jing Injection: 10-20ml each time, once daily.

4. High Blood Pressure (Hypertension)

High blood pressure is a blood pressure reading of 140/90 mmHg or higher. Once high blood pressure develops, it usually lasts a lifetime. The good news is that it can be treated and controlled. High blood pressure can cause heart failure, aneurysms, kidney failure, stroke, vision changes or even blindness. There are two levels of high blood pressure: stage 1 (140-159/90-99 mmHg) and stage 2 (160/100 mmHg or higher. There is an exception to the definition of high blood pressure. A blood pressure of 130/80 mmHg or higher is considered high blood pressure in people with diabetes and chronic kidney disease.

In many people with high blood pressure, a single specific cause is not known. This is called essential or primary high blood pressure. In some people, high blood pressure is the result of another medical problem or medicine. When the cause is known, this is called secondary high blood pressure.

About 65 million American adults—nearly 1 in 3—have high blood pressure. Over half of all Americans aged 60 and older have high blood pressure. In the United States, high blood pressure occurs more often in African Americans compared to other groups. Risk factors for developing high blood pressure include:

- Overweight
- A man over the age of 45
- A woman over the age of 55

- A family history of high blood pressure
- Prehypertension (blood pressure in the 120–139/80–89 mmHg range)
- Eating too much salt
- Drinking too much alcohol
- Not getting enough potassium in the diet
- Not doing enough physical activity
- Taking certain medicines
- Having long-lasting stress
- Smoking

Most people with high blood pressure have no signs or symptoms, even if blood pressure readings reach dangerously high levels. Although a few people with early-stage high blood pressure may have dull headaches, dizzy spells or a few more nosebleeds than normal, these signs and symptoms typically don't occur until high blood pressure has reached an advanced stage.

How is Hypertension Diagnosed by Conventional Western Medicine?

The only way to find out if a person has high blood pressure is to have his or her blood pressure measured. Both numbers in a blood pressure reading are important. A single high blood pressure reading usually isn't enough for a diagnosis. Diagnosis is based on more than one reading taken on more than one occasion. If any type of high blood pressure exists, routine tests, such as a urine test (urinalysis), blood tests and an electrocardiogram (ECG) may be recommended. More extensive testing isn't usually needed.

How is Hypertension Treated by Conventional Western Medicine?

Usually, the goal is to keep the blood pressure below 140/90 mmHg (130/80 mmHg for people with diabetes or chronic kidney disease).

Change to healthier habits, such as DASH (Dietary Approaches to Stop Hypertension) Eating Plan, losing excess weight and staying at a healthy weight, being physically active, quitting smoking and limiting alcohol intake, is the primary treatment. In addition, medication may be recommended to lower the blood pressure. Below are the types of medicine used to treat high blood pressure:

- Diuretics
- Beta blockers
- Angiotensin converting enzyme (ACE) inhibitors
- Angiotensin II receptor blockers (ARBs)

- Calcium channel blockers (CCBs)
- Alpha blockers
- Alpha-beta blockers
- Nervous system inhibitors
- Vasodilators

What Causes Hypertension According to Traditional Chinese Medicine?

1) Imbalanced Emotional Activity
2) Improper Food and Drink
3) Chronic Diseases and Overstrain
4) Weak Constitution

How is Hypertension Differentiated and Treated by Traditional Chinese Medicine?

1) <u>Hyperactivity of Liver Yang</u>

Symptoms: Dizziness, headache, dry mouth with bitter taste, flush complexion, conjunctival congestion, restlessness, irritability, constipation, dark urine, red tongue with thin and yellow coating, and taut, thready and forceful pulse.

Therapeutic Principle: To soothe liver and calm hyperactive yang.

Prescription: Modified Tian Ma Gou Teng Decoction.

Modifications: For pathogenic wind due to hyperactivity, add Cornu Saigae Tataricae powder (Ling Yang Jiao) 3g and Concha Margaritifera (Zheng Zhu Mu) 15g; for constipation, add Radix et Rhizoma Rhei (Da Huang) 6g and Natrii Sulfas (Mang Xiao) 10g; for insomnia, add Semen Ziziphi Spinosae (Suan Zao Ren) 15g and Radix Polygalae Tenuifoliae (Yuan Zhi) 10g.

2) <u>Internal Accumulation of Phlegm-Dampness</u>

Symptoms: Dizziness, headache, feeling of heaviness and tightness in the head, spleepiness, weakness, feeling of oppression in the chest, abdominal distention, poor appetite, dreamful sleep, vomiting, expectoration with abundant sputum, heaviness of extremities, chubby tongue with greasy coating, and soft and slippery pulse.

Therapeutic Principle: To resolve phlegm and clear turbidity.

Prescription: Modified Ban Xia Bai Zhu Tian Ma Decoction.

Modifications: For sensation of chest tightness, dyspnea, restlessness, vomiting, and red tongue with yellow and greasy coating, add Concretio Silicea Bambusae (Tian Zhu Huang) 5g and Rhizoma Coptidis (Huang Lian) 9g; for heaviness and numbness of the body, Rhizoma Arisaematis cum Bile (Dan Nan Xing) 5g and Bombyx Batryticatus (Jiang Can) 10g; for abdominal distention, poor appetite and diarrhea, add Fructus Amomi Villosi (Sha Ren) 5g, Herba Agastache seu Pogostemonis (Huo Xing) 9g and Massa Medicata Fermentata (Shen Qu) 10g.

3) Blood Stasis Blocking Collaterals

Symptoms: Lingering headache, which is localized; paroxysmal dizziness, numbness or paresthesias on one side of the body, feeling of oppression in the chest with occasional precordial chest pain, cyanosis of lips, purple tongue, and taut, thready and rough pulse.

Therapeutic Principle: To promote blood circulation and remove blood stasis.

Prescription: Modified Xue Fu Zhu Yu Decoction.

Modifications: For pronounced deficiency of qi, add Radix Astragali (Huang Qi) 12g and Rhizoma Dioscoreae (Shan Yao) 15g; for pronounced deficiency of yang, add Rhizoma Curculiginis Orchioidis (Xian Mao) 10g; for hyperactivity of fire due to deficiency of yin, add Carapax et Plastrum Testudinis (Gui Ban) 20g and Carapax Trionycis (Bie Jia) 20g.

4) Deficiency of Liver Yin and Kidney Yin

Symptoms: Dizziness, tinnitus, dry throat and eyes, feverish sensation in the chest, palms and soles, night sweating, insomnia, dreamful sleep, soreness and weakness of the lower back and knees, constipation, hot and dark urine, red tongue with little coating, and thready and rapid or thready and taut pulse.

Therapeutic Principle: To nourish the liver and the kidney, and soothe liver yang.

Prescription: Modified Qi Ju Di Huang Pill.

Modifications: For constipation, add Semen Cannabis Sativae (Huo Ma Ren) 12g.

5) Deficiency of Kidney Yang

Symptoms: Vertigo, headache, tinnitus, cold limbs, palpitation, shortness of breath, sore and weak loins and knees, seminal emission, impotence, nocturnal polyuria and frequent urination, diarrhea, pale and chubby tongue, and deep and weak pulse.

Therapeutic Principle: To warm and nourish kidney yang.

Prescription: Modified Ji Sheng Shen Qi Pill.

Modifications: For diarrhea, add Si Shen Pill; for oliguria and edema of lower extremities, add Semen Descurainiae seu Lepidii (Ting Li Zi) 10g.

What Kinds of Chinese Patent Drugs are Available to Treat Hypertension?

1) Song Ling Xue Mai Kang Pill: 4 pills each time, thrice daily.
2) Tian Ma Gou Teng Granule: 1 bag each time, thrice daily.

5. Atherosclerosis

Atherosclerosis is the hardening and narrowing of the arteries. It is caused by the slow buildup of plaque on the inside of walls of the arteries. Plaque is made up of fat, cholesterol, calcium, and other substances found in the blood. As it grows, the buildup of plaque narrows the inside of the artery and, in time, may restrict blood flow. Atherosclerosis can affect the arteries anywhere in the body and cause serious diseases and complications, such as coronary artery disease (CAD), cerebrovascular disease and peripheral arterial disease.

Diseases caused by atherosclerosis are the leading cause of illness and death in the United States

Atherosclerosis is a slow and complex disease that may start in childhood. Although the exact cause is unknown, researchers think that the buildup of plaque starts when the lining of the artery is damaged or injured. Risk factors that increase the risk of atherosclerosis include:

- High blood pressure
- High cholesterol
- Diabetes
- Obesity
- Smoking and using tobacco
- Age
- A family history of aneurysm or early heart disease
- Lack of physical activity

Atherosclerosis usually does not cause symptoms until it severely narrows or totally blocks an artery. The specific signs and symptoms depend on which arteries are affected.

- Affected coronary arteries cause symptoms of CAD
- Affected arteries that feed the brain cause symptoms of a stroke or a transient ischemic attack (TIA)
- Affected arteries in the legs, pelvis, or arms cause symptoms of peripheral arterial disease
- Affected arteries that feed the kidneys cause symptoms of renovascular hypertension

How is Atherosclerosis Diagnosed by Conventional Western Medicine?

Atherosclerosis is often diagnosed based on symptoms, complications, physical exams and tests, which include blood work, cholesterol levels, blood glucose level, ECG or EKG, chest x ray, ankle/brachial index, echocardiogram, CT scan, angiography, stress test, nuclear heart scanning, MRI and positron emission tomography (PET) scanning of the heart.

How is Atherosclerosis Treated by Conventional Western Medicine?

The goal of treatment is to reduce the symptoms and prevent the complications of atherosclerosis. Treatment can include: (1) lifestyle changes; (2) medicines to lower cholesterol and blood pressure, anticoagulants, and antiplatelet medicines such as aspirin; (3) special procedures and surgery, such as angioplasty, coronary artery bypass surgery, carotid artery surgery and bypass surgery of the leg arteries.

What Causes Atherosclerosis According to Traditional Chinese Medicine?

1) Improper Food and Drink
2) Internal Injury due to Seven Emotions
3) Overstrain and Overleisure
4) Deficiency of the Liver and the Kidney

How is Atherosclerosis Differentiated and Treated by Traditional Chinese Medicine?

1) <u>Internal Blockage of Turbid Phlegm</u>

Symptoms: Obesity, physical inactivity, sticky, greasy and insipid feeling in the mouth, pale tongue with white and thick or white and greasy coating, and deep and slow or slippery pulse.

Therapeutic Principle: To resolve phlegm and clear turbidity.

Prescription: Modified Dao Tan Decoction.

Modifications: For deficiency of the spleen and hyperactivity of phlegm with spiritlessness, fatigue, nausea, poor appetite and diarrhea, add fried Rhizoma Atractylodis Macrocephalae (Bai Zhu) 10g and Radix Codonopsitis Pilosulae (Dang Shen) 9g; for pronounced phlegm-heat with bitter taste in the mouth, and yellow and greasy tongue coating, add Caulis Bambusae in Taeniam (Zhu Ru) 10g; for constipation, add Radix et Rhizoma Rhei (Da Huang) 6g.

2) <u>Stagnation of Qi and Blood Stasis</u>

Symptoms: Irritable and restless temperament, distending and discomfort feeling in the chest and hypochondriac region, dizziness, dim tongue with ecchymosis and sublingual congested and tortuous veins, and taut or rough pulse.

Therapeutic Principle: To promote qi and blood circulation and remove blood stasis.

Prescription: Modified Xue Fu Zhu Yu Decoction.

Modifications: For pronounced distending pain in the chest and hypochondriac region, add Pericarpium Citri Reticulatae Viride (Qing Pi) 10g, Radix Curcumae (Yu Jin) 10g and Rhizoma Cyperi Rotundi (Xiang Fu) 10g; for vexation, and red tongue with yellow coating, Fructus Gardeniae Jasminoidis (Zhi Zi) 10g, Cortex Moutan Radicis (Mu Dan Pi) 10g and Fructus Meliae Toosendan (Chuan

Lian Zi) 10g; for lassitude, shortness of breath induced by exertion, sleepiness and indolence of speaking, sweating, pale and lusterless complexion, pale and dark tongue with ecchymosis, and thready and weak or rough pulse, add Bu Yang Huan Wu Decoction.

3) <u>Deficiency of the Liver and the Kidney</u>

Symptoms: Vertigo, headache, insomnia, amnesia, weak and sore loins and knees, baldness, loose teeth, deafness, tinnitus, retarded movements, spiritlessness, pale and dark tongue, and thready pulse.

Therapeutic Principle: To nourish the kidney and replenish essence.

Prescription: Modified Liu Wei Di Huang Pill.

Modifications: For feverish sensation in palms and soles, red tongue with little coating, use Zuo Gui Pill; for cold extremities and aversion to cold, use Jin Gui Shen Qi Pill or You Gui Pill.

What Kinds of Chinese Patent Drugs are Available to Treat Atherosclerosis?

1) Xue Zhi Kang Capsule: 2 capsules each time, twice daily.
2) Di Ao Xin Xue Kang Capsule: 1-2 capsule each time, thrice daily.
3) Yin Xing Ye Tablet: 2 tablets each time, thrice daily.
4) Jiao Gu Lan Zong Gan Tablet: 2-3 tablets each time, thrice daily.
5) Liu Wei Di Huang Pill: 4-6 pills each time, twice daily.

6. Coronary Atherosclerotic Heart Disease (Ischemic Heart Disease)

1) Angina Pectoris

Angina, also known as angina pectoris, is chest pain or discomfort that occurs when the heart muscle does not get enough blood. Angina may feel like pressure or a squeezing pain in the chest. The pain may also occur in the shoulders, arms, neck, jaw, or back. It may also feel like indigestion. Angina is caused by reduced blood flow to an area of the heart. This is most often due to coronary artery disease (CAD). Sometimes, other types of heart disease or uncontrolled high blood pressure can cause angina.

The three types of angina are stable, unstable, and variant (Prinzmetal's). Not all chest pain or discomfort is angina. Chest pain or discomfort can be caused by a heart attack, lung problems, heartburn, or a panic attack. However, all chest pain should be checked by a doctor. Stable angina is induced by physical exertion, emotional stress, heavy meals, smoking and exposure to very hot or cold temperature. Unstable angina is caused by blood clots that partially or totally block an artery. Variant angina is caused by a spasm in a coronary artery due to CAD, exposure to cold, emotional stress, medications (vasoconstricting), cigarette smoking and cocaine use.

More than 6 million people in the United States have angina. Pain and discomfort are the main symptoms of angina. These symptoms

- Are often described as pressure, squeezing, burning, or tightness in the chest
- Usually start in the chest behind the breastbone
- May also occur in the arms, shoulders, neck, jaw, throat, or back
- May feel like indigestion

Symptoms such as nausea, fatigue, shortness of breath, sweating, light-headedness, or weakness may also occur. Symptoms vary based on the type of angina.

How is Angina Diagnosed by Conventional Western Medicine?

Diagnosis of angina is made based on family or medical history, symptoms, physical examination and tests, which include ECG or EKG, stress test, chest x ray, nuclear heart scan, echocardiogram, cardiac catheterization, coronary angiography, a fasting lipoprotein profile and C-reactive protein (CRP) test.

How is Angina Treated by Conventional Western Medicine?

The main goals of treatment are to reduce the frequency and severity of symptoms, and prevent or lower the risk of heart attack and death. Treatment for angina includes lifestyle changes, medicine, special procedures, and cardiac rehabilitation. Lifestyle changes and medicine may be the only treatments needed if symptoms are mild and are not getting worse. Unstable angina is an emergency condition that requires treatment in the hospital.

Nitrates are the most commonly used medicines to treat angina. Other medicines that can be used to treat angina include beta blockers, calcium channel blockers and ACE inhibitors, medicines to lower cholesterol levels and high blood pressure, oral antiplatelet medicines, glycoprotein IIb-IIIa inhibitors and anticoagulants. When medicines and other treatments do not control angina, special (invasive) procedures may be needed. Two commonly used procedures are angioplasty and coronary artery bypass surgery.

What Causes Angina According to Traditional Chinese Medicine?

(1) Attack by Cold Pathogen

(2) Improper Food and Drink

(3) Imbalanced Emotional Activity

(4) Old Age and Physical Weakness

How is Angina Differentiated and Treated by Traditional Chinese Medicine?

(1) <u>Blood Stasis Blocking the Heart</u>

Symptoms: Localized stabbing chest pain aggravated at night or aggravated by temper, recurrent feeling of oppression in the chest, dark and purplish tongue with ecchymosis or sublingual congested and tortuous veins, and taut and rough or knot and intermittent pulse.

Therapeutic Principle: To promote blood circulation, remove blood stasis, dredge collaterals and relieve pain.

Prescription: Modified Xue Fu Zhu Yu Decoction.

Modifications: For severe chest pain, add Gummi Olibanum (Ru Xiang) 10g, Myrrha (Mo Yao) 10g, Radix Salviae Miltiorrhizae (Dan Shen) 10g and Radix Curcumae (Yu Jin) 10g; for feeling of oppression in the chest induced or aggravated by temper, add Rhizoma Cyperi Rotundi (Xiang Fu) 10g, Rhizoma Corydalis (Yan Hu Suo) 10g and Lignum Santali Albi (Tan Xiang) 2g; for white and greasy tongue coating, add Di Tan Decoction; for cold limbs, add Radix Aconiti Lateralis Praeparatae (Fu Zi) 10g, Ramulus Cinnamomi Cassiae (Gui Zhi) 10g, Rhizoma Alpiniae Officinarum (Gao Liang Jiang) 10g and Bulbus Allii Macrostemonis (Xie Bai) 10g; for shortness of breath, fatigue and spontaneous sweating, add Radix Ginseng (Ren Shen) 6g and Radix Astragali (Huang Qi) 12g.

(2) Turbid Phlegm Obstructing the Interior

Symptoms: Suffocative sensation and pain in the chest, chest pain radiating toward the shoulder and back, shortness of breath, abundant sputum, general heavy sensation, obesity, poor appetite, nausea, turbid and greasy tongue coating, and slippery pulse.

Therapeutic Principle: To activate yang, purge turbidity, eliminate phlegm and relieve stagnation.

Prescription: Gua Lou Xie Bai Ban Xia Decoction and Di Tan Decoction.

Modifications: For red tongue with yellow and greasy coating, and slippery and rapid pulse, remove Bulbus Allii Macrostemonis and add Rhizoma Coptidis (Huang Lian) 10g and Concretio Silicea Bambusae (Tian Zhu Huang) 5g; for dark and purple tongue with white and greasy coating, add Semen Pruni Persicae (Tao Ren) 10g, Flos Carthami Tinctorii (Hong Hua) 10g, Radix Salviae Miltiorrhizae (Dan Shen) 10g and Radix Notoginseng (San Qi) 9g; for fatigue and formless stool, add Radix Codonopsitis Pilosulae (Dang Shen) 9g, Rhizoma Atractylodis Macrocephalae (Bai Zhu) 10g and Semen Coicis (Yi Yi Ren) 20g.

(3) Stagnation of Yin Cold

Symptoms: Sudden stabbing chest pain radiating to the back, which is induced and aggravated by cold; cold limbs, spontaneous sweating of cold sweat, palpitation, shortness of breath, pale and red tongue with white coating, and deep and thready or deep and tense pulse.

Therapeutic Principle: To activate yang with pungent-warm herbs, remove obstruction and expel cold.

Prescription: Modified Zhi Shi Xie Bai Gui Zhi Decoction and Dang Gui Si Ni Decoction.

Modifications: For chest pain radiating to the back, chest stabbing pain, cold limbs, dyspnea and inability to lay flat, use Wu Tou Chi Shi Zhi Pill (change to decoction) and Su He Pill.

(4) <u>Deficiency of Qi and Blood Stasis</u>

Symptoms: Vague and tidal chest pain induced by overstrain, spiritlessness, lassitude, shortness of breath, indolence of speaking, palpitation, spontaneous sweating, dark, pale and chubby tongue with teeth marks, white and thin tongue coating, and slow, weak and forceless or knot and intermittent pulse.

Therapeutic Principle: To replenish qi, promote blood circulation, dredge collaterals and relieve pain.

Prescription: Modified Bu Yang Huan Wu Decoction.

Modifications: For severe chest pain, add Shi Xiao Powder; for abdominal distention and diarrhea, add Rhizoma Atractylodis Macrocephalae (Bai Zhu) 10g, Sclerotium Poriae Cocos (Fu Ling) 12g and Rhizoma Dioscoreae (Shan Yao) 20g; for aversion to cold and cold extremities, add Ramulus Cinnamomi Cassiae (Gui Zhi) 10g and Herba Epimedii (Yin Yang Huo) 12g; for turbid phlegm, add Fructus Trichosanthis (Gua Lou) 15g, Rhizoma Pinelliae Ternatae (Ban Xia) 10g and Rhizoma Acori Tatarinowii (Shi Chang Pu) 10g.

(5) <u>Deficiency of Qi and Yin</u>

Symptoms: Feeling of oppression in the chest, paroxysmal dull pain in the chest that is aggravated by exertion, palpitation, shortness of breath, lassitude, indolence of speaking, vertigo, vexation and dreamful sleep, or feverish sensation in palms and soles, red tongue with little coating, and thready, weak and forceless or knot and intermittent pulse.

Therapeutic Principle: To replenish qi, nourish yin, promote blood circulation and activate collaterals.

Prescription: Modified Sheng Mai Powder and Zhi Gan Cao Decoction.

Modifications: For blood stasis with severe chest pain, add Dan Shen Decoction; for phlegm-heat, add Wen Dan Decoction; for pale and lusterless complexion, pale lips and tongue, add Radix Angelicae Sinensis (Dang Gui) 10g, Radix Paeoniae Alba (Bai Shao Yao) 10g, Gelatinum Corii Asini (E Jiao) 10g and Arillus Longanae Euphoriae (Long Yan Rou) 12g; for deficiency of the heart and the spleen with poor appetite and insomnia, use Sheng Mai Powder and Gui Pi Decoction; for severe palpitation and insomnia, add Mastodi Ossis Fossilia (Long Gu) 20g, Concha Ostreae (Mu Li) 20g, Semen Ziziphi Spinosae (Suan Zao Ren) 15g and Caulis Polygoni Multiflori (Ye Jiao Teng) 20g.

(6) <u>Deficiency of Heart Yin and Kidney Yin</u>

Symptoms: Feeling of oppression or burning pain in the chest, palpitation, night sweating, restlessness, insomnia, sore and weak loins and knees, dizziness, tinnitus, red tongue with little coating, and deep, thready and rapid pulse.

Therapeutic Principle: To replenish yin, tonify the kidney, nourish the heart and tranquilize the mind.

Prescription: Modified Zuo Gui Pill.

Modifications: For palpitation, restlessness and insomnia, add Radix Ophiopogonis Japonici (Mai Dong) 12g, Fructus Schisandrae Chinensis (Wu Wei Zi) 5g, Semen Ziziphi Spinosae (Suan Zao Ren) 15g and Caulis Polygoni Multiflori (Ye Jiao Teng) 20g; for feeling of oppression in the chest and chest pain, add Radix Angelicae Sinensis (Dang Gui) 10g, Radix Salviae Miltiorrhizae (Dan Shen) 10g and Radix Curcumae (Yu Jin) 10g; for vertigo, numbness of tongue and extremities, and hot sensation of face, add Radix Polygoni Multiflori (He Shou Wu) 15g, Ramulus Uncariae cum Uncis (Gou Teng) 12g, Concha Haliotidis (Shi Jue Ming) 20g, Concha Ostreae (Mu Li) 20g and Carapax Trionycis (Bie Jia) 20g.

(7) <u>Deficiency of Heart Yang and Kidney Yang</u>

Symptoms: Palpitation, feeling of oppression in the chest, shortness of breath, chest pain radiating to the back, sweating, aversion to cold, cold limbs, edema of lower extremities, lumbago, pale complexion, pale or purple lips and nails, white and pale or dark and purple tongue, and deep and thready or deep, tinny and extremely faint pulse.

Therapeutic Principle: To replenish qi, activate yang, warm collaterals and relieve pain.

Prescription: Modified Shen Fu Decoction and You Gui Pill.

Modifications: For blood stasis, add Radix Salviae Miltiorrhizae (Dan Shen) 10g, Radix Curcumae (Yu Jin) 10g and Radix Notoginseng (San Qi) 10g; for cold stagnation, add Bulbus Allii Macrostemonis (Xie Bai) 10g, Ramulus Cinnamomi Cassiae (Gui Zhi) 10g and Herba cum Radice Asari (Xi Xin) 3g or add Su He Xiang Pill; for edema and oliguria, add Sclerotium Poriae Cocos (Fu Ling) 12g and Sclerotium Polypori Umbellati (Zhu Ling) 10g; for severe yang deficiency of the heart and the kidney, use Zhen Wu Decoction supplemented with Ramulus Cinnamomi Cassiae (Gui Zhi) 10g, Radix Stephaniae Tetrandrae (Fang Ji) 10g, Semen Descurainiae seu Lepidii (Ting Li Zi) 10g and Semen Plantaginis (Che Qian Zi) 9g; for chest pain radiating to the back, extremely cold extremities, purple lips, and tinny and extremely faint pulse, increase the dosage of Radix Ginseng Rubra and Radix Aconiti Lateralis Praeparatae, and add Mastodi Ossis Fossilia (Long Gu) 25g and Concha Ostreae (Mu Li) 25g.

What Kinds of Chinese Patent Drugs are Available to Treat Angina?

(1) Su Xiao Jiu Xin Pill: 4-6 pills each time, thrice daily. For acute onset, 10-15 pills each time.

(2) Guan Xin Su He Pill: 1 pill each time, 1-3 times daily.

(3) Tong Xin Luo Capsule: 2-4 capsules each time, thrice daily.

(4) Fu Fang Dan Shen Di Pill: 10 pills each time, thrice daily.

(5) She Xiang Bao Xin Pill: 1-2 pills each time, thrice daily.

(6) Xue Se Tong Injection: 200-400ml each time, once daily.

(7) Jing Zhi Guan Xin Granule (Guan Xin #2): 1 bag each time, thrice daily.

2) Myocardial Infarction (Heart Attack)

A heart attack occurs when the supply of blood and oxygen to an area of heart muscle is blocked, usually by a clot in a coronary artery. If treatment is not started quickly, the affected area of heart muscle begins to die. This injury to the heart muscle can lead to serious complications, and can even be fatal. Sudden death from heart attack is most often due to an arrhythmia (irregular heartbeat or rhythm) called ventricular fibrillation. If a person survives a heart attack, the injured area of the heart muscle is replaced by scar tissue. This weakens the pumping action of the heart and can lead to heart failure and other complications.

A heart attack is a life-threatening event. Each year, more than a million persons in the United States have a heart attack, and about half (515,000) of them die. About one-half of those who die do so within 1 hour of the start of symptoms and before reaching the hospital. Both men and women have heart attacks.

Most heart attacks are caused by a blood clot that blocks one of the coronary arteries. Coronary artery disease (CAD) is the most common underlying cause of a heart attack. A less common cause of heart attacks is a severe spasm of the coronary artery due to certain drugs (such as cocaine), emotional stress, exposure to cold and cigarette smoking. Risk factors of heart attack include:

- Age
- A family history of early heart disease
- A personal history of CAD: angina or chest pain, a previous heart attack and a surgical procedure (angioplasty, heart bypass)
- Smoking

- High blood pressure
- High blood cholesterol
- Overweight and obesity
- Being physically inactive
- Diabetes

    The warning signs and symptoms of a heart attack can include:

- Pressure, fullness or a squeezing pain in the center of the chest that lasts for more than a few minutes
- Pain extending beyond the chest to the shoulder, arm, back, or even to the teeth and jaw
- Increasing episodes of chest pain
- Prolonged pain in the upper abdomen
- Shortness of breath
- Sweating
- Impending sense of doom
- Lightheadedness or dizziness
- Fainting
- Nausea and vomiting
- Signs and symptoms vary from person to person. Some people have no symptoms ("silent" heart attack). The symptoms of angina can be similar to the symptoms of a heart attack.

How is Heart Attack Diagnosed by Conventional Western Medicine?

Diagnosis is made based on symptoms, medical and family history, and test results. Initial tests will be quickly followed by treatment if a person is having a heart attack. Tests used include: ECG or EKG, blood tests (troponin test, CK or CK-MB test and myoglobin test), nuclear heart scan, cardiac catheterization and coronary angiography.

How is Heart Attack Treated by Conventional Western Medicine?

A heart attack is a medical emergency. Delaying treatment can mean lasting damage to the heart or even death. The sooner treatment begins, the better the chances of recovering. Once heart attack is diagnosed, blood flow should be quickly restored to the heart by using thrombolytic drugs (clot busters), angioplasty and coronary artery bypass surgery, and the vital signs should be continuously monitored to detect and treat complications by ECG or EKG, a blood pressure monitor and pulse oximetry.

Several kinds of medicines can be used in treating heart attacks:

- Beta blockers
- Angiotensin-converting enzyme (ACE) inhibitors
- Nitrates, such as nitroglycerin
- Anticoagulants
- Antiplatelet medicines (such as aspirin and clopidigrel)
- Glycoprotein IIb-IIIa inhibitors
- Other medicines may be given to relieve pain and anxiety.
- Some medicines treat arrhythmias
- Oxygen therapy also may be given in the hospital.

What Causes Heart Attack According to Traditional Chinese Medicine?

(1) Inward Attack of Exogenous Pathogenic Cold

(2) Improper Diet

(3) Emotional Disharmony

(4) Aging and Debility

How is Heart Attack Differentiated and Treated by Traditional Chinese Medicine?

(1) Qi Stagnation and Blood Stasis

Symptoms: Severe chest pain, feeling of oppression in the chest, shortness of breath, restlessness, irritability, palpitation, abdominal distention, dark and bluish lips and nails, dark and purplish tongue with ecchymosis, and deep, taut and rough or knot and intermittent pulse.

Therapeutic Principle: To promote blood circulation, remove blood stasis, activate collaterals and relieve pain.

Prescription: Modified Xue Fu Zhu Yu Decoction.

Modifications: For severe chest pain, add Lignum Dalbergiae Odoriferae (Jiang Xiang) 5g, Radix Curcumae (Yu Jin) 10g and Rhizoma Corydalis (Yan Hu Suo) 10g.

(2) Accumulation of Pathogenic Cold in the Heart Vessel

Symptoms: Stabbing chest pain radiating to the back, oppressive and suffocative sensation in the chest, cold limbs, aversion to cold, spontaneous sweating of cold sweat, palpitation, shortness of breath, dark and purplish tongue with white and thin coating, and deep and thready or deep and tense pulse.

Therapeutic Principle: To dispel cold, remove obstruction, warm and activate yang with aromatic herbs.

Prescription: Modified Dang Gui Si Ni Decoction and Su He Xiang Pill.

Modifications: For persistent onset and cold limbs, use Wu Tou Chi Shi Zhi Pill; for severe blood stasis, add Rhizoma Ligustici Chuanxiong (Chuan Xiong) 10g, Radix Notoginseng (San Qi) 10g, Flos Carthami Tinctorii (Hong Hua) 10g and Radix Salviae Miltiorrhizae (Dan Shen) 10g.

(3) <u>Stagnation of Phlegm and Blood Stasis</u>

Symptoms: Severe stabbing chest pain, suffocative sensation in the chest, shortness of breath, abundant sputum, palpitation, abdominal distention, anorexia, nausea, vomiting, turbid and greasy tongue coating, and slippery pulse.

Therapeutic Principle: To resolve phlegm, promote blood circulation, regulate qi and relieve pain.

Prescription: Modified Gua Lou Xie Bai Ban Xia Decoction and Tao Hong Si Wu Decoction.

Modifications: For vexation, thirst, constipation, yellow and greasy tongue coating, and slippery and rapid pulse, add Radix Scutellariae Baicalensis (Huang Qin) 10g, Caulis Bambusae in Taeniam (Zhu Ru) 10g, Rhizoma Arisaematis cum Bile (Dan Nan Xing) 3g and Radix et Rhizoma Rhei (Da Huang) 6g; for nausea, vomiting and frequent hiccup, add Rhizoma Zingiberis Recens (Sheng Jiang) 10g, Rhizoma Pinelliae Ternatae (Ban Xia) 10g, Flos Inulae (Xuan Fu Hua) 10g and Cortex Magnoliae Officinalis (Hou Po) 10g; for aversion to cold, cold limbs and abdominal distention, add Rhizoma Zingiberis Recens (Sheng Jiang) 10g, Radix Aconiti Lateralis Praeparatae (Fu Zi) 10g and Radix Aucklandiae Lappae (Mu Xiang) 10g.

(4) <u>Deficiency of Qi and Blood Stasis</u>

Symptoms: Oppressive sensation in the chest, chest pain worsened by exertion, spiritlessness, lassitude, shortness of breath, indolence of speaking, palpitation, spontaneous sweating, dark, pale and bulgy tongue with teeth marks, white and thin tongue coating, and thready, weak and forceless or knot and intermittent pulse.

Therapeutic Principle: To replenish qi, promote blood circulation, remove stagnation and relieve pain.

Prescription: Modified Bu Yang Huan Wu Decoction.

Modifications: For severe chest pain, add Pollen Typhae (Pu Huang) 10g, Excrementum Trogopteri seu Pteromydis (Wu Ling Zhi) 10g and Radix Notoginseng (San Qi) 10g; for feeling of oppression in the chest, anorexia and greasy tongue coating, add Pericarpium Citri Reticulatae (Chen Pi) 6g, Rhizoma Pinelliae Ternatae (Ban Xia) 10g, Rhizoma Atractylodis Macrocephalae (Bai Zhu) 10g and Sclerotium Poriae Cocos (Fu Ling) 12g; for abdominal distention and constipation, add Radix et Rhizoma Rhei (Da Huang) 6g and Cortex Magnoliae Officinalis (Hou Po) 10g; for pronounced lassitude, poor appetite and diarrhea, add Radix Codonopsitis Pilosulae (Dang Shen) 9g, Rhizoma Atractylodis Macrocephalae (Bai Zhu) 10g, Sclerotium Poriae Cocos (Fu Ling) 12g and Fructus Amomi Villosi (Sha Ren) 5g.

(5) <u>Deficiency of Qi and Yin</u>

Symptoms: Feeling of oppression in the chest, chest pain, palpitation, shortness of breath, fatigue, restlessness, insomnia, spontaneous sweating, night sweating, dry mouth, tinnitus, sore and weak loins and knees, red tongue with little or peeled coating, and thready and rapid or knot and intermittent pulse.

Therapeutic Principle: To replenish qi, nourish yin, activate collaterals and relieve pain.

Prescription: Modified Sheng Mai Powder and Zuo Gui Decoction.

Modifications: For stabbing chest pain, add Radix Notoginseng (San Qi) 10g, Flos Carthami Tinctorii (Hong Hua) 10g, Radix Salviae Miltiorrhizae (Dan Shen) 10g and Semen Pruni Persicae (Tao Ren) 10g; for pronounced vexation and thirst, add Rhizoma Coptidis (Huang Lian) 10g and Rhizoma Anemarrhenae (Zhi Mu) 10g; for constipation, add Radix Scrophulariae Ningpoensis (Xuan Shen) 12g, Semen Cannabis Sativae (Huo Ma Ren) 12g, Radix Rehmanniae (Di Huang) 15g and Radix et Rhizoma Rhei (Da Huang) 6g; for palpitation, irritability and insomnia, add Radix Glycyrrhizae Uralensis (Gan Cao) 6g, Semen Ziziphi Spinosae (Suan Zao Ren) 15g, Semen Biotae Orientalis (Bai Zi Ren) 15g, Mastodi Ossis Fossilia (Long Gu) 20g and Concha Ostreae (Mu Li) 20g.

(6) <u>Deficiency of Yang and Fluid Retention</u>

Symptoms: Chest pain, feeling of oppression in the chest, dyspnea, palpitation, shortness of breath, fatigue, aversion to cold, cold limbs, edema of lower back and limbs, pale complexion, pale or bluish lips and nails, pale and chubby or dark and purplish tongue with slippery coating, and deep and thready pulse.

Therapeutic Principle: To warm yang, induce diuresis, activate collaterals and relieve pain.

Prescription: Modified Zhen Wu Decoction and Ting Li Da Zao Xie Fei Decoction.

Modifications: For severe chest pain, add Hirudo seu Whitmania (Shui Zhi) 5g, Lumbricus (Di Long) 10g and Flos Carthami Tinctorii (Hong Hua) 10g; for concurrent cold stagnation, add Bulbus Allii Macrostemonis (Xie Bai) 10g, Ramulus Cinnamomi Cassiae (Gui Zhi) 10g and Herba cum Radice Asari (Xi Xin) 3g; for severe edema, add Semen Plantaginis (Che Qian Zi) 9g, Herba Lycopi Lucidi (Ze Lan) 12g, Rhizoma Alismatis Orientalis (Ze Xie) 10g and Herba Leonuri Heterophylii (Yi

Mu Cao) 12g; for dyspnea, cough with sputum, add Semen Descurainiae seu Lepidii (Ting Li Zi) 10g and Cortex Mori Alba Radicis (Sang Bai Pi) 12g.

(7) <u>Prostration of Heart Yang</u>

Symptoms: Oppressive and suffocative sensation in the chest, frequent chest pain, extremely cold limbs, drenching sweat, pale complexion, cyanosis of lips, fingers and toes, restlessness, or delirium, or even syncope, purple tongue, and tinny and extremely faint pulse.

Therapeutic Principle: To restore yang from collapse and replenish qi

Prescription: Modified Shen Fu Long Mu Decoction.

Modifications: For concurrent yin prostration with irritability and sweating, add Radix Ophiopogonis Japonici (Mai Dong) 12g and Fructus Schisandrae Chinensis (Wu Wei Zi) 5g; for dark and purple lips, and thready and rough pulse, add Radix Salviae Miltiorrhizae (Dan Shen) 10g, Radix Notoginseng (San Qi) 10g and Ramulus Cinnamomi Cassiae (Gui Zhi) 10g.

What Kinds of Chinese Patent Drugs are Available to Treat Heart Attack?

(1) Su Xiao Jiu Xin Pill: 4-6 pills each time, thrice daily. For acute onset, 10-15 pills each time.
(2) Guan Xin Su He Pill: 1 pill each time, 1-3 times daily.
(3) Fu Fang Dan Shen Di Pill: 10 pills each time, thrice daily.
(4) Tong Xin Luo Capsule: 2-3 capsules each time, thrice daily.
(5) Xue Se Tong Injection: 200-400ml each time, once daily.
(6) Sheng Mai Injection: 20-60ml each time, once daily.
(7) Shen Fu Injection: 20-100ml each time, once daily.
(8) Shen Mai Injection: 10-60ml each time, once daily.

7. Rheumatic Valvular Heart Disease

Rheumatic heart disease results from single or repeated attacks of rheumatic fever that produce rigidity and deformity of valve cusps, fusion of the chordae tendinease. However, a history of rheumatic fever is obtainable in only 60% of patients with rheumatic heart disease. The heart valve is damaged by a disease process that generally begins with a strep throat caused by Streptococcus, and may eventually cause rheumatic fever.

During a first rheumatic fever attack, about half of people develop heart inflammation. Most people with rheumatic fever recover fully after six weeks. In some cases, however, one or more of the heart's valves may be scarred, resulting in stenosis or insufficiency (the two often coexist). A scarred heart valve may prevent adequate blood flow or not seal tightly, eventually causing congestive heart failure. If there's serious impairment to the function of affected heart valves, surgery may be needed to repair or replace the damaged valve or valves.

The most common symptoms of rheumatic fever may include:

- Joint inflammation
- Small nodules or hard, round bumps under the skin
- A change in neuromuscular movements
- Rash (a pink rash with odd edges that is usually seen on the trunk of the body or arms and legs)
- Fever
- Weight loss
- Fatigue
- Stomach pains

The first clue to rheumatic valvular disease is a murmur.

How is Rheumatic Heart Disease Diagnosed by Conventional Western Medicine?

Physical examination permits accurate diagnosis of most valve lesions. Echocardiography will reveal the condition of damaged valves, estimate the magnitude of regurgitation, and demonstrate the earliest stages of specific chamber enlargement.

How is Rheumatic Heart Disease Treated by Conventional Western Medicine?

The best treatment for rheumatic heart disease is prevention. Antibiotic therapy has sharply reduced the incidence and mortality rate of rheumatic fever and rheumatic heart disease. If inflammation of the heart has developed, bed rest may be needed. Medications are given to reduce the inflammation, as well as antibiotics to treat the Streptococcus infection. Other medications may be necessary to handle congestive heart failure.

With mitral valve disease, it is important to identify the onset of atrial fibrillation in order to institute anticoagulation. If heart valve damage occurs, surgical repair or replacement of the valve may be considered.

What Causes Rheumatic Heart Disease According to Traditional Chinese Medicine?

1) Weak Constitution and Deficiency of Anti-Pathogenic Qi
2) Attack by Exogenous Pathogenic Factors
3) Blood Stasis Blocking the Heart
4) Qi Deficiency of the Heart and the Lung
5) Deficiency of Yang and Fluid Retention

How is Rheumatic Heart Disease Differentiated and Treated by Traditional Chinese Medicine?

1) <u>Deficiency of Both Qi and Yin</u>

Symptoms: Palpitation, shortness of breath, lassitude, vertigo, pale and lusterless complexion, sweating on exertion, spontaneous sweating or night sweating, insomnia, dreamful sleep, dry mouth, red tongue with white and thin coating, and thready, rapid and forceless or hesitant, knot and intermittent pulse.

Therapeutic Principle: To replenish qi, nourish yin, tranquilize the heart and promote blood circulation.

Prescription: Modified Zhi Gan Cao Decoction.

Modifications: For palpitation and sweating, remove Ramulus Cinnamomi Cassiae and add Semen Biotae Orientalis (Bai Zi Ren) 15g, Mastodi Ossis Fossilia (Long Gu) 20g and Concha Ostreae (Mu Li) 20g; for insomnia and dreamful sleep, add Caulis Polygoni Multiflori (Ye Jiao Teng) 20g and Semen Ziziphi Spinosae (Suan Zao Ren) 15g; for oliguria and edema, add Semen Descurainiae seu Lepidii (Ting Li Zi) 10g, Sclerotium Poriae Cocos (Fu Ling) 12g and Rhizoma Alismatis Orientalis (Ze Xie) 10g.

2) <u>Deficiency of Qi and Blood Stasis</u>

Symptoms: Palpitation, shortness of breath, lusterless complexion, cyanosis of lips, jugular venous distention, distending and oppressive feeling in the chest and hypochondriac region, lump in the hypochondriac region, or blood-tinged sputum, tongue with ecchymosis, and thready and rough or knot and intermittent pulse.

Therapeutic Principle: To replenish qi, nourish the heart, promote blood circulation and activate collaterals.

Prescription: Modified Du Shen Decoction and Tao Ren Hong Hua Decoction.

Modifications: For suffocative sensation in the chest, remove Radix Rehmanniae and add Lignum Aquilariae Resinatum (Chen Xiang) 1g and Lignum Dalbergiae Odoriferae (Jiang Xiang) 5g; for turbid phlegm with distending pain in the chest, turbid and greasy tongue coating, add Fructus Trichosanthis (Gua Lou) 15g, Bulbus Allii Macrostemonis (Xie Bai) 10g and Rhizoma Pinelliae Ternatae (Ban Xia) 10g; for hemoptysis, add Radix Notoginseng (San Qi) 10g.

3) <u>Yang Deficiency of the Heart and the Kidney</u>

Symptoms: Palpitation, dyspnea, inability to lie flat, edema of the face and extremities, or ascites, hydrothorax, abdominal distention, cold limbs, diarrhea, oliguria, pale and chubby tongue with thin and white coating, and deep, thready and forceless or knot and intermittent pulse.

Therapeutic Principle: To warm and nourish the heart and the kidney, to replenish qi and induce diuresis.

Prescription: Modified Shen Fu Decoction and Wu Ling Powder.

Modifications: To promote blood circulation and remove blood stasis, add Herba Leonuri Heterophylii (Yi Mu Cao) 12g, Semen Pruni Persicae (Tao Ren) 10g and Flos Carthami Tinctorii (Hong Hua) 10g; for dyspnea, sweating and inability to lie flat, add Radix Ophiopogonis Japonici (Mai Dong) 12g, Fructus Schisandrae Chinensis (Wu Wei Zi) 5g and Mastodi Ossis Fossilia (Long Gu) 20g.

4) Deficiency of Yang and Fluid Retention

Symptoms: Dyspnea, abundant sputum, cough with pink and frothy sputum, pale complexion, cyanosis of lips, sweating, cold limbs, restlessness, irritability, dark and red tongue with white and greasy coating, and thready and hesitant pulse.

Therapeutic Principle: To warm the kidney, activate yang, purge heat from the lung and induce diuresis.

Prescription: Modified Zhen Wu Decoction and Ting Li Da Zao Xie Fei Decoction.

Modifications: For abundant sputum, add Fructus Perillae (Su Zi) 10g and Rhizoma Pinelliae Ternatae (Ban Xia) 10g; for distending pain in the chest, add Radix Salviae Miltiorrhizae (Dan Shen) 10g and Lignum Dalbergiae Odoriferae (Jiang Xiang) 5g.

5) Prostration of Heart Yang

Symptoms: Palpitation, irritability, dyspnea, shortness of breath, inability to lie flat, persistent sweating, spiritlessness, cyanosis of lips and nails, extremely cold limbs, pale tongue with white coating, and thready, tinny and extremely faint pulse.

Therapeutic Principle: To replenish yang and restore yang from collapse.

Prescription: Shen Fu Decoction and Sheng Mai Powder.

Modifications: To tranquilize the mind, add Mastodi Ossis Fossilia (Long Gu) 20g and Concha Ostreae (Mu Li) 20g; to restore yang from collapse, use Shen Fu Injection, Shen Fu Qi Injection or Sheng Mai Injection.

What Kinds of Chinese Patent Drugs are Available to Treat Rheumatic Heart Disease?

1) Tong Xin Luo Capsule: 2-4 capsules each time, thrice daily.
2) Zhen Yuan Capsule: 2-3 capsules each time, thrice daily.

3) Xin Bao Pill: 2-6 pills each time, thrice daily.

4) Sheng Mai Injection: 20-60ml each time, once daily.

5) Shen Fu Injection: 20-40ml each time, once daily.

8. Infective Endocarditis

Endocarditis is an infection of the inner lining of heart chambers. Endocarditis occurs when pathogens enter bloodstream, travel to the heart and attach to abnormal heart valves or damaged heart tissue. Bacteria are the cause of most cases, but fungi, viruses or other microorganisms also may be responsible.

Endocarditis is rare in people with healthy hearts. Most people who develop endocarditis have a diseased or damaged heart valve, an artificial heart valve or other heart defects. Those at risk of endocarditis are those who have:

- Damaged or artificial heart valves
- Congenital heart defects
- A history of endocarditis
- Intravenous drug users
- People who are hospitalized with IV tubes

Signs and symptoms may include:

- Fever
- Chills
- Weakness
- Fatigue
- Aching joints and muscles
- Night sweats
- Shortness of breath
- Paleness
- Persistent cough
- Swelling in the feet, legs or abdomen
- Unexplained weight loss
- Hematuria
- A new heart murmur

- Tenderness in the spleen
- Osler's nodes (red, tender spots under the skin of the fingers)
- Petechiae
- Sublingual hemorrhages
- Janeway lesions (painless erythematous lesions of the palms or soles)
- Roth spots (exudative lesions in the retina)

How is Infective Endocarditis Diagnosed by Conventional Western Medicine?

Diagnosis may be made based on medical history, signs and symptoms, physical exam (such as murmur) and various tests, which include blood tests (such as blood cultures), echocardiogram, transesophageal echocardiogram, ECG or EKG and chest X-ray.

How is Infective Endocarditis Treated by Conventional Western Medicine?

High doses of intravenous antibiotics may be needed in the hospital. Patients may need to take antibiotics for up to six weeks to clear up the infection. Blood tests may help identify the type of microorganism that's infecting the heart. Sometimes surgery is needed to treat persistent infections or replace a damaged valve. Endocarditis prophylactic antibiotics are recommended for certain cardiac lesions and procedures.

What Causes Infective Endocarditis According to Traditional Chinese Medicine?

1) Deficiency of Anti-Pathogenic Qi
2) Surgical Injury
3) Invasion of Toxic-Heat

How is Infective Endocarditis Differentiated and Treated by Traditional Chinese Medicine?

1) <u>Exterior Attack by Wind-Heat</u>

Symptoms: Fever, slight aversion to cold and wind, headache, general aching, no sweating or little sweating, stuffy sensation in the chest, palpitation, sore throat, cough with yellow sputum, slight thirst, red tongue tip, thin and yellow coating, and floating and rapid pulse.

Therapeutic Principle: To dispel wind, relieve heat, resolve exterior syndrome with pungent and cold herbs.

Prescription: Modified Yin Qiao Powder.

Modifications: For severe fever, add Fructus Gardeniae Jasminoidis (Zhi Zi) 10g, Radix Scutellariae Baicalensis (Huang Qin) 10g, Gypsum Fibrosum (Shi Gao) 30g and Radix Isatidis seu Baphicacanthi (Ban Lan Gen) 12g; for palpitation and stuffy feeling in the chest, add Fructus Citri Aurantii (Zhi Ke) 10g and Fructus Trichosanthis (Gua Lou) 15g; for headache, add Folium Mori Alba (Sang Ye) 10g,

Flos Chrysanthemi Morifolii (Ju Hua) 12g and Radix Angelicae Dahuricae (Bai Zhi) 10g; for joint pain, add Rhizoma et Radix Notopterygii (Qiang Huo) 10g and Radix Angelicae Pubescentis (Du Huo) 10g.

2) <u>Flaming Heat Attacking Qi Division/Level (qi fen)</u>

Symptoms: Severe fever, restlessness, thirst, sweating that does not relieve fever, palpitation, dyspnea, distending pain in the chest, dark urine, red tongue with dry and yellow coating, and slippery and rapid or full pulse.

Therapeutic Principle: To relieve fever, induce moisture, purge fire and remove toxic substance.

Prescription: Modified Bai Hu Decoction and Wu Wei Xiao Du Decoction.

Modifications: For palpitation and dyspnea, add Radix Ginseng (Ren Shen) 9g; for distending pain in the chest, add Radix Salviae Miltiorrhizae (Dan Shen) 10g, Semen Pruni Persicae (Tao Ren) 10g and Rhizoma Corydalis (Yan Hu Suo) 10g; for constipation, add Radix et Rhizoma Rhei (Da Huang) 6g and Natrii Sulfas (Mang Xiao) 12g.

3) <u>Heat Invading the Nutritive Division/Level (ying fen) of the Heart</u>

Symptoms: Persistent fever worsened at night, thirst without a desire to drink a lot, palpitation, stuffy sensation in the chest, ecchymosis, restlessness, irritability, delirium in severe cases, crimson tongue with little dry and yellow coating, and thready and rapid pulse.

Therapeutic Principle: To clear away ying heat, remove toxic substance, cool blood and promote blood circulation.

Prescription: Modified Qing Ying Decoction and Xi Jiao Di Huang Decoction.

Modifications: For high fever and constipation, add Radix et Rhizoma Rhei (Da Huang) 6g; for qi deficiency of the heart, add Radix Ginseng (Ren Shen) 9g; for delirium, add An Gong Niu Huang Pill; for convulsions and spasm, add Zi Xue Pill; for ecchymosis, hematemesis and epistaxis, add Cacumen Biotae Orientalis (Ce Bai Ye) 12g, Herba Ecliptae Prostratae (Han Lian Cao) 20g and Nodus Nelumbinis Nuciferae Rhizomatis (Ou Jie) 12g.

4) <u>Hyperactivity of Fire due to Deficiency of Yin</u>

Symptoms: Persistent low-grade fever, afternoon or night hectic fever, restlessness, palpitation, insomnia, dreamful sleep, stuffy sensation in the chest, shortness of breath, spontaneous sweating, night sweating, feverish sensation in palms and soles, flushed cheeks, dry mouth and throat, red tongue with little moisture, little or smooth and peeled tongue coating, and thready and rapid pulse.

Therapeutic Principle: To nourish yin, clear away heat, cool blood and promote blood circulation.

Prescription: Modified Qing Hao Bie Jia Decoction.

Modifications: For dark tongue with ecchymosis, rough or knot and intermittent pulse, add Radix Paeoniae Rubra (Chi Shao) 10g, Radix Salviae Miltiorrhizae (Dan Shen) 10g and Radix Rubiae Cordifoliae (Qian Cao) 12g; for severe dry mouth, vexation, red tongue and flushed cheeks, add Radix Ophiopogonis Japonici (Mai Dong) 12g, Herba Dendrobii (Shi Hu) 10g, Fructus Ligustri Lucidi (Nu Zhen Zi) 12 and Herba Ecliptae Prostratae (Han Lian Cao) 20g; for lassitude and indolence of speaking, add Radix Astragali (Huang Qi) 12g and Radix Pseudostellariae Heterophyllae (Tai Zi Shen) 15g; for palpitation and insomnia, add Semen Ziziphi Spinosae (Suan Zao Ren) 15g and Caulis Polygoni Multiflori (Ye Jiao Teng) 20g; for spontaneous sweating and night sweating, add Concha Ostreae (Mu Li) 20g, Fructus Tritici Aestivi Levis (Fu Xiao Mai) 20g and Radix Oryzae Glutinosae (Nuo Dao Gen Xu) 20g.

5) <u>Deficiency of Qi and Yin, and Blood Stasis</u>

Symptoms: Low-grade fever, fatigue, feverish sensation in the chest, palms and soles, shortness of breath on exertion, spontaneous or night sweating, palpitation, insomnia, dreamful sleep, or general aching, or dark, purple or red skin, or hemiplegia, dark and purple tongue with ecchymosis, and thready and rough pulse.

Therapeutic Principle: To replenish qi, nourish yin, promote blood circulation and remove stagnation.

Prescription: Modified Sheng Mai Powder and Bu Yang Huan Wu Decoction.

Modifications: For lusterless complexion, pale lips and tongue, palpitation and insomnia, add Radix Polygoni Multiflori (He Shou Wu) 20g, Gelatinum Corii Asini (E Jiao) 9g and Arillus Longanae Euphoriae (Long Yan Rou) 12g; for palpitation, remarkable insomnia and dreamful sleep, add Semen Ziziphi Spinosae (Suan Zao Ren) 15g, Semen Biotae Orientalis (Bai Zi Ren) 15g and Concha Margaritiferae (Zhen Zhu Mu) 20g; for night sweating and spontaneous sweating, add Concha Ostreae (Mu Li) 20g and Fructus Tritici Aestivi Levis (Fu Xiao Mai) 20g; for poor appetite and diarrhea, add Radix Codonopsitis Pilosulae (Dang Shen) 9g and Rhizoma Atractylodis Macrocephalae (Bai Zhu) 10g.

What Kinds of Chinese Patent Drugs are Available to Treat Infective Endocarditis?

1) Zi Xue Powder: 1.5-3g each time, twice daily.
2) An Gong Niu Huang Pill: 1 pill each time, once daily.
3) Yu Xing Cao Injection: 50-100ml each time, once daily.
4) Qing Kai Ling Injection: 20-40ml each time, once daily.
5) Sheng Mai Injection: 20-60ml each time, once daily.

9. Cardiomyopathy

Cardiomyopathy refers to diseases of the heart muscle that becomes enlarged or abnormally thick or rigid. In rare cases, the muscle tissue in the heart is replaced with scar tissue. As cardiomyopathy progresses, it can lead to heart failure, arrhythmias, fluid buildup in the lungs or legs, other severe complications, and, more rarely, endocarditis. The four main types of cardiomyopathy are:

- Dilated cardiomyopathy
- Hypertrophic cardiomyopathy
- Restrictive cardiomyopathy
- Arrhythmogenic right ventricular dysplasia (ARVD)

Cardiomyopathy can have a specific cause. Some types of cardiomyopathy can be inherited. In many cases, the cause is unknown. Dilated cardiomyopathy can be inherited. It also can be caused by ischemic cardiomyopathy, myocarditis, alcohol (alcoholic cardiomyopathy), peripartum complications, certain toxins (such as cobalt), certain drugs (such as cocaine, amphetamines, doxorubicin and daunorubicin) and diseases such as diabetes and thyroid disease. Hypertrophic cardiomyopathy can be inherited. It also can develop over time because of high blood pressure or aging. Often, the cause of hypertrophic cardiomyopathy is unknown. Restrictive cardiomyopathy is caused by hemochromatosis, amyloidosis, sarcoidosis, and connective tissue disorders. Arrythmogenic right ventricular dysplasia is thought to be an inherited disease.

Cardiomyopathy can affect people of all ages. However, certain age groups are more likely to have certain types of cardiomyopathy.

Some people with cardiomyopathy never have symptoms, and others have no symptoms in the early stages of the disease. As cardiomyopathy progresses, signs and symptoms of heart failure usually appear. These signs and symptoms include:

- Tiredness
- Weakness
- Shortness of breath after exercise or even at rest
- Swelling of the abdomen, legs, ankles, and feet

Other signs and symptoms can include dizziness, lightheadedness, fainting during exercise, arrhythmias, and heart murmur.

How is Cardiomyopathy Diagnosed by Conventional Western Medicine?

The diagnosis is based on a person's symptoms, medical and family history, physical exam and results on diagnostic tests and procedures. Diagnostic tests and procedures include ECG or EKG, holter monitor, echocardiogram, transesophageal echocardiography (TEE), stress test, chest x ray, blood tests, cardiac catheterization, coronary angiography and myocardial biopsy.

How is Cardiomyopathy Treated by Conventional Western Medicine?

People who have no symptoms may not need treatment. In some cases, dilated cardiomyopathy that comes on suddenly may even go away on its own. For other people with cardiomyopathy, treatment is necessary. Specific treatments depend on the type of cardiomyopathy, how severe the symptoms and complications are, and the age and overall health of the person. The main goals of treating cardiomyopathy are to:

- Manage any conditions that cause or contribute to the cardiomyopathy
- Control symptoms so that the person can live as normally as possible
- Stop the disease from getting worse
- Reduce complications and the chance of sudden cardiac death

Treatments for cardiomyopathy may include medicines, surgery, nonsurgical procedures, and lifestyle changes. Medicines include diuretics, angiotensin-converting enzyme (ACE) inhibitors, beta-blockers, calcium channel blockers, digoxin, anticoagulants, antiarrhythmia medicines, antibiotics and corticosteroids. Surgery includes septal myectomy, implanting devices and heart transplant

What Causes Cardiomyopathy According to Traditional Chinese Medicine?

1) Attack by Pathogenic Factors
2) Deficiency of Anti-Pathogenic Qi

How is Cardiomyopathy Differentiated and Treated by Traditional Chinese Medicine?

1) <u>Pathogenic Factors Attacking the Heart</u>

Symptoms: Fever, slight aversion to cold, sore throat, general aching, palpitation, distending pain in the chest, shortness of breath, fatigue, vexation, insomnia, red tongue tip, thin and yellow tongue coating, and floating and rapid or hesitant, knot and intermittent pulse.

Therapeutic Principle: To clear away heat, remove toxic substances and tranquilize the mind.

Prescription: Modified Yin Qiao Powder.

Modifications: For distending pain in the chest, add Gummi Olibanum (Ru Xiang) 10g, Myrrha (Mo Yao) 10g, Fructus Trichosanthis (Gua Lou) 15g, Radix Salviae Miltiorrhizae (Dan Shen) 10g and Semen Pruni Persicae (Tao Ren) 10g; for cough with sticky sputum, add Bulbus Fritillariae Thunbergii (Zhe Bei Mu) 10g and Concretio Silicea Bambusae (Tian Zhu Huang) 5g; for spiritlessness, shortness of breath, and red tongue with little coating, add Radix Astragali (Huang Qi) 12g, Radix Panacis Quinquefolii (Xi Yang Shen) 5g, Rhizoma Phragmitis Communis (Lu Gen) 20g and Radix Ophiopogonis Japonici (Mai Dong) 12g; for knot and intermittent pulse, add Radix Sophorae Flavescentis (Ku Shen) 6g, Radix Salviae Miltiorrhizae (Dan Shen) 10g, Radix Scrophulariae Ningpoensis (Xuan Shen) 10g and Radix Ginseng (Ren Shen) 6g.

2) <u>Deficiency of Qi and Blood Stasis</u>

Symptoms: Palpitation, shortness of breath, spiritlessness and fatigue on exertion, or spontaneous sweating, dreamful sleep, dim tongue with ecchymosis, and weak, rough or knot and intermittent pulse.

Therapeutic Principle: To replenish qi, nourish the heart, promote blood circulation and remove blood stasis.

Prescription: Modified Sheng Yu Decoction and Tao Hong Si Wu Decoction.

Modifications: For cough with sticky sputum, add Fructus Trichosanthis (Gua Lou) 15g, Bulbus Fritillariae Cirrhosae (Bei Mu) 10g, Rhizoma Pinelliae Ternatae (Ban Xia) 10g and Radix Asteris Tatarici (Zi Wan) 10g; for stuffy sensation in the chest, shortness of breath, and nocturnal paroxysmal dyspnea, add Semen Descurainiae seu Lepidii (Ting Li Zi) 10g, Herba Ephedrae (Ma Huang) 6g and Semen Armeniacae Amarum (Xing Ren) 10g; for oliguria and edema of lower extremities, remove Radix Rehmanniae and add Ramulus Cinnamomi Cassiae (Gui Zhi) 10g, Rhizoma Atractylodis Macrocephalae (Bai Zhu) 10g, Sclerotium Poriae Cocos (Fu Ling)12g, Rhizoma Alismatis Orientalis (Ze Xie) 10g, Sclerotium Polypori Umbellati (Zhu Ling) 10g and Herba Lycopi Lucidi (Ze Lan) 10g; for abundant sputum and stuffy sensation in the chest, add Fructus Trichosanthis (Gua Lou) 15g, Bulbus Allii Macrostemonis (Xie Bai) 10g and Rhizoma Pinelliae Ternatae (Ban Xia) 10g; for localized distending pain in the chest, add Gummi Olibanum (Ru Xing) 10g, Myrrha (Mo Yao) 10g, Lignum Aquilariae Resinatum (Chen Xiang) 1g and Radix Curcumae (Yu Jin) 10g or use Xue Fu Zhu Yu Decoction.

3) <u>Deficiency of Both Qi and Yin</u>

Symptoms: Postexertional palpitation and shortness of breath, lassitude, vertigo, flushed cheeks, spontaneous or night sweating, insomnia, dry mouth, red or pale and red tongue with white and thin coating, and thready, rapid and forceless or knot and intermittent pulse.

Therapeutic Principle: To replenish qi, nourish yin and tranquilize the mind.

Prescription: Modified Zhi Gan Cao Decoction and Tian Wang Bu Xin Pill.

Modifications: For pale complexion and severe sweating, add Radix Ginseng (Ren Shen) 6g and Radix Astragali (Huang Qi) 12g; for flushed complexion, red tongue with little coating, add Radix Rehmanniae Praeparatae (Shu Di Huang) 20g.

4) <u>Deficiency of Yang and Fluid Retention</u>

Symptoms: Palpitation, spontaneous sweating, cold limbs, spiritlessness, oliguria, edema of lower extremities, cough, dyspnea, inability to lie flat, cyanosis of lips and nails, pale and dark or purple and dark tongue with white and slippery coating, and deep and thready pulse.

Therapeutic Principle: To warm yang and induce diuresis.

Prescription: Modified Zhen Wu Decoction.

Modifications: For cyanosis of lips and tongue, add Radix Salviae Miltiorrhizae (Dan Shen) 10g, Radix Notoginseng (San Qi) 9g and Flos Carthami Tinctorii (Hong Hua) 10g; for abundant sputum and dyspnea, add Semen Descurainiae seu Lepidii (Ting Li Zi) 10g, Semen Pharbitidis (Qian Niu Zi) 10g and Fructus Zizyphi Jujubae (Da Zao) 20g.

5) <u>Prostration of Heart Yang</u>

Symptoms: Palpitation, dyspnea, shortness of breath, inability to lie flat, drenching sweat, spiritlessness, cyanosis of lips and nails, extremely cold limbs, pale tongue with white coating, and thready, tinny and extremely faint pulse.

Therapeutic Principle: To recuperate yang and restore yang from collapse.

Prescription: Modified Si Ni Decoction and Shen Fu Long Mu Decoction.

Modifications: This syndrome should be treated with the combination of decoction and intravenous injection with Shen Fu Injection (30-50ml each time, once daily) or Shen Fu Qi Injection (20-40ml each time, once daily).

What Kinds of Chinese Patent Drugs are Available to Treat Cardiomyopathy?

1) Yi Xin Shu Capsule: 4 capsules each time, thrice daily.
2) Shu Xin Oral Liquid: 1 little bottle each time, 2-3 times daily.
3) Huang Qi Sheng Mai Oral Liquid: 10ml each time, thrice daily.
4) Shen Fu Injection: 30-50ml each time, once daily.
5) Shen Fu Qi Injection: 20-40ml each time, once daily.

10. Viral Myocarditis

Myocarditis is an inflammation of the myocardium, the thick muscular layer of the heart wall. It can result in a variety of signs and symptoms, including vague chest pain, an abnormal heartbeat and congestive heart failure. Myocarditis may develop as a complication of an infectious disease, usually caused by a virus. Years ago, rheumatic fever was a common cause of myocarditis. But today there are usually other reasons for the condition. Most often it develops secondary to an underlying infection caused by viruses, bacteria, parasites and fungi. Myocarditis sometimes occurs when a person is exposed to certain chemicals (such as arsenic and hydrocarbons), medications that may cause an allergic or toxic reaction (such as penicillin, sulfonamide drugs, as well as cocaine) and systemic diseases.

Myocarditis can occur in people of all ages and is diagnosed more often in men than in women. Treatment of myocarditis depends on the underlying cause.

The signs and symptoms of myocarditis may vary, depending on the cause and the severity of the disease. The signs and symptoms may include:

- Vague chest pains
- A rapid or abnormal heartbeat (arrhythmia)
- Shortness of breath, particularly during physical activity
- Fluid retention, with swelling of the legs, ankles and feet
- Fatigue
- Fainting or a sudden loss of consciousness
- Other symptoms associated with a viral infection, such as a headache, body aches, joint pain, fever, a sore throat or diarrhea

Myocarditis can be accompanied by pericarditis, which may cause sharp pains over the center of the chest.

How is Myocarditis Diagnosed by Conventional Western Medicine?

Diagnosis is based on medical history, physical examination and one or more tests, including ECG or EKG, chest x ray, echocardiogram, blood tests and cardiac catheterization.

How is Myocarditis Treated by Conventional Western Medicine?

Treatment of myocarditis depends on the underlying cause and involves treating the underlying cause, arrhythmia and heart failure.

What Causes Viral Myocarditis According to Traditional Chinese Medicine?

1) Weak Constitution
2) Attack by Exogenous Seasonal Pathogenic Factors and Toxic-Heat
3) Internal Attack on the Stomach and Intestines by Heat-Dampness and Toxic-Heat

How is Viral Myocarditis Differentiated and Treated by Traditional Chinese Medicine?

1) <u>Toxic-Heat Disturbing the Heart</u>

Symptoms: Fever, slight aversion to cold, general aching, headache, nasal stuffiness, running nose, sore throat, thirst, dry mouth with bitter taste, dark urine, palpitation, shortness of breath, stuffy sensation in the chest or dull chest pain, red tongue with thin and yellow coating, and floating and rapid or knot and intermittent pulse.

Therapeutic Principle: To clear away heat, remove toxic substances and tranquilize the mind.

Prescription: Modified Yin Qiao Powder.

Modifications: For distending pain in the chest, add Gummi Olibanum (Ru Xiang) 10g, Myrrha (Mo Yao) 10g, Fructus Trichosanthis (Gua Lou) 15g, Radix Salviae Miltiorrhizae (Dan Shen) 10g and Semen Pruni Persicae (Tao Ren) 10g; for cough with sticky sputum, add Bulbus Fritillariae Thunbergii (Zhe Bei Mu) 10g and Concretio Silicea Bambusae (Tian Zhu Huang) 5g; for spiritlessness, shortness of breath, and red tongue with little coating, add Radix Astragali (Huang Qi) 12g, Radix Panacis Quinquefolii (Xi Yang Shen) 5g, Rhizoma Phragmitis Communis (Lu Gen) 20g and Radix Ophiopogonis Japonici (Mai Dong) 12g.

2) <u>Toxic-Dampness Attacking the Heart</u>

Symptoms: Fever, slight aversion to cold, nausea, vomiting, distending pain in the abdomen, diarrhea, lassitude, thirst, palpitation, stuffy sensation in the chest, or dull chest pain, red tongue with yellow and greasy coating, and soft and rapid or hesitant, knot and intermittent pulse.

Therapeutic Principle: To remove toxic substances, resolve dampness and tranquilize the mind.

Prescription: Modified Ge Gen Qin Lian Decoction and Gan Lu Xiao Du Powder.

Modifications: For severe vomiting, add Rhizoma Pinelliae Ternatae (Ban Xia) 10g, Caulis Bambusae in Taeniam (Zhu Ru) 10g and Folium Perillae Frutescentis (Su Ye) 10g; for severe abdominal pain, add Radix Aucklandiae Lappae (Mu Xiang) 10g, Radix Paeoniae Alba (Bai Shao Yao) 10g and Pericarpium Areca Catechu (Da Fu Pi) 10g.

3) <u>Deficiency of Heart Yin</u>

Symptoms: Palpitation, feeling of oppression in the chest, dry mouth, restlessness, insomnia, dreamful sleep, or low-grade fever and night sweating, feverish sensation in palms and soles, red tongue with little or no coating, and thready and rapid, or hesitant, knot and intermittent pulse.

Therapeutic Principle: To nourish yin, clear away heat and tranquilize the mind.

Prescription: Modified Tian Wang Bu Xin Pill.

Modifications: For low-grade fever, night sweating, and feverish sensation in palms and soles, add Radix Stellariae Dichotomae (Yin Chai Hu) 10g, Radix Cynanchi Atrati (Bai Wei) 10g and Cortex

Moutan Radicis (Mu Dan Pi) 10g; for vexation and insomnia, add Rhizoma Coptidis (Huang Lian) 9g and Caulis Polygoni Multiflori (Ye Jiao Teng) 20g; for turbid phlegm, add Bulbus Fritillariae Thunbergii (Zhe Bei Mu) 10g, Rhizoma Arisaematis cum Bile (Dan Nan Xing) 5g and Concretio Silicea Bambusae (Tian Zhu Huang) 5g.

4) <u>Deficiency of Both Qi and Yin</u>

Symptoms: Palpitation, distending pain in the chest, shortness of breath, fatigue, insomnia, dreamful sleep, spontaneous and night sweating, red tongue with little or thin coating, and thready, rapid and forceless or hesitant, knot and intermittent pulse.

Therapeutic Principle: To replenish qi, nourish yin and tranquilize the mind.

Prescription: Zhi Gan Cao Decoction and Sheng Mai Powder.

Modifications: For severe palpitation, add Mastodi Dentis Fossilia (Long Chi) 20g, Concha Ostreae (Mu Li) 20g, Concha Margaritiferae (Zhen Zhu Mu) 20g, Radix Polygalae Tenuifoliae (Yuan Zhi) 10g and Semen Ziziphi Spinosae (Suan Zao Ren) 15g; for severe deficiency of qi, add Radix Astragali (Huang Qi) 12g and Rhizoma Polygonati (Huang Jing) 12g; for chest pain, dark and purple tongue with ecchymosis, and knot and intermittent pulse, add Radix Salviae Miltiorrhizae (Dan Shen) 10g, Radix Paeoniae Rubra (Chi Shao) 10g, Hirudo seu Whitmania (Shui Zhi) 5g, Radix Curcumae (Yu Jin) 10g and Rhizoma Acori Tatarinowii (Shi Chang Pu) 10g.

5) <u>Deficiency of Both Yin and Yang</u>

Symptoms: Palpitation, shortness of breath, distending pain in the chest, dim and lusterless complexion, cyanosis of lips, cold limbs, aversion to cold, dyspnea and inability to lie flat in severe cases, cough with abundant sputum, insomnia, edema, diarrhea, pale and red tongue with white coating, and deep, thready and forceless or hesitant, knot and intermittent pulse.

Therapeutic Principle: To replenish qi, warm yang, nourish yin and activate collaterals.

Prescription: Modified Shen Fu Yang Rong Decoction.

Modifications: For severe edema, add Semen Plantaginis (Che Qian Zi) 10g, Sclerotium Poriae Cocos (Fu Ling) 12g and Sclerotium Polypori Umbellati (Zhu Ling) 10g; for dyspnea and inability to lie flat, add Semen Descurainiae seu Lepidii (Ting Li Zi) 10g and Fructus Perillae (Su Zi) 10g; for chest pain, dark and purple tongue, and knot and intermittent pulse, add Radix Salviae Miltiorrhizae (Dan Shen) 10g, Semen Pruni Persicae (Tao Ren) 10g, Hirudo seu Whitmania (Shui Zhi) 5g and Lumbricus (Di Long) 10g; for distending sensation in the chest and hypochondriac region, add Fructus Trichosanthis (Gua Lou) 15g and Bulbus Allii Macrostemonis (Xie Bai) 10g.

What Kinds of Chinese Patent Drugs are Available to Treat Viral Myocarditis?

1) Kong Bing Du Granule: 1-2 bags each time, 3-4 times daily.
2) Yu Ping Feng Granule: 1 bag each time, thrice daily.
3) Tian Wang Bu Xin Pill: 1 pill each time, twice daily.
4) Qing Kai Ling Injection: 20-40ml each time, once daily.
5) Sheng Mai Injection: 40-60ml each time, once daily.
6) Huang Qi Injection: 20-60ml each time, once daily.

11. Acute Pericarditis

Pericarditis is inflammation or infection of the pericardium, the thin sac-like membrane that surrounds the heart. There is a small amount of fluid between the inner and outer layers of the pericardium. When the pericardium becomes inflamed, the amount of fluid between its two layers increases, compressing the heart and interfering with the heart's ability to function properly. The causes of pericarditis are often hard to determine and they may include:

- Infection (viral, bacterial, fungal, parasitic)
- Heart attack or surgery
- Systemic inflammatory disorders, such as lupus and rheumatoid arthritis.
- Heart or chest trauma
- Other health disorders, such as kidney failure, AIDS, tuberculosis and cancer
- Certain medications, although this is unusual

Signs and symptoms often associated with pericarditis include:

- Chest pain. (1) Sharp, stabbing chest pain behind the breastbone or in the left side of the chest. The sharp pain may radiate to the left shoulder and neck. Lying down or inhaling deeply often intensifies the pain, and sitting up and leaning forward can often ease the pain. (2) Or dull, achy or pressure-like pain with varying intensity.
- Shortness of breath when reclining
- Low-grade fever
- Irritability
- An overall sense of weakness, fatigue or feeling sick
- Dry cough
- Abdominal or leg swelling
- Loss of appetite

- Irregular heartbeat
- Pericardial rub on physical exam

How is Pericarditis Diagnosed by Conventional Western Medicine?

Diagnosis is made based on a complete medical history, physical examination and tests, which may include blood tests, chest x-ray, echocardiography, CT scan and MRI.

How is Pericarditis Treated by Conventional Western Medicine?

The goal of treatment for pericarditis is to determine and eliminate the cause of the disease. Treatment may include: (1) rest and medications, such as analgesics and anti-inflammatory drugs; (2) pericardiocentesis to remove and drain the excess fluid; (3) pericardiectomy, a surgical procedure to remove the entire pericardium.

What Causes Acute Pericarditis According to Traditional Chinese Medicine?

1) Healthy Qi Deficiency
2) Infection of Contagious Toxicants
3) Attack by Pathogenic Factors
4) Up Attacking of Pericardium by Toxic Fluid due to Kidney Failure

How is Acute Pericarditis Differentiated and Treated by Traditional Chinese Medicine?

1) <u>Wind-Heat Attacking the Pericardium</u>

Symptoms: Fever, aversion to cold, thirst, dry throat, irritability, sweating, cough, palpitation, shortness of breath, distending pain in the chest, red tongue with thin and yellow coating, and floating and rapid or knot and intermittent pulse.

Therapeutic Principle: To dispel wind, clear away heat and release lung qi

Prescription: Modified Yin Qiao Powder.

Modifications: For severe toxic-heat, add Radix Scutellariae Baicalensis (Huang Qin) 10g, Folium Isatidis (Da Qing Ye) 15g and Radix Isatidis seu Baphicacanthi (Ban Lan Gen) 12g; for severe wind-heat, add Folium Mori Alba (Sang Ye) 10g and Flos Chrysanthemi Morifolii (Ju Hua) 12g; for severe dampness, add Rhizoma Alismatis Orientalis (Ze Xie) 10g and Semen Coicis (Yi Yi Ren) 15g; for severe phlegm-heat, add Bulbus Fritillariae Thunbergii (Bei Mu) 10g and Semen Trichosanthis (Gua Lou Zi) 12g.

2) <u>Deficiency of Yin and Internal Heat</u>

Symptoms: Afternoon fever, flushed cheeks, feverish sensation in the chest, palms and soles, spontaneous or night sweating, palpitation, shortness of breath, cough, blood-stained sputum, red tongue with little moisture, and thready and rapid or hesitant, knot and intermittent pulse.

Therapeutic Principle: To nourish yin, clear away heat, replenish deficiency and remove toxicants.

Prescription: Modified Yue Hua Pill.

Modifications: For low-grade fever, add Rhizoma Anemarrhenae (Zhi Mu) 10g, Cortex Phellodendri (Huang Bai) 10g, Radix Stellariae Dichotomae (Yin Chai Hu) 10g and Cortex Lycii Radicis (Di Gu Pi) 10g; for blood-stained sputum, add Herba Agrimoniae Pilosae (Xian He Cao) 12g, Cacumen Biotae Orientalis (Ce Bai Ye) 12g and Rhizoma Bletillae Striatae (Bai Ji) 10g.

3) <u>Accumulation of Toxic-Heat in the Pericardium</u>

Symptoms: Fever, red complexion, cough, dyspnea, irritability, anxiety, distending pain in the chest, palpitation, red tongue with yellow coating, and rapid and forceful pulse.

Therapeutic Principle: To clear away heat, remove toxic substances, promote blood circulation and relieve pain.

Prescription: Modified Xian Fang Huo Ming Decoction.

Modifications: For severe toxic-heat, add Radix Scutellariae Baicalensis (Huang Qin) 10g, Rhizoma Coptidis (Huang Lian) 10g and Cortex Phellodendri (Huang Bai) 10g; for dry mouth and vexation, add Radix Rehmanniae (Di Huang) 15g, Radix Scrophulariae Ningpoensis (Xuan Shen) 12g and Radix Ophiopogonis Japonici (Mai Dong) 12g.

4) <u>Blockage of Heart Vessel by Damp-Heat</u>

Symptoms: Fever, dyspnea, dry mouth with bitter taste, restlessness, red, swollen, hot and pain joints, palpitation, chest pain, dark urine, red tongue with turbid and yellow or greasy coating, and slippery and rapid pulse.

Therapeutic Principle: To clear away heat, eliminate dampness, remove stagnation and recuperate pulse.

Prescription: Modified Xuan Bi Decoction.

Modifications: For remarkable joint pain, add Ramulus Mori (Sang Zhi) 15g, Radix Gentianae Macrophyllae (Qin Jiao) 10g and Rhizoma Cyperi Rotundi (Xiang Fu) 10g; for qi stagnation and blood stasis, add Semen Pruni Persicae (Tao Ren) 10g, Flos Carthami Tinctorii (Hong Hua) 10g and Radix Salviae Miltiorrhizae (Dan Shen) 10g.

5) <u>Up Attacking of the Pericardium by Toxic Fluid due to Deficiency of Kidney Yang</u>

Symptoms: Dyspnea, chest pain, spiritlessness, lusterless complexion, sore and weak loins and limbs, aversion to cold, cold limbs, edema of lower extremities, a smell of urine in the mouth, oliguria, fluid retention in the pericardium, pale and chubby tongue with teeth marks, white and thin tongue coating, and deep and weak pulse.

Therapeutic Principle: To warm yang, nourish the kidney, induce diuresis and remove toxic substances.

Prescription: Modified Zhen Wu Decoction.

Modifications: For severe chest pain, add Rhizoma Corydalis (Yan Hu Suo) 10g and Rhizoma Cyperi Rotundi (Xiang Fu) 10g; for nausea and vomiting, add Herba Agastache seu Pogostemonis (Huo Xiang) 10g and Rhizoma Pinelliae Ternatae (Ban Xia) 10g.

6) <u>Accumulation of Turbid Dampness in the Pericardium</u>

Symptoms: Stuffy sensation in the chest, chest pain, abundant sputum, dyspnea, inability to lie flat, dizziness, palpitation, edema of extremities, oliguria, white and greasy tongue coating, and slippery and rapid or soft and rapid pulse.

Therapeutic Principle: To resolve dampness and fluid retention, and activate yang.

Prescription: Modified Ling Gui Zhu Gan Decoction and Ting Li Da Zao Xie Fei Decoction.

Modifications: For shortness of breath and fatigue, add Radix Astragali (Huang Qi) 12g and Radix Codonopsitis Pilosulae (Dang Shen) 9g; for severe chest pain, lump in hypochondriac region, dark and purple tongue, add Radix Notoginseng (San Qi) 10g, Semen Pruni Persicae (Tao Ren) 10g and Rhizoma Corydalis (Yan Hu Suo) 10g; for abdominal distention, anorexia and insipid mouth, add Pericarpium Citri Reticulatae (Chen Pi) 9g, Fructus Amomi Villosi (Sha Ren) 6g and Semen Raphani Sativi (Lai Fu Zi) 10g.

7) <u>Blockage of Heart Vessel by Qi Stagnation and Blood Stasis</u>

Symptoms: Localized stabbing chest pain, palpitation, dyspnea, dark and purple tongue with ecchymoses or petechiae, thin tongue coating, and deep and rough or knot and intermittent pulse.

Therapeutic Principle: To promote blood circulation, remove blood stasis, promote qi circulation and relieve pain.

Prescription: Modified Xue Fu Zhu Yu Decoction.

Modifications: To increase the function of relieving pain of the above prescription, add Rhizoma Corydalis (Yan Hu Suo) 10g; for fluid retention in the pericardium, distention in the chest and hypochondriac region, and vertigo, add Ling Gui Zhu Gan Decoction.

What Kinds of Chinese Patent Drugs are Available to Treat Acute Pericarditis?

1) Sheng Mai Oral Liquid: 10ml each time, thrice daily.
2) Qing Kai Ling Injection: 20-40ml each time, once daily.
3) Fu Fang Dan Shen Injection: 10-20ml each time, once daily.

12. Constrictive Pericarditis

Refer to Acute Pericarditis for etiology, symptoms, diagnosis and treatment in conventional Western Medicine.

What Causes Constrictive Pericarditis According to Traditional Chinese Medicine?

1) Deficiency of Healthy Qi
2) Infection of Contagious Toxicants
3) Attack by Pathogenic Factors
4) Up Attacking of Pericardium by Toxic Fluid due to Kidney Failure

How is Constrictive Pericarditis Differentiated and Treated by Traditional Chinese Medicine?

1) <u>Phlegm Accumulation and Blood Stasis</u>

Symptoms: Palpitation, dyspnea, shortness of breath, stuffy sensation in the chest, chest pain, distending pain in the hypochondriac region, cyanosis of lips, anorexia, edema of extremities, general heavy sensation, dark and purple tongue with ecchymosis, white and greasy tongue coating, and rough or knot and intermittent pulse.

Therapeutic Principle: To promote blood circulation, resolve phlegm, activate collaterals and relieve pain.

Prescription: Ge Xia Zhu Yu Decoction and Gua Lou Xie Bai Ban Xia Decoction, or Xue Fu Zhu Yu Decoction and Gua Lou Xie Bai Ban Xia Decoction.

Modifications: For severe stuffy sensation in the chest and chest pain, add Radix Curcumae (Yu Jin) 10g and Rhizoma Corydalis (Yan Hu Suo) 10g; for severe palpitation, add Semen Ziziphi Spinosae (Suan Zao Ren) 15g and Mastodi Dentis Fossilia (Long Chi) 20g; for remarkable edema, add Semen Plantaginis (Che Qian Zi) 10g and Sclerotium Polypori Umbellati (Zhu Ling) 10g.

2) <u>Deficiency of the Spleen and Fluid Retention</u>

Symptoms: Dyspnea, spiritlessness, fatigue, abdominal distention, anorexia, diarrhea, edema of lower extremities, pale tongue with white and greasy coating, and deep and slow or deep and weak pulse.

Therapeutic Principle: To invigorate the spleen, warm yang, promote circulation of qi and induce diuresis.

Prescription: Shi Pi Decoction.

Modifications: For severe deficiency of qi, add Radix Ginseng (Ren Shen) 6g and Radix Astragali (Huang Qi) 12g; for sputum, add Pericarpium Trichosanthis (Gua Lou Pi) 9g, Bulbus Allii Macrostemonis (Xie Bai) 9g and Rhizoma Pinelliae Ternatae (Ban Xia) 10g; for blood stasis, add Radix Ligustici Chuanxiong (Chuang Xiong) 9g, Radix Salviae Miltiorrhizae (Dan Shen) 10g and Lignum Dalbergiae Odoriferae (Jiang Xiang) 5g.

3) Yang Deficiency of the Heart and Kidney

Symptoms: Dyspnea, palpitation, pale complexion, sore lower back and knees, aversion to cold, cold limbs, edema of lower extremities, pale tongue with white coating, and deep, thready and forceless pulse.

Therapeutic Principle: To tonify the kidney, nourish the heart, warm yang and induce diuresis.

Prescription: Modified Zhen Wu Decoction.

Modifications: Add Radix Salviae Miltiorrhizae (Dan Shen) 10g, Herba Leonuri Heterophylii (Yi Mu Cao) 10g, Semen Plantaginis (Che Qian Zi) 9g and Rhizoma Alismatis Orientalis (Ze Xie) 9g to promote blood circulation and induce diuresis; for distending pain in the chest, add Rhizoma Cyperi Rotundi (Xiang Fu) 10g, Rhizoma Corydalis (Yan Hu Suo) 9g and Radix Notoginseng (San Qi) 9g.

13. Chronic Cor Pulmonale (Pulmonary Heart Disease)

Chronic cor pulmonale is defined as right heart hypertrophy and/or chronic right heart failure. Several different pathophysiologic mechanisms can lead to pulmonary hypertension and, subsequently, to cor pulmonale. These include (1) pulmonary vasoconstriction due to alveolar hypoxia or blood acidemia; (2) anatomic compromise of the pulmonary vascular bed secondary to lung disorders; (3) increased blood viscosity secondary to blood disorders; and (4) idiopathic primary pulmonary hypertension. The result is increased pulmonary arterial pressure. Cor pulmonale is most commonly caused by COPD. Other causes include:

- Repeated pulmonary emboli
- Pulmonary vasculitis
- Pulmonary veno-occlusive disease
- Congenital heart disease with left-to-right shunting
- Sickle cell disease
- High altitude disease with pulmonary vasoconstriction
- Primary pulmonary hypertension
- Parenchymal lung diseases (interstitial lung diseases, chronic obstructive lung diseases)
- Neuromuscular disorders (e.g., myasthenia gravis, poliomyelitis, amyotrophic lateral sclerosis)
- Obstructive and central sleep apnea
- Thoracic deformities (e.g., kyphoscoliosis)

Cor pulmonale is estimated to account for 6-7% of all types of adult heart disease in the United States. Development of cor pulmonale as a result of a primary pulmonary disease usually heralds a poorer prognosis.

Clinical manifestations of cor pulmonale generally are nonspecific:

- Chronic productive cough
- Exertional dyspnea
- Wheezing respirations
- Fatigue and weakness
- Edema
- Right upper quadrant pain
- Cyanosis
- Clubbing
- Distended neck veins
- Right ventricular heave or gallop
- Prominent lower sternal or epigastric pulsations
- Enlarged and tender liver

How is Chronic Cor Pulmonale Diagnosed by Conventional Western Medicine?

Diagnosis is made based on medical history, clinical findings and tests, which include lab tests (polycythemia is often present in cor pulmonale, the arterial oxygen saturation is below 85%), ECG or EKG, chest x ray, pulmonary function tests and pulmonary angiography. Essentials of diagnosis include:

- Symptoms and signs of COPD
- Elevated jugular venous pressure, parasternal lift, edema, hepatomegaly, ascites
- ECG or EKG shows tall, peaked P waves, right axis deviation, and right ventricular hypertrophy
- Chest x ray finding of enlarged right ventricle and pulmonary artery
- Echocardiogram or radionuclide angiography excludes primary left ventricular dysfunction.

How is Chronic Cor Pulmonale Treated by Conventional Western Medicine?

Medical therapy for chronic cor pulmonale is generally focused on treatment of the underlying pulmonary disease and improving oxygenation and right ventricle function. Oxygen, salt and fluid restriction, and diuretics are mainstays.

What Causes Chronic Cor Pulmonale According to Traditional Chinese Medicine?

1) Deficiency of the Lung, Spleen and Kidney
2) Invasion of Exogenous Pathogenic Factors
3) Stagnation of Phlegm and Blood Stasis

How is Chronic Cor Pulmonale Differentiated and Treated by Traditional Chinese Medicine?

1) <u>Retention of Turbid Phlegm in the Lung</u>

Symptoms: Cough with abundant white, sticky, greasy or foamy sputum, shortness of breath aggravated by exertion, abdominal distention, anorexia, lassitude, pale tongue with thin and greasy or turbid and greasy coating, and slippery pulse.

Therapeutic Principle: To strengthen the spleen, resolve phlegm and lower adverse flow of qi.

Prescription: Modified Su Zi Jiang Qi Decoction.

Modifications: For fullness in the chest, dyspnea and inability to lie flat, add Semen Descurainiae seu Lepidii (Ting Li Zi) 9g and Sclerotium Poriae Cocos (Fu Ling) 12g; for shortness of breath, fatigue and spontaneous sweating, add Rhizoma Atractylodis Macrocephalae (Bai Zhu) 10g and Radix Codonopsitis Pilosulae (Dang Shen) 9g; for marked blood stasis, add Radix Paeoniae Rubra (Chi Shao) 10g and Semen Pruni Persicae (Tao Ren) 9g.

2) <u>Accumulation of Phlegm-Heat in the Lung</u>

Symptoms: Dyspnea, coarse breathing sound, restlessness, fullness in the chest, cough with yellow or white, thick and sticky sputum that is difficult to be expectorated, or fever, slight aversion to cold, mild sweating, yellow urine, constipation, thirst, red tongue with yellow or yellow and greasy coating, and rapid or slippery pulse.

Therapeutic Principle: To clear away lung heat, resolve phlegm, lower adverse flow of qi and relieve dyspnea.

Prescription: Modified Yue Bi Jia Ban Xia Decoction.

Modifications: For excessive phlegm-heat with difficult expectoration, add Herba cum Radice Houttuyniae Cordatae (Yu Xing Cao) 15g, Pericarpium Trichosanthis (Gua Lou Pi) 9g and Bulbus Fritillariae Thunbergii (Bei Mu) 9g; for dry mouth and tongue, add Radix Trichosanthis (Tian Hua Fen) 10g, Rhizoma Anemarrhenae (Zhi Mu) 10g and Rhizoma Phragmitis Communis (Lu Gen) 15g; for wheezing in the throat, dyspnea and inability to lie flat, add Rhizoma Belamcandae Chinensis (She Gan) 9g and Semen Descurainiae seu Lepidii (Ting Li Zi) 9g; for marked blood stasis, add Radix Paeoniae Rubra (Chi Shao) 10g and Semen Pruni Persicae (Tao Ren) 9g.

3) <u>Pathogenic Phlegm Blocking the Heart Orifice</u>

Symptoms: Somnolence, delirium, restlessness, dull facial expression, lethargy, coma, or spasm of the limbs, cough, tachypnea, difficult expectoration, crimson or slight purple tongue with white and greasy or yellow and greasy coating, and thready, slippery and rapid pulse.

Therapeutic Principle: To resolve phlegm, induce resuscitation, calm wind and stop spasm.

Prescription: Modified Di Tan Decoction and An Gong Niu Huang Pill.

Modifications: For internal stirring-up of liver wind with spasm, add Ramulus Uncariae cum Uncis (Gou Teng) 12g, Buthus Martensi (Quan Xie) 3g and Cornu Saigae Tataricae (Ling Yang Jiao) 2g; for mucocutaneous bleeding, hemoptysis and hematochezia with bright red blood, add Cornu Bubali (Shui Niu Jiao) 9g, Folium Callicarpae Formosanae (Zi Zhu) 10g and Radix Rehmanniae (Di Huang) 15g.

4) <u>Deficiency of Yang and Overflow of Water</u>

Symptoms: Facial edema, edema of the lower extremities, or even anasarca, abdominal distention and fullness, ascites, palpitation, cough with thin and clear sputum, dyspnea, anorexia, oliguria, cold intolerance, purplish face and lips, dark and chubby tongue with white and slippery coating, deep and thready pulse.

Therapeutic Principle: To warm the kidney, strengthen the spleen and induce diuresis.

Prescription: Modified Zhen Wu Decoction and Wu Ling Powder.

Modifications: For severe blood stasis and marked cyanosis, add Herba Lycopi Lucidi (Ze Lan) 12g, Flos Carthami Tinctorii (Hong Hua) 9g and Cortex Acanthopanacis Radicis (Wu Jia Pi) 9g; for severe edema, add Radix Stephaniae Tetrandrae (Fang Ji) 9g, Semen Zanthoxyli (Jiao Mu) 3g and Semen Descurainiae seu Lepidii (Ting Li Zi) 9g.

5) <u>Deficiency of Lung Qi and Kidney Qi</u>

Symptoms: Shallow and short respiration patten, shortness of breath, weak voice, exertional dyspnea, inability to lie flat, cough with white, clear, thin and foamy sputum, sensation of stuffiness in the chest, palpitation, general coldness, sweating, pale or dark purple tongue, and deep, thready, tinny and forceless or knot and intermittent pulse.

Therapeutic Principle: To nourish the lung and kidney, lower the adverse flow of qi and relieve dyspnea.

Prescription: Modified Bu Fei Decoction.

Modifications: For failure of the kidney to arrest qi, add Semen Juglandis (Hu Tao Ren) 15g and Lignum Aquilariae Resinatum (Chen Xiang) 1.2g; for cold intolerance and pale tongue, add Cortex

Cinnamomi Cassiae (Rou Gui) 5g, Rhizoma Zingiberis Officinalis (Gan Jiang) 6g and Herba cum Radice Asari (Xi Xin) 3g.

6) <u>Qi Deficiency and Blood Stasis</u>

Symptoms: Dyspnea, cough, fatigue, shortness of breath, difficult expectoration, palpitation, sensation of stuffiness in the chest, dry mouth, dim complexion, cyanosis of lips and nails, listlessness, lassitude, dim tongue, and thready, rough and forceless pulse.

Therapeutic Principle: To replenish qi, promote blood circulation, stop cough and relieve phlegm.

Prescription: Modified Sheng Mai Powder and Xue Fu Zhu Yu Decoction.

Modifications: For abundant sputum and difficult expectoration, add Radix Asteris Tatarici (Zi Wan) 9g, Flos Farfarae (Kuan Dong Hua) 9g and Bulbus Fritillariae Cirrhosae (Bei Mu) 9g; for yin deficiency with lung heat and flushed face, add Radix Adenophorae (Sha Shen) 10g, Bulbus Lilii (Bai He) 15g and Rhizoma Polygonati Odorati (Yu Zhu) 10g.

What Kinds of Chinese Patent Drugs are Available to Treat Chronic Cor Pulmonale?

1) Ji Sheng Shen Qi Pill: 1 pill each time, thrice daily.
2) Gu Shen Ding Chuan Pill: 1.5-2.0g each time, 2-3 times each day.

Chapter 3: Disorders of the Gastrointestinal System

1. Chronic Gastritis

Gastritis is a term used to describe a group of conditions characterized by inflammation of the lining of the stomach. Gastritis may occur suddenly (acute gastritis), or it can occur slowly over time (chronic gastritis). In some cases, gastritis can lead to ulcers and an increased risk of stomach cancer. For most people, however, gastritis isn't serious and improves quickly with treatment. Gastritis usually develops when the stomach's protective layer becomes overwhelmed or damaged. A number of factors can contribute to or trigger gastritis, including:

- Infection of H. pylori bacteria
- Regular use of pain relievers
- Excessive alcohol use
- Bile reflux disease.
- Autoimmune response (autoimmune gastritis)
- Other diseases and conditions, including HIV/AIDS, Crohn's disease, parasitic infections, some connective tissue disorders and liver or kidney failure

The signs and symptoms of gastritis include:

- An epigastric gnawing or burning ache or pain that may be aggravated or relieved by meals
- Nausea
- Vomiting
- Loss of appetite
- Belching or bloating
- A feeling of fullness in the upper abdomen after eating
- Weight loss
- Occasional stomach bleeding

Acute gastritis occurs suddenly and is more likely to cause nausea and burning pain or discomfort in the upper abdomen. Chronic gastritis develops gradually and is more likely to cause a dull pain and a feeling of fullness or loss of appetite after a few bites of food. For many people, though, chronic gastritis causes no signs or symptoms at all.

How is Gastritis Diagnosed by Conventional Western Medicine?

Diagnosis is made based on medical history, physical exam and certain tests to pinpoint the exact cause. These tests include: blood tests (for the presence of H. pylori antibodies and anemia), breath test, stool tests, upper gastrointestinal endoscopy and upper gastrointestinal X-ray.

How is Gastritis Treated by Conventional Western Medicine?

Treatment of gastritis depends on the specific cause. Acute gastritis caused by NSAIDs or alcohol may be relieved by stopping use of those substances. Chronic gastritis caused by H. pylori infection is treated by eradicating the bacteria, using a combination of two antibiotics and a proton pump inhibitor. Sometimes bismuth (Pepto-Bismol) is added to the mix. Most gastritis treatment plans also include medications that treat stomach acid in order to reduce signs and symptoms and promote healing in the stomach. Medications to treat stomach acid include antacids, acid blockers and proton pump inhibitors.

What Causes Chronic Gastritis According to Traditional Chinese Medicine?

1) Improper Diet, Cigarette Smoking and Alcohol Indulgence
2) Internal Injury by Seven Emotions
3) Pathogenic Cold Attacking the Stomach
4) Deficiency of the Spleen and the Stomach

How is Chronic Gastritis Differentiated and Treated by Traditional Chinese Medicine?

1) <u>Pathogenic Cold Attacking the Stomach</u>

Symptoms: Sudden onset of gastric pain that is aggravated by pressure and coldness and alleviated by hot compression and warmth; absence of thirst, preference to hot drinks, white tongue coating, and taut and tense pulse.

Therapeutic Principle: To disperse cold, warm the stomach, regulate qi and relieve pain.

Prescription: Modified Liang Fu Pill and Zheng Qi Tian Xiang Powder.

Modifications: For severe stomach cold and gastric pain, add Cortex Cinnamomi Cassiae (Rou Gui) 3g and Radix Aconiti Lateralis Praeparatae (Fu Zi) 10g; for invasion of cold and dampness in summer with nausea, anorexia, and thick and greasy tongue coating, add Herba Agastache seu Pogostemonis (Huo Xiang) 10g, Rhizoma Atractylodis (Cang Zhu) 10g and Fructus Amomi Cardamomi (Bai Kou Ren) 3g.

2) <u>Disharmony between the Liver and Stomach</u>

Symptoms: Distending pain in the gastric area radiating to the hypochondriac region, which is aggravated by emotional disturbance and alleviated by belching or passing flatus; frequent belching, gastric discomfort sensation, acid regurgitation, pale and red tongue with thin and white coating, and taut pulse.

Therapeutic Principle: To soothe the liver, regulate qi, normalize the function of the stomach and relieve pain.

Prescription: Modified Chai Hu Shu Gan Powder.

Modifications: For severe pain, add Rhizoma Corydalis (Yan Hu Suo) 10g and Fructus Meliae Toosendan (Chuan Lian Zi) 10g; for frequent belching, add Lignum Aquilariae Resinatum (Chen Xiang) 1g, Calyx Diospyri Kaki (Shi Di) 10g and Caulis Perillae (Su Geng) 10g; for heat accumulation, add Radix Curcumae (Yu Jin) 10g and Fructus Meliae Toosendan (Chuan Lian Zi) 10g.

3) <u>Damp-Heat in the Spleen and Stomach</u>

Symptoms: Burning, discomfort and distending pain sensation in the gastric area, dry mouth with bitter taste, thirst without a desire to drink, general heavy sensation, dark urine, red tongue with yellow and greasy coating, and slippery pulse.

Therapeutic Principle: To clear away heat, remove turbidity, recuperate the spleen and regulate the stomach.

Prescription: Modified San Ren Decoction.

Modifications: For severe dampness, add Herba Agastache seu Pogostemonis (Huo Xiang) 10g and Herba Eupatorii (Pi Lan) 10g; for severe heat, add Rhizoma Coptidis (Huang Lian) 9g and Fructus Gardeniae Jasminoidis (Zhi Zi) 10g.

4) <u>Insufficiency of Stomach Yin</u>

Symptoms: Discomfort sensation and dull pain in the gastric area, dry mouth and throat, feverish sensation in the chest, palms soles, constipation, red tongue with little moisture, and thready pulse.

Therapeutic Principle: To nourish yin, regulate the stomach and relieve pain.

Prescription: Modified Yi Wei Decoction.

Modifications: For severe internal heat in the stomach, add Gypsum Fibrosum (Shi Gao) 30g and Rhizoma Anemarrhenae (Zhi Mu) 10g; for remarkable depletion of yin, add Radix Rehmanniae (Di Huang) 15g, Radix Paeoniae Alba (Bai Shao Yao) 10g and Herba Dendrobii (Shi Hu) 10g; for gastric discomfort sensation and regurgitation of acid, add Zuo Jin Pill.

5) <u>Blood Stasis Blocking the Collaterals of the Stomach</u>

Symptoms: Localized pricking or stabbing gastric pain aggravated by pressure or aggravated at night, or hematemesis, hemafecia, dim complexion, dark and purple tongue with ecchymosis, and taut and rough pulse.

Therapeutic Principle: To promote blood circulation, remove blood stasis, activate the collaterals, regulate the stomach and relieve pain.

Prescription: Modified Shi Xiao Powder and Dan Shen Decoction.

Modifications: For severe pain, add Rhizoma Corydalis (Yan Hu Suo) 10g, Radix Curcumae (Yu Jin) 10g and Radix Aucklandiae Lappae (Mu Xiang) 10g; for tarry stools, add Rhizoma Bletillae Striatae (Bai Ji) 10g and Radix Notoginseng (San Qi) 10g.

6) <u>Qi Deficiency of the Spleen and Stomach</u>

Symptoms: Distending sensation in the gastric area worsened by intake of food, anorexia, lassitude, diarrhea, pale and chubby tongue with thin and white coating, and deep and weak pulse.

Therapeutic Principle: To nourish the spleen, replenish qi, strengthen middle warmer and regulate the stomach.

Prescription: Modified Bu Zhong Yi Qi Decoction.

Modifications: For food retention, add Semen Raphani Sativi (Lai Fu Zi) 10g and Fructus Hordei Germinatus (Mai Ya) 12g; for deficiency of qi and blood, add Fructus Lycii (Gou Qi Zi) 10g; for bleeding, add Radix Notoginseng (San Qi) 10g and Rhizoma Bletillae Striatae (Bai Ji) 10g.

7) <u>Yang Deficiency of the Spleen and Stomach</u>

Symptoms: Lingering dull gastric pain that is relieved by warmth, pressure and intake of food; vomiting of clear fluid, anorexia, spiritlessness, lassitude, cold limbs, diarrhea, pale and chubby tongue with white and thin coating, and thready and weak pulse.

Therapeutic Principle: To replenish qi, warm middle warmer, invigorate the spleen and regulate the stomach.

Prescription: Modified Huang Qi Jian Zhong Decoction.

Modifications: For vomiting of abundant clear fluid, add Pericarpium Citri Reticulatae (Chen Pi) 6g, Rhizoma Pinelliae Ternatae (Ban Xia) 10g and Sclerotium Poriae Cocos (Fu Ling) 12g; for stomach cold with severe pain, add Rhizoma Alpiniae Officinarum (Gao Liang Jiang) 10g and Rhizoma Cyperi Rotundi (Xiang Fu) 10g; for chronic pain with blood stasis blocking the collaterals, add Flos Carthami Tinctorii (Hong Hua) 10g, Pollen Typhae (Pu Huang) 10g, Excrementum Trogopteri seu Pteromydis (Wu Ling Zhi) 10g and Radix Salviae Miltiorrhizae (Dan Shen) 10g; for tarry stools, add

Rhizoma Zingiberis Praeparatae (Pao Jiang) 10g, Rhizoma Bletillae Striatae (Bai Ji) 10g and Radix Sanguisorbae Officinalis (Di Yu) 12g.

8) <u>Yin Deficiency of the Spleen and Stomach</u>

Symptoms: Dull and burning pain in the gastric area, restlessness, thirst with a desire to drink, dry mouth and dry throat, discomfort and feverish sensation in the stomach, constipation, dizziness, insomnia, anorexia, or feverish sensation in palms and soles, red tongue with little or cracked or peeled coating, and thready and rapid pulse.

Therapeutic Principle: To nourish yin, clear away heat, strengthen the stomach and produce body fluid.

Prescription: Modified Yi Wei Decoction.

Modifications: For stomach heat, add Rhizoma Coptidis (Huang Lian) 5g and Folium Phyllostachydis Henonis (Zhu Ye) 10g; for poor appetite, add Pericarpium Citri Reticulatae (Chen Pi) 6g, Massa Medicata Fermentata (Shen Qu) 12g and Fructus Hordei Germinatus (Mai Ya) 12g; for severe pain, add Radix Paeoniae Alba (Bai Shao Yao) 10g and Radix Glycyrrhizae Uralensis (Gan Cao) 6g; for blood stasis, add Radix Salviae Miltiorrhizae (Dan Shen) 10g and Semen Pruni Persicae (Tao Ren) 10g.

What Kinds of Chinese Patent Drugs are Available to Treat Chronic Gastritis?

1) San Jiu Wei Tai Granule: 1 bag each time, 2-3 times daily.
2) Wei Su Granule: 15g each time, thrice daily.
3) Xiang Sha Yang Wei Pill: 9g each time, twice daily.

2. Peptic Ulcer

Peptic ulcer is a break in the gastric or duodenal mucosa that arises when the normal mucosal defensive factors are impaired or are overwhelmed by aggressive luminal factors such as acid and pepsin. The most common symptom of a peptic ulcer is pain. Depending on their location, peptic ulcers have different names: gastric ulcer, duodenal ulcer and esophageal ulcer.

The cause of most ulcers is Helicobacter pylori (H. pylori). H. pylori is a common gastrointestinal infection around the world. In the United States, one in five people younger than 30 and half the people older than 60 are infected. H. pylori may be transmitted from person to person by close contact, or through food and water. Other causes of peptic ulcer include regular use of pain relievers, smoking, excessive alcohol consumption and stress. Although stress per se isn't a cause of peptic ulcers, it's a contributing factor.

Burning pain is the most common peptic ulcer symptom. The pain typically may be felt anywhere from the navel to the breastbone, last from a few minutes to many hours, be worse when the stomach is empty, flare at night, often be temporarily relieved by eating certain foods or by taking an acid-reducing medication, come and go for a few days or weeks. Less often, ulcers may cause severe signs or symptoms such as the vomiting of blood that may appear red or black, tarry or black stools, nausea or vomiting, unexplained weight loss, and chest pain.

How is Peptic Ulcer Diagnosed by Conventional Western Medicine?

The following diagnostic tests may be ordered to detect an ulcer: upper gastrointestinal x ray and endoscopy with biopsy.

Other tests to determine the cause of ulcer include: (1) blood test. This test checks for the presence of H. pylori antibodies; (2) breath test. This procedure uses a radioactive carbon atom to detect H. pylori; and (3) stool antigen test. This test checks for H. pylori in stool samples.

How is Peptic Ulcer Treated by Conventional Western Medicine?

1) <u>Treatment of H. pylori associated ulcers</u>

The goal of treatment is to kill H. pylori and reduce the level of acid in the digestive system to relieve pain and encourage healing. Accomplishing these two goals requires the use of at least two, and sometimes three or four, of the following medications:

- Antibiotic medications, such as amoxicillin (Amoxil), clarithromycin (Biaxin) and metronidazole (Flagyl).
- Acid blockers, such as ranitidine (Zantac), famotidine (Pepcid), cimetidine (Tagamet) and nizatidine (Axid)
- Antacids
- Proton pump inhibitors
- Cytoprotective agents, such as sucralfate (Carafate), misoprostol (Cytotec) and bismuth subsalicylate (Pepto-Bismol)

2) <u>Treatment of NSAID associated ulcers</u>

Quit using NSAIDs and reduce acid levels through use of acid blockers, antacids or proton pump inhibitors or cytoprotective drugs.

3) <u>Treatment of refractory ulcers</u>

Refractory ulcers may be a result of:

- Not taking medications according to directions
- Some types of H. pylori are resistant to antibiotics

- Regular use of tobacco, alcohol or NSAIDs
- Extreme overproduction of stomach acid, such as occurs in Zollinger-Ellison syndrome
- An infection other than H. pylori
- Stomach cancer
- Other digestive diseases, including Crohn's disease or cancer

Treatment for refractory ulcers generally includes: (1) eliminating factors that may interfere with healing; (2) stronger doses of ulcer medications; (3) additional medications may be included; and (4) Surgery.

What Causes Peptic Ulcer According to Traditional Chinese Medicine?

1) Improper Diet
2) Internal Injury by Seven Emotions
3) Deficiency of the Spleen and the Stomach

How is Peptic Ulcer Differentiated and Treated by Traditional Chinese Medicine?

1) <u>Disharmony of the liver and Stomach</u>

Symptoms: Gastric distending pain radiating to the hypochondriac region, which is induced or aggravated by emotional disturbance; frequent sighing, belching, acid regurgitation, bitter taste in the mouth, pale and red tongue with white and thin coating, and taut pulse.

Therapeutic Principle: To soothe the liver, regulate qi, invigorate the spleen and normalize the function of the stomach.

Prescription: Modified Chai Hu Shu Gan Powder and Wu Mo Decoction.

Modifications: For severe pain, add Rhizoma Corydalis (Yan Hu Suo) 10g; for remarkable belching, add Lignum Aquilariae Resinatum (Chen Xiang) 1g and Calyx Diospyri Kaki (Shi Di) 10g; for remarkable acid regurgitation, add Rhizoma Coptidis (Huang Lian) 9g and Fructus Evodiae Rutaecarpae (Wu Zhu Yu) 3g.

2) <u>Deficiency of Spleen Yang and Stomach Yang</u>

Symptoms: Persistent dull epigastric pain alleviated by warmth and pressure, aversion to cold, cold limbs, vomiting of watery fluid, abdominal distention, diarrhea, chubby tongue with teeth marks on the margin, white coating, and slow pulse.

Therapeutic Principle: To warm the middle warmer, disperse cold, invigorate the spleen and warm the stomach.

Prescription: Modified Huang Qi Jian Zhong Decoction.

Modifications: For remarkable vomiting of watery fluid, add Rhizoma Pinelliae Ternatae (Ban Xia) 10g and Sclerotium Poriae Cocos (Fu Ling) 12g; for severe acid regurgitation, add Fructus Evodiae Rutaecarpae (Wu Zhu Yu) 3g and Os Sepiae seu Sepiellae (Wu Zei Gu) 10g.

3) <u>Insufficiency of Stomach Yin</u>

Symptoms: Epigastric dull pain, gastric discomfort, hunger without a desire to eat, dry mouth without a desire to drink, anorexia, non-productive vomiting, feverish sensation in palms and soles, constipation, red tongue with little moisture and coating, and thready and rapid pulse.

Therapeutic Principle: To invigorate the spleen, nourish yin, strengthen the stomach and relieve pain.

Prescription: Modified Yi Guan Decoction and Shao Yao Gan Cao Decoction.

Modifications: For constipation, add Semen Cannabis Sativae (Huo Mai Ren) 12g and Semen Biotae Orientalis (Bai Zi Ren) 15g; for spiritlessness and lassitude, add Radix Pseudostellariae Heterophyllae (Tai Zi Shen) 15g and Radix Astragali (Huang Qi) 12g; for belching, add Fructus Citri Medicae seu Wilsonii (Xiang Yuan) 9g and Fructus Citri Sarcodactyli (Fo Shou) 9g.

4) <u>Stagnation of Heat in the Liver and Stomach</u>

Symptoms: Burning and feverish sensation in the epigastrium, epigastric pain, distending sensation in the chest and hypochondriac region, acid regurgitation, dry mouth with bitter taste, restlessness, irritability, constipation, red tongue with yellow coating, and taut and rapid coating.

Therapeutic Principle: To clear away stomach heat, purge heat, soothe the liver and regulate qi.

Prescription: Modified Hua Gan Decoction and Zuo Jin Pill.

Modifications: For severe distending pain in the hypochondriac region, add Radix Curcumae (Yu Jin) 10g and Fructus Meliae Toosendan (Chuan Lian Zi) 10g; for yellow and greasy tongue coating, remove Pericarpium Citri Reticulatae Viride and add Herba Artemisiae Scopariae (Yin Chen Hao) 20g and Herba Agastache seu Pogostemonis (Huo Xiang) 9g.

5) <u>Blood Stagnation Blocking the Collaterals of the Stomach</u>

Symptoms: Localized pricking epigastric pain, cold limbs, sweating, hematemesis, or tarry stools, dark and purple tongue with ecchymosis, and rough pulse.

Therapeutic Principle: To promote blood circulation, remove blood stasis, activate the collaterals and normalize the function of the stomach.

Prescription: Modified Huo Luo Xiao Ling Pill and Dan Shen Decoction.

Modifications: For dry mouth and throat, add Radix Adenophorae (Sha Shen) 12g, Radix Ophiopogonis Japonici (Mai Dong) 12g and Radix Trichosanthis (Tian Hua Fen) 12g; for severe pain at night, add Aspongopus (Jiu Xiang Chong) 3g and Radix Notoginseng (San Qi) 9g.

What Kinds of Chinese Patent Drugs are Available to Treat Peptic Ulcer?

1) Wei Ke Ning Tablet: 3-5 tablets each time, 3-4 times daily.
2) Jian Wei Yu Yang Tablet: 4-6 tablets each time, 4 times daily.
3) Yin Xu Wei Tong Tablet: 6 tablets each time, thrice daily.
4) Xiao Jian Zhong Oral Liquid: 20ml each time, thrice daily.

3. Upper Gastrointestinal Bleeding (UGIB)

Upper gastrointestinal bleeding or hemorrhage (UGIB) refers to bleeding that arises in the lining of the upper gastrointestinal tract, or upper GI. There are approximately 350,000 hospitalizations a year in the United States for acute UGIB, with a mortality rate of 10%. The major causes of UGIB are duodenal ulcer hemorrhage (25%), gastric ulcer hemorrhage (20%), portal hypertension, Mallory-Weiss tears, vascular anomalies, gastric neoplasms, erosive gastritis and erosive esophagitis. Rare causes of UGIB include aortoenteric fistula, Dieulafoy lesion, hepatic tumor or vascular lesion, pancreatic malignancy or pseudoaneurysm.

Patients should be considered for upper endoscopy if blood loss from the upper gastrointestinal tract is suspected. Urgent endoscopy is indicated when patients present with hematemesis, melena, or postural changes in blood pressure. Primary surgical intervention should be considered in patients with a perforated visceral organ. In patients who are poor operative candidates, conservative treatment with nasogastric suction and broad-spectrum antibiotics can be instituted. Endoscopic clipping or sewing techniques have also been used in such patients.

The most common symptoms include weakness, dizziness, syncope associated with hematemesis (either bright red blood or coffee ground vomitus), melena (black stools with a rotten odor), and hematochezia (red or maroon stool).

How is UGIB Diagnosed by Conventional Western Medicine?

Essential of diagnosis includes:

- Hematemesis
- Melena
- Hematochezia in massive UGIB
- Assess volume status to determine severity of blood loss
- Endoscopy is diagnostic and therapeutic

How is UGIB Treated by Conventional Western Medicine?

Upper gastrointestinal bleeding is self-limited in 80% of patients. Treatment for upper gastrointestinal bleeding includes:

- Stabilization
- Blood replacement
- History and physical examination
- Upper endoscopy to identify the source of the bleeding, determine the risk of rebleeding and render therapy as needed
- Acute pharmacologic therapies: intravenous H_2 receptor antagonists, octreotide and vasopressin
- Other treatment: intra-arterial vasopressin or embolization, and surgery

What Causes UGIB According to Traditional Chinese Medicine?

1) Improper Diet
2) Internal Injury by Emotional Disturbance
3) Internal Injury by Overstrain

How is UGIB Differentiated and Treated by Traditional Chinese Medicine?

1) <u>Accumulation of Heat in the Stomach</u>

Symptoms: Hematemesis with purple dark or coffee ground or even bright red blood mixed with undigested food, tarry stools, dry mouth with a desire for cold drinks, epigastric distending sensation or burning pain, red tongue with yellow coating, and slippery and rapid pulse.

Therapeutic Principle: To clear away stomach heat, purge fire, remove blood stasis and stop bleeding.

Prescription: Modified Xie Xin Decoction and Shi Hui Powder.

Modifications: For belching, nausea and vomiting, add Ochra Haematitum (Dai Zhe Shi) 15g, Caulis Bambusae in Taeniam (Zhu Ru) 10g and Flos Inulae (Xuan Fu Hua) 10g; for injury of stomach yin by heat, add Radix Ophiopogonis Japonici (Mai Dong) 12g, Herba Dendrobii (Shi Hu) 12g and Radix Trichosanthis (Tian Hua Fen) 12g.

2) <u>Liver Fire Attacking the Stomach</u>

Symptoms: Hematemesis with bright red or dark purple blood, conjunctival congestion, bitter taste in the mouth, distending pain in the chest and hypochondriac region, restlessness, irritability, or jaundice, red tongue with yellow coating, and taut and rapid pulse.

Therapeutic Principle: To purge liver fire, clear away stomach heat, lower adverse flow of qi and stop bleeding.

Prescription: Modified Long Dan Xie Gan Decoction.

Modifications: Add Rhizoma Imperatae Cylindricae (Bai Mo Gen) 20g, Radix Rubiae Cordifoliae (Qian Cao) 12g and Herba Ecliptae Prostratae (Han Lian Cao) 20g to increase the haemostatic function; for acid regurgitation, add Os Sepiae seu Sepiellae (Wu Zi Gu) 10g and Bulbus Fritillariae Cirrhosae (Bei Mu) 10g; for constipation, add Radix Scrophulariae Ningpoensis (Xuan Shen) 12g and Radix Ophiopogonis Japonici (Mai Dong) 12g.

3) <u>Inability of the Spleen to Govern the Blood</u>

Symptoms: Hematemesis with dark colored blood, tarry loose stools, pale complexion, dizziness, palpitation, spiritlessness, lassitude, anorexia, pale and red tongue with thin and white coating, and thready and weak pulse.

Therapeutic Principle: To replenish qi, invigorate the spleen, nourish blood and stop bleeding.

Prescription: Modified Gui Pi Decoction.

Modifications: For deficient coldness in the spleen and the stomach, use Bai Ye Decoction; for large amount of bleeding, add Charred Radix Sanguisorbae Officinalis (Di Yu Tan) 12g, Cacumen Biotae Orientalis (Ce Bai Ye) 12g and Hominis Crinis Carbonisatus (Xue Yu Tan) 9g.

4) <u>Collapse of Qi Following Blood Prostration</u>

Symptoms: Hematemesis with copious amount of blood, tarry stools, pale complexion, drenching sweat, extremely cold limbs, vertigo, palpitation, irritability, dry mouth, delirium, coma, pale and red tongue, and thready, rapid and forceless or tinny and thready pulse.

Therapeutic Principle: To replenish qi and blood, and restore yang from collapse.

Prescription: Modified Du Shen Decoction or Si Wei Hui Yang Decoction.

What Kinds of Chinese Patent Drugs are Available to Treat UGIB?

1) Yun Nan Bai Yao Powder: 1g each time, 4 times daily.
2) Shen Mai Injection: 40-100ml each time, once daily.
3) Shen Fu Injection: 50-100ml each time, once daily.

4. Ulcerative Colitis (UC)

Ulcerative colitis is a disease that causes inflammation and ulcers in the lining of the rectum and colon. Ulcerative colitis is classified as ulcerative proctitis, pancolitis, distal colitis (or left-sided or limited) and fulminant colitis. When the inflammation occurs in the rectum and lower part of the colon it is called ulcerative proctitis. If the entire colon is affected it is called pancolitis. If only the left side of the colon is affected it is called limited or distal colitis.

Ulcerative colitis is an inflammatory bowel disease (IBD), the general name for diseases that cause inflammation in the small intestine and colon. It can be difficult to diagnose because its symptoms are similar to other intestinal disorders and to another type of IBD called Crohn's disease. But ulcerative colitis usually affects only the innermost lining of the colon and rectum. Crohn's disease, on the other hand, can occur anywhere in the digestive tract, often spreading deep into the layers of affected tissues.

More than 500,000 Americans have ulcerative colitis. Ulcerative colitis can occur in people of any age, but it usually starts between the ages of 15 and 30, and less frequently between 50 and 70 years of age. It affects men and women equally and appears to run in families. A higher incidence of ulcerative colitis is seen in Whites and people of Jewish descent. People living in an urban area or in an industrialized country are more likely to develop ulcerative colitis. People living in Northern climates also seem to have a greater risk of ulcerative colitis.

Many theories exist about what causes ulcerative colitis. Ulcerative colitis is not caused by emotional distress or sensitivity to certain foods or food products, but these factors may trigger symptoms in some people. The possible causes of ulcerative colitis include immune system, heredity, environment and antibiotics.

There's no known medical cure for ulcerative colitis, but therapies are available that may dramatically reduce the signs and symptoms of ulcerative colitis and even bring about a long-term remission.

The most common symptoms of ulcerative colitis are abdominal pain and bloody diarrhea. Other symptoms may include:

- Anemia
- Fatigue
- Weight loss
- Loss of appetite
- Rectal bleeding
- Loss of body fluids and nutrients
- Skin lesions
- Joint pain
- Growth failure (specifically in children)
- Fevers
- Nausea
- Abdominal cramps
- Arthritis, inflammation of the eye, liver disease, and osteoporosis

How is Ulcerative Colitis Diagnosed by Conventional Western Medicine?

A physical exam and medical history are usually the first step. To help confirm a diagnosis of ulcerative colitis, one or more of the following tests and procedures may be included: blood tests (anemia, low serum albumin), stool sample tests (negative stool culture), colonoscopy or sigmoidoscopy, barium enema, small bowel X-ray and CT scans.

How is Ulcerative Colitis Treated by Conventional Western Medicine?

Treatment for ulcerative colitis depends on the severity of the disease. The goal of medical treatment is to reduce the inflammation that triggers the signs and symptoms. In the best cases, this may lead not only to symptom relief but also to long-term remission. Treatment for ulcerative colitis usually involves either drug therapy or surgery. Medications include: (1) anti-inflammatory drugs, such as sulfasalazine (Azulfidine), mesalamine (Asacol, Rowasa) and olsalazine (Dipentum), balsalazide (Colazal), corticosteroids; (2) immune system suppressors, such as azathioprine (Imuran) and mercaptopurine (Purinethol), cyclosporine (Neoral, Sandimmune), infliximab (Remicade). (3) **Nicotine** patches; (4) other medications may be given to relax the patient or to relieve pain, diarrhea, or infection.

About 25 to 40 percent of ulcerative colitis patients eventually need surgery to have their colons removed because of massive bleeding, severe illness, rupture of the colon, or risk of cancer.

What Causes Ulcerative Colitis According to Traditional Chinese Medicine?

1) Improper Diet
2) Emotional Disturbance
3) Deficiency of the Spleen and the Stomach
4) Deficiency of Kidney Yang

How is Ulcerative Colitis Differentiated and Treated by Traditional Chinese Medicine?

1) <u>Internal Accumulation of Damp-Heat</u>

Symptoms: Bloody, purulent and mucous diarrhea, tenesmus, burning pain in the abdomen, fever, feverish sensation in the anus, scanty dark urine, red tongue with yellow and greasy coating, and slippery and rapid or soft and rapid pulse.

Therapeutic Principle: To clear away heat and promote diuresis.

Prescription: Modified Bai Tou Weng Decoction.

Modifications: For significant toxic-heat, add Herba Portulacae (Ma Chi Xian) 12g and Patriniae Herba cum Radice (Bai Jiang Cao) 12g; for significant hematochezia, add Cortex Moutan Radicis (Mu

Dan Pi) 10g and Radix Sanguisorbae Officinalis (Di Yu) 12g; for remarkable abdominal pain and tenesmus, add Radix Aucklandiae Lappae (Mu Xiang) 10g and Semen Areca Catechu (Bing Lang) 10g.

2) <u>Deficiency of the Spleen and Stomach</u>

Symptoms: Lingering, recurrent and fluctuating diarrhea, mucous, purulent and bloody stools, anorexia, abdominal distention, weak extremities, spiritlessness, indolence of speaking, pale and chubby tongue with teeth marks on the margin, thin and white tongue coating, and thready and weak or soft and slow pulse.

Therapeutic Principle: To invigorate the spleen, replenish qi, promote transportation and relieve diarrhea.

Prescription: Modified Shen Ling Bai Zhu Powder.

Modifications: For persistent diarrhea, add Bu Zhong Yi Qi Decoction; for abundant mucus in the stools, add Rhizoma Pinelliae Ternatae (Ban Xia) 10g.

3) <u>Yang Deficiency of the Spleen and Kidney</u>

Symptoms: Chronic diarrhea, abdominal pain alleviated by warmth and pressure, abdominal distention, lumbago, weak knees, anorexia, cold limbs, spiritlessness, indolence of speaking, pale tongue with teeth marks, white and moist coating, and deep and thready pulse.

Therapeutic Principle: To warm the kidney, strengthen the spleen and relieve diarrhea.

Prescription: Modified Si Shen Pill.

Modifications: May add Li Zhong Pill to warm spleen yang; For significant lumbago and cold limbs, add Radix Aconiti Lateralis Praeparatae (Fu Zi) 10g and Cortex Cinnamomi Cassiae (Rou Gui) 3g; for severe diarrhea, add Semen Dolichoris Lablab (Bian Dou) 20g, Rhizoma Dioscoreae (Shan Yao) 15g and Fructus Terminaliae Chebulae (He Zi) 9g.

4) <u>Qi Stagnation of the liver and Deficiency of the Spleen</u>

Symptoms: Abdominal pain closely followed by diarrhea, which is induced or aggravated by depression, anger, anxiety or stress; abdominal pain relieved after diarrhea, anorexia, distending pain in the chest and hypochondriac region, belching, spiritlessness, indolence of speaking, pale tongue with white coating, and taut or taut and thready pulse.

Therapeutic Principle: To soothe the liver and strengthen the spleen.

Prescription: Modified Tong Xie Formula.

Modifications: For damp-heat, add Radix Pulsatillae Chinensis (Bai Tou Weng) 10g, Rhizoma Coptidis (Huang Lian) 9g and Herba Portulacae (Ma Chi Xian) 10g; for distending pain in the chest, hypochondriac region and abdomen, add Radix Bupleuri (Chai Hu) 10g, Fructus Citri Aurantii (Zhi Ke)

10g and Rhizoma Cyperi Rotundi (Xiang Fu) 10g; for stagnation, add Pollen Typhae (Pu Huang) 10g and Radix Salviae Miltiorrhizae (Dan Shen) 10g; for chronic diarrhea, add Fructus Pruni Mume (Wu Mei) 20g and Fructus Terminaliae Chebulae (He Zi) 10g.

5) Deficiency of Yin Blood

Symptoms: Constipation or little purulent and bloody stools, dull abdominal pain, low-grade fever in the afternoon, night sweating, feverish sensation in the chest, palms and soles, vertigo, spiritlessness, indolence of speaking, red tongue with little coating, and thready and rapid pulse.

Therapeutic Principle: To nourish yin, replenish blood, clear away heat and resolve dampness.

Prescription: Modified Zhu Che Pill.

Modifications: For severe heat, add Rhizoma Anemarrhenae (Zhi Mu) 10g and Radix et Rhizoma Rhei (Da Huang) 6g.

6) Qi Stagnation and Blood Stasis

Symptoms: Abdominal pain, diarrhea, difficult defecation, hematochezia with dark purple or black stools, distending sensation in the chest and hypochondriac region, lump in the abdomen, dim complexion, squamous and dry skin, purple tongue with ecchymoses or petechiae, and taut and rough pulse.

Therapeutic Principle: To remove blood stasis and activate the collaterals.

Prescription: Modified Ge Xia Zhu Yu Decoction.

Modifications: For damp-heat, add Radix Pulsatillae Chinensis (Bai Tou Weng) 10g, Rhizoma Coptidis (Huang Lian) 9g and Herba Portulacae (Ma Chi Xian) 10g; for dampness due to deficiency of the spleen, add Radix Codonopsitis Pilosulae (Dang Shen) 9g, Rhizoma Atractylodis (Cang Zhu) 10g and Cortex Magnoliae Officinalis (Hou Po) 10g; for qi stagnation of the liver, add Radix Bupleuri (Chai Hu) 10g, Rhizoma Cyperi Rotundi (Xiang Fu) 10g and Radix Curcumae (Yu Jin) 10g.

What Kinds of Chinese Patent Drugs are Available to Treat Ulcerative Colitis?

1) Gu Ben Yi Chang Tablet: 8 tablets each time, thrice daily.
2) Bu Pi Yi Chang Pill: 6g each time, thrice daily.

5. Crohn's Disease (CD)

Crohn's disease is an ongoing disorder that causes inflammation of the digestive tract. The swelling extends deep into the lining of the affected organ and all layers of the intestine may be involved. An estimated 500,000 Americans have Crohn's disease.

Crohn's disease begins with inflammation, most often in ileum or in the colon. Crohn's disease can develop in several places simultaneously, with healthy tissue in between. What triggers inflammation in Crohn's disease is not quite known, but some possible causes include: (1) immune system reacts abnormally in people with Crohn's disease, mistaking bacteria, foods, and other substances for being foreign; (2) heredity. About 20 percent of people with Crohn's disease have a parent, sibling or child who also has the disease; (3) environment. Crohn's disease occurs more often among people living in cities and industrial nations. The course of Crohn's disease varies greatly. Some people have long periods of remission, sometimes years, when they are free of symptoms. Or some people may have recurrent episodes of abdominal pain, diarrhea, and sometimes fever or bleeding. However, the disease usually recurs at various times over a person's lifetime.

The most common symptoms of Crohn's disease are abdominal pain, often in the lower right area, and diarrhea. Rectal bleeding, weight loss, arthritis, skin problems, and fever may also occur. Bleeding may be serious and persistent, leading to anemia. Children with Crohn's disease may suffer delayed development and stunted growth. Signs and symptoms of Crohn's disease can range from mild to severe and may develop gradually or come on suddenly, without warning.

How is Crohn's Disease Diagnosed by Conventional Western Medicine?

Crohn's disease is diagnosed only after ruling out other possible causes for the signs and symptoms. To help confirm a diagnosis of Crohn's disease, one or more of the following tests and procedures may be included: blood tests, colonoscopy, flexible sigmoidoscopy, barium enema, small bowel x ray, CT scan and capsule endoscopy.

Essentials of diagnosis include: insidious onset; intermittent bouts of low-grade fever, diarrhea and right lower quadrant pain; right lower quadrant mass and tenderness; perianal disease with abscess or fistulas; radiographic evidence of ulceration, structuring or fistulas of the small intestine or colon.

How is Crohn's Disease Treated by Conventional Western Medicine?

Treatment may include drugs, nutrition supplements, surgery, or a combination of these options. The goals of treatment are to control inflammation, correct nutritional deficiencies, and relieve symptoms. Treatment for Crohn's disease depends on the location and severity of disease, complications, and the person's response to previous medical treatments when treated for reoccurring symptoms. Someone with Crohn's disease may need medical care for a long time, with regular doctor visits to monitor the condition. Drug therapy includes anti-Inflammation drugs, cortisone or steroids, immune system suppressors, Infliximab (Remicade), antibiotics, anti-diarrheal and fluid replacements.

Two-thirds to three-quarters of patients with Crohn's disease will require surgery at some point in their lives. Surgery is used either to relieve symptoms that do not respond to medical therapy or to correct complications. However, surgery does not eliminate the disease.

What Causes Crohn's Disease According to Traditional Chinese Medicine?

1) Attack by Exogenous Pathogenic Factors
2) Improper Diet
3) Emotional Disturbance
4) Deficiency of the Spleen and Stomach

How is Crohn's Disease Differentiated and Treated by Traditional Chinese Medicine?

1) <u>Retention of Damp-Cold in the Spleen</u>

Symptoms: Abdominal pain, diarrhea, sensation of fullness and lump in the abdomen, which is alleviated by warmth and pressure; anorexia, insipid mouth, or vomiting, distending sensation in the head, general aching and heavy sensation, dim complexion, white and greasy tongue coating, and soft or slow pulse.

Therapeutic Principle: To resolve dampness, disperse cold, strengthen the spleen and regulate the middle warmer.

Prescription: Modified Wei Ling Decoction.

Modifications: For remarkable dampness, add Semen Coicis (Yi Yi Ren) 15g and Fructus Amomi Villosi (Sha Ren) 5g; for remarkable coldness, add Rhizoma Zingiberis Officinalis (Gan Jiang) 10g; for severe coldness, add Radix Aconiti Lateralis Praeparatae (Fu Zi) 10g; for vomiting, add Flos Caryophylli (Ding Xiang) 3g and Fructus Evodiae Rutaecarpae (Wu Zhu Yu) 3g; for belching, add Rhizoma Pinelliae Ternatae (Ban Xia) 10g.

2) <u>Damp-Heat in the Spleen and Stomach</u>

Symptoms: Abdominal pain and lump, diarrhea with foul smell, feverish sensation in the anus, bitter taste and odor in the mouth, fever, oliguria, yellow and greasy tongue coating, and soft and rapid pulse.

Therapeutic Principle: To clear away heat and promote diuresis.

Prescription: Modified Ge Gen Qin Lian Decoction.

Modifications: For abdominal lump, anorexia and remarkable dampness, add Rhizoma Atractylodis (Cang Zhu) 10g and Herba Agastache seu Pogostemonis (Huo Xiang) 10g; for severe fever, add Cortex Phellodendri (Huang Bai) 10g and Fructus Gardeniae Jasminoidis (Zhi Zi) 10g; for abdominal pain, add Radix Aucklandiae Lappae (Mu Xiang) 10g and Fructus Citri Aurantii Immaturus (Zhi Shi) 10g.

3) <u>Toxic-Heat Damaging the Bowel</u>

Symptoms: Right lower quadrant abdominal pain and tender mass, fever, constipation, yellow tongue coating, and rapid pulse.

Therapeutic Principle: To clear away heat, remove toxic substances, loosen the bowel and relieve stagnation.

Prescription: Modified Wu Wei Xiao Du Decoction and Xiao Cheng Qi Decoction.

Modifications: For severe toxic heat, add Herba cum Radice Houttuyniae Cordatae (Yu Xing Cao) 20g and Fructus Forsythiae Suspensae (Lian Qiao) 10g; for abscesses, add Semen Coicis (Yi Yi Ren) 20g, Cortex Moutan Radicis (Mu Dan Pi) 10g, Semen Benincasae Hispidae (Dong Gua Zi) 12g and Semen Pruni Persicae (Tao Ren) 10g; for constipation, add Natrii Sulfas (Mang Xiao) 10g; for abdominal pain, add Radix Paeoniae Rubra (Chi Shao) 10g and Radix Paeoniae Alba (Bai Shao Yao) 10g.

4) <u>Blood Stasis Accumulating in the Bowel</u>

Symptoms: Hard and fixed abdominal mass, localized abdominal pain, recurrent diarrhea, dark complexion, ecchymosis of the tongue, and rough pulse.

Therapeutic Principle: To promote qi circulation, remove lump, promote blood circulation and remove blood stasis.

Prescription: Modified Xue Fu Zhu Yu Decoction.

Modifications: For remarkable abdominal pain, add Pollen Typhae (Pu Huang) 10g and Excrementum Trogopteri seu Pteromydis (Wu Ling Zhi) 10g; for severe diarrhea, add Semen Dolichoris Lablab (Bian Dou) 20g and Rhizoma Dioscoreae (Shan Yao) 20g.

5) <u>Deficiency of the Spleen</u>

Symptoms: Watery diarrhea, dim complexion, weight loss, pale lips, edema, anorexia, spiritlessness, pale tongue, and deep, thready and forceless pulse.

Therapeutic Principle: To nourish the spleen and resolve edema.

Prescription: Modified Bu Zhong Yi Chi Decoction.

Modifications: For deficiency of the spleen with chronic diarrhea and tenesmus, add Fructus Citri Aurantii (Zhi Ke) 10g and Radix Puerariae (Ge Gen) 15g; for dampness, add Sclerotium Poriae Cocos (Fu Ling) 12g.

What Kinds of Chinese Patent Drugs are Available to Treat Crohn's Disease?

1) Fu Ke Ning Tablet: 5 tablets each time, thrice daily.
2) Jin Fo Zhi Tong Pill: 6g each time, thrice daily.
3) Yun Dan Bai Yao: 0.5g each time, thrice daily.

6. Gastric Carcinoma

Although the gastric carcinoma is a leading cause of cancer death worldwide, its incidence has declined dramatically in the United States and Western Europe in the last 60 years. Types of stomach cancer include adenocarcinomas, lymphomas and carcinoid tumors. The causes of stomach cancer aren't clear. Researchers have made progress in pinpointing factors that lead to cancer. These factors include H. pylori infection, nitrates and nitrites, salted, smoked or pickled foods and red meat, tobacco and alcohol use.

Stomach cancer is more readily treated when caught early. Unfortunately, by the time stomach cancer causes symptoms, it's often at an advanced stage and may have spread beyond the stomach. A few changes in lifestyle can reduce the risk of stomach cancer. Risk factors for stomach cancer include H. pylori infection, sex, age, diet, tobacco use, previous stomach surgery, stomach polyps, familial cancer syndromes, pernicious anemia, family history, type A blood, country of origin, and obesity.

One early sign of stomach cancer include microscopic internal bleeding, fatigue due to anemia, heartburn and abdominal pain. Signs and symptoms of advanced stomach cancer include:

- Epigastric discomfort that may not be relieved by food or antacids
- Abdominal discomfort aggravated by eating
- Black, tarry stools
- Vomiting blood
- Vomiting after meals
- Weakness and fatigue
- Unintended weight loss
- Feeling of fullness after meals, even when eating less than normal

However, other more common conditions, especially peptic ulcers, can cause similar problems.

How is Gastric Carcinoma Diagnosed by Conventional Western Medicine?

To help diagnose stomach cancer and rule out other possibilities, one or more of the following diagnostic tests may be recommended: upper endoscopy, stomach x ray (barium upper GI series), endoscopic ultrasound, CT scan, MRI and chest x ray. Essentials of diagnosis include: (1) dyspeptic symptoms with weight loss in patients over age 40; (2) iron deficiency anemia and occult blood in stools; (3) abnormality detected on upper GI series or endoscopy.

How is Gastric Carcinoma Treated by Conventional Western Medicine?

The kind of treatment for stomach cancer depends on the location of the cancer, how advanced it is, and the overall health and preferences of patients. The goal of treatment is to eliminate the cancer completely, or prevent the tumor from growing. In some cases, palliative care may be best. Treatment options include the following: surgery, chemotherapy, radiation therapy, antibiotics, targeted drug therapy and clinical trials.

What Causes Gastric Carcinoma According to Traditional Chinese Medicine?

1) Improper Diet
2) Emotional Disturbance
3) Weak Constitution

How is Gastric Carcinoma Differentiated and Treated by Traditional Chinese Medicine?

1) <u>Stagnation of Phlegm and Qi</u>

Symptoms: Sensation of fullness, distention or pain in the epigastrium, early satiety, anorexia, or dysphagia, vomiting of sputum and saliva, white and greasy tongue coating, and taut and slippery pulse.

Therapeutic Principle: To regulate qi, resolve phlegm, promote digestion and remove stagnation.

Prescription: Modified Hai Zao Yu Hu Decoction.

Modifications: For distending pain in the epigastrium, add Radix Bupleuri (Chai Hu) 10g, Fructus Citri Sarcodactyli (Fo Shou) 10g and Radix Curcumae (Yu Jin) 10g; for difficult swallowing and vomiting of sputum, saliva and food, add Flos Inulae (Xuan Fu Hua) 10g and Ochra Haematitum (Dai Zhe Shi) 15g; for burning pain in the epigastrium and dry mouth with bitter taste, add Herba Hedyotis Diffusae (Bai Hua She She Cao) 30g, Taraxaci Mongolici Herba cum Radice (Pu Gong Ying) 15g, Herba Scutellaria Barbatae (Ban Zhi Lian) 15g and Herba Solani Nigri (Long Kui) 20g.

2) <u>Incoordination between the Liver and Stomach</u>

Symptoms: Epigastric distention, intermittent vague pain radiating to the hypochondriac region, frequent belching, or dysphagia, red tongue with thin and white or thin and yellow coating, and taut pulse.

Therapeutic Principle: To soothe the liver, regulate the function of the stomach, lower the adverse flow of qi and relieve pain.

Prescription: Modified Chai Hu Shu Gan Powder.

Modifications: For bitter taste in the mouth, dry mouth, distending and burning sensation in the epigastrium, remove Radix Angelicae Sinensis (Dang Gui), Radix Bupleuri (Chai Hu) and Rhizoma Zingiberis Recens (Sheng Jiang), and add Fructus Evodiae Rutaecarpae (Wu Zhu Yu) 3g, Rhizoma Coptidis (Huang Lian) 9g and Radix Scutellariae Baicalensis (Huang Qin) 10g; for constipation and impassable flatus, Semen Trichosanthis (Gua Lou Zi) 12g, Semen Pruni (Yu Li Ren) 10g and Semen Cannabis Sativae (Huo Ma Ren) 12g.

3) <u>Deficiency Cold of the Spleen and Stomach</u>

Symptoms: Lingering vague epigastric pain, which is alleviated by warmth, pressure and intake of warm food, and aggravated by intake of cold food; vomiting of clear fluid, diarrhea, or vomiting of retained food, pale and lusterless complexion, spiritlessness, lassitude, cold limbs, pale and chubby tongue with teeth marks, and white, moist and slippery coating; deep and thready or deep and slow pulse.

Therapeutic Principle: To warm the middle warmer, expel cold, strengthen the spleen and replenish qi.

Prescription: Modified Li Zhong Decoction and Si Jun Zi Decoction.

Modifications: For diarrhea, add Rhizoma Dioscoreae (Shan Yao) 15g, Fructus Psoraleae Corylifoliae (Bu Gu Zhi) 10g and Semen Myristicae Fragrantis (Rou Dou Kou) 10g; for epigastric distention, belching, vomiting, thick, white and greasy tongue coating, add Herba Agastache seu Pogostemonis (Huo Xiang) 9g, Rhizoma Atractylodis (Cang Zhu) 10g and Fructus Amomi Tsao-Ko (Cao Guo) 5g.

4) <u>Stomach Heat Damaging Yin</u>

Symptoms: Postprandial epigastric discomfort, distending pain and burning sensation, acid regurgitation, dry mouth with a desire for cold drinks, feverish sensation in the chest, palms and soles, constipation, dark urine, crimson tongue with little or yellow and dry or peeled coating, and thready and rapid pulse.

Therapeutic Principle: To clear away heat, regulate the function of the stomach, nourish yin and moisten dryness.

Prescription: Modified Yu Nu Decoction.

Modifications: Add Herba Hedyotis Diffusae (Bai Hua She She Cao) 30g, Flos Lonicerae (Jin Yin Hua) 15g and Rhizoma Paridis (Zao Xiu) 9g to relieve heat and remove toxicants; for nausea, belching and vomiting of sputum and saliva, remove Rhizoma Anemarrhenae and add Rhizoma Pinelliae Ternatae (Ban Xia) 10g and Rhizoma Coptidis (Huang Lian) 9g; for abdominal distending pain, add

Radix Aucklandiae Lappae (Mu Xiang) 10g, Pericarpium Areca Catechu (Da Fu Pi) 10g and Rhizoma Corydalis (Yan Hu Suo) 10g; for constipation, add Radix et Rhizoma Rhei (Da Huang) 6g.

5) <u>Internal Blockage of Toxic Blood Stasis</u>

Symptoms: Localized severe epigastric pain radiating to the back, which is aggravated by pressure; epigastric lump, squamous and dry skin, dark or black eye sockets, dark and purple tongue with ecchymosis and sublingual varicosis, and taut and rough pulse.

Therapeutic Principle: To regulate qi, promote blood circulation, remove blood stasis and relieve pain.

Prescription: Modified Ge Xia Zhu Yu Decoction.

Modifications: For burning sensation in the stomach, add Herba Taraxaci Mongolici (Pu Gong Ying) 20g, Fructus Gardeniae Jasminoidis (Zhi Zi) 10g; for hematemesis and melena, add Rhizoma Bletillae Striatae (Bai Ji) 10g and Radix Sanguisorbae Officinalis (Di Yu) 12g.

6) <u>Accumulation of Phlegm and Dampness in the Stomach</u>

Symptoms: Epigastric distention, vomiting of sputum and saliva, dysphagia, insipid mouth, anorexia, alternate constipation and diarrhea, chubby tongue with teeth marks, white, thick and greasy tongue coating, and slippery pulse.

Therapeutic Principle: To dry dampness, strengthen the spleen, resolve phlegm and regulate the function of the stomach.

Prescription: Modified Kai Yu Er Chen Decoction.

Modifications: For shortness of breath and fatigue, Radix Astragali (Huang Qi) 12g and Radix Codonopsitis Pilosulae (Dang Shen) 9g; for frequent vomiting, add Rhizoma Zingiberis Recens (Sheng Jiang) 10g and Herba Agastache seu Pogostemonis (Huo Xiang) 10g.

7) <u>Deficiency of Qi and Blood</u>

Symptoms: Spiritlessness, lassitude, lusterless complexion, shortness of breath, indolence of speaking, dyspnea on exertion, spontaneous sweating, emaciation, pale tongue with teeth marks on the margin, thin and white tongue coating, and deep, thready and forceless or deficiency, large and forceless.

Therapeutic Principle: To replenish qi, nourish blood, strengthen the spleen and invigorate the kidney.

Prescription: Modified Ba Zhen Decoction.

Modifications: For dry mouth and feverish sensation in the chest, palms and soles, add Radix Adenophorae (Sha Shen) 12g and Radix Ophiopogonis Japonici (Mai Dong) 12g; for palpitation and insomnia, add Concha Margaritiferae (Zhen Zhu Mu) 15g and Fructus Ziziphi Jujubae (Da Zao) 20g.

What Kinds of Chinese Patent Drugs are Available to Treat Gastric Carcinoma?

1) Xi Huang Pill: 3g each time, thrice daily.
2) Liu Shen Pill: 20 pills each time, thrice daily.
3) Mu Xiang Shun Qi Pill: 6g each time, twice daily.

7. Carcinoma of Esophagus

Esophageal cancer usually develops in people between age 50 and 70. The overall ratio of men to women is 3:1. Esophageal cancer starts in the inner layer of the esophagus and can occur almost anywhere along the length of the esophagus. The types of esophageal cancer include squamous cell carcinoma, adenocarcinoma and other types such as sarcoma, lymphoma, small cell carcinoma and spindle cell carcinoma. In addition, breast cancer or lung cancer can metastasize through the bloodstream or lymph system to the esophagus.

Contributing factors that can lead to esophageal cancer include heavy alcohol consumption, tobacco use, chronic acid reflux, exposure to silica dust, diet, and obesity. The risk of cancer is also increased in patients with achalasia, esophageal webs and tylosis. A vast majority of esophageal adenocarcinomas develop as a complication of Barrett's esophagus due to chronic gastroesophageal reflux. Survival rates have improved in part because close monitoring of Barrett's esophagus can help detect cancer early. Even more important is that diet and lifestyle changes can significantly reduce the chances of developing cancer.

Usually, there are no signs and symptoms of esophageal cancer in the early stages of the disease. The symptoms of advanced esophageal cancer may include:

- Solid food dysphagia
- Sometimes odynophagia (pain on swallowing)
- Severe, unintentional weight loss.
- Pain in the throat, in the mid-chest or between the shoulder blades
- Hoarseness, a chronic cough and sometimes coughing of blood

How is Carcinoma of Esophagus Diagnosed by Conventional Western Medicine?

Diagnosis is made based on symptoms, physical exam and diagnostic tests such as barium esophagram and upper endoscopy.

Esophageal cancers are staged using the numbers 0 through IV. In general, the higher the number the more advanced the cancer. To help stage esophageal cancer, one or more of these staging tests may be performed: bronchoscopy, CT scan, endoscopic ultrasound, and positron emission tomography (PET) scan. If a person is at high risk of esophageal cancer, screening testes, such as regular endoscopic examinations and biopsies, may be recommended.

How is Carcinoma of Esophagus Treated by Conventional Western Medicine?

Treatment for esophageal cancer depends on the type, location and stage of cancer as well as on the age, overall health and personal preferences. The goal of treatment is to eliminate the cancer completely or prevent the tumor from growing. In some cases, an approach called palliative care may be best.

Treatment options include surgery (esophagectomy, esophagogastrectomy), chemotherapy, radiation therapy, photodynamic therapy, gene therapy, immunotherapy and clinical trials. Combinations of surgery, chemotherapy and radiation may be more effective than any single treatment.

What Causes Carcinoma of Esophagus According to Traditional Chinese Medicine?

1) Emotional Disturbance
2) Improper Diet
3) Deficiency of Healthy Qi

How is Carcinoma of Esophagus Differentiated and Treated by Traditional Chinese Medicine?

1) <u>Stagnation of Phlegm and Qi</u>

Symptoms: Dysphagia, substernal fullness, distention or pain that is alleviated by ease of mind and aggravated by meals, belching or hiccup, or regurgitation of sputum, saliva and undigested food, dry mouth, irritability, red tongue with thin and greasy coating, and taut and slippery pulse.

Therapeutic Principle: To relieve stagnation, resolve phlegm, moisten dryness and lower adverse flow of qi.

Prescription: Modified Qi Ge Powder.

Modifications: For dysphagia, add Fructus Citri Aurantii (Zhi Ke) 10g, Pericarpium Trichosanthis (Gua Lou Pi) 10g and Concha Arcae (Wa Leng Zi) 15g; for chest fullness, add Exocarpium Citri Rubrum (Ju Hong) 10g, Radix Bupleuri (Chai Hu) 10g, Fructus Citri Aurantii (Zhi Ke) 10g, Fructus Akebia (Ba Yue Zha) 10g and Rhizoma Pinelliae Ternatae (Ban Xia) 10g; for frequent belching and vomiting of sputum and saliva, add Flos Inulae (Xuan Fu Hua) 10g, Ochra Haematitum (Dai Zhe Shi) 15g, Rhizoma Pinelliae Ternatae (Ban Xia) 10g, Pericarpium Citri Reticulatae (Chen Pi) 6g and

Caulis Bambusae in Taeniam (Zhu Ru) 10g; for dry mouth and throat, add Radix Rehmanniae (Di Huang) 15g, Radix Scrophulariae Ningpoensis (Xuan Shen) 12g, Radix Ophiopogonis Japonici (Mai Dong) 12g and Radix Trichosanthis (Tian Hua Fei) 12g.

2) Consumption of Body Fluid by Heat Accumulation

Symptoms: Substernal pain on swallowing, dysphagia for solid food but not for liquids, progressive weight loss, feverish sensation in the chest, palms and soles, dry mouth and throat, constipation, red and dry tongue with crackles, and thready and rapid pulse.

Therapeutic Principle: To clear away heat, disperse mass, nourish yin and moisten dryness.

Prescription: Modified Wu Zhi An Zhong Decoction.

Modifications: For dysphagia for solid food and liquids, remove Succus Bambosae (Zhu Li) and add Caulis Bambusae in Taeniam (Zhu Ru) 10g, Folium Eriobotryae Japonicae (Pi Pa Ye) 12g, Rhizoma Phragmitis Communis (Lu Gen) 20g and Radix Trichosanthis (Tian Hua Fen) 12g; for constipation, add Semen Cannabis Sativae (Huo Ma Ren) 12g and Radix Polygoni Multiflori (He Shou Wu) 15g; for abdominal distention, dyschezia and severe heat in the stomach and intestine, add Da Huang Gan Cao Decoction.

3) Internal Stagnation of Phlegm and Blood

Symptoms: Localized substernal pricking or stabbing pain, solid food dysphagia, postprandial vomiting, or even dysphagia for liquids, or vomiting of sputum, saliva, clear fluid, or foul smelling undigested food; emaciation, spiritlessness, squamous and dry skin, pale and purple tongue with greasy coating, and thready and rough pulse.

Therapeutic Principle: To nourish blood, remove blood stasis, disperse mass and relieve stagnation.

Prescription: Modified Tong You Decoction.

Modifications: For qi stagnation and blood stasis with chest distending pain, add Xue Fu Zhu Yu Decoction; for dysphagia, add Fructus Citri Aurantii (Zhi Ke) 10g, Pericarpium Trichosanthis (Gua Lou Pi) 10g, Semen Canavaliae (Dao Dou) 12g, Radix Scrophulariae Ningpoensis (Xuan Shen) 12g and Radix Platycodi Grandiflori (Jie Gen) 9g; for vomiting during meals, add Flos Inulae (Xuan Fu Hua) 10g, Ochra Haematitum (Dai Zhe Shi) 15g, Succus Bambosae (Zhu Li) 30g and Rhizoma zingiberis officinalis (Shen Jiang) 10g; for vomiting of sputum and saliva, add Rhizoma Pinelliae Ternatae (Ban Xia) 10g, Pumex (Fu Hai Shi) 9g, Bulbus Fritillariae Cirrhosae (Chuan Bei Mu) 10g, Exocarpium Citri Grandis Rubrum (Hua Ju Hong) 10g and Pseudobulbus Cremastrae seu Pleiones (Shan Ci Gu) 5g; for severe substernal pain, add Pericarpium Citri Reticulatae Viride (Qing Pi) 10g, Radix

Aucklandiae Lappae (Mu Xiang) 10g, Rhizoma Corydalis (Yan Hu Suo) 10g and Excrementum Trogopteri seu Pteromydis (Wu Ling Zhi) 10g.

4) <u>Depletion of Yin and Deficiency of Blood</u>

Symptoms: Sensation of dryness, roughness and pain in the chest, dysphagia for solid food and liquids, emaciation, dry and squamous skin, feverish sensation in the chest, palms and soles, constipation with dry and hard stools, or infrequent defecation, red tongue with little moisture, and thready, rapid and forceless pulse.

Therapeutic Principle: To nourish yin, replenish blood, disperse mass and relieve stagnation.

Prescription: Modified Sha Shen Mai Dong Decoction.

Modifications: For internal heart due to yin deficiency, add Rhizoma Anemarrhenae (Zhi Mu) 10g and Radix Stellariae Dichotomae (Yin Chai Hu) 10g.

5) <u>Deficiency of Qi and Yang</u>

Symptoms: Chronic dysphagia, pale complexion with edema, spiritlessness, cold limbs, shortness of breath, regurgitation of clear fluid, edema of the lower limbs, abdominal distention, even difficult urination and defecation, pale and chubby tongue with white coating, and thready and weak pulse.

Therapeutic Principle: To warm and nourish the spleen and kidney, replenish qi and restore yang from collapse.

Prescription: Modified Bu Qi Yun Pi Decoction.

Modifications: For vomiting with inability to eat, add Flos Inulae (Xuan Fu Hua) 10g and Ochra Haematitum (Dai Zhe Shi) 15g; for deficiency of qi and yin, add Herba Dendrobii (Shi Hu) 10g, Radix Ophiopogonis Japonici (Mai Dong) 12g and Radix Adenophorae (Sha Shen) 12g; for excess syndrome of phlegm stagnation, add Semen Malvae (Dong Kui Zi) 12g, Spica Prunellae Vulgaris (Xia Ku Cao) 12g and Herba Hedyotis Diffusae (Bai Hua She She Cao) 20g.

What Kinds of Chinese Patent Drugs are Available to Treat Carcinoma of Esophagus?

1) Mei Hua Dian She Pill: 2-3 pills each time, twice daily.
2) Liu Shen Pill: 10 pills each time, 4 times daily.
3) Xi Huang Pill: 3g each time, twice daily.

8. Carcinoma of the Large Intestine (Colon Cancer, Colorectal Carcinoma)

Colon cancer and rectal cancer are often referred to as colorectal cancers, and they make up the second-leading cause of cancer-related deaths in the United States. Most cases of colon cancer begin as small, benign clumps of cells called adenomatous polyps. Over time some of these polyps become cancerous. So it's important to get regular screening tests to help prevent colon cancer. Polyps can occur anywhere in the large intestine. They are either mushroom-shaped or flat and may be large or small. There are also several different types of colon polyps. Among the most common are: adenomas, hyperplastic polyps and inflammatory polyps. Risk factors for colon and rectal cancers include:

- Age. Colon and rectal cancers can occur at any age, however, about 90 percent of people with the disease are older than 50
- Inflammatory bowel disease
- Family history
- Diet
- A sedentary lifestyle
- Diabetes
- Smoking
- Alcohol
- A personal history of colorectal cancer or polyps

Despite the relatively high number of cases and deaths, screening tests, along with diet and lifestyle changes, can dramatically reduce the overall risk of developing colon cancer.

Adenocarcinomas grow slowly and may be present for several years before symptoms appear. Signs and symptoms depend upon tumor location. Proximal colon cancer may cause fecal occult blood and anemia; distal colon cancer may have changes in bowel habits and hematochezia. Warning signs and symptoms may include:

- A change in the bowel habits
- Narrow stools
- Rectal bleeding or blood in the stool
- Persistent abdominal discomfort, such as cramps, gas or pain
- Abdominal pain with a bowel movement
- A feeling that the bowel doesn't empty completely
- Unexplained weight loss

How is Colon Cancer Diagnosed by Conventional Western Medicine?

Most colon cancers develop from adenomatous polyps. Screening is extremely important for detecting polyps before they become cancerous. Common screening and diagnostic procedures include the following:

- Digital rectal exam
- Fecal occult (hidden) blood test
- Flexible sigmoidoscopy
- Barium enema
- Colonoscopy
- Genetic testing
- New technologies, such as virtual colonoscopy

How is Colon Cancer Treated by Conventional Western Medicine?

The type of treatment will depend largely on the stage of colon cancer. The treatment options are surgery, chemotherapy, radiation, monoclonal antibody therapy and follow-up care.

What Causes Colon Cancer According to Traditional Chinese Medicine?

1) Constitutional Deficiency of the Spleen and Kidney
2) Improper Diet
3) Accumulation of Toxic Heat
4) Fire and Dampness Flowing Downwards to the Intestines
5) Deficiency of Healthy Qi

How is Colon Cancer Differentiated and Treated by Traditional Chinese Medicine?

1) <u>Accumulation of Toxic Damp-Heat</u>

Symptoms: Abdominal distention, abdominal pain aggravated by pressure, blood stained stools, tenesmus, or fever, stuffy sensation in the chest, anorexia, burning sensation in the anus, crimson tongue with yellow and greasy coating, and taut and rapid or taut and slippery pulse.

Therapeutic Principle: To clear away heat, promote diuresis, remove toxic substances and eliminate mass.

Prescription: Modified Di Yu Powder.

Modifications: For severe abdominal pain, add Radix Paeoniae Alba (Bai Shao Yao) 10g and Radix Glycyrrhizae Uralensis (Gan Cao) 6g; for stuffy sensation in the chest, anorexia and abdominal distention, add Semen Armeniacae Amarum (Xin Ren) 10g, Radix Platycodi Grandiflori (Jie Gen) 9g, Fructus Crataegi (Shan Zha) 10g, Fructus Meliae Toosendan (Chuan Lian Zi) 10g, Fructus Citri Aurantii (Zhi Ke) 10g, Radix Aucklandiae Lappae (Mu Xiang) 9g and Semen Areca Catechu (Bing Lang) 10g.

2) <u>Stagnation of Toxic Substances and Blood Stasis</u>

Symptoms: Localized pricking abdominal pain aggravated by pressure, palpable abdominal mass, abdominal tenderness, hematochezia with pus, fever or no fever, dark and purple tongue with ecchymosis, thin and yellow tongue coating, and rough or thready and rapid pulse.

Therapeutic Principle: To promote blood circulation, remove blood stasis and toxic substances and disperse mass.

Prescription: Modified Ge Xia Zhu Yu Decoction.

Modifications: For severe purulent and bloody stools, add Radix Pulsatillae Chinensis (Bai Tou Weng) 10g, Herba Portulacae (Ma Chi Xian) 12g, Radix Notoginseng (San Qi) 10g, Herba Agrimoniae Pilosae (Xian He Cao) 12g and Radix Sanguisorbae Officinalis (Di Yu) 12g; for fever, add Radix Sophorae Flavescentis (Ku Shen) 9g, Rhizoma Smilacis Glabrae (Tu Fu Ling) 20g, Taraxaci Mongolici Herba cum Radice (Pu Gong Ying) 15g and Herba cum Radice Violae (Zi Hua Di Ding) 15g.

3) <u>Yang Deficiency of the Spleen and Kidney</u>

Symptoms: Dim complexion, shortness of breath, indolence of speaking, aversion to cold, cold limbs, abdominal pain that is relieved by warmth, anorexia or chronic diarrhea and dysentery, pale and chubby tongue with white coating, and deep, thready and weak pulse.

Therapeutic Principle: To warm and nourish the spleen and kidney, promote diuresis and relieve diarrhea.

Prescription: Modified Fu Zi Li Zhong Decoction and Si Shen Pill.

Modifications: For anorexia, add Fructus Crataegi (Shan Zha) 12g, Fructus Hordei Germinatus (Mai Ya) 12g and Endothelium Corneum Gigeriae Galli (Ji Nei Jin) 10g; for severe diarrhea, add Fructus Terminaliae Chebulae (He Zi) 10g, Pericarpium Papaveris (Ying Su Ke) 10g, Semen Plantaginis (Che Qian Zi) 10g and Acaciae seu Uncariae Pasta (Er Cha) 2g; for shortness of breath and fatigue, add Radix Astragali (Huang Qi) 12g and Radix Ginseng (Ren Shen) 6g.

4) <u>Deficiency of Qi and Blood</u>

Symptoms: Palpitation, shortness of breath, lusterless complexion, pale lips and nails, emaciation, lassitude, anorexia, prolapse of anus, pale tongue with thin and white coating, and deep and thready pulse.

Therapeutic Principle: To replenish qi and blood, nourish the kidney and strengthen the spleen.

Prescription: Modified Ba Zhen Decoction.

Modifications: For cold limbs, add Cortex Cinnamomi Cassiae (Rou Gui) 3g, Rhizoma Zingiberis Officinalis (Gan Jiang) 10g and Radix Glycyrrhizae Uralensis (Gan Cao) 6g; for prolapse of anus, add Rhizoma Cimicifugae (Sheng Ma) 10g, Radix Bupleuri (Chai Hu) 10g, Fructus Schisandrae Chinensis

(Wu Wei Zi) 3g and Fructus Citri Aurantii (Zhi Ke) 10g; for poor appetite, add Fructus Crataegi (Shan Zha) 12g, Fructus Hordei Germinatus (Mai Ya) 12g and Endothelium Corneum Gigeriae Galli (Ji Nei Jin) 10g.

5) Hyperactivity of Fire due to Yin Deficiency

Symptoms: Emaciation, feverish sensation in the chest, palms, and soles, vertigo, weak and sore loins and knees, bitter taste in the mouth, dry throat, or constipation, red tongue with no or little coating, and thready and weak or thready and rapid pulse.

Therapeutic Principle: To replenish the liver and kidney, nourish yin and clear away heat.

Prescription: Modified Zhi Bai Di Huang Decoction.

Modifications: For severe heat syndrome, add Fructus Gardeniae Jasminoidis (Zhi Zi) 10g and Herba Artemisiae Apiaceae seu Annuae (Qing Hao) 10g; for vertigo, add Magnetitum (Ci Shi) 10g, Concha Haliotidis (Shi Jue Ming) 20g, Rhizoma Acori Tatarinowii (Shi Chang Pu) 10g and Radix Curcumae (Yu Jin) 10g; for insomnia, add Rhizoma Coptidis (Huang Lian) 9g and Cortex Cinnamomi Cassiae (Rou Gui) 3g.

9. Primary Carcinoma of the Liver

Primary liver cancer begins in the cells of the liver itself. New cases of primary liver cancer are increasing in the United States and are likely to continue to increase for the next two decades. Most cancers found in the liver are metastatic cancers. Because liver cancer is rarely discovered early and is difficult to control with current treatments, the prognosis is often poor.

Several types of liver cancer exist, each with its own set of causes. Types of primary liver cancer include hepatocellular carcinoma (HCC), cholangiocarcinoma, hepatoblastoma, and angiosarcoma or hemangiosarcoma. The causes of liver cancer include:

- Hepatitis B and C
- Cirrhosis
- Long-term exposure to aflatoxins
- Vinyl chloride and thorium dioxide (Thorotrast)
- Arsenic
- Primary biliary cirrhosis
- Ulcerative colitis

Liver cancer can affect people of all ages and races, but certain factors may increase the risk. Men are twice as likely to develop liver cancer as women are. Asian-Americans have the highest rate of liver cancer in the United States due to high rates of chronic hepatitis B infection. American blacks and Hispanics are more likely to develop liver cancer than whites are, but their risk is more moderate than it is for immigrants from Asian countries where hepatitis B infection is endemic. In the United States, liver cancer occurs most often in people age 60 and older. Other risk factors include:

- Chronic infection with HBV or HCV
- Cirrhosis
- Diabetes.
- Certain gene mutations
- Exposure to aflatoxins
- Excessive alcohol consumption.
- Smoking

Most people don't have signs and symptoms in the early stages of liver cancer. Symptoms of advanced liver cancer may include:

- Loss of appetite and weight
- Abdominal pain, especially in the upper right quadrant, that may radiate into the back and shoulder
- Nausea and vomiting
- General weakness and fatigue
- Hepatomegaly
- Abdominal swelling (ascites)
- Jaundice

How is Liver Cancer Diagnosed by Conventional Western Medicine?

Although AFP screening can detect small tumors in some people, most liver cancer isn't diagnosed early. Diagnosis is made based on medical history, physical exam, and one or more of the following tests, such as ultrasonography, CT scan, MRI, liver biopsy and blood tests.

How is Liver Cancer Treated by Conventional Western Medicine?

Treatments for primary liver cancer depend on the stage of the disease as well as patient's age, overall health, feelings and personal preferences. The goal of any treatment is to eliminate the cancer completely or prevent the tumor from growing. In some cases the treatment option is palliative care.

Standard therapies for adult liver cancer primarily include surgery, radiation therapy and chemotherapy. Other treatments may include alcohol injections, electric current therapy, cryosurgery or cryotherapy, liver transplantation and clinical trials.

What Causes Primary Liver Cancer According to Traditional Chinese Medicine?

1) Stagnation of Liver Qi due to Emotional Disturbance

2) Dysfunction of the Spleen in Transformation and Transportation due to Improper Diet and Overstrain

3) Qi Stagnation and Blood Stasis

4) Accumulation of Phlegm

5) Toxic Heat Accumulation

6) Incoordination between the Liver, Spleen and Kidney

How is Primary Liver Cancer Differentiated and Treated by Traditional Chinese Medicine?

1) <u>Qi Stagnation and Blood Stasis</u>

Symptoms: Distending pain in the hypochondriac region, fixed and localized abdominal mass, distention and fullness in the abdomen and hypochondrium, anorexia, lassitude, belching, acid regurgitation, loose stools, red or crimson tongue with ecchymosis, thin and white or thin and yellow tongue coating, and taut or rough pulse.

Therapeutic Principle: To soothe the liver, regulate qi, promote blood circulation and remove blood stasis.

Prescription: Modified Xiao Yao Powder and Tao Hong Si Wu Decoction.

Modifications: For insufficiency of spleen qi, add Radix Astragali (Huang Qi) 12g and Radix Codonopsitis Pilosulae (Dang Shen) 9g; for anorexia, add Fructus Crataegi (Shan Zha) 12g, Fructus Hordei Germinatus (Mai Ya) 12g and Endothelium Corneum Gigeriae Galli (Ji Nei Jin) 10g.

2) <u>Accumulation of Damp-Heat</u>

Symptoms: Firm or hard mass and pricking pain in the hypochondriac region, abdominal distention and fullness, progressive jaundice, dim and lusterless complexion, squamous and dry skin, or high fever, dysphoria with thirst, dry throat, bitter taste in the mouth, dark urine, dry and black stools, red tongue with ecchymosis, yellow and greasy tongue coating, and taut and rapid or rough pulse.

Therapeutic Principle: To clear away heat, resolve dampness, remove stasis, normalize the function of gallbladder and remove toxic substances.

Prescription: Modified Yin Chen Hao Decoction and Bie Jia Jian Pill.

Modifications: For severe pain in the liver area, add Gummi Olibanum (Ru Xiang) 10g, Myrrha (Mo Yao) 10g, Rhizoma Corydalis (Yan Hu Suo) 10g and Radix Curcumae (Yu Jin) 10g; for remarkable ascites, add Semen Pharbitidis (Qian Niu Zi) 10g, Herba Lycopi Lucidi (Ze Lan) 12g and Pericarpium Areca Catechu (Da Fu Pi) 10g.

3) <u>Yin Deficiency of the Liver and Kidney</u>

Symptoms: Enlarged abdomen with mass, abdominal distention and fullness, emaciation, hectic fever, night sweating, vertigo, weak and sore loins and knees, dull pain in the hypochondriac region, oliguria, constipation, red tongue with little or smooth, peeled or cracked coating, and taut and thready or thready and rapid pulse.

Therapeutic Principle: To nourish yin, soothe the liver and disperse mass.

Prescription: Modified Zi Shui Qing Gan Decoction and Bie Jia Jian Pill.

Modifications: For deficiency of qi, add Radix Astragali (Huang Qi) 12g and Radix Pseudostellariae Heterophyllae (Tai Zi Shen) 15g; for low-grade fever, add Herba Artemisiae Apiaceae seu Annuae (Qing Hao) 10g, Radix Stellariae Dichotomae (Yin Chai Hu) 10g and Cortex Lycii Radicis (Di Gu Pi) 10g.

What Kinds of Chinese Patent Drugs are Available to Treat Primary Liver Cancer?

1) Gan Fu Le Tablet: 10 tablets each time, thrice daily.
2) Fu Fang Mu Ji Granule: 1 bag each time, thrice daily.
3) Lian Hua Tablet: 6-8 tablets each time, thrice daily.

10. Hepatic Cirrhosis

Cirrhosis is the end result of hepatocellular injury that leads to both fibrosis and nodular regeneration throughout the liver. As fibrosis and nodular regeneration replace normal tissue, blood flow through the liver is affected. This makes it increasingly difficult for the liver to carry out essential functions, such as detoxifying harmful substances, purifying blood and manufacturing vital nutrients.

Excessive use of alcohol and chronic infection with the hepatitis C virus are the leading causes of cirrhosis. Chronic alcoholism is the primary cause of cirrhosis in the United States. Alcoholic cirrhosis usually occurs after a decade or more of heavy drinking, although the amount of alcohol that can injure the liver varies from person to person. Other factors can cause liver scarring include chronic hepatitis B, autoimmune disorder, nonalcoholic steatohepatitis, inherited diseases, blocked or inflamed bile ducts, and prolonged exposure to toxic materials.

Cirrhosis rarely causes signs and symptoms in its early stages. But as liver function deteriorates, cirrhosis may cause a number of signs, symptoms and complications:

- Anorexia

- Weight loss
- Nausea and occasional vomiting
- Spider nevi, palmar erythema, glossitis and cheilosis
- Easy bruising
- Weakness
- Fatigue
- Jaundice
- Abdominal pain
- Itching
- Possible fever
- Bleeding from engorged veins in the esophagus or intestines
- Loss of libido, impotence, or sterility
- Menstrual abnormalities
- Ascites, pleural effusion, or peripheral edema
- Encephalopathy
- Hepatomegaly or splenomegaly

How is Hepatic Cirrhosis Diagnosed by Conventional Western Medicine?

Diagnosis is made based on medical history, physical exam and certain tests such as liver blood tests, bilirubin test, ultrasound, CT scan, MRI and liver biopsy.

How is Hepatic Cirrhosis Treated by Conventional Western Medicine?

Specific treatment for cirrhosis depends on the underlying cause. Although liver damage from cirrhosis is irreversible, treatment can often help prevent further damage and reduce complications. The most important principle of treatment is abstinence from alcohol and other substances that harm the liver. Nutrition is also often a key part of therapy. In the presence of fluid retention, sodium restriction should be applied. Vitamin supplementation is also desirable.

In addition to treating the cause of cirrhosis, complications should be treated and prevented. Complications of cirrhosis include portal hypertension, varices, bruising and bleeding, fluid retention, itching, hepatic encephalopathy, Jaundice, osteoporosis, liver cancer and liver failure.

What Causes Hepatic Cirrhosis According to Traditional Chinese Medicine?

1) Improper Diet and Binge
2) Emotional Disturbance

3) Infection and Fluke

4) Transformation from Other Disorders.

How is Hepatic Cirrhosis Differentiated and Treated by Traditional Chinese Medicine?

1) <u>Stagnation of Qi and Dampness</u>

Symptoms: Abdominal enlargement, distention and fullness that is soft by palpation, distending pain in the hypochondriac region, anorexia, postprandial distention that is alleviated by belching or passing flatus, oliguria, thin, white and greasy tongue coating, and taut pulse.

Therapeutic Principle: To soothe the liver, regulate qi, invigorate the spleen and promote diuresis.

Prescription: Modified Chai Hu Shu Gan Powder and Wei Ling Decoction.

Modifications: For severe abdominal distention, add Radix Aucklandiae Lappae (Mu Xiang) 10g, Pericarpium Areca Catechu (Da Fu Pi) 10g and Lignum Aquilariae Resinatum (Chen Xiang) 1g; for hypochondriac pain, add Radix Salviae Miltiorrhizae (Dan Shen) 10g, Rhizoma Corydalis (Yan Hu Suo) 10g and Fructus Meliae Toosendan (Chuan Lian Zi) 10g; for anorexia and diarrhea, add Rhizoma Zingiberis Officinalis (Gan Jiang) 10g and Radix Aconiti Lateralis Praeparatae (Fu Zi) 10g.

2) <u>Retention of Cold-Damp in the Spleen</u>

Symptoms: Enlargement, distention and fullness in the abdomen, which feels like a bag full of water; edema in severe cases, aversion to cold, physical inactivity, spiritlessness, abdominal distention that is relieved by warmth, anorexia, diarrhea, oliguria, white and slippery or white and greasy tongue coating, and slow or deep and slow pulse.

Therapeutic Principle: To warm the middle warmer, dispel cold, promote qi circulation and induce diuresis.

Prescription: Modified Shi Pi Decoction.

Modifications: For remarkable edema and oliguria, add Sclerotium Poriae Cocos (Fu Ling) 12g, Cortex Cinnamomi Cassiae (Rou Gui) 3g and Rhizoma Alismatis Orientalis (Ze Xie) 10g; for abdominal distention and fullness, add Fructus Citri Aurantii (Zhi Ke) 10g and Fructus Amomi Villosi (Sha Ren) 5g; for hypochondriac pain, add Rhizoma Corydalis (Yan Hu Suo) 10g, Rhizoma Cyperi Rotundi (Xiang Fu) 10g and Pericarpium Citri Reticulatae Viride (Qing Pi) 10g.

3) <u>Accumulation of Damp-Heat in the Spleen</u>

Symptoms: Hard abdominal enlargement, fullness and distention, dysphoria with feverish sensation, bitter taste in the mouth, thirst without a desire to drink, or jaundice, oliguria with yellow urine, constipation, or dyschezia with loose stool, red tongue with yellow and greasy or gray and black coating, and taut, slippery and rapid pulse.

Therapeutic Principle: To clear away heat, eliminate dampness and promote diuresis.

Prescription: Modified Zhong Man Fen Xiao Pill and Yin Chen Hao Decoction.

Modifications: For jaundice, remove Radix Ginseng (Ren Shen), Fructus Amomi Villosi (Sha Ren) and Rhizoma Zingiberis Officinalis (Gan Jiang), and add Rhizoma Polygoni Cuspidati (Hu Zhang) 20g and Herba Lysimachiae (Jin Qian Cao) 20g; for difficult urination and oliguria with dark urine, add Herba Verbenae (Ma Bian Cao) 20g and Talcum (Hua Shi Fen) 10g; for severe abdominal distention, persistent ascites, oliguria and constipation, add Zhou Che Pill, Radix Euphorbia Kansui (Gan Sui) 0.5g or Yu Gong Powder.

4) <u>Blood Stasis in the Liver and Spleen</u>

Symptoms: Abdominal enlargement, distention and fullness, varicosis on the abdominal wall, pricking pain in the hypochondriac region and abdomen, darkish gray or black complexion, hypochondriac mass, spider nevi or red threads on the upper half of the body, palmar erythema (mottled redness of the thenar and hypothenar eminences), dry mouth without a desire to drink, or melena, dark and purple tongue with ecchymosis, and thready and rough pulse.

Therapeutic Principle: To promote blood circulation, remove blood stasis, regulate qi circulation and resolve masses.

Prescription: Modified Tiao Ying Decoction.

Modifications: For hypochondriac mass, add Rhizoma Sparganii Stoloniferi (San Leng) 10g, Rhizoma Curcumae Ezhu (E Zhu) 10g and Squama Manitis Pentadactylae (Chuan Shan Jia) 10g; for melena, add Pollen Typhae (Pu Huang) 10g, Radix Notoginseng (San Qi) 10g and Radix Rubiae Cordifoliae (Qian Cao) 12g; for severe ascites, add Sclerotium Polypori Umbellati (Zhu Ling) 10g, Semen Plantaginis (Che Qian Zi) 9g and Herba Verbenae (Ma Bian Cao) 20g; for persistent ascites after the above treatment, use Zhou Che Pill.

5) <u>Yang Deficiency of the Spleen and Kidney</u>

Symptoms: Enlargement, distention and fullness in the abdomen, which looks like the abdomen of a frog in a supine position; malaise, aversion to cold, pale and yellow or pale and lusterless complexion, epigastric stuffiness, anorexia, edema of the lower limbs, difficult urination, oliguria, pale and chubby tongue with white and slippery coating, and deep, slow and forceless pulse.

Therapeutic Principle: To warm the kidney, nourish the spleen, regulate qi circulation and induce diuresis.

Prescription: Modified Fu Zi Li Zhong Decoction and Wu Ling Powder.

Modifications: For varicosis of the abdominal wall, add Radix Salviae Miltiorrhizae (Dan Shen) 10g and Hirudo seu Whitmania (Shui Zhi) 5g; for malaise, lassitude, shortness of breath and indolence of speaking, add Radix Astragali (Huang Qi) 12g, Semen Coicis (Yi Yi Ren) 15g and Semen Dolichoris Lablab (Bian Dou) 20g; for lusterless complexion, aversion to cold, weak and sore loins and knees, use Ji Sheng Shen Qi Pill.

6) <u>Yin Deficiency of the Liver and Kidney</u>

Symptoms: Abdominal enlargement, distention and fullness, dilated superficial veins of the abdomen and thorax in severe cases, dark and gloomy complexion, dry mouth and tongue, dysphoria, insomnia, gingival hemorrhage and atrophy, occasional epistaxis, oliguria, crimson tongue with little moisture and coating, and taut, thready and rapid pulse.

Therapeutic Principle: To nourish the liver and kidney, regulate qi circulation and induce diuresis.

Prescription: Modified Yi Guan Decoction and Ge Xia Zhu Yu Decoction.

Modifications: For bitter taste in the mouth, dry mouth and throat, add Herba Dendrobii (Shi Hu) 10g, Radix Adenophorae (Sha Shen) 10g, Radix Scrophulariae Ningpoensis (Xuan Shen) 10g and Rhizoma Imperatae Cylindricae (Bai Mao Gen) 20g; for bleeding of the gums and epistaxis, add Cacumen Biotae Orientalis (Ce Bai Ye) 10g, Nodus Nelumbinis Nuciferae Rhizomatis (Ou Jie) 12g and Herba Agrimoniae Pilosae (Xian He Cao) 12g; for oliguria, add Semen Plantaginis (Che Qian Zi) 9g, Talcum (Hua Shi Fen) 10g and Sclerotium Polypori Umbellati (Zhu Ling) 10g; for vertigo and flushed face, add Carapax et Plastrum Testudinis (Gui Ban) 20g, Carapax Trionycis (Bie Jia) 20g and Concha Ostreae (Mu Li) 20g; for hectic fever and night sweating, Radix Stellariae Dichotomae (Yin Chai Hu) 10g, Cortex Lycii Radicis (Di Gu Pi) 10g and Herba Artemisiae Apiaceae seu Annuae (Qing Hao) 10g.

What Kinds of Chinese Patent Drugs are Available to Treat Hepatic Cirrhosis?

1) Da Huang Zhe Chong Pill: 5 pills (3g) each time, thrice daily.
2) Bie Jia Jian Pill: 7 pills each time, thrice daily.
3) Hu Dan Tablet: 4 tablets each time, thrice daily.
4) Wu Pi Pill: 9g each time, twice daily.

11. Hepatic Encephalopathy/Hepatic Coma

Hepatic encephalopathy is a state of disordered central nervous system function resulting from failure of the liver to detoxify noxious agents of gut origin because of hepatocellular dysfunction and portosystemic shunting. Ammonia, which is a byproduct of protein digestion, is the most readily identified toxin that can damage the brain, leading to changes in mental state, behavior and personality. Symptoms of hepatic encephalopathy include forgetfulness, confusion and mood changes, and in advanced cases, delirium and coma. Many factors can cause hepatic encephalopathy. These factors include:

- Enhanced sensitivity of central nervous system neurons to GABA, an inhibitory neurotransmitter
- Increased circulating levels of endogenous benzodiazepines
- Bleeding into the intestinal tract
- Alkalosis
- Medications containing ammonium or amino compounds
- Paracentesis with attendant hypovolemia
- Hepapic or systemic infection

In patients with progressive hepatic encephalopathy, there is a gradual decrease in level of consciousness, intellectual capacity, and logical behavior along with development of specific neurological deficits.

How is Hepatic Encephalopathy Diagnosed by Conventional Western Medicine?

Hepatic encephalopathy is diagnosed by excluding a variety of metabolic disorders, toxic ingestions, or intracranial processes with similar neuropsychiatric symptoms. Brain imaging or electroencephalography, lumbar puncture with cerebrospinal fluid analysis, venous or serum ammonia level, arterial ammonia concentration, complete blood cell count, electrolyte levels, renal function, and body fluid culture may be required for diagnosis.

How is Hepatic Encephalopathy Treated by Conventional Western Medicine?

Treatment of hepatic encephalopathy includes:

- Withhold dietary protein
- Control gastrointestinal bleedings
- Purge blood from the gastrointestinal tract
- Control ammonia-producing intestinal flora by lactulos or neomycin sulfate
- Avoid narcotics, tranquilizers, and sedatives
- Medications such as oxazepam and flumazenil

What Causes Hepatic Encephalopathy According to Traditional Chinese Medicine?

1) Attack by Exogenous Pathogenic Factors
2) Improper Diet
3) Chronic Diseases not Treated Properly

4) Collapse of Yin and Yang

How is Hepatic Encephalopathy Differentiated and Treated by Traditional Chinese Medicine?

1) <u>Turbid Phlegm Disturbing the Mind</u>

Symptoms: Apathetic and dull expression, drowsiness, delirium, and ultimately lethargy and coma; wheezing sound in the throat, stuffiness in the chest and epigastrium, pale complexion, acid regurgitation, copious amount of sputum, white and greasy tongue coating, and soft and thready pulse.

Therapeutic Principle: To resolve turbidity, remove toxic substances, cause resuscitation and regain consciousness.

Prescription: Modified Chang Pu Yu Jin Decoction.

Modifications: For coma, add Su He Xiang Pill; for abdominal distention and oliguria, add Lignum Aquilariae Resinatum (Chen Xiang) 1g, Succinum (Hu Po) 2g and Herba Verbenae (Ma Bian Cao) 20g.

2) <u>Phlegm-Heat Obstructing the Mind</u>

Symptoms: Fever, flushed face, irritability, delirium, ultimately coma, dyspnea, or enlarged abdomen, jaundice, oliguria, constipation, red tongue with yellow and greasy coating, and slippery and rapid pulse.

Therapeutic Principle: To clear away heat, resolve phlegm, resuscitate the mind and regain consciousness.

Prescription: Modified An Gong Niu Huang Pill and Huang Lian Wen Dan Decoction.

Modifications: For cramps of the extremities, replace the above prescription with Zi Xue Pill; for dyschezia, add Radix et Rhizoma Rhei (Da Huang) 6g and Natrii Sulfas (Mang Xiao) 10g; for hematemesis and epistaxis, add Fructus Gardeniae Jasminoidis (Zhi Zi) 9g, Radix et Rhizoma Rhei (Da Huang) 6g and Radix Notoginseng (San Qi) 9g; for jaundice, add Herba Artemisiae Scopariae (Yin Chen Hao) 15g and Rhizoma Polygoni Cuspidati (Hu Zhang) 15g.

3) <u>Hyperactivity of Toxic-Heat</u>

Symptoms: High fever, irritability, drowsiness, delirium, extremities cramps, jaundice, hypochondriac and abdominal pain, nausea, vomiting, hematemesis, epistaxis, dry mouth, thirst, dark yellow urine, crimson tongue with dry and yellow coating, and taut and rapid pulse.

Therapeutic Principle: To clear away heat, remove toxic substances, cool blood and resuscitate the mind.

Prescription: Modified Xi Jiao Di Huang Decoction.

Modifications: For cramps of the extremities, add Cornu Saigae Tataricae (Ling Yang Jiao) 2g, Ramulus Uncariae cum Uncis (Gou Teng) 12g and Concha Haliotidis (Shi Jue Ming) 20g or use Zi Xue Pill; for severe jaundice, add Yin Chen Hao Decoction; for dry mouth and thirst, add Radix Trichosanthis (Tian Hua Fen) 12g, Radix Ophiopogonis Japonici (Mai Dong) 10g and Rhizoma Imperatae Cylindricae (Bai Mao Gen) 20g.

4) Deficiency of Yang and Qi

Symptoms: Lethargy or coma, no response to calls or circumstances, pale complexion, cyanosis of lips, extremely cold limbs, weak breathing, drenching sweat, jaundice, abdominal distention, oliguria or no urination, fecal incontinence, pale and dark tongue with moist, white and slippery coating, and tinny and extremely faint pulse.

Therapeutic Principle: To replenish qi, recuperate yang and restore yang from collapse.

Prescription: Modified Shen Fu Long Mu Decoction.

Modifications: For dry mouth with a desire to drink, red tongue with little moisture, use Sheng Mai Decoction.

What Kinds of Chinese Patent Drugs are Available to Treat Hepatic Encephalopathy?

1) Xing Nao Jing Injection: 4ml each time intramuscularly, 1-4 times daily; or 20ml each time intravenously, 1-2 times daily.
2) Qing Kai Ling Injection: 40ml each time intravenously, once daily.

12. Viral Hepatitis

Hepatitis is the inflammation of the liver and can result in liver cell damage and destruction. It has many different origins or causes. It can be caused by many drugs and toxic agents as well as by numerous viruses. There are six main types of the hepatitis virus that have been identified, including hepatitis A, B, C, D, E, and G. Hepatitis is communicable. In some cases, liver failure or death can occur. However, not everyone who is infected will experience symptoms.

In the United States, one-third of Americans will be exposed to hepatitis A each year. There are 60,000 hepatitis B infections and 26,000 hepatitis C infections will occur each year. The following are the most common symptoms for hepatitis, however, each person may experience symptoms differently and some people may experience no symptoms at all:

- Flu-like symptoms or symptoms of upper respiratory infection
- Fever
- Nausea and vomiting

- Aversion to smoking
- Decreased appetite
- Malaise
- Abdominal pain or discomfort
- Diarrhea
- Joint pain
- Sore muscles
- Itchy red hives on skin
- Dark colored urine and jaundice
- Hepatomegaly and liver tenderness on physical exam

How is Hepatitis Diagnosed by Conventional Western Medicine?

In addition to a complete medical history and examination, other tests may be recommended to determine the extent of the disease, such as blood test, ultrasound and liver biopsy. Blood testing includes tests for liver function, antibodies, cellular blood counts, bleeding times, electrolytes, and other chemicals.

How is Hepatitis Treated by Conventional Western Medicine?

Treatment for hepatitis varies depending on the underlying cause of the disease. The goal of treatment is to stop damage to the liver and alleviate symptoms. Treatment may include one, or more, of the following:

- Supportive care, such as healthy diet and rest
- Medications to help control itching
- Avoiding alcohol and drugs
- Preventing the spread of the disease
- Antiviral or immunomodulator medications, such as interferon
- Frequent blood testing to determine its progression
- Hospitalization may be required in more severe cases
- Liver transplantation may be recommended for end-stage liver failure

Proper hygiene is the key to preventing the spread of hepatitis. Other preventative measures include vaccinations, routinely screened blood transfusions for hepatitis B and C, and immunoglobulin.

What Causes Hepatitis According to Traditional Chinese Medicine?

1) Infection of Exogenous Pathogenic Damp-Heat

2) Retention of Damp-Heat in the Interior

3) Incoordination between the Liver and Spleen

How is Hepatitis Differentiated and Treated by Traditional Chinese Medicine?

1) <u>Damp-Heat Retention</u>

Symptoms: Jaundice, fever, thirst, lassitude, anorexia, dark and yellow urine, constipation, yellow and greasy tongue coating, taut and rapid or soft and rapid pulse.

Therapeutic Principle: To clear away heat, remove toxic substance, promote diuresis and relieve jaundice.

Prescription: Modified Yin Chen Hao Decoction.

Modifications: For aversion to cold, fever, headache, malaise, thin and yellow tongue coating, and floating pulse, use Herba Ephedrae (Ma Huang) 9g, Fructus Forsythiae Suspensae (Lian Qiao) 12g, Herba Plantaginis (Che Qian Cao) 12g, Semen Coicis (Yi Yi Ren) 15g and Semen Phaseoli (Chi Xiao Dou) 20g, Radix Isatidis seu Baphicacanthi (Ban Lan Gen) 15g and Radix Glycyrrhizae Uralensis (Gan Cao) 6g; for nausea, vomiting and poor appetite, add ginger prepared Rhizoma Pinelliae Ternatae (Ban Xia) 10g, Pericarpium Citri Reticulatae (Ju Pi) 9g, Caulis Bambusae in Taeniam (Zhu Ru) 10g and Massa Medicata Fermentata (Shen Qu) 10g.

2) <u>Dampness Stagnation in the Spleen</u>

Symptoms: Epigastric stuffiness, abdominal distention, nausea, vomiting, anorexia, general weakness, hypochondriac pain, or jaundice, diarrhea, insipid or sticky mouth, white, greasy and slight yellow tongue coating, and soft and slippery pulse.

Therapeutic Principle: To invigorate the spleen, remove dampness, and regulate qi and middle warmer.

Prescription: Modified Yin Chen Wei Ling Decoction.

Modifications: For thick and greasy tongue coating, remarkable abdominal distention and epigastric stuffiness, add Herba Agastache seu Pogostemonis (Huo Xiang) 10g and Herba Eupatorii (Pi Lan) 10g; for abdominal distention, epigastric stuffiness, jaundice, spiritlessness, lassitude, aversion to cold, cold limbs, insipid mouth without a desire to drink, pale tongue with white and greasy coating, soft and slow or deep and slow pulse, use Herba Artemisiae Scopariae (Yin Chen Hao) 30g, Radix Aconiti Lateralis Praeparatae (Fu Pian) 10g, Rhizoma Zingiberis Officinalis (Gan Jiang) 6g, Radix Glycyrrhizae Uralensis (Gan Cao) 6g, Rhizoma Atractylodis Macrocephalae (Bai Zhu) 10g, Radix Paeoniae Alba (Bai Shao Yao) 10g, Sclerotium Poriae Cocos (Fu Ling) 15g and Semen Coicis (Yi Yi Ren) 20g.

3) <u>Stagnation of Liver Qi</u>

Symptoms: Distention, stuffiness and pain in the chest and hypochondrium, epigastric fullness, abdominal distention, frequent belching and passing flatus, anorexia, bitter taste in the mouth, thin and white or yellow tongue coating, and taut pulse.

Therapeutic Principle: To disperse stagnant liver qi, regulate qi and relieve pain.

Prescription: Modified Chai Hu Shu Gan Powder.

Modifications: For distending pain in the hypochondrium, belching, stuffy sensation in the chest, insipid mouth, lassitude, anorexia, abdominal distention and diarrhea, use Radix Bupleuri (Chai Hu) 9g, Radix Angelicae Sinensis (Dang Gui) 10g, Radix Paeoniae Alba (Bai Shao Yao) 10g, Sclerotium Poriae Cocos (Fu Ling) 12g, Radix Curcumae (Yu Jin) 10g, Rhizoma Atractylodis Macrocephalae (Bai Zhu) 10g, Semen Coicis (Yi Yi Ren) 15g, Fructus Germinatus Oryzae Sativae (Gu Ya) 15g and Fructus Hordei Germinatus (Mai Ya) 15g.

4) <u>Blood Stasis Obstructing the Collaterals</u>

Symptoms: Dark and gloomy complexion, or spider nevi, hepatomegaly and splenomegaly with hard texture, stabbing hypochondriac pain, bright red palms, frequent epistaxis and gingival hemorrhage, low-grade fever that is worse at night, dysmenorrheal with dark colored clots, dark purple tongue with ecchymosis, deep, thready and rough pulse.

Therapeutic Principle: To promote blood circulation, remove blood stasis, eliminate stagnation and dredge the collaterals.

Prescription: Modified Ge Xia Zhu Yu Decoction.

Modifications: For localized stabbing hypochondriac pain, palpable masses in the hypochondriac region, epistaxis and gingival hemorrhage, use Cornu Bubali (Shui Niu Jiao) 15g, Radix Rehmanniae (Di Huang) 15g, Radix Paeoniae Rubra (Chi Shao) 15g, Herba Hedyotis Diffusae (Bai Hua She She Cao) 30g, Rhizoma Polygoni Cuspidati (Hu Zhang) 30g, Cortex Moutan Radicis (Mu Dan Pi) 10g, Radix Bupleuri (Chai Hu) 10g, Sclerotium Poriae Cocos (Fu Ling) 10g, and Fructus Lycii (Gou Qi Zi) 10g.

5) <u>Insufficiency of the Liver and Spleen</u>

Symptoms: Shortness of breath, indolence of speaking, lassitude, lusterless complexion, anorexia, postprandial abdominal distention, dull pain in the hypochondrium, vertigo, dry eyes, emaciation, edema of the face, occasional diarrhea, pale tongue with white coating, and thready and weak pulse.

Therapeutic Principle: To nourish the liver and support the spleen.

Prescription: Modified Gui Shao Liu Jun Zi Decoction.

Modifications: For dull pain in the hypochondrium, epigastric stuffiness and abdominal distention, and thready and taut pulse, add Radix Bupleuri (Chai Hu) 9g and Fructus Citri Aurantii (Zhi Ke) 10g.

6) <u>Yin Deficiency of the Liver and Kidney</u>

Symptoms: Dull hypochondriac pain aggravated by exertion, vertigo, tinnitus, dry eyes, mouth and throat, insomnia, dreamfulness, feverish sensation in the chest, palms and soles, fore and weak loins and knees, little menses or amenorrhea, red small tongue with little moisture and coating or with cracks, and thready and rapid pulse.

Therapeutic Principle: To nourish blood, soothe the liver, replenish yin and tonify the kidney.

Prescription: Modified Yi Guan Decoction.

Modifications: For emaciation, dysphoria, dry mouth, sweating on exertion, vertigo and dry eyes, use Radix Pseudostellariae Heterophyllae (Tai Zi Shen) 15g, Radix Ophiopogonis Japonici (Mai Dong) 12g, Radix Paeoniae Alba (Bai Shao Yao) 12g, Fructus Lycii (Gou Qi Zi) 12g and Rhizoma Dioscoreae (Shan Yao) 15g; for epistaxis and gingival hemorrhage, add Herba Ecliptae Prostratae (Han Lian Cao) 12g and Rhizoma Imperatae Cylindricae (Bai Mao Gen) 15g.

7) <u>Yang Deficiency of the Spleen and Kidney</u>

Symptoms: Aversion to cold, preference to warmth, cold limbs, cold pain in the lower abdomen, lower back and knees; malaise, dull pain in the hypochondrium, anorexia, diarrhea with undigested food, or even fecal incontinence, abdominal fullness, oliguria, no edema of the lower extremities, pale and chubby tongue, and deep, thready and forceless or deep and slow pulse.

Therapeutic Principle: To invigorate the spleen, replenish qi, warm the kidney and nourish yang.

Prescription: Modified Fu Zi Li Zhong Decoction and Jin Gui Shen Qi Pill.

Modifications: For cold and sore loins and knees, deep, thready and weak pulse, add Herba Epimedii (Yin Yang Huo) 10g, Rhizoma Curculiginis Orchioidis (Xian Mao) 10g, Radix Morindae officinalis (Ba Ji Tian) 10g and Fructus Psoraleae Corylifoliae (Bu Gu Zhi) 10g; for abdominal distention, edema of the limbs and oliguria, add Semen Plantaginis (Che Qian Zi) 10g and Rhizoma Alismatis Orientalis (Ze Xie) 10g.

What Kinds of Chinese Patent Drugs are Available to Treat Hepatitis?

1) Ao Tai Le Granule: 15g each time, thrice daily.
2) Jiang Gan Le Granule: 15g each time, twice daily.
3) Ji Gu Cao Capsule: 4 capsules each time, thrice daily.
4) Gan Yan Ling Injection: 4ml each time intramuscularly, once daily.

13. Cholecystitis

Cholecystitis is inflammation of the gall bladder. Cholecystitis is usually caused by a gallstone in the cystic duct and is associated with gallstones in over 90% cases. Other causes of cholecystitis may include the following:

- Bacterial infection in the bile duct system
- Tumor of the pancreas or liver
- Decreased blood supply to the gallbladder
- Gallbladder "sludge"

Cholecystitis can occur suddenly or gradually over many years. The acute attack is often precipitated by a large or fatty meal. A typical acute attack of cholecystitis may gradually subside over a period of 12-18 hours. The following are the most common symptoms of gallstones. However, each individual may experience symptoms differently. Symptoms may include:

- Intense, sudden and steady pain in the epigastrium or right hypochondrium, which is often worse with deep breaths and extends to lower part of right shoulder blade
- Recurrent painful attacks for several hours after meals
- Nausea
- Vomiting
- Rigid abdominal muscles on right side
- Fever
- Chills
- Jaundice
- Itching
- Loose, light-colored bowel movements
- Abdominal bloating

How is Cholecystitis Diagnosed by Conventional Western Medicine?

In addition to a complete medical history and medical examination, diagnostic procedures for cholecystitis may include the following:

- Ultrasound or sonography
- Hepatobiliary scintigraphy
- Cholangiography

- Percutaneous transhepatic cholangiography (PTC)
- Endoscopic retrograde cholangiopancreatography (ERCP)
- Computed tomography scan (CT or CAT scan)

How is Cholecystitis Treated by Conventional Western Medicine?

Treatment for acute cholecystitis usually involves a hospital stay and a conservative regimen including withholding of oral feedings, intravenous alimentation, analgesics, and antibiotics. Sometimes, the gallbladder is surgically removed (cholecystectomy). Other treatment options may include:

- Oral dissolution therapy (drugs made from bile acid are used to dissolve the stones)
- Medications to prevent the formation of gallstones
- Low-fat diet
- Pain management

The overall prognosis for cholecystitis is favorable. In some individuals, complications may arise if other organs are involved.

What Causes Cholecystitis According to Traditional Chinese Medicine?

1) Prolonged Stagnation of Liver Qi due to Worry, Pensiveness and Anger
2) Blockage of the Gallbladder due to Stagnation of Damp-Heat
3) Deficiency with Impairment, Overstrain
4) Cold Invasion
5) Stagnation of Qi Causing Blood Stasis that Further Blocks the Collaterals

How is Cholecystitis Differentiated and Treated by Traditional Chinese Medicine?

1) <u>Qi Stagnation of the Liver and Gallbladder</u>

Symptoms: Right hypochondriac distending pain and fullness, which radiates to the right shoulder and is aggravated by anger; chest stuffiness, frequent sighing and belching with foul odor, acid regurgitation, white and greasy tongue coating, and taut and large pulse.

Therapeutic Principle: To soothe the liver, increase bile secretion, regulate qi and promote descending.

Prescription: Modified Chai Hu Shu Gan Powder.

Modifications: For constipation, add Radix et Rhizoma Rhei Praeparatae (Zhi Da Huang) 6g and Semen Areca Catechu (Bing Lang) 10g; for abdominal distention and fullness, add Cortex Magnoliae Officinalis (Hu Pu) 10g and Semen Alpiniae Katsumadai (Cao Dou Kou) 3g; for bitter taste in the mouth and dysphoria, add Radix Astragali (Huang Qi) 10g and Fructus Gardeniae Jasminoidis (Zhi Zi) 10g; for belching and vomiting, add Ochra Haematitum (Dai Zhe Shi) 15g and Semen Raphani

Sativi (Lai Fu Zi) 10g; for liver qi stagnation impairing the spleen, anorexia and diarrhea, add Sclerotium Poriae Cocos (Fu Ling) 12g, Rhizoma Atractylodis Macrocephalae (Bai Zhu) 10g and Rhizoma Dioscoreae (Shan Yao) 12g.

2) <u>Qi Stagnation and Blood Stasis</u>

Symptoms: Severe localized stabbing pain in the right hypochondrium, which is aggravated by pressure, sallow complexion, dry mouth with bitter taste, dark purple tongue with ecchymosis on the margin, taut, thready and rough pulse.

Therapeutic Principle: To soothe the liver, regulate qi, promote blood circulation and relieve pain.

Prescription: Modified Chai Hu Shu Gan Powder and Shi Xiao Powder.

Modifications: For severe right hypochondriac pain, add Rhizoma Corydalis (Yan Hu Suo) 10g; for acid regurgitation and vomiting, add Caulis Bambusae in Taeniam (Zhu Ru) 10g; for constipation, add Radix et Rhizoma Rhei (Da Huang) 6g; for concurrent damp-heat, add Herba Artemisiae Scopariae (Yin Chen Hao) 15g and Fructus Gardeniae Jasminoidis (Zhi Zi) 10g; for deficiency of the spleen and stomach, add Radix Codonopsitis Pilosulae (Dang Shen) 10g and Rhizoma Dioscoreae (Shan Yao) 10g; for gall stone, add Spora Lygodii Japonici (Hai Jin Sha) 15g and Endothelium Corneum Gigeriae Galli (Ji Nei Jin) 10g.

3) <u>Accumulation of Heat in the Gallbladder</u>

Symptoms: Burning pain in the right hypochondrium, bitter taste in the mouth, dry throat, flushed face with red eyes, constipation, oliguria, dysphoria, insomnia, irritability, red tongue with dry, yellow and thick coating, and taut and rapid pulse.

Therapeutic Principle: To clear away heat in the liver and gallbladder, relieve stagnation and relieve pain.

Prescription: Modified Qing Dan Decoction.

Modifications: For dysphoria and insomnia, add Radix Salviae Miltiorrhizae (Dan Shen) 12g and Semen Ziziphi Spinosae (Suan Zao Ren) 10g; for jaundice, add Herba Artemisiae Scopariae (Yin Chen Hao) 15g and Fructus Citri Aurantii (Zhi Ke) 10g; for thirst with a desire to drink, add Radix Trichosanthis (Tian Hua Fen) 15g and Radix Ophiopogonis Japonici (Mai Dong) 10g; for nausea, add Rhizoma Pinelliae Ternatae (Ban Xia) 6g and Caulis Bambusae in Taeniam (Zhu Ru) 10g.

4) <u>Damp-Heat in the Liver and Gallbladder</u>

Symptoms: Right hypochondriac distention, fullness and pain, chest stuffiness, anorexia, nausea, vomiting, bitter taste in the mouth, restlessness, dyschezia, or jaundice, red tongue with yellow and greasy coating, and taut and slippery pulse.

Therapeutic Principle: To soothe the liver, increase bile secretion and clear away damp-heat.

Prescription: Modified Da Chai Hu Decoction and Yin Chen Hao Decoction.

Modifications: For palpable and tender mass in the right hypochondrium, add Rhizoma Ligustici Chuanxiong (Chuan Xiong) 10g and Radix Salviae Miltiorrhizae (Dan Shen) 30g; for severe qi stagnation, add Rhizoma Cyperi Rotundi (Xiang Fu) 10g and Fructus Meliae Toosendan (Chuan Lian Zi) 10g; for dry mouth and dysphoria with feverish sensation, add Herba Dendrobii (Shi Hu) 10g and Radix Adenophorae (Sha Shen) 15g; for gall stone, add Spora Lygodii Japonici (Hai Jin Sha) 12g, Squama Manitis Pentadactylae (Chuan Shan Jia) 12g, Herba Lysimachiae (Jin Qian Cao) 15g and Endothelium Corneum Gigeriae Galli (Ji Nei Jin) 10g; for deep yellow urine, add Talcum (Hua Shi Fen) 10g, Semen Plantaginis (Che Qian Zi) 10g and Medulla Tetrapanacis Papyriferi (Tong Cao) 6g; for severe dampness with white and greasy tongue coating, remove Radix et Rhizoma Rhei and Fructus Gardeniae Jasminoidis, and add Sclerotium Poriae Cocos (Fu Ling) 10g, Fructus Amomi Cardamomi (Bai Kou Ren) 3g and Fructus Amomi Villosi (Sha Ren) 3g.

5) <u>Yin Deficiency and Liver Qi Stagnation</u>

Symptoms: Dull pain or slight burning pain in the right hypochondrium, dry mouth and throat, irritability, feverish sensation in the chest, vertigo, low-grade fever in the afternoon, red tongue with little coating, and thready and rapid pulse.

Therapeutic Principle: To nourish yin, clear away heat, soothe the liver, and increase bile secretion.

Prescription: Modified Yi Guan Decoction.

Modifications: For dysphoria and insomnia, add Semen Ziziphi Spinosae (Suan Zao Ren) 10g, Semen Biotae Orientalis (Bai Zi Ren) 10g and Caulis Polygoni Multiflori (Ye Jiao Teng) 12g; for burning pain in the right epigastrium, add Radix Paeoniae Alba (Bai Shao Yao) 12g and Radix Glycyrrhizae Uralensis (Gan Cao) 3g; for irritability, add Fructus Gardeniae Jasminoidis (Zhi Zi) 10g, Pericarpium Citri Reticulatae Viride (Qing Pi) 6g and Concha Margaritiferae (Zhen Zhu Mu) 20g.

6) <u>Yang Deficiency and Liver Qi Stagnation</u>

Symptoms: Intermittent dull distending pain in the right hypochondrium, distention and fullness in the abdomen, vomiting of clear fluid, aversion to cold, cold limbs, spiritlessness, shortness of breath, lassitude, pale tongue with white and greasy coating, and taut, weak and forceless pulse.

Therapeutic Principle: To warm yang, replenish qi, regulate the liver and increase bile secretion.

Prescription: Modified Li Zhong Pill.

Modifications: For cold pain in the abdomen, add Fructus Evodiae Rutaecarpae (Wu Zhu Yu) 3g, Radix Linderae Strychnifoliae (Wu Yao) 10g; for gall stone, add Herba Lysimachiae (Jin Qian Cao)

15g and Endothelium Corneum Gigeriae Galli (Ji Nei Jin) 10g.

What Kinds of Chinese Patent Drugs are Available to Treat Cholecystitis?

1) Shu Gan Zhi Tong Bolus: 1 bolus each time, thrice daily.
2) Dan Shi Tong Capsule: 4-6 capsules each time, thrice daily.
3) Jia Wei Xiao Yao Pill: 6g each time, 2-3 times each day.
4) Long Dan Xie Gan Pill: 6g each time, 2-3 times each day.

14. Acute Pancreatitis

Pancreatitis is the inflammation and autodigestion of the pancreas. Autodigestion is a process whereby pancreatic enzymes destroy its own tissue leading to inflammation. The inflammation may be acute or ongoing chronic. The exact pathogenesis is not known, but may include edema or obstruction of the ampulla of Vater, resulting in reflux of bile into pancreatic ducts or direct injury to the acinar cells. Acute pancreatitis usually involves a single attack, after which the pancreas returns to normal. Severe acute pancreatitis can be life threatening. In chronic pancreatitis, permanent damage occurs to the pancreas and its function, often leading to fibrosis. The causes of pancreatitis include the following:

- Gallstones that block the pancreatic duct
- Hypercalcemia, hyperlipidemias
- Alcohol abuse or a heavy meal
- Abdominal trauma or surgery
- Drugs, including sulfonamides and thiazides
- Kidney failure
- Lupus
- Infections such as mumps, hepatitis A or B, or salmonella
- Cystic fibrosis
- Presence of a tumor
- Pancreas divisum (a congenital anomaly)
- A venomous sting from a scorpion

The following are the most common symptoms of pancreatitis. However, each individual may experience symptoms differently. Symptoms may include:

- Epigastric abdominal pain that may radiate to the back or chest

- Nausea
- Vomiting
- Weakness, sweating, and anxiety
- Rapid pulse rate
- Malaise
- Fever
- Swelling in the upper abdomen
- Ascites
- Hypotension
- Tachycardia, pallor, and cool clammy skin
- Mild jaundice

How is Acute Pancreatitis Diagnosed by Conventional Western Medicine?

In addition to a complete medical history and physical examination, diagnostic procedures for pancreatitis may include abdominal x-ray, various blood tests, ultrasound, endoscopic retrograde cholangiopancreatography (ERCP), CT or CAT scan, and ECG or EKG. Essentials of diagnosis for acute pancreatitis include:

- Abrupt onset of deep epigastric pain with radiation to the back
- Nausea, vomiting, fever, sweating, and weakness
- Abdominal tenderness and distention
- Leukocytosis, elevated serum amylase and lipase
- History of previous episodes, often related to alcohol intake

How is Acute Pancreatitis Treated by Conventional Western Medicine?

The overall goal for treatment of pancreatitis is to rest the pancreas and allow it to recover from the inflammation. Treatment may include:

- Hospitalization for observation and intravenous feeding
- Bed rest or light activity only
- Placement of a nasogastric tube
- Surgery
- Antibiotics
- Avoiding alcohol
- Pain management

- Frequent blood tests to monitor electrolytes and kidney function
- No food by mouth for several days

Acute pancreatitis is self-limiting; up to 90 percent of individuals recover from acute pancreatitis without any complications.

What Causes Acute Pancreatitis According to Traditional Chinese Medicine?

1) Internal Injury by Emotional Disturbance
2) Improper Diet
3) Damp-Heat in the Liver and Gallbladder
4) Ascarid (Roundworm) Invading the Bile Ducts and Qi Regurgitation of the Liver and Gallbladder.

How is Acute Pancreatitis Differentiated and Treated by Traditional Chinese Medicine?

1) <u>Qi Stagnation of the Liver</u>

Symptoms: Abrupt epigastric pain that radiates into the hypochondrium or right shoulder and back, nausea, vomiting, dry mouth with bitter taste, dyschezia, pale red tongue with thin and white coating, and taut and thready or tense pulse.

Therapeutic Principle: To disperse stagnant liver qi, increase bile secretion, promote qi circulation and relieve pain.

Prescription: Modified Xiao Chai Hu Decoction.

Modifications: For severe pain, add Rhizoma Corydalis (Yan Hu Suo) 10g and Fructus Meliae Toosendan (Chuan Lian Zi) 10g; for dyschezia, add Natrii Sulfas (Mang Xiao) 10g, Semen Raphani Sativi (Lai Fu Zi) 10g and Cortex Magnoliae Officinalis (Hou Po) 10g; for food retention, belching with foul smell and acid regurgitation, add Fructus Crataegi (Shan Zha) 10g, Fructus Hordei Germinatus (Mai Ya) 12g and Semen Areca Catechu (Bing Lang) 10g; for fever, add Flos Lonicerae (Jin Yin Hua) 12g, Fructus Forsythiae Suspensae (Lian Qiao) 10g and Taraxaci Mongolici Herba cum Radice (Pu Gong Ying) 20g.

2) <u>Damp-Heat in the Liver and Gallbladder</u>

Symptoms: Epigastric distending pain aggravated by pressure, hypochondriac pain, or fever, nausea, vomiting, jaundice, scanty and dark urine, dyschezia, red tongue with thin and yellow or yellow and greasy coating, and taut and rapid pulse.

Therapeutic Principle: To clear away damp-heat from the liver and gallbladder.

Prescription: Modified Qing Yi Decoction and Long Dan Xie Gan Decoction.

Modifications: For remarkable jaundice, add Herba Artemisiae Scopariae (Yin Chen Hao) 15g, Rhizoma Polygoni Cuspidati (Hu Zhang) 15g and Herba Lysimachiae (Jin Qian Cao) 20g; for nausea and vomiting, add Caulis Bambusae in Taeniam (Zhu Ru) 10g, Pericarpium Citri Reticulatae (Chen Pi) 6g and Folium Eriobotryae Japonicae (Pi Pa Ye) 12g; for gall stone, add Herba Lysimachiae (Jin Qian Cao) 20g, Spora Lygodii Japonici (Hai Jin Sha) 10g and Endothelium Corneum Gigeriae Galli (Ji Nei Jin) 10g; for infection of roundword with severe cutting pain in the abdomen and hypochondrium, use No.2 Qing Yi Decoction.

3) <u>Heat Accumulation in the Stomach and Bowel</u>

Symptoms: Abdominal pain aggravated by pressure, fever, dry mouth with bitter taste, abdominal distention, constipation, scanty and yellow urine, red tongue with yellow and greasy coating, and deep and excess or slippery and rapid pulse.

Therapeutic Principle: To clear away heat, loosen the bowel, promote qi circulation, and relieve pain.

Prescription: Modified Da Cheng Qi Decoction.

Modifications: For severe pain, add Pollen Typhae (Pu Huang) 10g, Excrementum Trogopteri seu Pteromydis (Wu Ling Zhi) 10g and Rhizoma Corydalis (Yan Hu Suo) 10g; for jaundice, add Herba Artemisiae Scopariae (Yin Chen Hao) 15g and Rhizoma Polygoni Cuspidati (Hu Zhang) 15g; for persistent high fever, add Wu Wei Xiao Du Decoction.

What Kinds of Chinese Patent Drugs are Available to Treat Acute Pancreatitis?

1) Mu Xiang Bing Lang Pill: 3-6g each time, 2-3 times daily.
2) Zhi Zi Jin Hua Pill: 6g each time, twice daily.

15. Chronic Pancreatitis

Pancreatitis is the inflammation and autodigestion of the pancreas. Autodigestion is a process that pancreatic enzymes destroy its own tissue leading to inflammation. The inflammation may be acute or ongoing chronic. The exact pathogenesis is not known, but may include edema or obstruction of the ampulla of Vater, resulting in reflux of bile into pancreatic ducts or direct injury to the acinar cells. In chronic pancreatitis, permanent damage occurs to the pancreas and its function, often leading to fibrosis.

Chronic pancreatitis may be self-limiting, but may resolve after several attacks and with a greater risk of developing long-term problems such as diabetes, chronic pain, diarrhea, ascites, biliary cirrhosis, bile duct obstruction, or pancreatic cancer. The causes of pancreatitis include the following:

- Gallstones that block the pancreatic duct
- Severe malnutrition

- Alcohol abuse or a heavy meal
- Untreated hyperparathyroidism
- Abdominal trauma or surgery
- Drugs, including sulfonamides and thiazides
- Kidney failure
- Lupus
- Infections such as mumps, hepatitis A or B, or salmonella
- Cystic fibrosis
- Presence of a tumor
- Congenital anomaly

The following are the most common symptoms of pancreatitis. However, each individual may experience symptoms differently. Symptoms may include:

- Persistent or recurrent epigastric and left upper quadrant pain with referral to the upper left lumbar region
- Nausea, vomiting, anorexia, constipation, flatulence, and weight loss
- Steatorrhea (bulky, foul and fatty stools)
- Malaise
- Fever
- Swelling in the upper abdomen
- Ascites
- Hypotension
- Mild jaundice

How is Chronic Pancreatitis Diagnosed by Conventional Western Medicine?

In addition to a complete medical history and physical examination, diagnostic procedures for pancreatitis may include abdominal x-ray, various blood tests, ultrasound, endoscopic retrograde cholangiopancreatography (ERCP), CT or CAT scan, and ECG or EKG.

How is Chronic Pancreatitis Treated by Conventional Western Medicine?

The overall goal for treatment of pancreatitis is to rest the pancreas and allow it to recover from the inflammation. Treatment may include:

- Hospitalization for observation and intravenous feeding

- Bed rest or light activity only
- Placement of a nasogastric tube
- Surgery
- Antibiotics
- Avoiding alcohol
- Pain management
- Frequent blood tests to monitor electrolytes and kidney function
- No food by mouth for several days

Individuals with chronic pancreatitis may also require:

- Enzyme supplements to aid in food digestion.
- Insulin (if diabetes develops).
- Small high-protein meals.
- Medications (i.e., H2-blockers) to decrease gastric acid production in the stomach.

What Causes Chronic Pancreatitis According to Traditional Chinese Medicine?

1) Improper Diet
2) Emotional Disturbances
3) Yang Deficiency of the Spleen and Stomach
4) Internal Stagnation of Blood

How is Chronic Pancreatitis Differentiated and Treated by Traditional Chinese Medicine?

1) <u>Damp-Heat in the Spleen and Stomach</u>

Symptoms: Epigastric distending pain radiating to hypochondrium, which is aggravated by pressure; nausea, vomiting, epigastric stuffiness, anorexia, dry mouth with bitter taste, no desire to drink much, foul smelling loose stools, dyschezia, red tongue with yellow or yellow and greasy coating, and taut, slippery and rapid pulse.

Therapeutic Principle: To clear away heat and eliminate dampness.

Prescription: Modified Qing Zhong Decoction.

Modifications: For severe pain, add Fructus Meliae Toosendan (Chuan Lian Zi) 10g, Rhizoma Corydalis (Yan Hu Suo) 10g and Radix Curcumae (Yu Jin) 10g; for hypochondriac pain and dyschezia, use Da Chai Hu Decoction; for hyperactivity of pathogenic heat with bitter taste in the mouth, dysphoria and fever, add Radix Scutellariae Baicalensis (Huang Qin) 10g, Taraxaci Mongolici

Herba cum Radice (Pu Gong Ying) 20g and Herba cum Radice Houttuyniae Cordatae (Yu Xing Cao) 20g.

2) <u>Stagnation of Liver Qi and Deficiency of the Spleen</u>

Symptoms: Distending pain in the epigastrium and hypochondrium, or occasional severe pain, which radiates to the chest and back, lassitude, belching, anorexia, abdominal distention, loose stools, dark and pale tongue with thin and white coating, taut, thready and weak pulse.

Therapeutic Principle: To disperse stagnant liver qi, replenish qi and strengthen the spleen.

Prescription: Modified Chai Shao Liu Jun Zi Decoction.

Modifications: For sensation of stuffiness in the chest and epigastrium, white and greasy tongue coating, add Rhizoma Atractylodis (Cang Zhu) 10g, Cortex Magnoliae Officinalis (Hou Po) 10g and Herba Agastache seu Pogostemonis (Huo Xiang) 9g; for anorexia, add Massa Medicata Fermentata (Shen Qu) 10g, Fructus Hordei Germinatus (Mai Ya) 12g and Rhizoma Acori Tatarinowii (Shi Chang Pu) 10g.

3) <u>Internal Retention of Blood Stasis</u>

Symptoms: Localized pricking pain in the epigastrium and middle abdomen, which is worse at night; sallow complexion, or tender mass in the abdomen, emaciation, anorexia, nausea, vomiting, or diarrhea, dark purple tongue with ecchymosis, and taut and rough pulse.

Therapeutic Principle: To promote blood circulation and qi circulation, remove blood stasis and relieve pain.

Prescription: Modified Ge Xia Zhu Yu Decoction.

Modifications: For abdominal mass and extreme weakness, add Squama Manitis Pentadactylae (Chuan Shan Jia) 10g, Carapax Trionycis (Bie Jia) 20g, Rhizoma Sparganii Stoloniferi (San Leng) 10g and Rhizoma Curcumae Ezhu (E Zhu) 10g; for chronic disease with sallow complexion and emaciation, add Radix Angelicae Sinensis (Dang Gui) 15g and Radix Astragali (Huang Qi) 15g.

4) <u>Deficiency Cold in the Spleen and Stomach</u>

Symptoms: Intermittent dull pain in the epigastrium, which is alleviated by warmth and pressure; sallow complexion, cold limbs, shortness of breath, indolence of speaking, anorexia, nausea, vomiting, diarrhea, pale red tongue with teeth marks and white coating, deep, thready and forceless pulse.

Therapeutic Principle: To replenish qi, warm yang, strengthen the spleen and normalize the function of the stomach.

Prescription: Modified Huang Qi Jian Zhong Decoction.

Modifications: For severe abdominal pain, use Da Jian Zhong Decoction; for diarrhea, add Rhizoma Atractylodis Macrocephalae (Bai Zhu) 10g, Rhizoma Dioscoreae (Shan Yao) 15g and Semen Nelumbinis Nuciferae (Lian Zi) 10g; for cold limbs, use Li Zhong Decoction.

What Kinds of Chinese Patent Drugs are Available to Treat Chronic Pancreatitis?

1) Xin Fu Qi Tong Pill: 1 pill each time, twice daily.
2) Shan Zha Nei Xiao Pill: 6g each time, twice daily.
3) Jiu Qi Nian Tong Pill: 6-9g each time, twice daily.

Chapter 4: Disorders of the Kidney and Urinary Tract

1. Acute Glomerulonephritis (AGN)

Glomerulonephritis is an inflammatory process primarily involving the glomerulus, though at times the renal vasculature, interstitium, and tubular epithelium may also be affected. During glomerulonephritis, the kidney's ability to filter urine is impaired. Glomerulonephritis can be acute, referring to a sudden attack of inflammation, or chronic, which comes on gradually. Glomerular disease can be part of a systemic disease, such as lupus or diabetes, or it can be a disease by itself, i.e., primary glomerulonephritis.

Glomerulonephritis is one disorder that can lead to kidney failure. There are many causes of glomerulonephritis. They include those related to infections, immune diseases, vasculitis and conditions that scar the glomeruli. However, the exact cause is initially unknown. Here are some of the known causes:

- Systemic lupus erythematosus (SLE) or lupus
- Polyarteritis nodosa
- Wegener's granulomatosis
- A gene on the X chromosome passed on from carrier mothers
- Streptococcal infection (acute poststreptococcal glomerulonephritis, or APSGN)
- Bacterial endocarditis
- Viral infections
- Goodpasture's syndrome
- IgA nephropathy (Berger's disease and Henoch-Schönlein purpura)
- Bacterial endocarditis Viral infections
- High blood pressure
- Diabetic kidney disease
- Focal segmental glomerulosclerosis.

Complications of glomerulonephritis may include acute kidney failure, chronic kidney failure, high blood pressure and nephrotic syndrome.

The following are the most common symptoms of glomerulonephritis. However, each individual may experience symptoms differently. Symptoms may include:
- Hematuria
- Proteinuria
- Sore throat
- Diminished urine output
- Fatigue from anemia or kidney failure
- Lethargy
- Increased breathing effort
- Headache
- Hypertension
- Edema
- Seizures
- Rash, especially over the buttocks and legs
- Weight loss
- Joint pain
- Pale skin color

How is Glomerulonephritis Diagnosed by Conventional Western Medicine?

In addition to a thorough physical examination and complete medical history, the following diagnostic tests may be recommended: throat culture, urine tests, blood tests, ECG or EKG, renal ultrasound, chest x-ray and renal biopsy.

How is Glomerulonephritis Treated by Conventional Western Medicine?

Treat the underlying cause of glomerulonephritis. If glomerulonephritis is caused by a streptococcal infection, then treatment will be focused on curing the infection and treating the symptoms associated with the infection. Unfortunately, glomerulonephritis caused by a different reason cannot be cured. Therefore, treatments focus on slowing the progression of the disease and preventing complications. Treatment for glomerulonephritis may include:
- Fluid restriction
- Decreased protein diet

- Decreased salt and potassium diet
- Medication, such as diuretics, blood pressure medications, phosphate binders, and immunosuppressive agents
- Plasma exchange therapy
- Dialysis
- Kidney transplantation.

What Causes AGN According to Traditional Chinese Medicine?

1) Dysfunction of the Lung to Facilitates the Circulation of Fluid due to the Attack by Exogenous Pathogenic Wind
2) Accumulation of Damp-Heat due to the Invasion of Toxic Heat
3) Stagnation of Spleen Qi due to the Attack by Dampness
4) Weak Constitution

How is AGN Differentiated and Treated by Traditional Chinese Medicine?

1) Stage of Acute Onset

(1) <u>Wind-Cold Attacking the Lung</u>

Symptoms: Severe aversion to cold, fever, cough, shortness of breath, edema of the face or anasarca, luster complexion, pale tongue with thin and white coating, and floating and tense or deep and thready.

Therapeutic Principle: To dispel wind, disperse cold, release lung qi and promote diuresis.

Prescription: Modified Ma Huang Decoction and Wu Ling Powder.

Modifications: For severe cough and dyspnea, Semen Descurainiae seu Lepidii (Ting Li Zi) 10g and Semen Sinapis Albae (Bai Jie Zi) 10g; for sweating and aversion to wind, replace the prescription with modified Fang Ji Huang Qi Decoction.

(2) <u>Wind-Heat Attacking the Lung</u>

Symptoms: Fever without aversion to cold, or severe fever with little chill, sore throat, dry mouth, thirst, edema of the face, oliguria with dark urine, red tongue with thin and yellow coating, and floating and rapid or thready and rapid pulse.

Therapeutic Principle: To clear away heat, dispel wind, release lung qi and promote diuresis.

Prescription: Modified Yue Bi Jia Zhu Decoction.

Modifications: May add Herba Spirodelae (Fu Ping) 10g, Rhizoma Alismatis Orientalis (Ze Xie) 10g and Sclerotium Poriae Cocos (Fu Ling) 12g to release lung qi and promote diuresis; for sore throat, add Radix Isatidis seu Baphicacanthi (Ban Lan Gen) 12g, Radix Platycodi Grandiflori (Jie Geng) 9g and Fructus Forsythiae Suspensae (Lian Qiao) 10g; for severe fever, dark urine or hematuria, add Rhizoma Imperatae Cylindricae (Bai Mao Gen) 20g, Herba seu Radix Cirsii Japonici (Da Ji) 10g and Herba Cephalanoploris (Xiao Ji) 15g; for severe cough and dyspnea, add Radix Peucedani (Qian Hu) 9g and Semen Armeniacae Amarum (Xing Ren) 10g; for urinary frequency, urgency and dysuria, add Radix Rehmanniae (Di Huang) 15g, Herba Polygoni Avicularis (Bian Xu) 12g, Herba Dianthi (Qu Mai) 10g, Folium Phyllostachydis Henonis (Zhu Ye) 12g and Herba Commelinae (Ya Zhi Cao) 20g.

(3) <u>Invasion of Toxic Heat</u>

Symptoms: Unhealed skin boil, or skin scab or crusts, edema of the face or anasarca, dry mouth with bitter taste, oliguria with dark urine, or even hematuria, red tongue with thin and yellow or yellow greasy coating, and slippery and rapid or thready and rapid pulse.

Therapeutic Principle: To clear away heat, remove toxic substances, eliminate dampness and subside swelling.

Prescription: Modified Ma Huang Lian Qiao Chi Xiao Dou Decoction and Wu Wei Xiao Du Decoction.

Modifications: For remarkable dampness with skin erosion, add Radix Sophorae Flavescentis (Ku Shen) 10g and Rhizoma Smilacis Glabrae (Tu Fu Ling) 30g; for hyperactivity with skin itching, add Cortex Dictamni Radicis (Bai Xian Pi) 10g and Fructus Kochiae Scopariae (Di Fu Zi) 12g; for severe red swelling, add Cortex Moutan Radicis (Mu Dan Pi) 10g and Radix Paeoniae Rubra (Chi Shao) 12g; for dyschezia, add Radix et Rhizoma Rhei (Da Huang) 6g and Natrii Sulfas (Mang Xiao) 10g; for severe edema, add Cortex Poriae Cocos (Fu Ling Pi) 12g and Pericarpium Areca Catechu (Da Fu Pi) 10g.

(4) <u>Deficiency of the Spleen and Kidney</u>

Symptoms: Pitted edema of the lower extremities, general heaviness, abdominal stuffiness and distention, anorexia, lumbago, oliguria, shortness of breath, fatigue, pale tongue with white and greasy coating, and soft and slow pulse.

Therapeutic Principle: To strengthen the spleen, eliminate dampness, activate yang and induce diuresis.

Prescription: Modified Wu Pi Decoction and Wu Ling Powder.

Modifications: For severe edema of the upper body, add Herba Ephedrae (Ma Huang) 6g, Semen Armeniacae Amarum (Xing Ren) 10g and Semen Descurainiae seu Lepidii (Ting Li Zi) 10g; for severe edema of the lower body, add Semen Zanthoxyli (Jiao Mu) 5g and Radix Stephaniae Tetrandrae (Fang Ji) 10g; for cold limbs, deep and slow pulse, add Radix Aconiti Lateralis Praeparatae (Fu Zi) 10g and

Rhizoma Zingiberis Officinalis (Gan Jiang) 10g; for palpitation, anxiety, stuffy chest, cyanosis, cold limbs, difficult urination, severe edema, dark tongue with white coating, tinny, knot and intermittent pulse, use Zhen Wu Decoction supplemented with Fructus Citri Aurantii Immaturus (Zhi Shi) 10g and Radix Salviae Miltiorrhizae (Dan Shen)10g; for malaise, sleepiness, acid regurgitation, even urine odor in the mouth, and oliguria, add Radix Aconiti Lateralis Praeparatae (Fu Zi) 10g, Radix et Rhizoma Rhei Praeparatae (Zhi Da Huang) 6g, Rhizoma Coptidis (Huang Lian) 9g and Rhizoma Pinelliae Ternatae (Ban Xia) 10g.

(5) <u>Insufficiency of the Lung and Kidney</u>

Symptoms: Lassitude, edema of lower extremities, lumbago, oliguria, dark red throat, or low-grade fever, slight red tongue with little coating, and thready or thready and rapid pulse.

Therapeutic Principle: To replenish qi, induce diuresis and subside swelling.

Prescription: Modified Fang Ji Huang Qi Decoction.

Modifications: For remarkable lassitude and lumbago, add Cortex Eucommiae Ulmoidis (Du Zhong) 12g, Radix Achyranthis Bidentatae (Niu Xi) 12g, Radix Dipsaci Asperi (Xu Duan) 15g and Rhizoma Dioscoreae (Shan Yao) 15g; for dark red throat, or low-grade fever, add Bai He Gu Jin Decoction.

2) Stage of Convalescence

(1) <u>Deficiency of Spleen Qi</u>

Symptoms: Lassitude, anorexia, sallow complexion, pale and red tongue with white coating, and thready and weak pulse.

Therapeutic Principle: To strengthen the spleen and replenish qi.

Prescription: Modified Shen Ling Bai Zhu Powder.

Modifications: For edema of lower extremities, add Rhizoma Alismatis Orientalis (Ze Xie) 10g and Semen Plantaginis (Che Qian Zi) 9g; for aversion to cold and cold limbs, add Semen Trigonellae Foeni-graeci (Hu Lu Ba) 10g and Cortex Cinnamomi Cassiae (Rou Gui) 3g; for anorexia, add Fructus Germinatus Oryzae Sativae (Gu Ya) 12g, Massa Medicata Fermentata (Shen Qu) 12g and Fructus Crataegi (Shan Zha) 12g.

(2) <u>Qi and Yin Deficiency of the Lung and Kidney</u>

Symptoms: Low-grade fever, dry throat, cough with little sputum, spiritlessness, vertigo, sore and weak loins and knees, feverish sensation in palms and soles, red tongue tip with thin and little coating, thready or thready and rapid pulse.

Therapeutic Principle: To nourish the lung and kidney, and replenish qi and yin.

Prescription: Modified Shen Qi Di Huang Decoction.

Modifications: For low-grade fever, dry throat, cough with little sputum, add Bai He Gu Jin Decoction; for liability to exogenous pathogenic factors, add Yu Ping Feng Powder and Cordyceps Sinensis (Dong Chong Xia Cao) 10g.

What Kinds of Chinese Patent Drugs are Available to Treat AGN?

1) Jin Shui Bao Capsule: 3 capsules each time, thrice daily.
2) Shen Yan Xiao Zhong Tablet: 2-4 tablets each time, thrice daily.
3) Qing Kai Ling Injection: 40ml each time, once daily.

2. Rapidly Progressive Glomerulonephritis (RPGN)

Rapidly progressive glomerulonephritis can be defined as any glomerular disease associated with rapid progressive loss of renal function over days or weeks. Rapidly progressive glomerulonephritis should be considered if the renal biopsy reveals the presence of crescents in 50% or more glomeruli. The causes of rapidly progressive glomerulonephritis can be categorized according to the immunofluorescence patterns found on renal biopsy. Since the prognosis and treatment depend on the cause, early renal biopsy and immunofluorescence studies should be done before the start of medical therapy.

For symptoms, diagnosis and treatment please refer to acute glomerulonephritis.

What Causes RPGN According to Traditional Chinese Medicine?

1) Weak Constitution
2) Improper Diet
3) Overstrain
4) Internal Injury by Seven Emotions

How is RPGN Differentiated and Treated by Traditional Chinese Medicine?

1) <u>Retention of Pathogenic Factors in the Triple Warmer</u>

Symptoms: Edema, fever, sore throat, scanty and dark urine, or vomiting, sensation of stuffiness in the chest, oliguria, vertigo, headache, red tongue with yellow and greasy coating, and slippery or slippery and rapid pulse.

Therapeutic Principle: To dispel wind, clear away heat, induce diuresis and remove toxic substance.

Prescription: Modified Ma Huang Lian Qiao Chi Xiao Dou Decoction and Huang Lian Wen Dan Decoction.

Modifications: For remarkable edema, add Sclerotium Polypori Umbellati (Zhu Ling) 10g, Sclerotium Poriae Cocos (Fu Ling) 12g and Rhizoma Alismatis Orientalis (Ze Xie) 10g; for sore throat, add Flos Lonicerae (Jin Yin Hua) 15g, Radix Isatidis seu Baphicacanthi (Ban Lan Gen) 12g and Radix Platycodi Grandiflori (Jie Geng) 9g.

2) <u>Deficiency of Yin and Hyperactivity of Yang</u>

Symptoms: Vertigo, headache, oliguria, nausea, vomiting, lassitude, sore and weak loins and knees, convulsion, drowsiness, red tongue with greasy coating, and taut and thready pulse.

Therapeutic Principle: To nourish yin, suppress hyperactivity of yang, tonify the kidney and eliminate dampness.

Prescription: Modified Ling Jiao Gou Teng Decoction.

Modifications: For deficiency of blood, add Radix Angelicae Sinensis (Dang Gui) 12g; for remarkable edema, add Rhizoma Alismatis Orientalis (Ze Xie) 10g and Semen Plantaginis (Che Qian Zi) 9g; for severe heat, add Gypsum Fibrosum (Shi Gao) 30g; for constipation, add Fructus Citri Aurantii Immaturus (Zhi Shi) 10g and Radix et Rhizoma Rhei (Da Huang) 6g.

3) <u>Deficiency of the Spleen and Overflow of Water</u>

Symptoms: Edema, malaise, lassitude, anorexia, loose stools, pale and chubby tongue with white and slippery coating, and taut and soft pulse.

Therapeutic Principle: To replenish qi and induce diuresis.

Prescription: Modified Bu Zhong Yi Qi Decoction and Wu Ling Powder.

Modifications: For edema and abdominal distention, add Pericarpium Areca Catechu (Da Fu Pi) 10g and Stylus Zeae Mays (Yu Mi Xu) 20g; for remarkable anorexia and loose stools, add Semen Coicis (Yi Yi Ren) 15g and Rhizoma Atractylodis (Cang Zhu) 10g.

4) <u>Blood Stasis and Fluid Retention</u>

Symptoms: Dizziness, distending pain in the head, difficult urination, peripheral edema, dark and gloomy or black complexion, localized soreness in the lower back, dark purple tongue with ecchymosis and petechiae, white and thin tongue coating, and rough pulse.

Therapeutic Principle: To promote blood and fluid circulation.

Prescription: Modified Tiao Ying Decoction.

Modifications: For oliguria with dark urine, add Talcum (Hua Shi Fen) 10g and Folium Pyrrosiae (Shi Wei) 10g; for low voice, shortness of breath and fatigue, add Radix Astragali (Huang Qi) 12g and Radix Codonopsitis Pilosulae (Dang Shen) 10g.

5) <u>Invasion of the Heart by Kidney Water</u>

Symptoms: Oliguria, peripheral edema, irritating cough, dyspnea, palpitation, stuffy sensation in the chest, cyanosis, irritability, inability to lie flat, dark tongue wit greasy coating, and tinny, knot and intermittent pulse.

Therapeutic Principle: To purge the lung and induce diuresis.

Prescription: Modified Ji Jiao Li Huang Pill.

Modifications: For anorexia, thick and greasy tongue coating, add Rhizoma Atractylodis (Cang Zhu) 10g, Herba Agastache seu Pogostemonis (Huo Xiang) 10g and Herba Eupatorii (Pei Lan) 10g; for severe edema of lower extremities, add Semen Plantaginis (Che Qian Zi) 9g, Sclerotium Polypori Umbellati (Zhu Ling) 10g and Stylus Zeae Mays (Yu Mi Xu) 20g; for nausea and vomiting, add Rhizoma Coptidis (Huang Lian) 9g, Rhizoma Pinelliae Ternatae (Ban Xia) 10g, Caulis Bambusae in Taeniam (Zhu Ru) 10g and Pericarpium Citri Reticulatae (Chen Pi) 9g; for constipation, add Fructus Citri Aurantii Immaturus (Zhi Shi) 10g and Semen Areca Catechu (Bing Lang) 12g.

6) <u>Internal Retention of Toxic Turbidity</u>

Symptoms: Headache, vertigo, or drowsiness, stuffy sensation in the chest, nausea, bitter taste or urine foul odor in the mouth, anorexia, constipation, abdominal distention and fullness, edema, difficult urination, pale red tongue with thick and greasy coating, and deep and slow pulse.

Therapeutic Principle: To eliminate dampness and turbidity.

Prescription: Modified Wen Dan Decoction.

Modifications: For epigastric discomfort and stuffiness, add Caulis Perillae (Su Geng) 10g and Fructus Citri Sarcodactyli (Fo Shou) 10g; for tinnitus, add Radix Curcumae (Yu Jin) 10g and Rhizoma Acori Tatarinowii (Shi Chang Pu) 10g; for frequent vomiting, add Ochra Haematitum (Dai Zhe Shi) 15g and Rhizoma Zingiberis Recens (Sheng Jiang) 10g; for abdominal distention and diarrhea, add Rhizoma Zingiberis Officinalis (Gan Jiang) 9g and Semen Myristicae Fragrantis (Rou Dou Kou) 10g; for toxicant invading the blood division/level (xue fen), or internal wind hyperactivity of the liver, add Cornu Saigae Tataricae (Ling Yang Jiao) 3g, Bombyx Batryticatus (Jiang Can) 10g and Cortex Moutan Radicis (Mu Dan Pi) 10g.

What Kinds of Chinese Patent Drugs are Available to Treat RPGN?

1) Qing Kai Ling Injection: 40ml each time, once daily.
2) Sheng Mai Injection: 40ml each time, once daily.

3. Chronic Glomerulonephritis (CGN)

Chronic glomerulonephritis sometimes develops after a bout of acute glomerulonephritis. In some people there's no history of kidney disease at all, and the first indication of chronic glomerulonephritis is chronic kidney failure. Infrequently, chronic glomerulonephritis runs in families. In many cases, the cause is not known.

For symptoms, diagnosis and treatment please refer to acute glomerulonephritis.

What Causes CGN According to Traditional Chinese Medicine?

1) Weak Constitution
2) Internal Injury of the Spleen and Stomach by Improper Diet and Overstrain
3) Stagnation of the Blood and Qi due to Emotional Disturbance
4) Dysfunction of the Lung to Facilitates the Circulation of Fluid due to the Attack by Exogenous Pathogenic Wind
5) Accumulation of Damp-Heat in the Triple Warmer
6) Stagnation of Spleen Qi due to the Attack by Dampness

How is CGN Differentiated and Treated by Traditional Chinese Medicine?

1) Causes (so-called Root or Principal Aspects)

(1) <u>Qi Deficiency of the Spleen and Kidney</u>

Symptoms: Lumbago, spiritlessness, lassitude, or edema, anorexia, or epigastric distention, diarrhea, urinary frequency, or nocturia, pale tongue with teeth marks, thin and white tongue coating, and theady pulse.

Therapeutic Principle: To replenish qi, strengthen the spleen and nourish the kidney.

Prescription: Modified Yi Gong Powder.

Modifications: For deficiency of the spleen and retention of dampness with anorexia, abdominal distention, add Rhizoma Atractylodis (Cang Zhu) 10g, Herba Agastache seu Pogostemonis (Huo Xiang) 10g, Herba Eupatorii (Pi Lan) 10g and Pericarpium Citri Reticulatae (Chen Pi) 9g; for deficiency of the spleen with loose stools, add Semen Dolichoris Lablab (Bian Dou) 20g and Semen Euryales Ferocis (Qian Shi) 12g; for remarkable edema, add Semen Plantaginis (Che Qian Zi) 10g and Sclerotium Polypori Umbellati (Zhu Ling) 10g.

(2) <u>Qi Deficiency of the Lung and Kidney</u>

Symptoms: Edema of the face or peripheral edema, lassitude, shortness of breath, indolence of speaking, spontaneous sweating, increased susceptibility to cold, lumbago, sallow complexion, pale tongue with white and moist coating, and thready and weak pulse.

Therapeutic Principle: To nourish the lung and kidney.

Prescription: Modified Yu Ping Feng Powder and Jin Gui Shen Qi Pill.

Modifications: For wind-cold, use modified Ma Huang Decoction; for wind-heat, use modified Yin Qiao Powder; for severe edema of the face, dry and sore throat, use modified Ma Huang Lian Qiao Chi Xiao Dou Decoction; for severe edema, oliguria and constipation, use Ji Jiao Li Huang Pill and Wu Ling Powder; for proteinuria, add Semen Euryales Ferocis (Qian Shi) 12g and Fructus Rosae Laevigatae (Jin Ying Zi) 15g; for hematuria, add Herba Ecliptae Prostratae (Han Lian Cao) 15g, Rhizoma Imperatae Cylindricae (Bai Mao Gen) 20g and Radix Rubiae Cordifoliae (Qian Cao) 12g.

(3) <u>Yang Deficiency of the Spleen and Kidney</u>

Symptoms: Anasarca, pale complexion, aversion to cold, cold limbs, cold pain in the lower back and spine, spiritlessness, anorexia, loose stools, seminal emission, impotence, premature ejaculation, or abnormal menstruation, pale, tender and chubby tongue with teeth marks, and deep and thready or deep, slow and forceless pulse.

Therapeutic Principle: To warm and nourish the spleen and kidney.

Prescription: Modified Fu Zi Li Zhong Pill or Ji Sheng Shen Qi Pill.

Modifications: For severe deficiency of kidney yang with cold limbs and diarrhea, add Herba Epimedii (Yin Yang Huo) 12g and Fructus Psoraleae Corylifoliae (Bu Gu Zhi) 10g; for remarkable edema, use Shi Pi Decoction and Zhen Wu Decoction; for hydrothorax, cough, belching and inability to lie flat, add Ting Li Da Zao Decoction; for ascites, add Wu Pi Decoction.

(4) <u>Yin Deficiency of the Liver and Kidney</u>

Symptoms: Dryness or fuzziness of the eyes, vertigo, tinnitus, feverish sensation in the chest, palms and soles, dry mouth and throat, lumbago, seminal emission, or abnormal menstruation, red tongue with little coating, and taut and thready or thready and rapid pulse.

Therapeutic Principle: To nourish the liver and kidney.

Prescription: Modified Qi Ju Di Huang Pill.

Modifications: For severe deficiency of liver yin, add Radix Angelicae Sinensis (Dang Gui) 10g and Radix Paeoniae Alba (Bai Shao Yao) 10g; for concurrent deficiency of heart yin, add Semen Biotae Orientalis (Bai Zi Ren) 15g, Semen Ziziphi Spinosae (Suan Zao Ren) 15g and Fructus Schisandrae Chinensis (Wu Wei Zi) 3g; for concurrent deficiency of lung yin, add Tuber Asparagi Cochinchinensis (Tian Dong) 10g, Radix Ophiopogonis Japonici (Mai Dong) 12g and Fructus Schisandrae Chinensis (Wu Wei Zi) 3g; for hyperactivity of liver yang, add Rhizoma Gastrodiae Elatae (Tian Ma) 10g, Ramulus Uncariae cum Uncis (Gou Teng) 12g and Bombyx Batryticatus (Jiang Can) 10g; for damp-heat in the Lower Triple Warmer, add Rhizoma Anemarrhenae (Zhi Mu) 10g, Cortex Phellodendri (Huang Bai) 10g and Folium Pyrrosiae (Shi Wei) 10g; for hematuria, remove Radix Rehmanniae Praeparata, and add Radix Rehmanniae (Di Huang) 15g, Herba seu Radix Cirsii Japonici (Da Ji) 12g, Herba Cephalanoploris (Xiao Ji) 15g and Rhizoma Imperatae Cylindricae (Bai Mao Gen) 20g; for constipation, add Radix et Rhizoma Rhei (Da Huang) 6g.

(5) Deficiency of Qi and Yin

Symptoms: Lusterless complexion, shortness of breath, fatigue, or liability to cold, low-grade fever in the afternoon, or feverish sensation in palms and soles, lumbago, or edema, dry mouth and throat, or dark red throat, sore throat, red tongue with little coating, and thready or weak pulse.

Therapeutic Principle: To replenish qi and nourish yin.

Prescription: Modified Shen Qi Di Huang Decoction.

Modifications: For constipation, add Radix Scrophulariae Ningpoensis (Xuan Shen) 10g, Semen Biotae Orientalis (Bai Zi Ren) 15g and Radix et Rhizoma Rhei (Da Huang) 6g; for chronic sore throat, and dark red throat, add Radix Adenophorae (Sha Shen) 10g, Radix Ophiopogonis Japonici (Mai Dong) 12g, Semen Pruni Persicae (Tao Ren) 10g and Radix Paeoniae Rubra (Chi Shao) 10g; for anorexia and abdominal distention, add Fructus Amomi Villosi (Sha Ren) 5g and Radix Aucklandiae Lappae (Mu Xiang) 10g; for deficiency of kidney qi, add Semen Cuscutae Chinensis (Tu Si Zi) 12g and Fructus Rubi Chingii (Fu Pen Zi) 10g; for dry mouth and throat, dry cough with little sputum, oliguria with dark urine, and constipation, replace the prescription with Ren Shen Gu Ben Pill.

2) Manifestation (so-called Branch or Secondary Aspects)

(1) Water and Dampness

Symptoms: Edema of the face or extremities, white or white and greasy tongue coating, and slow or deep and slow pulse.

Therapeutic Principle: To induce diuresis and subside swelling.

Prescription: Modified Wu Ling Powder and Wu Pi Decoction.

Modifications: For pathogenic wind with edema of upper body, add Radix Saposhnikoviae Divaricatae (Fang Feng) 10g and Rhizoma et Radix Notopterygii (Qiang Huo) 10g; for edema of the lower body, add Radix Stephaniae Tetrandrae (Fang Zi) 10g and Semen Coicis (Yi Yi Ren) 15g; for concurrent cold syndrome, add Radix Aconiti Lateralis Praeparatae (Fu Zi) 10g and Rhizoma Zingiberis Officinalis (Gan Jiang) 10g; for heat syndrome, add Medulla Tetrapanacis Papyriferi (Tong Cao) 3g and Talcum (Hua Shi Fen) 10g.

(2) Damp-Heat

Symptoms: Edema of the face and extremities, fever, sweating, dry mouth without desire to drink, stuffiness in the chest and epigastrium, abdominal distention and fullness, anorexia, oliguria, loose stools and dyschezia, red tongue with yellow and greasy coating, and slippery and rapid pulse.

Therapeutic Principle: To clear away heat and eliminate dampness.

Prescription: Modified San Ren Decoction.

Modifications: For accumulation of damp-heat in the Upper Warmer manifesting cough with yellow sputum, add modified Xing Ren Hua Shi Decoction; for retention of damp-heat in the Middle Warmer with abdominal distention, stuffiness and fullness, add modified Huang Lian Wen Dan Decoction; for retention of damp-heat in the Lower Warmer, use modified Ba Zheng Powder; for remarkable sore and swollen throat, use modified Yin Qiao Powder.

(3) <u>Blood Stasis</u>

Symptoms: Black or dim and gloomy complexion, localized soreness or pricking pain in the lower back, squamous and dry skin, numbness of the extremities, dark purple tongue with ecchymosis, or thready and rough pulse.

Therapeutic Principle: To promote blood circulation and remove blood stasis.

Prescription: Modified Xue Fu Zhu Yu Decoction.

Modifications: For concurrent deficiency of qi and yang, replace the prescription with modified Gui Zhi Fu Ling Pill

(4) <u>Turbid Dampness</u>

Symptoms: Anorexia, nausea or vomiting, sticky and greasy feeling in the mouth, abdominal distention, general heaviness, drowsiness, edema, oliguria, spiritlessness, greasy tongue coating, and deep and thready or deep and slow pulse.

Therapeutic Principle: To strengthen the spleen, eliminate dampness and purge turbidity.

Prescription: Modified Wei Ling Decoction.

Modifications: For severe nausea and vomiting, add Rhizoma Zingiberis Recens (Sheng Jiang) 10g and Caulis Bambusae in Taeniam (Zhu Ru) 10g; for constipation, add Radix et Rhizoma Rhei (Da Huang) 6g and Herba Serissae (Liu Yue Xue) 12g.

What Kinds of Chinese Patent Drugs are Available to Treat CGN?

1) Bao Shen Kang Tablet: 3-4 tablets each time, thrice daily.
2) Shen Fu Kang Capsule: 4-6 capsules each time, thrice daily.
3) Shen Yan Shu Tablet: 6 tablets each time, thrice daily.

4. Latent Glomerulonephritis (LGN)

Latent glomerulonephritis can be defined as a group of glomerular diseases with different pathologic types due to different causes and pathogenetic mechanisms. Latent glomerulonephritis is characterized by mild persistent or intermittent asymptomatic hematuria and/or proteinuria, and normal kidney functions.

For symptoms, diagnosis and treatment please refer to acute glomerulonephritis.

What Causes LGN According to Traditional Chinese Medicine?

1) Pensiveness Damaging the Spleen
2) Weak Constitution
3) Overstrain Injuring the Kidney
4) Attack by Toxic Heat or Damp-Heat

How is LGN Differentiated and Treated by Traditional Chinese Medicine?

1) <u>Hyperactivity of Heat in the Lower Warmer</u>

Symptoms: History of syndromes by exogenous pathogenic factors, abrupt onset of bright red hematuria or proteinuria, burning sensation in the urethra, dark urine, dysphoria, thirst, flushed face, aphthous stomatitis, insomnia, dreamful sleep, red tongue, and rapid pulse.

Therapeutic Principle: To clear away heat, purge fire, cool blood and stop bleeding.

Prescription: Modified Xiao Ji Decoction.

Modifications: For chronic hematuria and deficiency of qi and yin, remove Talcum and Medulla Tetrapanacis Papyriferi, and add Radix Pseudostellariae Heterophyllae (Tai Zi Shen) 15g, Radix Astragali (Huang Qi) 12g and Gelatinum Corii Asini (E Jiao) 9g; for severe burning pain in the urethra, difficult urination and dark urine, add Folium Pyrrosiae (Shi Wei) 10g, Herba Taraxaci Mongolici (Pu Gong Ying) 20g and Radix Notoginseng (San Qi) 10g; for fever and sore throat, add modified Yin Qiao Powder; for remarkable proteinuria, add Folium Pyrrosiae (Shi Wei) 10g and Herba Pteridis Multifidae (Feng Wei Cao) 15g.

2) <u>Hyperactivity of Fire due to Deficiency of Yin</u>

Symptoms: Oliguria with dark urine, vertigo, tinnitus, spiritlessness, feverish sensation in palms and soles, flushed cheeks, hectic fever, weak and sore loins and knees, red tongue, and thready and rapid pulse.

Therapeutic Principle: To nourish yin, purge fire, cool blood and stop bleeding.

Prescription: Modified Zhi Bai Di Huang Pill.

Modifications: For severe deficiency of kidney yin, add Fructus Lycii (Gou Qi Zi) 10g and Herba Ecliptae Prostratae (Han Lian Cao) 15g; for deficiency of qi, add Radix Pseudostellariae Heterophyllae (Tai Zi Shen) 15g and Radix Astragali (Huang Qi) 12g; for severe heat, add Herba Taraxaci Mongolici (Pu Gong Ying) 20g and Herba Pteridis Multifidae (Feng Wei Cao) 15g; for concurrent blood stasis, add Radix Salviae Miltiorrhizae (Dan Shen) 10g and Herba Leonuri Heterophylii (Yi Mu Cao) 12g; for remarkable proteinuria, add Cortex Lycii Radicis (Di Gu Pi) 10g, Folium Mahoniae (Shi Da Gong Lao) 12g and Carapax Trionycis (Bie Jia) 15g.

3) Blockage of the Collaterals by Blood Stasis

Symptoms: Dark purple urine with blood clod, black or dark and gloomy complexion, localized pain or pricking pain in the lower back, dark purple tongue with ecchymosis or petechiae, and rough pulse.

Therapeutic Principle: To promote blood circulation and activate collaterals.

Prescription: Modified Xue Fu Zhu Yu Decoction.

Modifications: For severe blood stasis, add Radix Salviae Miltiorrhizae (Dan Shen) 10g, Radix Notoginseng (San Qi) 9g, Pollen Typhae (Pu Huang) 10g and Hominis Crinis Carbonisatus (Xue Yu Tan) 10g; for concurrent deficiency of the kidney, remove Radix Rehmanniae, and add Radix Rehmanniae Praeparatae (Shu Di Huang) 15g, Cortex Eucommiae Ulmoidis (Du Zhong) 12g and Radix Dipsaci Asperi (Xu Duan) 15g; for severe lumbago, replace the prescription with Shen Tong Zhu Yu Decoction; for remarkable proteinuria, add Bombyx Batryticatus (Jiang Can) 10g, Buthus Martensi (Quan Xie) 3g and Rhizoma Curcumae Ezhu (E Zhu) 10g.

4) Deficiency of Spleen Qi

Symptoms: Hematuria or proteinuria, lusterless complexion, lassitude, anorexia, shortness of breath, low voice, or gingival hemorrhage, pale tongue, and thready and weak pulse.

Therapeutic Principle: To nourish the spleen and replenish blood.

Prescription: Modified Gui Pi Decoction.

Modifications: For remarkable hematuria, add Rhizoma Imperatae Cylindricae (Bai Mao Gen) 20g, Pollen Typhae (Pu Huang) 10g and Nodus Nelumbinis Nuciferae Rhizomatis (Ou Jie) 12g; for concurrent blood stasis, add San Qi Powder; for lingering hemorrhage, add Fructus Corni Officinalis (Shan Zhu Yu) 10g, Fructus Schisandrae Chinensis (Wu Wei Zi) 3g and Halloysitum Rubrum (Chi Shi Zhi) 12g; for remarkable proteinuria, add Radix Astragali (Huang Qi) 12g, Semen Euryales Ferocis (Qian Shi) 12g and Fructus Rosae Laevigatae (Jin Ying Zi) 12g.

5) Deficiency of Kidney Qi

Symptoms: Pale red hematuria or proteinuria, vertigo, tinnitus, malaise, lumbago, pale tongue, deep, thready and forceless pulse.

Therapeutic Principle: To nourish the kidney, replenish and arrest kidney qi, and stop bleeding.

Prescription: Modified Wu Bi Shan Yao Pill.

Modifications: For remarkable hematuria, add Herba Agrimoniae Pilosae (Xian He Cao) 12g, Pollen Typhae (Pu Huang) 10g, Flos Sophorae Japonicae (Huai Hua) 12g and Folium Callicarpae Formosanae (Zi Zhu) 12g; for lumbago, aversion to cold and timidity, add Cornu Cervi (Lu Jiao) 10g and Rhizoma Cibotii Barometz (Gou Ji) 12g; for remarkable proteinuria, add Fructus Rubi Chingii (Fu Pen Zi) 10g, Fructus Rosae Laevigatae (Jin Ying Zi) 12g and Fructus Alpinae Oxyphyllae (Yi Zhi Ren) 10g.

What Kinds of Chinese Patent Drugs are Available to Treat LGN?

1) Shen Yan Kang Fu Tablet: 8 tablets each time, thrice daily.
2) Shen Fu Kang Capsule: 1.2-1.8g each time, thrice daily.
3) Shen Yan Shu Capsule: 1.5g each time, thrice daily.
4) Huang Qi Injection: 20-40ml each time, once daily.
5) Jin Shui Bao Capsule: 3-4 capsules each time, thrice daily.

5. Nephrotic Syndrome (NS)

Nephrotic syndrome is a glomerular disorder characterized by very high levels of protein in the urine, low levels of protein albumin in the blood due to its severe loss in the urine, edema and ascites, and high cholesterol levels in the blood. Nephrotic syndrome results from damage to the kidneys' glomeruli.

Nephrotic syndrome can develop from gradual progression of a mild loss of protein in the urine (sometimes called microalbuminuria), or it can develop suddenly. Nephrotic syndrome can occur at any age. In children, it is most common between the ages of 18 months and 4 years, and more boys than girls are affected. In older people, both sexes are more equally affected.

In adults, about one-third of patients with nephritic syndrome will have a systemic disease such as diabetes mellitus, amyloidosis, or lupus. The remainder will be categorized as having idiopathic nephritic syndrome due to one of four forms of glomerular diseases: minimal change disease (lipoid nephrosis, nil disease), focal glomerular sclerosis, membranous glomerulonephritis, and membranoproliferative glomerulonephritis. There is a rare nephrotic syndrome present in the first week of life called "congenital nephrotic syndrome." Congenital nephrotic syndrome is inherited by an autosomal recessive gene. The outcome for this type of nephrotic syndrome is extremely poor.

The following are the most common symptoms of nephrotic syndrome. However, each individual may experience symptoms differently. Symptoms may include:

- Fatigue and malaise

- Decreased appetite
- Weight gain and facial swelling
- Abdominal swelling, fullness or pain
- Feeling bloated or tight
- Foamy urine
- Peripheral edema, ascites or anasarca
- Pale fingernail beds
- Dull hair

How is Nephrotic Syndrome Diagnosed by Conventional Western Medicine?

Diagnosis is made based on a thorough physical examination, complete medical history and diagnostic tests, such as urine tests, blood tests, microscopic analysis, renal ultrasound and renal biopsy. Essentials of diagnosis include: (1) urine protein excretion $> 3.5g/1.73m^2$ per 24 hours; (2) hypoalbuminemia (serum albumin $< 3.0g/dL$); (3) peripheral edema, or anasarca with ascites; and (4) hypercholesterolemia (fasting level $> 200mg/dL$).

How is Nephrotic Syndrome Treated by Conventional Western Medicine?

During the initial episode of nephrotic syndrome, a patient may require hospitalization to be monitored for edema, blood pressure and breathing problems. Some management problems are common to all patients with nephritic syndrome regardless of the cause, such as protein loss, peripheral edema and ascites, hyperlipidemia and hypercoagulable state. Medications may be required to treat initial symptoms and during relapses, including: corticosteroids, immunosuppressive drug therapy, diuretics, intravenous (IV) albumin and dietary management. If thrombosis is detected, heparin therapy followed by warfarin is necessary for at least 6 months.

What Causes Nephrotic Syndrome According to Traditional Chinese Medicine?

1) Attack by Exogenous Pathogenic Wind
2) Invasion of Toxic Substances from Skin Carbuncle Ulcers
3) Invasion of Water and Dampness
4) Improper Diet
5) Internal Injury of Overstrain and Sex Indulgence
6) Internal Obstruction of Blood Stasis

How is Nephrotic Syndrome Differentiated and Treated by Traditional Chinese Medicine?

1) <u>Invasion by Pathogenic Wind and Overflow of Water</u>

Symptoms: Edema of eyelids at the beginning, progressive edema of the extremities and ultimate anasarca, luster complexion, pitted edema (the depressed part of the skin is easily resumed by itself), fever, sore throat, cough, difficult urination, thin and white tongue coating, and floating pulse.

Therapeutic Principle: To dispel wind, relieve exterior syndrome, release lung qi and induce diuresis.

Prescription: Modified Yue Bi Jia Zhu Decoction.

Modifications: For wind-heat syndrome, add Radix Isatidis seu Baphicacanthi (Ban Lan Gen) 12g, Radix Platycodi Grandiflori (Jie Gen) 9g, Flos Lonicerae (Jin Yin Hua) 15g and Fructus Forsythiae Suspensae (Lian Qiao) 10g; for wind-cold syndrome, remove Gypsum Fibrosum, and add Folium Perillae Frutescentis (Su Ye) 10g, Ramulus Cinnamomi Cassiae (Gui Zhi) 10g and Radix Saposhnikoviae Divaricatae (Fang Feng) 10g; for severe edema, add Rhizoma Imperatae Cylindricae (Bai Mao Gen) 20g, Herba Spirodelae (Fu Ping) 10g, Rhizoma Alismatis Orientalis (Ze Xie) 10g and Sclerotium Poriae Cocos (Fu Ling) 12g.

2) <u>Retention of Toxic Dampness</u>

Symptoms: Edema of the eyelids, progressive anasarca, carbuncle ulcers, aversion to wind, fever, difficult urination, red tongue with thin and yellow coating, and floating and rapid or slippery and rapid pulse.

Therapeutic Principle: To release lung qi, remove toxic substance, eliminate dampness and subside swelling.

Prescription: Modified Ma Huang Lian Qiao Chi Xiao Dou Decoction and Wu Wei Xiao Du Decoction.

Modifications: For severe dampness, add Radix Sophorae Flavescentis (Ku Shen) 9g and Rhizoma Smilacis Glabrae (Tu Fu Ling) 30g; for itch, add Cortex Dictamni Radicis (Bai Xian Pi) 9g and Fructus Kochiae Scopariae (Di Fu Zi) 12g; for red swelling, add Cortex Moutan Radicis (Mu Dan Pi) 10g and Radix Paeoniae Rubra (Chi Shao) 10g.

3) <u>Retention of Water and Dampness</u>

Symptoms: Pitted anasarca, chest stuffiness, abdominal distention, general heavy sensation, drowsiness, anorexia, acid regurgitation, oliguria, white and greasy tongue coating, and soft and slow pulse.

Therapeutic Principle: To strengthen the spleen, eliminate dampness, activate yang and induce diuresis.

Prescription: Modified Wu Pi Decoction and Wei Ling Decoction.

Modifications: For severe edema and dyspnea, add Herba Ephedrae (Ma Huang) 6g, Semen Armeniacae Amarum (Xing Ren) 10g, Semen Descurainiae seu Lepidii (Ting Li Zi) 10g and Fructus Zizyphi Jujubae (Da Zao) 20g.

4) Internal Accumulation of Damp-Heat

Symptoms: Remarkable edema with strained skin, abdominal enlargement, stuffiness and fullness, chest stuffiness, dysphoria with feverish sensation, bitter taste in the mouth, dry mouth, constipation, oliguria with dark urine, red tongue with yellow and greasy coating, and deep and rapid or soft and rapid pulse.

Therapeutic Principle: To clear away heat, eliminate dampness, induce diuresis and subside swelling.

Prescription: Modified Shu Zao Decoction.

Modifications: For hoarse breathing voice, dyspnea with inability to lie flat, and severe edema, use Si Ling Powder or Wu Pi Decoction combined with Ting Li Da Zao Xie Fei Decoction; for chronic damp-heat transforming into dryness that impairs yin, use Zhu Ling Decoction; for hematuria, add Rhizoma Imperatae Cylindricae (Bai Mao Gen) 20g, Radix Rubiae Cordifoliae (Qian Cao) 10g, Radix Euphorbiae Pekinensis (Da Ji) 3g and Herba Cephalanoploris (Xiao Ji) 15g.

5) Spleen Deficiency and Dampness Retention

Symptoms: Pitted edema (the depressed part of the skin is not easily resumed), abdominal distention, anorexia, sallow complexion, spiritlessness, fatigue, oliguria with clear urine, loose stools, pale tongue with white and greasy or white and slippery coating, and deep and slow or deep and weak pulse.

Therapeutic Principle: To invigorate the spleen, warm spleen yang, induce diuresis and subside swelling.

Prescription: Modified Shi Pi Decoction.

Modifications: For oliguria, add Ramulus Cinnamomi Cassiae (Gui Zhi) 9g and Rhizoma Alismatis Orientalis (Ze Xie) 10g; for severe qi deficiency, add Radix Codonopsitis Pilosulae (Dang Shen) 10g and Radix Astragali (Huang Qi) 12g.

6) Deficiency of Kidney Yang

Symptoms: Generalized pitted edema (the depressed part of the skin does not resume itself), palpitation, dyspnea, cold pain and soreness in the lower back, oliguria or polyuria, spiritlessness, cold limbs, aversion to cold, cold limbs, dark complexion, pale and chubby tongue with white coating, and deep and thready or deep, slow and forceless pulse.

Therapeutic Principle: To warm the kidney, activate yang.

Prescription: Modified Ji Sheng Shen Qi Pill and Zhen Wu Decoction.

Modifications: For palpitation, cyanosis of lips, deficiency and rapid or knot and intermittent pulse, add Ramulus Cinnamomi Cassiae (Gui Zhi) 10g, Radix Glycyrrhizae Uralensis (Gan Cao) 6g and Radix Salviae Miltiorrhizae (Dan Shen) 10g; for dyspnea, sweating, deficiency, float and rapid pulse, add Radix Ginseng (Ren Shen) 6g, Gecko (Ge Jie) 5g, Fructus Schisandrae Chinensis (Wu Wei Zi) 5g and Fructus Corni Officinalis (Shan Zhu Yu) 10g.

7) <u>Deficiency of Kidney Yin</u>

Symptoms: Recurrent and persistent edema, spiritlessness, lumbago, seminal emission, dry mouth and throat, feverish sensation in the chest, palms and soles, red tongue, and thready and weak pulse.

Therapeutic Principle: To nourish kidney yin and induce diuresis.

Prescription: Modified Zuo Gui Pill supplemented with Rhizoma Alismatis Orientalis (Ze Xie) 10g, Sclerotium Poriae Cocos (Fu Ling) 12g and Semen Malvae (Dong Kui Zi) 12g.

Modifications: Add Radix Salviae Miltiorrhizae (Dan Shen) 10g, Rhizoma Ligustici Chuanxiong (Chuan Xiong) 10g, Radix Paeoniae Rubra (Chi Shao) 10g and Herba Lycopi Lucidi (Ze Lan) 10g to promote blood circulation and remove blood stasis, and ultimately promote fluid and water circulation.

What Kinds of Chinese Patent Drugs are Available to Treat Nephrotic Syndrome?

1) Shen Yan Xiao Zhong Tablet: 5 tablets each time, thrice daily.
2) Lei Gong Teng Duo Gan Tablet: 20mg each time, thrice daily.
3) Bai Ling Capsule: 4 capsules each time, thrice daily.
4) Huang Qi Injection: 20-40ml each time, once daily.

6. Acute Tubulointerstitial Nephritis (Acute Interstitial Nephritis, AIN)

Acute interstitial nephritis is an immune-mediated inflammatory disorder of the renal tubulointerstitium, initiated by medications, infection, and other causes. Acute tubulointerstitial nephritis more accurately describes this disease entity, because the renal tubules, as well as the interstitium, are involved. 15 percent of cases of acute renal failure are caused by acute interstitial nephritis. Clinical features are essentially those of acute renal failure from any cause. There are no specific history, physical examination, or laboratory findings that distinguish acute interstitial nephritis from other causes of acute renal failure. Classic findings of fever, rash, and eosinophilia are found in less that 30% of patients. Diagnostic studies such as urine eosinophils and renal gallium 67 scanning provide suggestive evidence, but they are unable to reliably confirm or exclude the diagnosis of acute interstitial nephritis. Renal biopsy remains the gold standard for diagnosis.

The most frequent causes of AIN include drug reactions (antibiotics and NSAIDs), systemic infections, and immune or neoplastic disorders. Most patients with AIN in whom offending medications are withdrawn early can be expected to recover normal or near-normal renal function within a few weeks. Prognosis for those who remain on the precipitating medication for three or more weeks is poor.

Patients with AIN typically present with nonspecific symptoms of acute renal failure, including oliguria, malaise, anorexia, or nausea and vomiting, with acute or subacute onset. The clinical presentation can range from asymptomatic elevation in creatinine or blood urea nitrogen (BUN) or abnormal urinary sediment, to generalized hypersensitivity syndrome with fever, rash, occasional flank pain, eosinophilia, and oliguric renal failure.

The classic triad of low-grade fever, skin rash, and arthralgias was primarily described with methicillin (Staphcillin)-induced AIN, but it was present only about one third of the time.

How is AIN Diagnosed by Conventional Western Medicine?

Renal biopsy is the only definitive method of establishing the diagnosis of AIN; other laboratory features, e.g. hematuria and peripheral blood eosinophilia, are used to provide suggestive evidence of AIN, to guide conservative management, or to permit empiric treatment with steroids. Imaging tests include ultrasound and gallium scan.

How is AIN Treated by Conventional Western Medicine?

All medications that are likely to cause AIN must be discontinued. If there is significant renal impairment, treatment with steroids typically is required. Stronger immunosuppressive agents may be needed if there is no response to the steroids. Corticosteroids appear to provide some benefit in terms of clinical improvement and return of renal function, but no controlled clinical trials have been conducted to confirm this.

What Causes AIN According to Traditional Chinese Medicine?

1) Infection of Damp-Heat and Toxic Heat
2) Weak Constitution

How is AIN Differentiated and Treated by Traditional Chinese Medicine?

1) Primary Aspect

(1) <u>Yin Deficiency and Hyperactivity of Fire</u>

Symptoms: Weak and sore loins and knees, dysphoria with feverish sensation in the chest, palms and soles, vertigo, tinnitus, night sweating, dry mouth and throat, constipation, oliguria with dark urine, hematuria, red tongue with little coating, and thready and rapid pulse.

Therapeutic Principle: To nourish yin, purge fire, cool blood and stop hemorrhage.

Prescription: Modified Zhi Bai Di Huang Decoction and Xiao Ji Decoction.

Modifications: For dysphoria with feverish sensation in the chest, palms and soles, add Radix Ophiopogonis Japonici (Mai Dong) 12g, Radix Scrophulariae Ningpoensis (Xuan Shen) 12g and Cortex Lycii Radicis (Di Gu Pi) 12g; for constipation, add Radix et Rhizoma Rhei (Da Huang) 6g; for hectic fever and night sweating, add Carapax et Plastrum Testudinis (Gui Ban) 20g and Carapax Trionycis (Bie Jia) 20g; for insomnia and dreamful sleep, add Semen Biotae Orientalis (Bai Zi Ren) 15g and Semen Ziziphi Spinosae (Suan Zao Ren) 15g.

(2) <u>Qi Deficiency of the Spleen and Kidney</u>

Symptoms: Sallow and lusterless complexion, spiritlessness, fatigue, weak and sore loins and knees, heel pain, abdominal distention, anorexia, or nausea and vomiting, nocturnal polyuria and urinary frequency, or polyuria with clear urine, pale and chubby tongue with thin and white coating, and deep, thready and forceless pulse.

Therapeutic Principle: To strengthen the spleen and nourish the kidney.

Prescription: Modified Si Jun Zi Decoction and Ji Sheng Shen Qi Pill.

Modifications: For seniors with extreme deficiency of kidney qi and yang, add Radix Panacis Quinquefolii (Xi Yang Shen) 5g, Cordyceps Sinensis (Dong Chong Xia Cao) 10g, Semen Cuscutae Chinensis (Tu Si Zi) 12g and sliced Cornu Cervi (Lu Jiao) 10g; for abdominal distention, white and greasy tongue coating, add Fructus Amomi Villosi (Sha Ren) 5g, Rhizoma Atractylodis (Cang Zhu) 10g and Semen Coicis (Yi Yi Ren) 12g; for sallow complexion, shortness of breath and fatigue, add Radix Astragali (Huang Qi) 12g and Radix Angelicae Sinensis (Dang Gui) 10g.

2) Secondary Aspect

(1) <u>Attack by Exterior Wind-Heat</u>

Symptoms: Fever, slight aversion to cold, sweating, headache, thirst, dry throat, red tongue tip and margin, thin and slight yellow tongue coating, and floating and rapid pulse.

Therapeutic Principle: To clear away heat and relieve exterior syndrome.

Prescription: Modified Ma Huang Lian Qiao Chi Xiao Dou Decoction.

Modifications: For proteinuria, add Radix Astragali (Huang Qi) 12g, Fructus Rosae Laevigatae (Jin Ying Zi) 15g and Semen Cuscutae Chinensis (Tu Si Zi) 12g; for severe hematuria, add Herba Agrimoniae Pilosae (Xian He Cao) 12g and Rhizoma Imperatae Cylindricae (Bai Mao Gen) 20g; for oliguria, add Cortex Poriae Cocos (Fu Ling Pi) 12g and Semen Plantaginis (Che Qian Zi) 9g; for vomiting, add Herba Agastache seu Pogostemonis (Huo Xiang) 10g, Caulis Bambusae in Taeniam (Zhu Ru) 10g and Rhizoma Coptidis (Huang Lian) 9g.

Hyperactivity of Toxic Heat

Symptoms: Chill, high fever, lumbago, headache, drowsiness, dry mouth with preference to drink, skin rash, oliguria with dark and hot urine, difficult urination, constipation, crimson tongue with dry and yellow coating, and taut, slippery and rapid pulse.

Therapeutic Principle: To clear away heat, remove toxic substance, cool blood and resolve rash.

Prescription: Modified Qing Wen Bai Du Decoction.

Modifications: For constipation, abdominal pain or jaundice, add Radix et Rhizoma Rhei (Da Huang) 9g; for nausea, vomiting, abdominal distention and fullness, add Rhizoma Pinelliae Ternatae (Ban Xia) 10g, Pericarpium Citri Reticulatae (Chen Pi) 9g and Fructus Citri Aurantii Immaturus (Zhi Shi) 10g; for skin rash, add Radix Lithospermi seu Macrotomiae (Zi Cao) 10g, Herba seu Radix Cirsii Japonici (Da Ji) 12g and Herba Cephalanoploris (Xiao Ji) 15g; for lumbago, add Cortex Eucommiae Ulmoidis (Du Zhong) 12g and Radix Achyranthis Bidentatae (Huai Niu Xi) 12g; for joint pain, add Fructus Chaenomelis (Mu Gua) 10g and Semen Coicis (Yi Yi Ren) 20g.

(2) Retention of Damp-Heat

Symptoms: Lumbago, epigastric stuffiness, anorexia, no desire for drink, dark yellow and hot urine, urination with burning sensation, or dysuria, or difficult urination, loose stools, dyschezia, yellow and greasy tongue coating, soft and rapid or slippery and rapid pulse.

Therapeutic Principle: To clear away heat, eliminate dampness, purge fire and treat stranguria.

Prescription: Modified Si Miao Pill.

Modifications: For bitter taste in the mouth, add Radix Gentianae (Long Dan Cao) 5g and Rhizoma Coptidis (Huang Lian) 9g; for nausea, add Caulis Bambusae in Taeniam (Zhu Ru) 10g and Rhizoma Pinelliae Ternatae (Ban Xia) 10g; for abdominal distention and anorexia, add Fructus Amomi Cardamomi (Bai Kou Ren) 5g and Fructus Amomi Villosi (Sha Ren) 5g; for severe lumbago, add Cortex Eucommiae Ulmoidis (Du Zhong) 12g and Radix Achyranthis Bidentatae (Huai Niu Xi) 12g; for blood stasis, add Semen Pruni Persicae (Tao Ren) 10g, Flos Carthami Tinctorii (Hong Hua) 10g and Rhizoma Ligustici Chuanxiong (Chuan Xiong) 10g.

(3) Spread of Turbid Dampness

Symptoms: Anorexia, nausea and vomiting, general heavy sensation, drowsiness, cloudy consciousness, or coma, oliguria, diarrhea or constipation, pale and chubby or dry and red tongue with greasy or black coating, thready and taut or taut and slippery pulse.

Therapeutic Principle: To clear away heat, eliminate dampness and regulate Triple Warmer.

Prescription: Modified Chang Pu Yu Jin Decoction, Er Chen Decoction, or Fu Ling Pi Decoction.

Modifications: For deficiency of the spleen with anorexia, add Radix Codonopsitis Pilosulae (Dang Shen) 10g and Rhizoma Atractylodis Macrocephalae (Bai Zhu) 10g; for irritability, red tongue and bitter taste in the mouth, add Rhizoma Coptidis (Huang Lian) 10g, Herba Lophatheri Gracilis (Dan Zhu Ye) 12g and Rhizoma Anemarrhenae (Zhi Mu) 10g.

What Kinds of Chinese Patent Drugs are Available to Treat AIN?

Shen Fu Kang Capsule: 4-6 capsules each time, thrice daily.

7. Chronic Tubulointerstitial Nephritis (Chronic Interstitial Nephritis, CTIN or CIN)

Kidney diseases that involve structures in the kidney outside the glomerulus are broadly referred to as tubulointerstitial. These diseases generally involve tubules and/or the interstitium of the kidney and spare the glomeruli. Chronic tubulointerstitial nephritis CTIN) is characterized by interstitial scarring, fibrosis, and tubule atrophy, resulting in progressive chronic renal insufficiency. The causes of CTIN are numerous. The most common cause is prolonged obstruction of the urinary tract, followed by reflux nephropathy. The causes of tubulointerstitial nephritis include:

- Drugs, such as analgesics, lithium, cyclosporine, tacrolimus
- Heavy metals
- Obstructive uropathy, nephrolithiasis, and reflux disease
- Immunologic diseases, such as lupus, sarcoidosis, vasculitis, chronic transplant nephropathy
- Neoplasia, such as myeloma, leukemia, amyloidosis
- Atherosclerotic kidney disease
- Metabolic diseases, such as hypercalcemia, cystinosis, potassium depletion, hyperoxaluria
- Genetics, such as Alport syndrome, medullary cystic disease
- Miscellaneous such as Balkan endemic nephropathy

In CTIN, prognosis depends on the cause and on the ability to recognize and stop the process before irreversible fibrosis occurs. Many genetic (cystic kidney disease), metabolic (cystinosis), and toxic (heavy metal) causes may not be modifiable, in which case CTIN usually evolves to end-stage renal disease.

Polyuria and nocturia are the most frequent clinical complaints. Some individuals may also have a salt-wasting defect, putting them at risk for significant volume depletion following sodium restriction or the use of diuretics.

How is CTIN Diagnosed by Conventional Western Medicine?

Diagnosis is based on history, physical examination, laboratory and imaging tests. Urinalysis is non-specific. The most characteristic laboratory finding is evidence for tubular dysfunction (polyuria and sodium wasting) out of proportion to the degree of renal impairment and an inability to acidify the urine in association with hyperchloremic metabolic acidosis.

How is CTIN Treated by Conventional Western Medicine?

Treatment depends upon identifying the underlying disorders and the degree of interstitial fibrosis that has developed. Once there is evidence for loss of parenchyma, treatment is then directed toward management of medical complications. Treatment of chronic tubulointerstitial Nephritis includes:

- Withdrawal of drugs and heavy metals
- Relieve the obstruction of the urinary tract
- Medical treatment, such as potassium dietary restriction or sodium and bicarbonate supplements, and chelation therapy
- Surgical removal of urinary tract obstructions
- Dialysis
- Kidney transplantation

What Causes CTIN According to Traditional Chinese Medicine?

1) Weak Zang Organs
2) Deficiency of the Kidney Essence
3) Infection of Damp-Heat and Other Pathogenic Factors

How is CTIN Differentiated and Treated by Traditional Chinese Medicine?

1) Primary Aspect

(1) Yin Deficiency of the Liver and Kidney

Symptoms: Vertigo, headache, thirst with a desire to drink, dysphoria with feverish sensation in the chest, palms and soles, numbness or even slight tremor of extremities, emaciation, constipation, oliguria, dark urine, red tongue with little coating, and taut and thready pulse.

Therapeutic Principle: To replenish blood, soothe the liver, nourish yin and tonify the kidney.

Prescription: Modified San Jia Fu Mai Decoction.

Modifications: For fever, add Herba Artemisiae Apiaceae seu Annuae (Qing Hao) 10g and Radix Cynanchi Atrati (Bai Wei) 10g; for palpitation, add Semen Ziziphi Spinosae (Suan Zao Ren) 15g and Mastodi Dentis Fossilia (Long Chi) 20g.

(2) Qi and Yin Deficiency of the Spleen and kidney

Symptoms: Lusterless complexion, shortness of breath, fatigue, sore loins and weak knees, dry mouth without a desire to drink, oliguria with yellow urine, nocturnal polyuria with clear urine, pale tongue with teeth marks, or slight red tongue with little coating, and deep and thready or thready and rapid pulse.

Therapeutic Principle: To nourish the spleen and kidney, and replenish qi and yin.

Prescription: Modified Liu Wei Di Huang Pill and Bu Zhong Yi Qi Decoction.

Modifications: For loose stools, add Rhizoma Atractylodis Macrocephalae (Bai Zhu) 12g, Semen Nelumbinis Nuciferae (Lian Zi) 12g and Semen Euryales Ferocis (Qian Shi) 12g; for anorexia and food retention, add Fructus Crataegi (Shan Zha) 12g, Fructus Hordei Germinatus (Mai Ya) 12g, Massa Medicata Fermentata (Shen Qu) 12g and Fructus Citri Aurantii (Zhi Ke) 10g; for deficiency and collapse of qi, double the amount of Radix Astragali (Huang Qi); for chest fullness and fatigue, add Rhizoma Atractylodis (Cang Zhu) 10g and Radix Aucklandiae Lappae (Mu Xiang) 10g.

(3) Yang Deficiency of the Spleen and Kidney

Symptoms: Lassitude, anorexia, abdominal distention, sore loins and weak knees, cold limbs, loose and soft stools, nocturnal polyuria with clear urine, pale tongue with teeth marks, and deep and thready pulse.

Therapeutic Principle: To warm and nourish the spleen and kidney.

Prescription: Modified Jin Gui Shi Qi Pill.

Modifications: For seniors with deficiency of kidney yang, add Radix Ginseng Rubra (Hong Shen) 10g, sliced Cornu Cervi (Lu Jiao) 10g and Cordyceps Sinensis (Dong Chong Xia Cao) 10g; for anemia, deficiency of qi and blood, add Radix Angelicae Sinensis (Dang Gui) 12g and Placenta Hominis (Zi He Che) 3g; for kidney deficiency with lumbago, add Radix Morindae officinalis (Ba Ji Tian) 12g, Herba Cistanches (Rou Cong Rong) 15g, Cortex Eucommiae Ulmoidis (Du Zhong) 12g and Herba Taxilli (Sang Ji Sheng) 15g.

2) Secondary Aspect

(1) Attack by Toxic Heat

Symptoms: Chill, high fever, lumbago, oliguria with dark and hot urine, difficult urination, dry mouth with a desire to drink, or vague skin rash, or jaundice, or abdominal distention and pain, nausea, vomiting, constipation, or joint pain, crimson tongue with dry, yellow and abundant coating, and taut, slippery and rapid pulse.

Therapeutic Principle: To nourish yin, purge fire, cool blood and stop hemorrhage.

Prescription: Modified Zhi Bai Di Huang Pill and Xiao Ji Decoction.

Modifications: For damp-heat, difficult urination with hot urine, add Herba Taraxaci Mongolici (Pu Gong Ying) 20g, Herba Dianthi (Qu Mai) 10g, Herba Polygoni Avicularis (Bian Xu) 12g and Herba Plantaginis (Che Qian Cao) 12g; for deficiency of yin with smooth and red tongue, feverish sensation in palms and soles, add Herba Dendrobii (Shi Hu) 12g, Radix Ophiopogonis Japonici (Mai Dong) 12g, Radix Scrophulariae Ningpoensis (Xuan Shen) 12g and Carapax Trionycis (Bie Jia) 20g; for deficiency of the spleen with spiritlessness, lassitude and lusterless complexion, add Radix Astragali (Huang Qi) 12g, Radix Angelicae Sinensis (Dang Gui) 12g and Radix Pseudostellariae Heterophyllae (Tai Zi Shen) 15g.

(2) <u>Invasion of Pathogenic Factors</u>

Symptoms: Dysphoria, dry mouth, thirst, lumbago, fever, constipation, oliguria with dark urine, red tongue with little coating, and thready and rapid pulse.

Therapeutic Principle: To clear away heat, remove toxic substance, induce diuresis and nourish yin.

Prescription: Modified Qing Xin Lian Zi Decoction.

Modifications: For kidney damaged by drugs, add Semen Phaseoli Radiati (Lu Dou) 20g, Rhizoma Smilacis Glabrae (Tu Fu Ling) 30g and Radix Saposhnikoviae Divaricatae (Fang Feng) 10g; for fever, add Radix Bupleuri (Chai Hu) 10g and Herba Menthae Haplocalycis (Bo He) 10g; for severe qi deficiency, increase the dosage of Radix Astragali (Huang Qi), and add Radix Pseudostellariae Heterophyllae (Tai Zi Shen) 20g; for severe deficiency of yin, add Radix Rehmanniae (Di Huang) 20g and Radix Scrophulariae Ningpoensis (Xuan Shen) 12g.

(3) <u>Retention of Water and Dampness</u>

Symptoms: Pale complexion, cold pain in the lower back and knees, edema of extremities, difficult urination, pale tongue with thin coating, and deep and slow pulse.

Therapeutic Principle: To eliminate dampness, relieve swelling, warm yang and regulate qi.

Prescription: Modified Wu Pi Decoction and Zhen Wu Decoction.

Modifications: For deficiency of kidney yang, add Semen Cuscutae Chinensis (Tu Si Zi) 12g, Radix Morindae officinalis (Ba Ji Tian) 12g, Herba Epimedii (Yin Yang Huo) 12g and sliced Cornu Cervi (Lu Jiao) 10g; for deficiency of spleen yang, add Radix Codonopsitis Pilosulae (Dang Shen) 10g, Rhizoma Pinelliae Ternatae (Ban Xia) 10g, Rhizoma Atractylodis (Cang Zhu) 10g and Radix Glycyrrhizae

Uralensis (Gan Cao) 6g; for oliguria, add Herba Lycopi Lucidi (Ze Lan) 12g, Semen Coicis (Yi Yi Ren) 20g, Semen Plantaginis (Che Qian Zi) 9g and Sclerotium Polypori Umbellati (Zhu Ling) 10g.

What Kinds of Chinese Patent Drugs are Available to Treat CTIN?

Jin Shui Bao Capsule: 3-5 capsules each time, thrice daily.

8. Diabetic Nephropathy (DN)

Diabetic nephropathy, also known as Kimmelstiel-Wilson syndrome and intercapillary glomerulonephritis, is a complication of diabetes. Diabetic nephropathy is a clinical syndrome characterized by persistent albuminuria, a relentless decline in the glomerular filtration rate (GFR), and elevated arterial blood pressure. Diabetic nephropathy is the most common cause of chronic kidney failure and end-stage kidney disease in the United States. People with both type 1 and type 2 diabetes are at risk. The risk is higher if blood-glucose levels are poorly controlled.

The earliest detectable change in the course of diabetic nephropathy is a thickening in the glomerulus, resulting in microalbuminuria. The glomeruli and kidneys are typically normal or increased in size initially. As diabetic nephropathy progresses, increasing numbers of glomeruli are destroyed. Protein may appear in the urine for 5 to 10 years before other symptoms develop. High blood pressure often accompanies diabetic nephropathy. Over time, the kidney's ability to function starts to decline. Diabetic nephropathy may eventually lead to chronic kidney failure. The disorder continues to progress toward end-stage kidney disease.

The exact cause of diabetic nephropathy is unknown, but various postulated mechanisms are hyperglycemia (causing hyperfiltration and renal injury), advanced glycosylation products, and activation of cytokines.

Early stage diabetic nephropathy has no symptoms. Symptoms develop late in the disease and may be a result of kidney failure or eliminating high amounts of protein in the urine. Symptoms may include:

- Fatigue
- Foamy appearance or excessive frothing of the urine
- Frequent hiccups
- Malaise
- Generalized itching
- Headache
- Nausea and vomiting

- Poor appetite
- Edema of the legs
- Edema, usually around the eyes in the mornings; general edema may occur with late-stage disease
- Unintentional weight gain (from fluid build up)
- Symptoms associated with other associated disorders, such as hypertension, diabetic retinopathy, peripheral vascular occlusive disease, diabetic neuropathy, nonhealing skin ulcers and osteomyelitis

How is Diabetic Nephropathy Diagnosed by Conventional Western Medicine?

Diagnosis is made based on medical history, physical exam and diagnostic tests. The first laboratory abnormality is a positive microalbuminuria test. The diagnosis is suspected when a routine urinalysis shows proteinuria of someone with diabetes. Serum creatinine and BUN eventually may increase as kidney damage gets worse. A kidney biopsy confirms the diagnosis. The biopsy may be done if there is any doubt in the diagnosis, and to study the extent of the disease.

How is Diabetic Nephropathy Treated by Conventional Western Medicine?

The goals of treatment are to slow the progression of kidney damage and control related complications. The treatment of diabetic nephropathy may include:

- Medical care such as glycemic control, hypertension treatment, ACE inhibitors or angiotensin receptor blockers, medications to manage diabetes, and antibiotics to treat urinary tract and other infections
- Diet
- Renal replacement therapies, such as hemodialysis, peritoneal dialysis, kidney transplantation, or combined kidney-pancreas transplantation
- Activity: No restriction in activity is necessary for people with diabetic nephropathy

What Causes Diabetic Nephropathy According to Traditional Chinese Medicine?

1) Congenital Insufficiency
2) Improper Diet
3) Emotional Disturbance

How is Diabetic Nephropathy Differentiated and Treated by Traditional Chinese Medicine?

1) <u>Deficiency of Qi and Yin</u>

Symptoms: Lusterless complexion, emaciation, dry mouth with a desire to drink, dry throat, shortness of breath, fatigue, constipation, or increased susceptibility to cold, low-grade fever in the afternoon, or feverish sensation in palms and soles, slight red tongue with little coating, and thready and rapid or weak pulse.

Therapeutic Principle: To replenish qi and nourish yin.

Prescription: Modified Shen Qi Di Huang Decoction.

Modifications: For remarkable qi deficiency, use Wu Zi Yan Zong Pill supplemented with Radix Codonopsitis Pilosulae (Dang Shen) 10g and Radix Astragali (Huang Qi) 12g; for remarkable yin deficiency, add Da Bu Yuan Decoction; for exterior syndromes, add Flos Lonicerae (Jin Yin Hua) 15g, Fructus Forsythiae Suspensae (Lian Qiao) 10g and Radix Astragali (Huang Qi) 12g.

2) <u>Yin Deficiency of the Liver and Kidney</u>

Symptoms: Dry eyes, blurred vision, vertigo, tinnitus, dysphoria with feverish sensation in the chest, palms and soles, dry mouth and throat, sore and weak loins and knees, nocturnal seminal emission, or abnormal menstruation, red tongue with little coating, and taut and thready or thready and rapid pulse.

Therapeutic Principle: To nourish the liver and kidney.

Prescription: Modified Gui Shao Di Huang Decoction.

Modifications: For yin deficiency and hyperactivity of yang, add Carapax et Plastrum Testudinis (Gui Ban) 20g, Haliotidis Concha (Shi Yue Ming) 20g and Concha Ostreae (Mu Li) 20g, or replace the prescription with San Jia Fu Mai Decoction; for damp-heat, add Si Miao Pill.

3) <u>Qi Deficiency of the Spleen and Kidney</u>

Symptoms: Edema of the face and extremities, sallow complexion, anorexia, loose stools, shortness of breath, fatigue, increase susceptibility to cold, lumbago, pale tongue with teeth marks on margin and tip, white and moist tongue coating, and thready and weak pulse.

Therapeutic Principle: To strengthen the spleen and kidney.

Prescription: Modified Shui Lu Er Xian Pill. Or Bu Zhong Yi Qi Decoction supplemented with Fructus Rosae Laevigatae (Jin Ying Zi) 15g, Fructus Psoraleae Corylifoliae (Bu Gu Zhi) 10g and Semen Cuscutae Chinensis (Tu Si Zi) 12g.

Modifications: For remarkable edema, add Wu Ling Powder.

4) <u>Yang Deficiency of the Spleen and Kidney</u>

Symptoms: Remarkable edema, pale complexion, aversion to cold, cold limbs, lumbago, or weakness of the lower extremities, spiritlessness, anorexia, or loose stools, seminal emission, impotence, premature ejaculation, or abnormal menstruation, pale, tender and chubby tongue with deep teeth marks on margin, deep and thready or deep, slow and forceless pulse.

Therapeutic Principle: To warm and nourish the spleen and kidney.

Prescription: Modified Zhen Wu Decoction.

Modifications: For severe deficiency of kidney yang, add Cornu Cervi (Lu Jiao) 10g; for severe diarrhea, add fried Rhizoma Dioscoreae (Shan Yao) 20g, Semen Dolichoris Lablab (Bai Bian Dou) 20g and Pericarpium Punicae Granati (Shi Liu Pi) 10g.

5) Deficiency of Yin and Yang

Symptoms: Black complexion, aversion to cold, cold limbs, urinary frequency with turbid urine, lumbago, impotence in severe cases, or abnormal menstruation, dry mouth with a desire to drink, or edema, constipation or diarrhea, dark or red tongue with white coating, and deep, thready and forceless pulse.

Therapeutic Principle: To nourish yin and yang.

Prescription: Modified Shen Qi Pill.

Modifications: For blood stasis, add Herba Lycopi Lucidi (Ze Lan) 12g, Semen Pruni Persicae (Tao Ren) 10g, Flos Carthami Tinctorii (Hong Hua) 10g and Rhizoma Ligustici Chuanxiong (Chuan Xiong) 10g; for dampness, add Radix Achyranthis Bidentatae (Niu Xi) 12g, Semen Plantaginis (Che Qian Zi) 10g, Sclerotium Polypori Umbellati (Zhu Ling) 10g, Semen Phaseoli (Chi Xiao Dou) 15g and Exocarpium Benincasae Hispidae (Dong Gua Pi) 15g; for nausea, vomiting, yellow and greasy tongue coating, add Rhizoma Coptidis (Huang Lian) 9g, Caulis Bambusae in Taeniam (Zhu Ru) 10g and Radix et Rhizoma Rhei Praeparatae (Zhi Da Huang) 6g.

What Kinds of Chinese Patent Drugs are Available to Treat Diabetic Nephropathy?

Lei Gong Teng Duo Gan Tablet: 20mg each time, thrice daily.

9. Lupus Nephritis (LN)

Lupus nephritis is an inflammation of the kidney caused by systemic lupus erythematosus (SLE). There are five types of lupus nephritis: I (normal), II (minimal or mesangial proliferative), III (focal and segmental proliferative), IV (diffuse proliferative) and V (membranous).

Some people with SLE may have no symptoms of kidney disease. However, patients may present with either a nephrotic or a nephritic clinical picture. Lupus nephritis may cause weight gain, high blood pressure, dark urine, or swelling around the eyes, legs, ankles, or fingers.

How is Lupus Nephritis Diagnosed by Conventional Western Medicine?

Diagnosis may require urine and blood tests and x rays of the kidneys, as well as a renal biopsy. Serologic evidence of activity includes increased levels of antinuclear antibodies and antibodies to double-stranded DNA, and reduced levels of C3, C4 and CH50. The best markers for following the activity of renal disease are the serum creatinine levels, urine protein excretion, and microscopic examination of the urinary sediment.

How is Lupus Nephritis Treated by Conventional Western Medicine?

Treatment depends on the symptoms. Medicines can decrease swelling, lower blood pressure, and decrease inflammation by suppressing the immune system. Patients may need to limit protein, sodium, and potassium intake in their diet. Oral steroids are of benefit in treating lupus nephritis. Cytotoxic drugs appear to improve the outlook for long-term renal survival in those with type IV lupus nephritis.

What Causes Lupus Nephritis According to Traditional Chinese Medicine?

1) Congenital Insufficiency
2) Internal Injury by Seven Emotions
3) Attack by Exogenous Pathogenic Factors, Especially Toxic Heat

How is Lupus Nephritis Differentiated and Treated by Traditional Chinese Medicine?

1) <u>Hyperactivity of Toxic Heat</u>

Symptoms: Acute progressive stage of lupus nephritis, bright red rash over the face, trunk or the extremities (areas exposed to sunlight), sustained high fever, dysphoria, flushed face, thirst, or even madness, delirium or other psychosis, coma, convulsion, or hematuria, cutaneous discoid lupus (erythematous papule or plaque), dark urine, constipation, crimson tongue with yellow coating, and taut, thready and rapid or slippery and rapid pulse.

Therapeutic Principle: To clear away heat, remove toxic substance and cool blood.

Prescription: Modified Xi Jiao Di Huang Decoction and Wu Wei Xiao Du Decoction.

Modifications: For drowsiness and delirium, add An Gong Niu Huang Pill or Zi Xue Pill; for convulsion and madness, add Cornu Saigae Tataricae (Ling Yang Jiao) 2g, Ramulus Uncariae cum Uncis (Gou Teng) 12g and Concha Margaritiferae (Zhen Zhu Mu) 20g; for constipation, add Radix et Rhizoma Rhei (Da Huang) 6g.

2) <u>Retention of Damp-Heat</u>

Symptoms: Onset stage of lupus nephritis, muscular and joint moving pain of the extremities, or multiple red, swollen, hot, aching and tender joints that are accompanied by stiffness; fever, bright red skin rash or discoid lupus (erythematous papule or plaque) or purpura, red tongue with dry and yellow or greasy and yellow coating, and slippery and rapid pulse.

Therapeutic Principle: To clear away heat, eliminate dampness, promote blood circulation and remove blood stasis.

Prescription: Modified Si Miao Pill and Hua Ban Decoction.

Modifications: For severe damp-heat, add Rhizoma Coptidis (Huang Lian) 9g, Radix Rhapontici seu Echinops (Lou Lu) 10g and Semen Coicis (Yi Yi Ren) 20g; for joint pain, add Radix Gentianae Macrophyllae (Qin Jiao) 10g, Zaocys Dhumnades (Wu Shao She) 9g, Radix et Caulis Jixueteng (Ji Xue Teng) 12g, Rhizoma Polygoni Cuspidati (Hu Zhang) 15g and Radix Clematidis (Wei Ling Xian) 10g; for severe blood stasis, add Radix et Rhizoma Rhei (Da Huang) 5g, Rhizoma Curcumae Ezhu (E Zhu) 10g, Radix Salviae Miltiorrhizae (Dan Shen) 10g, Semen Pruni Persicae (Tao Ren) 10g and Flos Carthami Tinctorii (Hong Hua) 10g.

3) Yin Deficiency of the Liver and Kidney

Symptoms: Sub-acute or chronic stage of lupus nephritis, dry eyes, feverish sensation in palms and soles, dry mouth and throat, alopecia, loose teeth, sore and weak loins and knees, or chronic low-grade fever, flushed cheeks, night sweating, vertigo, tinnitus, constipation, red tongue with little coating, and taut and thready or thready and rapid pulse.

Therapeutic Principle: To nourish the liver and kidney.

Prescription: Modified Qi Ju Di Huang Pill and Er Zhi Pill.

Modifications: For yellow or hot urine or hematuria, add Cortex Phellodendri (Huang Bai) 10g, Rhizoma Anemarrhenae (Zhi Mu) 10g, Herba seu Radix Cirsii Japonici (Da Ji) 12g and Herba Cephalanoploris (Xiao Ji) 15g; for slight edema of lower extremities, add Radix Achyranthis Bidentatae (Niu Xi) 12g, Semen Plantaginis (Che Qian Zi) 9g and Radix Stephaniae Tetrandrae (Fang Ji) 10g; for remarkable blood stasis with dark lips, purple tongue with ecchymosis or petechiae, add Radix Salviae Miltiorrhizae (Dan Shen) 10g and Herba Lycopi Lucidi (Ze Lan) 12g; for vertigo, add Ramulus Uncariae cum Uncis (Gou Teng) 12g, Magnetitum (Ci Shi) 15g.

4) Yang Deficiency of the Spleen and Kidney

Symptoms: Chronic stage of lupus nephritis, or corticosteroids tapering stage, lassitude, aversion to cold, cold limbs, edema of the face and extremities, remarkable edema of the lower limbs, sore and weak loins and knees, heel pain, anorexia, abdominal distention, diarrhea, moist and chubby or pale and chubby tongue with teeth marks on margin, deep and thready or deep, slow and forceless pulse.

Therapeutic Principle: To strengthen the spleen and warm the kidney.

Prescription: Shi Pi Decoction and Zhen Wu Decoction.

Modifications: For deficiency of kidney qi, use Wu Zi Yan Zong Pill supplemented with Radix Codonopsitis Pilosulae (Dang Shen) 9g and Radix Astragali (Huang Qi) 15g.

5) Deficiency of Qi and Yin

Symptoms: Stage of convalescence, lassitude, anorexia, spiritlessness, palpitation, shortness of breath on exertion, lumbago, alopecia, dry mouth, aversion to cold and wind, spontaneous sweating and night sweating, constipation, pale or red tongue with thin and white coating, and thready and weak or thready and rapid pulse.

Therapeutic Principle: To replenish qi and nourish yin.

Prescription: Modified Shen Qi Di Huang Decoction.

Modifications: For deficiency of Yin and Yang, use Di Huang Yin Zi; for blood stasis, add Radix Salviae Miltiorrhizae (Dan Shen) 10g, Herba Lycopi Lucidi (Ze Lan) 12g, Herba Leonuri Heterophylii (Yi Mu Cao) 12g, Lumbricus (Di Long) 10g, Rhizoma Ligustici Chuanxiong (Chuan Xiong) 10g, Herba Scutellaria Barbatae (Ban Zhi Lian) 15g and Herba Hedyotis Diffusae (Bai Hua She She Cao) 20g; for turbid phlegm, add Rhizoma Pinelliae Ternatae (Ban Xia) 10g, Bulbus Fritillariae Cirrhosae (Bei Mu) 10g, Fructus Trichosanthis (Gua Lou) 10g and Rhizoma Arisaematis cum Bile (Dan Nan Xing) 3g; for retention of dampness, add Semen Plantaginis (Che Qian Zi) 9g, Radix Stephaniae Tetrandrae (Fang Ji) 10g and Radix Achyranthis Bidentatae (Niu Xi) 12g.

What Kinds of Chinese Patent Drugs are Available to Treat Lupus Nephritis?

1) San Teng Syrup: 10-15ml each time, thrice daily.
2) Fu Fang Qin Jiao Tablet: 4-6 tablets each time, 2-3 times daily.
3) Lang Chuang Pill: 2 pills each time, twice daily.
4) Lei Gong Teng Duo Gan Tablet: 20mg each time, thrice daily.

10. Urinary Tract Infection (UTI)

Urinary tract infection (UTI) is an infection along the urinary tract. UTI are uncommon in children younger than 3 to 5 years. Women are most at risk of developing a UTI as a result of a shorter urinary tract. In fact, half of all women will develop a UTI during their lifetimes, and many will experience more than one. Uncircumcised males are more likely to develop UTI than circumcised males.

Urinary tract infections typically occur when bacteria enter the urinary tract through the urethra and begin to multiply. Most infections arise from Escherichia coli (E. coli) bacteria, which normally live in the colon. Risk factors for UTI include:

- Sex. Women are most at risk of developing a UTI due to a shorter urethra, sexual intercourse that can irritate the urethra, diaphragms use, spermicidal agents, and menopause, which makes tissues of the vagina, urethra and the base of the bladder become thinner and more fragile

- Anything that impedes the flow of urine, such as an enlarged prostate in men or a kidney stone
- Diabetes and other chronic illnesses
- Medications that lower immunity, such as chronic cortisone therapy or chemotherapy for cancer
- Prolonged use of catheters in the bladder

The following are the most common symptoms of UTI. However, each individual may experience symptoms differently. Symptoms may include:

- Urinary urgency
- Incontinence during day and/or night
- Frequent urination
- A burning sensation when urination
- Painful or difficult urination
- Discomfort above the pubic bone
- Hematuria
- Foul smelling urine
- Nausea and/or vomiting
- Fever, chills
- Pain in the back or flank
- Fatigue
- Postvoid dribbling

Each type of UTI may result in more specific signs and symptoms, depending on which part of the urinary tract is infected:

- Acute pyelonephritis. Kidney infection can cause upper back and flank pain, high fever, shaking chills, and nausea or vomiting
- Cystitis. Cystitis may result in pelvic pressure, lower abdomen discomfort, frequent, painful urination and strong-smelling urine
- Urethritis. Inflammation or infection of the urethra leads to burning with urination. In men, urethritis may cause penile discharge

How is UTI Diagnosed by Conventional Western Medicine?

Diagnosis is made based on physical examination and a description of symptoms. Other studies may include urinalysis, urine culture, renal ultrasound and voiding cystourethrography (VCUG).

How is UTI Treated by Conventional Western Medicine?

Treatment for UTI may include: (1) Antibiotics, such as amoxicillin (Amoxil, Trimox), nitrofurantoin (Furadantin, Macrodantin), trimethoprim (Proloprim) and the antibiotic combination of trimethoprim and sulfamethoxazole (Bactrim, Septra); (2) a heating pad or medications to relieve pain; (3) increased fluid intake.

What Causes UTI According to Traditional Chinese Medicine?

1) Damp-Heat in the Urinary Bladder
2) Heat Accumulation in the Liver and Gallbladder
3) Deficiency of the Spleen and Kidney
4) Insufficiency of the Kidney Yin

How is UTI Differentiated and Treated by Traditional Chinese Medicine?

1) <u>Damp-Heat in the Urinary Bladder</u>

Symptoms: Urinary frequency, burning and pricking pain, dark yellow urine, lower abdominal distending pain, or pain in loins aggravated by pressure, or fever with aversion to cold, or bitter taste in the mouth, constipation, red tongue with thin, yellow and greasy coating, and slippery and rapid pulse.

Therapeutic Principle: To clear away heat, eliminate dampness and treat stranguria.

Prescription: Modified Ba Zheng Powder.

Modifications: For urinary stones, add Folium Pyrrosiae (Shi Wei) 10g, Endothelium Corneum Gigeriae Galli (Ji Nei Jin) 10g, Herba Lysimachiae (Jin Qian Cao) 20g and Radix Curcumae (Yu Jin) 10g; for high fever, add Flos Lonicerae (Jin Yin Hua) 15g, Radix Scutellariae Baicalensis (Huang Qin) 10g and Cortex Phellodendri (Huang Bai) 10g; for thick and greasy tongue coating, add Semen Coicis (Yi Yi Ren) 20g and Fructus Gardeniae Jasminoidis (Zhi Zi) 10g.

2) <u>Accumulation of Heat in the Liver and Gallbladder</u>

Symptoms: Difficult urination with burning sensation and stabbing pain, distending pain in the lower abdomen, occasional hematuria, irritability, bitter and sticky sensation in the mouth, or alternate fever and chill, fullness in the chest and hypochondrium, dark red tongue with ecchymosis, and taut or taut and thready pulse.

Therapeutic Principle: To soothe the liver, regulate qi, clear away heat and treat stranguria.

Prescription: Modified Dan Zhi Xiao Yao Powder and Shi Wei Powder.

Modifications: For severe distention, fullness and pain in the lower abdomen, add Fructus Citri Aurantii Immaturus (Zhi Shi) 10g and Fructus Meliae Toosendan (Chuan Lian Zi) 10g; for hematuria, add Herba Cephalanoploris (Xiao Ji) 20g and Rhizoma Imperatae Cylindricae (Bai Mao Gen) 20g; for qi deficiency, weakness, frequent, dripping and difficult urination with clear urine, add Bu Zhong Yi Qi Decoction.

3) Deficiency of the Spleen and Kidney

Symptoms: Intermittent dripping urination aggravated or induced by exertion, burning sensation in the urethra, or dysuria, lusterless complexion, spiritlessness, lassitude, shortness of breath, indolence of speaking, weak and sore loins and knees, anorexia, dry mouth without desire to drink, pale tongue with thin and white coating, deep and thready pulse.

Therapeutic Principle: To strengthen the spleen and nourish the kidney.

Prescription: Modified Wu Bi Shan Yao Pill.

Modifications: For deficiency of the spleen and collapse of spleen qi with prolapse of anus, shortness of breath and indolence of speaking, add Radix Ginseng (Ren Shen) 6g, Radix Astragali (Huang Qi) 12g, Rhizoma Atractylodis Macrocephalae (Bai Zhu) 10g, Radix Glycyrrhizae Uralensis (Gan Cao) 6g, Rhizoma Cimicifugae (Sheng Ma) 10g and Radix Bupleuri (Chai Hu) 10g; for pale and lusterless complexion, cold extremities, lumbago, lassitude, pale tongue with white and moist coating, deep, thready and rapid pulse, add Radix Aconiti Lateralis Praeparatae (Fu Zi) 10g and Cortex Cinnamomi Cassiae (Rou Gui) 3g.

4) Insufficiency of Kidney Yin

Symptoms: Frequent, difficult and painful urination, turbid, dark and yellow urine, weak and sore loins and knees, feverish sensation in palms and sores, vertigo, tinnitus, weak extremities, dry mouth, thirst, red tongue with little coating, and thready and rapid pulse.

Therapeutic Principle: To nourish yin, tonify the kidney, clear away heat and treat stranguria.

Prescription: Modified Zhi Bai Di Huang Pill.

Modifications: For urination with burning sensation and stabbing pain, add Herba Polygoni Avicularis (Bian Xu) 12g, Herba Dianthi (Qu Mai) 10g and Talcum (Hua Shi Fen) 12g; for hectic fever, add Herba Artemisiae Apiaceae seu Annuae (Qing Hao) 10g and Carapax Trionycis (Bie Jia) 20g; for deficiency of qi and yin with shortness of breath and fatigue, add Radix Ginseng (Ren Shen) 6g and Rhizoma Atractylodis Macrocephalae (Bai Zhu) 10g.

What Kinds of Chinese Patent Drugs are Available to Treat UTI?

1) Suo Quan Pill: 10g each time, thrice daily.
2) Fen Qing Wu Lin Pill: 15g each time, thrice daily.
3) San Jin Tablet: 3 tablets each time, 3-4 times.

11. Urinary Stone Disease (Urolithiasis)

Urolithiasis is the medical term used to describe stones occurring in the urinary tract. Other frequently used terms are urinary tract stone disease, kidney stones and nephrolithiasis. Terms that describe the location of the stone in the urinary tract are also used. For example, a ureteral stone (or ureterolithiasis) is a kidney stone found in the ureter.

Kidney stones are one of the most common disorders of the urinary tract. In 2000, patients made 2.7 million visits to health care providers and more than 600,000 patients went to emergency rooms for kidney stone problems. Most people who develop kidney stones are between 20 and 70 years of age. Men are more likely to develop kidney stones than are women. In addition, white Americans are at higher risk of kidney stones than are black Americans.

Urinary calculi are polycrystalline aggregates composed of varying amounts of crystalloid and a small amount of organic matrix. There are five major types of urinary stones: calcium oxalate, calcium phosphate, struvite, uric acid, and cystine. The most common type of stone contains calcium in combination with either oxalate or phosphate. Most small kidney stones pass into the bladder without causing any permanent damage. It's important to determine the underlying cause to prevent from forming more stones in the future. A number of factors can cause changes in the urine, including the effects of heredity, diet and fluid intake, drugs, climate or geographic factors, lifestyle and certain medical conditions.

Kidney stones often do not cause any symptoms unless a kidney stone is large, causes a blockage or infection. Then the most common symptom is an intense, colicky pain that may fluctuate in intensity over periods of 5 to 15 minutes. The pain usually starts in the back or the flank. As the stone moves down the ureter toward the bladder, the pain may radiate to the lower abdomen, groin and genital structures on that side. Other signs and symptoms may include:

- Hematuria
- Cloudy or foul-smelling urine
- Nausea and vomiting
- Persistent urge to urinate
- Burning sensation during urination
- Fever and chills if an infection is present

How is Urolithiasis Diagnosed by Conventional Western Medicine?

Sometimes "silent" kidney stones are found on x rays taken during a routine medical exam, but many kidney stones are diagnosed after a person complains of severe kidney pain, chronic urinary tract infections or hematuria. If kidney stones are suspected, one or more of the following tests may be ordered: blood analysis, urinalysis, abdominal X-ray, ultrasound, intravenous pyelography (IVP), and spiral CT scan.

How is Urolithiasis Treated by Conventional Western Medicine?

Most kidney stones can pass through the urinary system by drinking plenty of water (2 to 3 quarts a day) and by staying physically active.

Stones that can't be treated with more conservative measures, either because they're too large to pass on their own or because they cause bleeding, kidney damage or ongoing urinary tract infection, may need the following procedures: extracorporeal shock wave lithotripsy (ESWL), percutaneous nephrolithotomy, ureteroscopic stone removal, and parathyroid surgery.

What Causes Urolithiasis According to Traditional Chinese Medicine?

1) External Invasion of Damp-Heat
2) Improper Diet
3) Retention of Damp-Heat in the Urinary Bladder

How is Urolithiasis Differentiated and Treated by Traditional Chinese Medicine?

1) <u>Damp-Heat at the Lower Warmer</u>

Symptoms: Frequent urination with burning sensation and pricking pain, dark yellow urine, difficult urination with episodic interruption or with stones, or acute colic in the flank that radiates into the lower abdomen, testicle or labium, or chill and fever, bitter taste in the mouth, nausea, vomiting, yellow and greasy tongue coating, and slippery and rapid pulse.

Therapeutic Principle: To clear away heat, eliminate dampness, treat stranguria and remove stones.

Prescription: Modified Ba Zheng Powder.

Modifications: For hematuria, add Herba Cephalanoploris (Xiao Ji) 15g, Nodus Nelumbinis Nuciferae Rhizomatis (Ou Jie) 10g, Pollen Typhae (Pu Huang) 10g and Folium Pyrrosiae (Shi Wei) 10g; for foul, yellow and turbid urine, accompanied by conjunctival congestion, bitter taste in the mouth, vexation and irritability, add Radix Gentianae (Long Dan Cao) 6g and Radix Scutellariae Baicalensis (Huang Qin) 10.

2) <u>Qi Stagnation and Blood Stasis</u>

Symptoms: Difficult and dripping urination, with blood clot, lower abdominal distending or pricking pain, or even colic in the flank and abdomen, dark purple tongue with ecchymoses or petechiae, and deep and taut or rough pulse.

Therapeutic Principle: To promote qi and blood circulation, treat stranguria and eliminate stones.

Prescription: Modified Chen Xiang Powder and Xue Fu Zhu Yu Decoction.

Modifications: For chest stuffiness and hypochondriac distending sensation, add Radix Bupleuri (Chai Hu) 6g and Rhizoma Cyperi Rotundi (Xiang Fu) 6g; for remarkable blood stasis and severe colic, add Gummi Olibanum (Ru Xiang) 9g and Myrrha (Mo Yao) 9g.

3) Qi Deficiency of the Spleen and Kidney

Symptoms: Intermittent dripping urination aggravated on exertion, or tiny stones in urine, sore and weak loins and knees, spiritlessness, fatigue, pale tongue, and thready and weak pulse.

Therapeutic Principle: To strengthen the spleen, nourish the kidney, replenish qi and remove stones.

Prescription: Modified Wu Bi Shan Yao Pill.

Modifications: For sinking qi of the Middle Warmer with distending and sinking sensation in the lower abdomen, and dripping urination, add Rhizoma Cimicifugae (Sheng Ma) 10g and Radix Bupleuri (Chai Hu) 9g.

4) Yin Deficiency of the Liver and Kidney

Symptoms: Sore loins and weak knees, vertigo, tinnitus, hectic fever, night sweating, flushed cheeks, red lips, dry mouth, sore throat, dripping urination even with tiny stones, red tongue with little or no coating, and deep, thready and rapid pulse.

Therapeutic Principle: To nourish yin, clear away heat, reinforce the kidney and remove stones.

Prescription: Modified Liu Wei Di Huang Pill.

Modifications: For deficiency of qi and hyperactivity of fire, add Rhizoma Anemarrhenae (Zhi Mu) 10g and Cortex Phellodendri (Huang Bai) 10g; for hyperactivity of liver yang with vertigo, add Fructus Lycii (Gou Qi Zi) 10g and Flos Chrysanthemi Morifolii (Ju Hua) 10g.

5) Deficiency of Kidney Yang

Symptoms: Sore loins and weak knees, lassitude, aversion to cold, cold limbs, pale complexion, urinary difficulty and urinary frequency, or dripping urination, pale tongue, and deep and thready pulse.

Therapeutic Principle: To warm kidney yang, treat stranguria and remove stones.

Prescription: Modified Jin Gui Shen Qi Pill.

Modifications: For edema of the lower extremities, add Radix Stephaniae Tetrandrae (Fang Ji) 10g, Semen Coicis (Yi Yi Ren) 20g and Semen Plantaginis (Che Qian Zi) 10g.

What Kinds of Chinese Patent Drugs are Available to Treat Urolithiasis?

1) Pai Shi Granule: 1 bag each time, thrice daily.

2) Jin Qian Cao Granule: 1 bag each time, thrice daily.

12. Acute Renal Failure (ARF)

Acute renal failure, also known as acute kidney failure, is defined as a sudden decrease in renal function resulting in the retention of urea nitrogen and creatinine in the blood. Causes of acute renal failure are generally categorized in relation to where and how they affect the kidneys:

<u>Prerenal:</u> Prerenal problems are among the most common causes of acute renal failure. Extremely low blood pressure, poor heart function, and low blood volume may leave the kidneys with an insufficient blood supply to function properly.

<u>Renal:</u> Conditions that may affect the structure and function of the kidney itself, potentially leading to acute renal failure, include: (1) disorders that reduce blood supply in the kidneys, such as atheroembolic kidney disease and idiopathic thrombocytopenic purpura; (2) hemolytic uremic syndrome; (3) inflammation in the kidneys; (4) toxic injury.

<u>Postrenal:</u> Postrenal causes of acute renal failure are generally related to obstruction of the flow of urine after it leaves the kidneys on the way out of the body. This may occur at the level of the ureters (ureter obstruction), or at the bladder level (bladder or urethral obstruction).

Acute renal failure almost always occurs in connection with another medical condition or event. In fact, most people who experience acute renal failure are already in the hospital for other reasons. Medical conditions that increase the risk of acute renal failure include:

- Chronic infection
- Diabetes
- High blood pressure
- Heart failure
- Various blood disorders
- Immune disorders, such as lupus, IgA nephropathy and scleroderma
- Kidney diseases
- Liver diseases
- Prostate gland enlargement
- Bladder outlet obstruction

Acute renal failure is reversible. However, if acute renal failure occurs in the context of severe chronic illness, the outcome is often worse. The following are the most common symptoms of acute renal failure. However, symptoms of acute renal failure depend largely on the underlying cause, and each individual may experience symptoms differently.

- Oliguria, although occasionally urine output remains normal
- Fluid retention, causing edema in the legs, ankles or feet
- Drowsiness
- Anorexia, nausea and malaise
- Shortness of breath
- Fatigue
- Confusion
- Seizures or coma in severe cases
- Chest pain related to pericarditis

How is ARF Diagnosed by Conventional Western Medicine?

In addition to a physical examination and complete medical history, the following diagnostic tests may be ordered: blood tests, urine tests, chest x-ray, bone scan, renal ultrasound, ECG or EKG, and renal biopsy.

How is ARF Treated by Conventional Western Medicine?

Treatment of acute renal failure depends on the underlying cause. The first goal is to treat the illness or injury that originally damaged the kidneys. Once that's under control, the focus will be on preventing the accumulation of excess fluids and wastes while the kidneys heal. Treatment may include:

- Hospitalization
- Administration of intravenous fluids in large volumes
- Diuretic therapy or medications to increase urine output
- Close monitoring of important electrolytes such as potassium, sodium, and calcium
- Medications to control blood pressure
- Specific diet requirements
- Dialysis

What Causes ARF According to Traditional Chinese Medicine?

1) Six Exogenous Pathogenic Factors
2) Improper Diet
3) Injury by an Accident
4) Impaired Kidney by Drugs

How is ARF Differentiated and Treated by Traditional Chinese Medicine?

1) Stage of Oliguria

(1) Hyperactivity of Toxic Heat

Symptoms: Abrupt onset of oliguria, or even anuresis, persistent fever, dry mouth with a desire to drink, headache, general aching, irritability, crimson tongue with dry and yellow coating, and rapid pulse.

Therapeutic Principle: To purge fire and remove toxic substance.

Prescription: Modified Huang Lian Jie Du Decoction.

Modifications: For constipation, add Radix et Rhizoma Rhei (Da Huang) 6g and Fructus Citri Aurantii Immaturus (Zhi Shi) 10g; for nausea and vomiting, add Rhizoma Pinelliae Ternatae (Ban Xia) 10g, Pericarpium Citri Reticulatae (Chen Pi) 9g and Caulis Bambusae in Taeniam (Zhu Ru) 10g; for syndrome induced by snake bite or wasp bite, add Herba Hedyotis Diffusae (Bai Hua She She Cao) 30g, Lobeliae Chinensis Herba cum Radice (Ban Bian Lian) 15g, Spica Prunellae Vulgaris (Xia Ku Cao) 12g and Radix Glycyrrhizae Uralensis (Gan Cao) 6g.

(2) Retention of Toxic Fire

Symptoms: Dripping urination, urinary difficulty, or hematuria, or anuresis, high fever, delirium, hematemesis, epistaxis, dark purple or bright red rash, dark purple tongue with prickles or with dry and yellowing coating, thready and rapid pulse.

Therapeutic Principle: To clear away heat, remove toxic substance, promote blood circulation and remove blood stasis.

Prescription: Modified Qing Wen Bai Du Decoction.

Modifications: For dysphoria and delirium, add Rhizoma Coptidis (Huang Lian) 9g, Folium Phyllostachydis Henonis (Zhu Ye) 10g and Rhizoma Acori Tatarinowii (Shi Chang Pu) 10g, or add An Gong Niu Huang Pill; for cough and dyspnea, add Radix Scutellariae Baicalensis (Huang Qin) 10g, Cortex Mori Alba Radicis (Sang Bai Pi) 12g and Radix Ophiopogonis Japonici (Mai Dong) 12g; for dyschezia, add Radix et Rhizoma Rhei (Da Huang) 6g and Semen Pruni Persicae (Tao Ren) 10g; for hyperactive heat affecting blood, add Rhizoma Imperatae Cylindricae (Bai Mao Gen) 20g, Cornu Bubali (Shui Niu Jiao) 10g and Folium Callicarpae Formosanae (Zi Zhu) 12g.

(3) Accumulation of Damp-Heat

Symptoms: Oliguria, anuresis, nausea, vomiting, foul odor of urine in the mouth, fever, dry mouth without a desire to drink, headache, irritability, or even unconsciousness and convulsion in severe cases, yellow and greasy tongue coating, and slippery and rapid pulse.

Therapeutic Principle: To clear away heat, promote diuresis, lower adverse flow of qi and eliminate turbidity.

Prescription: Modified Huang Lian Wen Dan Decoction.

Modifications: For severe edema, add Herba Lycopi Lucidi (Ze Lan) 12g and Sclerotium Polypori Umbellati (Zhu Ling) 10g; for retention of dampness in Triple Warmer with thick and greasy tongue coating, add Herba Eupatorii (Pei Lan) 10g, Fructus Amomi Villosi (Sha Ren) 5g, Fructus Amomi Cardamomi (Bai Kou Ren) 5g, Semen Coicis (Yi Yi Ren) 20g and Rhizoma Atractylodis (Cang Zhu) 10g.

(4) <u>Collapse of Qi and Consumption of Phlegm</u>

Symptoms: Oliguria or anuresis, cold and damp sweat, extremely weak respiration, or cough, tachypnea, dark bluish lips and nails, thready and rapid or deep pulse.

Therapeutic Principle: To replenish qi, nourish yin, restore yang from collapse.

Prescription: Modified Sheng Mai Decoction and Shen Fu Decoction.

Modifications: For remarkable blood stasis with cyanosis of lips and nails, add Radix Angelicae Sinensis (Dang Gui) 10g and Radix Salviae Miltiorrhizae (Dan Shen) 10g; for excessive loss of blood and deficiency of blood, use modified Dang Gui Bu Xue Decoction.

2) Stage of Polyuria

(1) <u>Deficiency of Qi and Yin</u>

Symptoms: Sallow complexion, general fatigue, dry throat with a desire to drink, feverish sensation in palms and soles, polyuria with clear urine, red tongue with little coating, or pale tongue with teeth marks, and thready pulse.

Therapeutic Principle: To replenish qi and nourish yin.

Prescription: Modified Shen Qi Di Huang Decoction.

Modifications: For deficiency of qi, add Radix Ginseng (Ren Shen) 9g, Rhizoma Atractylodis Macrocephalae (Bai Zhu) 12g and Rhizoma Dioscoreae (Shan Yao) 20g; for deficiency of yin, add Radix Adenophorae (Sha Shen) 10g, Fructus Lycii (Gou Qi Zi) 12g and Rhizoma Anemarrhenae (Zhi Mu) 10g; for lingering damp-heat with fever and greasy tongue coating, add Radix Scutellariae Baicalensis (Huang Qin) 10g, Fructus Forsythiae Suspensae (Lian Qiao) 12g, Talcum (Hua Shi Fen) 10g, Semen Coicis (Yi Yi Ren) 20g, Fructus Amomi Kravanh (Bai Dou Kou) 5g and Herba Agastache seu Pogostemonis (Huo Xiang) 9g.

(2) <u>Deficiency of Kidney Yin</u>

Symptoms: Sore lumbar region and weak knees, polyuria, dripping urination, dry mouth with a desire to drink, feverish sensation in palms and soles, red tongue with little coating, and thready pulse.

Therapeutic Principle: To nourish yin and tonify the kidney.

Prescription: Modified Liu Wei Di Huang Pill.

Modifications: For polyuria and dripping urination, add Ootheca Mantidis (Sang Piao Xiao) 10g, Fructus Rosae Laevigatae (Jin Ying Zi) 15g and Semen Euryales Ferocis (Qian Shi) 12g; for dysphoria with feverish sensation in the chest, palms and soles, add Rhizoma Anemarrhenae (Zhi Mu) 10g, Carapax Trionycis (Bie Jia) 20g and Radix Paeoniae Rubra (Chi Shao) 12g.

What Kinds of Chinese Patent Drugs are Available to Treat ARF?

1) Dong Chong Xia Cao Powder: 3-5g each time, 2-3 times each day.
2) Qing Kai Ling Injection: 20-40ml each time, once daily.
3) Sheng Mai Injection: 40ml each time, once daily.

13. Chronic Renal Failure (CRF)

Renal failure refers to temporary or permanent damage to the kidneys, which results in loss of normal kidney function. Chronic failure progresses slowly over at least three months and can lead to permanent renal failure. Progressive kidney damage most often results from a chronic illness over a period of years. High blood pressure and diabetes are the most common causes of chronic renal failure. Common causes include:

- Diabetes
- Hypertension
- Obstructive nephropathy due to an enlarged prostate, kidney stones or tumors, or by vesicoureteral reflux
- Kidney diseases, such as polycystic kidney disease, pyelonephritis, glomerulonephritis and tubulointerstitial nephritis
- Kidney (renal) artery stenosis due to atherosclerosis or fibromuscular dysplasia
- Toxins, such as carbon tetrachloride, and lead

Signs and symptoms of chronic renal failure are often nonspecific. Because the kidneys are highly adaptable and able to compensate for lost function, signs and symptoms of chronic renal failure may not appear until irreversible damage has occurred. Signs and symptoms may include:

- High blood pressure
- Unexplained weight loss

- Anemia
- Nausea, vomiting or anorexia
- Malaise
- Fatigue and weakness
- Headaches that seem unrelated to any other cause
- Decreased mental sharpness
- Muscle twitches and cramps
- Bloody or tarry stools
- Yellowish-brown cast to the skin
- Persistent pruritus, easy bruisability
- Metallic taste in mouth, urinous breath
- Epistaxis
- Dyspnea, shortness of breath, irritability
- Edema
- Recurrent urinary tract infections
- Stunted growth in children

How is CRF Diagnosed by Conventional Western Medicine?

In addition to a physical examination and complete medical history, the following diagnostic tests may be ordered: blood tests, urine tests, chest x-ray, renal ultrasound, CT scan, MRI, ECG or EKG, and renal biopsy. Bilateral small kidneys on ultrasound are diagnostic. Radiologic evidence of renal osteodystrophy confirms the diagnosis.

How is CRF Treated by Conventional Western Medicine?

The main goal of treatment of chronic renal failure is to halt or delay progression of the disease. Chronic renal failure can progress to end-stage kidney disease, where the kidneys function at a fraction of normal capacity. At this point, dialysis or a kidney transplant is needed.

Chronic renal failure has no cure, but treatment can help control signs and symptoms, reduce complications, and slow the progress of the disease. Treatment of chronic renal failure depends on the degree of kidney function that remains. Treatment may include:

- Treating the underlying condition
- Treating complications
- Specific diet restrictions

- Dialysis, such as hemodialysis, peritoneal dialysis, continuous ambulatory peritoneal dialysis, and continuous cycling peritoneal dialysis
- Kidney transplantation

What Causes CRF According to Traditional Chinese Medicine?

1) Chronic Kidney Diseases
2) Infection of Exogenous Pathogenic Factors
3) Improper Diet
4) Overstrain and Sex Indulgence

How is CRF Differentiated and Treated by Traditional Chinese Medicine?

1) Primary Aspect: Deficiency Syndromes

(1) <u>Qi Deficiency of the Spleen and Kidney</u>

Symptoms: Lassitude, shortness of breath, indolence of speaking, anorexia, abdominal distention, sore loins and weak knees, diarrhea, insipid mouth without a desire to drink, pale tongue with teeth marks, white or white and greasy tongue coating, and deep and thready pulse.

Therapeutic Principle: To replenish qi, strengthen the spleen and nourish the kidney.

Prescription: Modified Liu Jun Zi Decoction.

Modifications: For deficiency of kidney qi, Herba Epimedii (Yin Yang Huo) 12g, Semen Cuscutae Chinensis (Tu Si Zi) 12g, Cortex Eucommiae Ulmoidis (Du Zhong) 12g and Herba Taxilli (Sang Ji Sheng) 15g; for deficiency of the spleen with retention of dampness, add Rhizoma Atractylodis (Cang Zhu) 10g, Herba Agastache seu Pogostemonis (Huo Xiang) 9g, Herba Eupatorii (Pei Lan) 10g and Semen Coicis (Yi Yi Ren) 20g; for deficiency of the spleen with loose stools, add Semen Dolichoris Lablab (Bian Dou) 20g, Semen Euryales Ferocis (Qian Shi) 12g and Flos Sophorae Japonicae (Huai Hua) 12g; for constipation, add Radix et Rhizoma Rhei Praeparatae (Zhi Da Huang) 9g; for remarkable edema, add Semen Plantaginis (Che Qian Zi) 9g, Rhizoma Alismatis Orientalis (Ze Xie) 10g and Sclerotium Polypori Umbellati (Zhu Ling) 10g.

(2) <u>Yang Deficiency of the Spleen and Kidney</u>

Symptoms: Pale or dim and black complexion, pitted edema of lower extremities, spiritlessness, lassitude, anorexia, loose stools, or diarrhea, insipid and sticky sensation in the mouth without a desire to drink, sore and weak loins and knees or cold pain in the lumbar region, aversion to cold, cold limbs, nocturnal urinary frequency and polyuria with clear urine, pale, chubby and tender tongue with remarkable teeth marks, and deep and weak pulse.

Therapeutic Principle: To warm and nourish the spleen and kidney.

Prescription: Modified Ji Sheng Shen Qi Pill.

Modifications: For abdominal cold pain or loose stools, add Rhizoma Zingiberis Officinalis (Gan Jiang) 10g, Rhizoma Atractylodis Macrocephalae (Bai Zhu) 12g and Ramulus Cinnamomi Cassiae (Gui Zhi) 10g; for severe edema, add Sclerotium Polypori Umbellati (Zhu Ling) 10g, Stylus Zeae Mays (Yu Mi Xu) 20g, Cortex Mori Alba Radicis (Sang Bai Pi) 12g and Herba Lycopi Lucidi (Ze Lan) 12g.

(3) Deficiency of Qi and Yin

Symptoms: Lusterless complexion, spiritlessness, fatigue, sore loins and weak knees, dry mouth and lips without much desire to drink, or feverish sensation in palms and soles, constipation or diarrhea, nocturnal polyuria with clear urine, pale tongue with teeth marks, and deep and thready pulse.

Therapeutic Principle: To replenish qi, nourish yin, strengthen the spleen and tonify the kidney.

Prescription: To Shen Qi Di Huang Decoction.

Modifications: For deficiency of heart qi and yin with palpitation and shortness of breath, add Radix Ophiopogonis Japonici (Mai Dong) 12g, Fructus Schisandrae Chinensis (Wu Wei Zi) 5g, Radix Salviae Miltiorrhizae (Dan Shen) 10g and Radix Glycyrrhizae Uralensis (Gan Cao) 6g; for constipation, add Semen Cannabis Sativae (Huo Ma Ren) 12g or Radix et Rhizoma Rhei Praeparatae (Zhi Da Huang) 6g.

(4) Yin Deficiency of the Liver and Kidney

Symptoms: Vertigo, headache, tinnitus, dry eyes or blurred vision, dry mouth and throat, thirst with preference to drinks, or without much desire to drink, sore loins and weak knees, constipation, oliguria with yellow urine, high blood pressure, slight red tongue with thin and white or little coating, and taut or thready and taut pulse.

Therapeutic Principle: To nourish the kidney and soothe the liver.

Prescription: Modified Qi Ju Di Huang Decoction.

Modifications: For remarkable vertigo and headache, tinnitus and high blood pressure, add Ramulus Uncariae cum Uncis (Gou Teng) 12g, Spica Prunellae Vulgaris (Xia Ku Cao) 12g and Concha Ostreae (Mu Li) 20g.

(5) Deficiency of Yin and Yang

Symptoms: General fatigue, lassitude, aversion to cold, cold limbs, or feverish sensation in palms and soles, dry mouth with a desire to drink, sore and weak loins and knees, diarrhea, dark yellow urine or polyuria with clear urine, moist and chubby tongue with teeth marks and white coating, and deep and thready pulse.

Therapeutic Principle: To warm kidney yang and nourish yin.

Prescription: Modified Jin Gui Shen Qi Pill.

Modifications: For nausea, vomiting, anorexia and abdominal distention, add Rhizoma Dioscoreae (Shan Yao) 20g, Sclerotium Poriae Cocos (Fu Ling) 12g, Semen Coicis (Yi Yi Ren) 20g, Rhizoma Atractylodis Macrocephalae (Bai Zhu) 10g, Rhizoma Pinelliae Ternatae (Ban Xia) 10g, Pericarpium Citri Reticulatae (Chen Pi) 9g, Rhizoma Coptidis (Huang Lian) 9g and Folium Perillae Frutescentis (Su Ye) 10g.

2) Secondary Aspect: Excess Syndromes

(1) <u>Turbid Dampness Syndrome</u>

Symptoms: Nausea, vomiting, stuffiness in the chest, anorexia, or insipid, sticky and greasy sensation in the mouth, or an odor of urine in the mouth.

Therapeutic Principle: To regulate Middle Warmer, lower adverse of qi, eliminate dampness and turbidity.

Prescription: Modified Xiao Ban Xia Jia Fu Ling Decoction.

Modifications: For severe turbid dampness with white and greasy tongue coating, add Rhizoma Atractylodis (Cang Zhu) 10g, Fructus Amomi Villosi (Sha Ren) 5g, Fructus Amomi Cardamomi (Bai Kou Ren) 5g and Semen Coicis (Yi Yi Ren) 20g; for oliguria, add Rhizoma Alismatis Orientalis (Ze Xie) 10g, Semen Plantaginis (Che Qian Zi) 9g and Stylus Zeae Mays (Yu Mi Xu) 20g.

(2) <u>Damp-Heat Syndrome</u>

Symptoms: Dry mouth, bitter taste in the mouth, or even foul odor in the mouth, frequent nausea, and yellow and greasy tongue coating (damp-heat in Middle Warmer); dark yellow urine or difficult urination, frequent urination, urinary urgency and dysuria (damp-heat in Lower Warmer).

Therapeutic Principle: To clear and regulate the Middle Warmer for damp-heat in Middle Warmer; clear away heat and resolve dampness for damp-heat in Lower Warmer.

Prescription: Modified Huang Lian Wen Dan Decoction for damp-heat in Middle Warmer; modified Si Miao Pill for damp-heat in Lower Warmer.

Modifications: For remarkable nausea, add Folium Perillae Frutescentis (Su Ye) 10g and Ochra Haematitum (Dai Zhe Shi) 20g; for urinary frequency and urgency, add Herba Taraxaci Mongolici (Pu Gong Ying) 20g, Herba Plantaginis (Che Qian Cao) 12g, Herba Polygoni Avicularis (Bian Xu) 12g and Rhizoma Smilacis Glabrae (Tu Fu Ling) 30g.

(3) <u>Water and Qi Syndrome</u>

Symptoms: Edema of the face and extremities, or anasarca, or even hydrothorax and ascites.

Therapeutic Principle: To induce diuresis and eliminate swelling.

Prescription: Modified Wu Pi Decoction or Wu Ling Powder.

Modifications: For deficiency of qi with retention of water and fluid, use modified Fang Ji Huang Qi Decoction; for insufficiency of kidney yang, use modified Ji Sheng Shen Qi Pill or Zhen Wu Decoction.

(4) <u>Blood Stasis Syndrome</u>

Symptoms: Dim or black complexion, or dark purple lips, localized pain in the lumbar region, or numbness of extremities, dark purple tongue with petechiae or ecchymosis, and rough or thready and rough pulse.

Therapeutic Principle: To promote blood circulation and remove blood stasis.

Prescription: Modified Tao Hong Si Wu Decoction.

Modifications: For deficiency of qi and blood stasis, add Radix Astragali (Huang Qi) 15g; for chronic blood stasis, add Da Huang Zhe Chong Pill.

(5) <u>Liver Wind Syndrome</u>

Symptoms: Headache, dizziness, wriggly feet and hands, muscular tic, spasm and convulsion.

Therapeutic Principle: To calm the liver to stop wind.

Prescription: Modified Tian Ma Gou Teng Decoction.

Modifications: For yin deficiency of the liver and kidney, add Fructus Lycii (Gou Qi Zi) 12g, Fructus Corni Officinalis (Shan Zhu Yu) 12g, Radix Polygoni Multiflori (He Shou Wu) 20g, Radix Paeoniae Alba (Bai Shao Yao) 10g and Carapax Trionycis (Bie Jia) 20g.

What Kinds of Chinese Patent Drugs are Available to Treat CRF?

1) Niao Du Qing Granule: 1 bag each time, thrice daily.
2) Shen Shuai Ning Capsule: 4-6 capsules each time, 3-4 times each day.

Chapter 5: Hematology

1. Anemia

1) Iron Deficiency Anemia (IDA)

The most common cause of anemia is iron deficiency. Iron is needed to form hemoglobin. Iron is mostly stored in the body in the hemoglobin. About 30 percent of iron is also stored as ferritin and hemosiderin in the bone marrow, spleen, and liver.

Iron deficiency anemia can be caused by:

- Iron deficient diet
- Increased requirements. Children, adolescents, pregnancy and lactation can cause iron deficiency if increased iron requirements are not met
- Decreased absorption of iron due to gastrointestinal tract abnormalities
- Blood loss due to GI bleeding, menstrual bleeding, or injury
- Hemoglobinuria
- Iron sequestration due to pulmonary hemosiderosis

The following are the most common symptoms of iron deficiency anemia. However, each individual may experience symptoms differently. Symptoms may include:

- Extreme fatigue, weakness
- Pale skin
- Shortness of breath, headache, dizziness
- Cold hands and feet
- Inflammation or soreness of the tongue
- Tachycardia
- Brittle nails
- Pica (unusual cravings for non-nutritive substances, such as ice, dirt or pure starch)
- Poor appetite, especially in infants and children
- An uncomfortable tingling or crawling feeling in the legs

How is IDA Diagnosed by Conventional Western Medicine?

In addition to a complete medical history and physical examination, diagnostic procedures for iron deficiency anemia may include blood tests, bone marrow aspiration and/or biopsy.

How is IDA Treated by Conventional Western Medicine?

Treatment may include:

- Iron-rich diet. Eating a diet with iron-rich foods can help treat iron deficiency anemia
- Iron supplements. Iron supplements can be taken over several months to increase iron levels in the blood
- Treating causes other than poor diet. If iron supplements alone don't increase blood-iron levels in adults, it's likely the anemia is due to more than an iron-poor diet. It may be due to a source of bleeding or an iron-absorption problem that need to be investigated and treated. Depending on the cause, iron deficiency anemia treatment may involve: (1) medications, such as oral contraceptives to lighten heavy menstrual flow; (2) antibiotics and other medications to treat peptic ulcers; (3) surgery to remove a bleeding polyp, a tumor or a fibroid
- Blood transfusions. If iron deficiency anemia is severe, blood transfusions can help replace iron and hemoglobin quickly

What Causes IDA According to Traditional Chinese Medicine?

(1) Improper Diet

(2) Chronic Bleeding

(3) Chronic Diseases and Weak Constitution

(4) Infection of Parasites

How is IDA Differentiated and Treated by Traditional Chinese Medicine?

(1) <u>Deficiency of the Spleen and Stomach</u>

Symptoms: Sallow complexion, pale lips and nails, spiritlessness, fatigue, anorexia, loose stools, nausea, vomiting, pale tongue with thin and greasy coating, and thready and weak pulse.

Therapeutic Principle: To strengthen the spleen, regulate the stomach, replenish qi and nourish yin.

Prescription: Modified Xiang Sha Liu Jun Zi Decoction and Dang Gui Bu Xue Decoction.

Modifications: For diarrhea, add Semen Coicis (Yi Yi Ren) 15g and Rhizoma Dioscoreae (Shan Yao) 20g; for nausea, add Caulis Bambusae in Taeniam (Zhu Ru) 10g and Rhizoma Zingiberis Recens (Sheng Jiang) 9g.

(2) <u>Deficiency of the Heart and Spleen</u>

Symptoms: Pale complexion, lassitude, vertigo, palpitation, insomnia, shortness of breath, indolence of speaking, anorexia, dry hair and alopecia, brittle nails, pale and chubby tongue with thin coating, and soft and thready pulse.

Therapeutic Principle: To replenish qi and blood, nourish the heart and tranquilize the mind.

Prescription: Modified Gui Pi Decoction or modified Ba Zhen Decoction.

Modifications: For severe palpitation and insomnia, add Caulis Polygoni Multiflori (Ye Jiao Teng) 20g, Cortex Albizziae Julibrissin (He Huan Pi) 9g, Mastodi Ossis Fossilia (Long Gu) 20g and Concha Ostreae (Mu Li) 20g; for severe anemia, add Radix Polygoni Multiflori (He Shou Wu) 15g and Gelatinum Corii Asini (E Jiao) 9g.

(3) <u>Yang Deficiency of the Spleen and Kidney</u>

Symptoms: Pale complexion, cold limbs, sore and weak knees, spiritlessness, tinnitus, pale lips and nails, or general edema, or even ascites, diarrhea, polyuria with clear urine, impotence, or amenorrhea, pale tongue with teeth marks, and deep and thready pulse.

Therapeutic Principle: To warm and nourish the spleen and kidney.

Prescription: Modified Ba Zhen Decoction and Wu Bi Shan Yao Pill.

Modifications: For qi stagnation and deficiency of the spleen with remarkable abdominal distention, add Radix Aucklandiae Lappae (Mu Xiang) 10g and Fructus Citri Aurantii Immaturus (Zhi Shi) 10g; for aversion to cold and cold limbs, add Radix Aconiti Lateralis Praeparatae (Fu Zi) 10g and Ramulus Cinnamomi Cassiae (Gui Zhi) 9g.

(4) <u>Accumulation of Parasites</u>

Symptoms: Sallow and lusterless complexion, abdominal distention, craving for meals, hunger, nausea, vomiting, or loose stools, pica (an unusual craving for specific foods, such as raw rice, dirt, tea, ice cubes etc), spiritlessness, weak extremities, shortness of breath, vertigo, pale tongue with white coating, and deficiency and weak pulse.

Therapeutic Principle: To eliminate parasites and stagnation, replenish qi and blood.

Prescription: Modified Hua Chong Pill and Ba Zhen Decoction.

Modifications: For abdominal distending pain, add Radix Aucklandiae Lappae (Mu Xiang) 10g and Rhizoma Corydalis (Yan Hu Suo) 10g.

What Kinds of Chinese Patent Drugs are Available to Treat IDA?

(1) Xiao Wen Zhong Pill: 1.5-3g each time, thrice daily.

(2) Fa Mu Pill: 1.5-3g each time, thrice daily.

(3) Jiang Fan Pill: 1.5-3g each time, thrice daily.

(4) Zao Fan Pill: 1 pill each time, twice daily.

2) Aplastic Anemia (AA)

Aplastic anemia is a condition of bone marrow failure that arises from injury to or abnormal expression of the stem cell, resulting in pancytopenia (reduced number of red cells, white cells, and platelets). A reduced number of red blood cells can cause the hemoglobin to drop. A reduced number of white blood cells can cause the patient to be susceptible to infection. A reduced number of platelets can cause the blood not to clot as easily.

There are a number of causes of aplastic anemia. About half of cases of aplastic anemia occur sporadically for no known reason (idiopathic). Other causes are secondary, resulting from a previous illness or disorder. Causes of aplastic anemia may include:

- High-dose radiation and chemotherapy treatments
- Exposure to toxic chemicals
- Use of certain drugs
- Autoimmune disorders
- Viral infections
- Pregnancy
- Posthepatitis
- Paroxysmal nocturnal hemoglobinuria
- Unknown factors
- Congenital (rare)

Aplastic anemia can come on suddenly or develop slowly over weeks or months. The illness may be brief, or it may become chronic. Without treatment, it may progress and become fatal. The following are the most common symptoms of aplastic anemia. However, each individual may experience symptoms differently. Symptoms may include:

- Fatigue
- Shortness of breath with exertion
- Tachycardia
- Pale skin
- Frequent or prolonged infections
- Unexplained or easy bruising
- Nosebleeds and bleeding gums

- Prolonged bleeding from cuts
- Skin rash or petechiae
- Dizziness, nausea
- Headache
- Fever
- Hepatosplenomegaly

How is Aplastic Anemia Diagnosed by Conventional Western Medicine?

In addition to a complete medical history and physical examination, diagnostic procedures for aplastic anemia may include blood tests and bone marrow aspiration and/or biopsy.

How is Aplastic Anemia Treated by Conventional Western Medicine?

Aplastic anemia is a serious illness and treatment usually depends on the underlying cause. For certain causes, recovery can be expected after treatment, however, relapses can occur. Treatments for aplastic anemia may include observation for mild cases, blood transfusions, medications and, in severe cases, bone marrow transplantation. Following is a list of treatments for aplastic anemia:

- Blood transfusion (both red blood cells and platelets)
- Preventative antibiotic therapy
- Meticulous hand washing
- Special care to food preparation (such as only eating cooked foods)
- Bone marrow stimulants
- Bone marrow transplantation
- Immunosuppressive therapy
- Hormones

What Causes Aplastic Anemia According to Traditional Chinese Medicine?

(1) Weak Constitution and Deficiency of Kidney Essence
(2) Disturbance of Seven Emotions and Impairment of Five Zang Organs
(3) Improper Diet and Impairment of the Spleen and Stomach
(4) The Six Climatic Causes Impairing the Liver, Spleen and Kidney
(5) Exogenous Pathogenic Factors Invading Blood and Marrow
(6) Chronic Diseases and Blood Stasis

How is Aplastic Anemia Differentiated and Treated by Traditional Chinese Medicine?

(1) <u>Deficiency of Kidney Yin</u>

Symptoms: Pale complexion, pale lips and nails, palpitation, fatigue, flushed cheeks, night sweating, feverish sensation in palms and soles, thirst with a desire to drink, sore and weak loins and knees, remarkable hemorrhage, constipation, pale tongue with thin coating, or red tongue with little coating, and thready and rapid pulse.

Therapeutic Principle: To nourish yin and blood, tonify the kidney and replenish qi.

Prescription: Modified Zuo Gui Pill and Dang Gui Bu Xue Decoction.

Modifications: For deficiency of qi, add Radix Pseudostellariae Heterophyllae (Tai Zi Shen) 15g and Rhizoma Polygonati (Huang Jing) 12g; for remarkable deficiency of yin, add Fructus Ligustri Lucidi (Nu Zhen Zi) 12g and Herba Ecliptae Prostratae (Han Lian Cao) 20g; for constipation, add Fructus Citri Aurantii Immaturus (Zhi Shi) 10g and Semen Cannabis Sativae (Huo Ma Ren) 12g.

(2) Deficiency of Kidney Yang

Symptoms: Cold limbs, shortness of breath, indolence of speaking, pallor, pale lips and nails, loose stools, edema of the face and extremities, hemorrhage that is not remarkable, pale, chubby and tender tongue with thin and white coating, and thready and forceless pulse.

Therapeutic Principle: To tonify the kidney, activate yang, replenish qi and nourish blood.

Prescription: Modified You Gui Pill and Dang Gui Bu Xue Decoction.

Modifications: For diarrhea, add Radix Codonopsitis Pilosulae (Dang Shen) 10g, Rhizoma Atractylodis Macrocephalae (Bai Zhu) 10g and Sclerotium Poriae Cocos (Fu Ling) 12g; for remarkable edema, add Ramulus Cinnamomi Cassiae (Gui Zhi) 9g, Semen Plantaginis (Che Qian Zi) 9g and Rhizoma Alismatis Orientalis (Ze Xie) 10g.

(3) Deficiency of Kidney Yin and Kidney Yang

Symptoms: Pale complexion, lassitude, vertigo, palpitation, feverish sensation in palms and soles, sore and weak loins and knees, aversion to cold, cold limbs, gingival hemorrhage, epistaxis, or ecchymosis, pale tongue with white coating, and thready and forceless pulse.

Therapeutic Principle: To nourish yin, activate yang, replenish qi and enrich blood.

Prescription: Modified Zuo Gui Pill, You Gui Pill and Dang Gui Bu Xue Decoction.

Modifications: For remarkable yin deficiency, add Fructus Ligustri Lucidi (Nu Zhen Zi) 12g and Herba Ecliptae Prostratae (Han Lian Cao) 20g; for remarkable yang deficiency, add Fructus Psoraleae Corylifoliae (Bu Gu Zhi) 10g and Radix Morindae officinalis (Ba Ji Tian) 12g; for blood stasis, add Semen Pruni Persicae (Tao Ren) 10g, Flos Carthami Tinctorii (Hong Hua) 10g and Radix et Caulis Jixueteng (Ji Xue Teng) 10g.

(4) Deficiency of the Kidney and Blood Stasis

Symptoms: Palpitation, shortness of breath, general fatigue, dim complexion, vertigo, tinnitus, sore and weak loins and knees, skin ecchymosis, scaly dry skin, hypochondriac pain, hemorrhage that is not remarkable, dark purple tongue with ecchymoses or petechiae, and thready or rough pulse.

Therapeutic Principle: To nourish the kidney and promote blood circulation.

Prescription: Modified Liu Wei Di Huang Pill and Tao Hong Si Wu Decoction, or Jin Gui Shen Qi Pill and Tao Hong Si Wu Decoction.

Modifications: For remarkable hemorrhage, add Radix Notoginseng (San Qi) 9g, Hominis Crinis Carbonisatus (Xue Yu Tan) 10g and Pollen Typhae (Pu Huang) 10g.

(5) <u>Deficiency of Qi and Blood</u>

Symptoms: Pale and lusterless complexion, pale lips, vertigo, palpitation, shortness of breath and fatigue aggravated on exertion, pale tongue with thin and white coating, and thready and weak pulse.

Therapeutic Principle: To replenish qi and nourish blood.

Prescription: Modified Ba Zhen Decoction.

Modifications: For remarkable deficiency of qi, add Radix Astragali (Huang Qi) 12g and Rhizoma Dioscoreae (Shan Yao) 20g; for qi deficiency affecting yang, add Gelatinum Cornu Cervi (Lu Jiao Jiao) 9g and Fructus Psoraleae Corylifoliae (Bu Gu Zhi) 10g.

(6) <u>Retention of Toxic Heat</u>

Symptoms: High fever, thirst, sore throat, epistaxis, gingival hemorrhage, subcutaneous purpura, ecchymosis, palpitation, red and dry tongue with yellow coating, full and rapid pulse.

Therapeutic Principle: To clear away heat, cool blood, remove toxic substance and nourish yin.

Prescription: Modified Qing Wen Bai Du Decoction.

Modifications: For persistent high fever, dysphoria and cloudy consciousness, use An Gong Niu Huang Pill for enema; for severe toxic heat syndrome, increase the dosage of Cornu Rhinocerotis (Xi Jiao), Radix Rehmanniae (Di Huang) and Cortex Moutan Radicis (Mu Dan Pi).

What Kinds of Chinese Patent Drugs are Available to Treat Aplastic Anemia?

(1) Liu Wei Di Huang Pill: 6-9g each time, twice daily.

(2) Jin Gui Shen Qi Pill: 6-9g each time, twice daily.

(3) Yi Shen Sheng Xue Tablet: 4g each time, thrice daily.

(4) Zai Zhang Sheng Xue Tablet: 5 tablets each time, thrice daily.

3) Hemolytic Anemia (HA)

Hemolytic anemia is a disorder in which the red blood cells are destroyed faster than the bone marrow can produce them. There are two types of hemolytic anemia: intrinsic and extrinsic. In intrinsic anemia, the destruction of the red blood cells is caused by a defect within the red blood cells themselves due to membrane defects, glycolytic defects, oxidation vulnerability and hemoglobinopathies. Intrinsic hemolytic anemias are often inherited, such as sickle cell anemia and G6PD deficiency. In extrinsic anemia, red blood cells are produced healthy but are later destroyed due to infections, medications, leukemia or lymphoma, autoimmune disorders, microangiopathic conditions, hypersplenism, burns and various tumors.

Some types of extrinsic hemolytic anemia are temporary and resolve over several months. Other types can become chronic with periods of remissions and recurrence. The following are the most common symptoms of hemolytic anemia. However, each individual may experience symptoms differently. Symptoms may include:

- Paleness or lusterlessness of the skin
- Jaundice
- Dark colored urine
- Fever, chill
- Weakness, shortness of breath
- Dizziness
- Confusion
- Intolerance to physical activity
- Hepatosplenomegaly
- Tachycardia
- Heart murmur

How is Hemolytic Anemia Diagnosed by Conventional Western Medicine?

Diagnosis is made based on complete medical history, physical examination, and diagnostic tests, such as blood tests, urine tests, and bone marrow aspiration and/or biopsy.

How is Hemolytic Anemia Treated by Conventional Western Medicine?

The treatment for hemolytic anemia varies depending on the cause of the illness. Treatment may include:

- Discontinuing medications and chemicals that cause hemolytic anemia
- Discontinuing fava beans in patients with a G-6-PD deficiency
- Treatment of the causative diseases
- Blood transfusions

- Folic acid, mineral supplements
- Iron replacement
- Corticosteroids
- Immune globulin
- Splenectomy
- Immunosuppressive therapy

What Causes Hemolytic Anemia According to Traditional Chinese Medicine?

(1) Congenital Insufficiency

(2) Accumulation of Damp-Heat

(3) Improper Diet

(4) Qi Stagnation and Blood Stasis

How is Hemolytic Anemia Differentiated and Treated by Traditional Chinese Medicine?

(1) <u>Retention of Damp-Heat</u>

Symptoms: Jaundice, sallow complexion, reddish brown or dark urine, or fever, abdominal distention, anorexia, constipation or loose stools, red tongue with yellow and greasy coating, and soft and rapid pulse.

Therapeutic Principle: To clear away heat, eliminate dampness, replenish qi and nourish blood.

Prescription: Modified Yin Chen Wu Ling Powder.

Modifications: For abdominal distention and anorexia, add Rhizoma Dioscoreae (Shan Yao) 20g, Pericarpium Citri Reticulatae (Chen Pi) 9g and Fructus Amomi Villosi (Sha Ren) 5g; for deficiency of qi and blood, add Radix Codonopsitis Pilosulae (Dang Shen) 9g, Radix Angelicae Sinensis (Dang Gui) 10g and Radix Astragali (Huang Qi) 12g.

(2) <u>Deficiency of Both Qi and Blood</u>

Symptoms: Sallow complexion, shortness of breath, fatigue, vertigo, palpitation, spiritlessness, indolence of speaking, pale lips, dark urine, jaundice in sclera, pale tongue with thin and white coating, and thready pulse.

Therapeutic Principle: To replenish qi, nourish blood, induce diuresis and resolve jaundice.

Prescription: Modified Gui Pi Decoction.

Modifications: For anorexia and loose stools, add Pericarpium Citri Reticulatae (Chen Pi) 9g and Semen Coicis (Yi Yi Ren) 20g; for jaundice, add Herba Artemisiae Scopariae (Yin Chen Hao) 20g, Herba Artemisiae Apiaceae seu Annuae (Qing Hao) 10g and Rhizoma Alismatis Orientalis (Ze Xie) 10g.

(3) Deficiency of the Spleen and Kidney

Symptoms: Lusterless complexion, vertigo, tinnitus, sore and weak loins and knees, anorexia, loose stools; dysphoria with feverish sensation in the chest, palms and soles, red tongue with little coating, thready and rapid pulse (remarkable deficiency of yin); aversion to cold, cold limbs, chubby tongue with teeth marks and white coating, thready and weak pulse (remarkable deficiency of yang).

Therapeutic Principle: To nourish the spleen and kidney.

Prescription: Modified Shi Quan Da Bu Decoction.

Modifications: For remarkable deficiency of yin, add Radix Polygoni Multiflori (He Shou Wu) 15g, Fructus Ligustri Lucidi (Nu Zhen Zi) 12g and Radix Scrophulariae Ningpoensis (Xuan Shen) 12g; for remarkable deficiency of yang, add Herba Epimedii (Yin Yang Huo) 12g and Radix Aconiti Lateralis Praeparatae (Fu Zi) 10g.

(4) Qi Stagnation and Blood Stasis

Symptoms: Dim complexion, localized abdominal mass, distention and pain in the abdomen, dark tongue with ecchymosis, thin and white tongue coating, and thready and rough pulse.

Therapeutic Principle: To promote circulation of qi and blood.

Prescription: Modified Ge Xia Zhu Yu Decoction.

Modifications: For severe abdominal distending pain, add Radix Aucklandiae Lappae (Mu Xiang) 10g, Pericarpium Citri Reticulatae (Chen Pi) 9g and Rhizoma Corydalis (Yan Hu Suo) 10g.

What Kinds of Chinese Patent Drugs are Available to Treat Hemolytic Anemia?

(1) He Che Da Zao Pill: 1 pill each time, 2-3 times each day.

(2) Wu Zi Yan Zong Pill: 1 pill each time, 2-3 times each day.

(3) Fu Fang San Huang Tang Mixture: 10-20ml each time, twice daily.

2. Leukemia

Leukemia is cancer of the blood and develops in the bone marrow and lymphatic system. In leukemia, the bone marrow, for an unknown reason, begins to make white blood cells that do not mature correctly, but continue to reproduce themselves. These abnormal cells reproduce very quickly and do not function as healthy white blood cells to help fight infection. When the immature white blood cells (blasts), begin to crowd out other healthy cells in the bone marrow, the individual will experience the symptoms of leukemia.

Leukemia can occur at any age, although it is the most common form of cancer in childhood. It affects approximately 27,000 adults and 3,520 children each year in the United States. Leukemia occurs slightly more frequently in males than in females, and is more commonly seen in Caucasian children than in African-American children, or children of other races.

The exact cause of leukemia is unknown. It seems to develop from a combination of genetic and environmental factors. An alteration or defect in the immune system may increase the risk for developing leukemia. Factors such as exposure to certain viruses, environmental factors, chemical exposures, and various infections have been associated with damage to the immune system. The major types of leukemia include:

- Acute lymphocytic leukemia (ALL)
- Acute myelogenous leukemia (AML)
- Chronic lymphocytic leukemia (CLL)
- Chronic myelogenous leukemia (CML)
- Other chronic myeloid disorders

The stem cell matures into either the lymphoid or myeloid cells. The lymphoid cells mature into either B-lymphocytes or T-lymphocytes. If the leukemia is among these cells, it is called acute lymphocytic leukemia (ALL). The more mature the cell, the more difficult it is to treat. The myeloid cells develop into platelets, red blood cells, and specialized white blood cells called neutrophils and macrophages. There are many classifications of AML. The type of leukemia is determined by the stage of development when the normal cells become leukemia cells.

Prognosis greatly depends on the extent of the disease, disease response to treatment, genetics, age and overall health, tolerance of patients to specific medications, procedures, or therapies, and new developments in treatment. Signs and symptoms for each type of leukemia differ, but the following are the most common symptoms of leukemia. Each individual may experience symptoms differently.

- Anemia
- Fever or chills
- Persistent fatigue, weakness
- Frequent infections
- Loss of appetite or weight
- Swollen lymph nodes, enlarged liver or spleen
- Easy bleeding or bruising
- Shortness of breath, dyspnea
- Petechiae

- Excessive sweating, especially at night
- Bone and joint pain or tenderness
- Abdominal distress

The severity of signs and symptoms depends on the number of abnormal blood cells and where they collect. The early symptoms of leukemia may be overlooked because they may resemble symptoms of the flu and other common illnesses. With acute leukemia (ALL or AML), these symptoms may occur suddenly in a matter of days or weeks. With chronic leukemia (CML or CLL), these symptoms may develop slowly over months to years.

How is Leukemia Diagnosed by Conventional Western Medicine?

In addition to a complete medical history and physical examination, diagnostic procedures for leukemia may include:

- Bone marrow aspiration and/or biopsy
- Complete blood count (CBC)
- Additional blood tests
- CT scan
- MRI
- X ray
- Ultrasound
- Lymph node biopsy
- Spinal tap (lumbar puncture)
- Cytogenetic analysis

How is Leukemia Treated by Conventional Western Medicine?

Treatment usually begins by addressing the presenting symptoms such as anemia, bleeding, and/or infection. Treatment for leukemia is complex. It depends on many factors, including age and overall health of the patients, the type of leukemia and whether it has spread to other parts of the body. Treatment for leukemia may include the following:

- Chemotherapy
- Biological therapy (immunotherapy)
- Kinase inhibitors
- Other drug therapy, such as arsenic trioxide and all-trans retinoic acid (ATRA)
- Radiation therapy

- Bone marrow transplantation
- Stem cell transplant
- Clinical trials
- Blood transfusions (red blood cells, platelets)
- Antibiotics to prevent or treat infections
- Supportive care
- Continuous follow-up care

What Causes Leukemia According to Traditional Chinese Medicine?

1) Prolonged Retention of Toxic Heat and Disturbance of Essence and Marrow
2) Deficiency of Healthy Qi
3) Accumulation of Pathogenic Turbidity and Internal Blockage of Blood Stasis

How is Leukemia Differentiated and Treated by Traditional Chinese Medicine?

1) Acute Leukemia

Acute leukemia is a malignancy of the hematopoietic progenitor cell. There are two types of acute leukemia: acute lymphocytic leukemia (ALL) and acute myelogenous leukemia (AML). With acute leukemia, symptoms may occur suddenly in a matter of days or weeks.

ALL comprises 80% of the acute leukemia of childhood. The peak incidence is between 3 and 7 years of age. However, ALL is also seen in adults and comprises approximately 20% of adult acute leukemia. AML is chiefly an adult disease with median age at presentation of 50 years and an increasing incidence with advanced age.

(1) <u>Hyperactivity of Toxic Heat</u>

Symptoms: High fever, thirst, abundant sweat, irritability, headache, flushed face, general aching, aphthous stomatitis, swollen and sore throat, swelling, distention and pain in the face, or cough with yellow sputum, cellulitis (hot and red skin swelling), perianal abscess, constipation, dark urine, or hematemesis, epistaxis, hematochezia, hematuria, rash, or cloudy consciousness, delirium, crimson tongue with yellow coating, and large pulse.

Therapeutic Principle: To clear away heat, remove toxic substance, cool blood and stop bleeding.

Prescription: Modified Huang Lian Jie Du Decoction and Qing Ying Decoction.

Modifications: For accompanied dampness, add Herba Artemisiae Scopariae (Yin Chen Hao) 20g, Herba Agastache seu Pogostemonis (Huo Xiang) 9g and Semen Coicis (Yi Yi Ren) 15g; for bone and joint pain, add Excrementum Trogopteri seu Pteromydis (Wu Ling Zhi) 10g, Gummi Olibanum (Ru Xiang) 10g, Myrrha (Mo Yao) 10g and Pollen Typhae (Pu Huang) 10g; for hemorrhage, add Herba

Agrimoniae Pilosae (Xian He Cao) 12g, Cacumen Biotae Orientalis (Ce Bai Ye) 12g and Herba Cephalanoploris (Xiao Ji) 15g.

(2) <u>Accumulation of Phlegm-Heat</u>

Symptoms: Abdominal mass, enlarged lymph nodes in the lower jaw, axillae and neck, copious amount of sputum, heavy sensation of the head, anorexia, fever, weak extremities, vexation, bitter taste in the mouth, vertigo, bone pain, pricking pain and stuffiness in the chest, thirst without desire to drink, dark purple tongue with ecchymoses or petechiae, yellow and greasy tongue coating, slippery and rapid or deep, thready and rough pulse.

Therapeutic Principle: To clear away heat, resolve phlegm, promote blood circulation and dismiss mass.

Prescription: Modified Wen Dan Decoction and Tao Hong Si Wu Decoction.

Modifications: For hard abdominal mass, add Carapax Trionycis (Bie Jia) 20g, Squama Manitis Pentadactylae (Chuan Shan Jia) 10g, Thallus Laminariae (Kun Bu) 12g, Herba Sargassi (Hai Zao) 12g, Rhizoma Sparganii Stoloniferi (San Leng) 10g and Rhizoma Curcumae Ezhu (E Zhu) 10g.

(3) <u>Deficiency of Yin and Hyperactivity of Fire</u>

Symptoms: Cutaneous ecchymosis, epistaxis, gingival hemorrhage, fever, or dysphoria with feverish sensation in the chest, palms and soles, dry mouth with bitter taste, night sweating, fatigue, lassitude, dim complexion, red tongue with yellow coating, and thready and rapid pulse.

Therapeutic Principle: To nourish yin, purge fire, cool blood and remove toxic substance.

Prescription: Modified Zhi Bai Di Huang Pill and Er Zhi Pill.

Modifications: For severe hyperactive fire, add Herba Hedyotis Diffusae (Bai Hua She She Cao) 30g, Herba Scutellaria Barbatae (Ban Zhi Lian) 15g and Herba Taraxaci Mongolici (Pu Gong Ying) 15g.

(4) <u>Deficiency of Both Qi and Yin</u>

Symptoms: Low-grade fever, spontaneous sweating, night sweating, shortness of breath, fatigue, lusterless complexion, dizziness, sore and weak loins and knees, feverish sensation in palms and soles, cutaneous ecchymoses, petechiae, epistaxis, gingival hemorrhage, pale tongue with teeth marks, and deep and thready pulse.

Therapeutic Principle: To replenish qi, nourish yin, clear way heat and remove toxic substance.

Prescription: Modified Wu Yin Decoction.

Modifications: For concurrent blood stasis, bone pain, chest pain and abdominal mass, add Semen Pruni Persicae (Tao Ren) 10g, Flos Carthami Tinctorii (Hong Hua) 10g, Carapax Trionycis (Bie Jia)

20g, Rhizoma Sparganii Stoloniferi (San Leng) 10g, Rhizoma Curcumae Ezhu (E Zhu) 10g and Extremitas Radicis Angelicae Sinensis (Dang Gui Wei) 12g; for enlarged lymph nodes, add Herba Sargassi (Hai Zao) 12g, Bulbus Fritillariae Cirrhosae (Bei Mu) 10g, Pseudobulbus Cremastrae seu Pleiones (Shan Ci Gu) 5g, Rhizoma Dioscoreae Bulbiferae (Huang Yao Zi) 10g, Concha Ostreae (Mu Li) 30g and Concha Meretricis seu Cyclinae (Hai Ge Qiao) 15g; for severe toxic heat, add Herba Hedyotis Diffusae (Bai Hua She She Cao) 30g, Herba Scutellaria Barbatae (Ban Zhi Lian) 15g and Herba Taraxaci Mongolici (Pu Gong Ying) 15g.

(5) Retention of Damp-Heat

Symptoms: Fever, sweating that does not relieve fever, general heavy sensation, abdominal distention, anorexia, joint pain, dyschezia, or diarrhea, burning sensation in anus, difficult urination with dark urine, red tongue with yellow and greasy coating, and slippery and rapid pulse.

Therapeutic Principle: To clear away heat, remove toxic substance, eliminate dampness and resolve turbidity.

Prescription: Modified Ge Gen Qin Lian Decoction.

Modifications: For severe heat at Triple Warmer and sustained high fever, add Fructus Gardeniae Jasminoidis (Zhi Zi) 10g and Radix Gentianae (Long Dan Cao) 5g; for sore limbs, add Rhizoma et Radix Notopterygii (Qiang Huo) 9g, Herba Taxilli (Sang Ji Sheng) 15g and Herba Agastache seu Pogostemonis (Huo Xiang) 9g; for difficult, painful and dripping urination, add Herba Plantaginis (Che Qian Cao) 12g and Caulis Akebiae (Mu Tong) 5g.

2) Chronic Myelogenous Leukemia (CML)

Chronic myelogenous leukemia (CML), also known as chronic granulocytic leukemia, is a myeloproliferative disorder characterized by increased proliferation of the granulocytic cell line without the loss of their capacity to differentiate. Consequently, the peripheral blood cell profile shows an increased number of granulocytes and their immature precursors, including occasional blast cells. In the United States, CML accounts for 20% of all leukemias affecting adults. It typically affects middle-aged individuals. Although uncommon, the disease also occurs in younger individuals.

(1) Deficiency of Yin and Interior-Heat

Symptoms: Low-grade fever, abundant sweat, or night sweating, vertigo, vexation, flushed face, dry mouth with bitter taste, emaciation, feverish sensation in palms and soles, cutaneous ecchymosis, epistaxis, gingival hemorrhage, smooth and red tongue with little coating, and thready and rapid pulse.

Therapeutic Principle: To nourish yin, clear away heat, remove toxic substance and stagnation.

Prescription: Modified Qing Hao Bie Jia Decoction.

Modifications: For severe heat, add Rhizoma Paridis (Zao Xiu) 10g and Radix Sophorae Subprostratae (Shan Dou Gen) 10g; for hemorrhage, add Cortex Moutan Radicis (Mu Dan Pi) 10g, Radix Rubiae Cordifoliae (Qian Cao) 12g, Herba Cephalanoploris (Xiao Ji) 15g and Herba Agrimoniae Pilosae (Xian He Cao) 12g.

(2) <u>Internal Blockage of Blood Stasis</u>

Symptoms: Emaciation, dim complexion, sternal tenderness, hard and tender mass in hypochondrium (splenomegaly), cutaneous ecchymosis, epistaxis, gingival hemorrhage, hematuria, or hematochezia, dark purple tongue, and thready and rough pulse.

Therapeutic Principle: To promote circulation of blood and remove blood stasis.

Prescription: Modified Ge Xia Zhu Yu Decoction.

Modifications: For severe hypochondriac mass, add Carapax Trionycis (Bie Jia) 20g, Squama Manitis Pentadactylae (Chuan Shan Jia) 10g and Concha Ostreae (Mu Li) 20g; for remarkable bleeding, add powdered Radix Notoginseng (San Qi) 10g.

(3) <u>Deficiency of Both Qi and Blood</u>

Symptoms: Sallow or pale complexion, vertigo, blurred vision, palpitation, fatigue, weakness, shortness of breath, indolence of speaking, spontaneous sweating, anorexia, pale tongue with thin and white coating, and thready and weak pulse.

Therapeutic Principle: To nourish blood and replenish qi.

Prescription: Modified Ba Zhen Decoction.

Modifications: For epistaxis and muscular hemorrhage, add Radix Astragali (Huang Qi) 10g, Radix Rubiae Cordifoliae (Qian Cao) 12g, Herba Agrimoniae Pilosae (Xian He Cao) 12g and Gelatinum Corii Asini (E Jiao) 10g; for low-grade fever and dry mouth, add Herba Ecliptae Prostratae (Han Lian Cao) 15g and Radix Ophiopogonis Japonici (Mai Dong) 12g.

(4) <u>Retention of Toxic Heat</u>

Symptoms: Severe fever or high fever, sweating, thirst with a desire for cold drinks, epistaxis, ecchymosis, or hematochezia and hematuria, general aching, bone pain, gradual enlargement of a mass that is hard, localized and painful (splenomegaly) in the left hypochondrium, lassitude, spiritlessness, weight loss, red tongue with yellow coating, and rapid pulse.

Therapeutic Principle: To clear away heat and remove toxic substances.

Prescription: Modified Qing Ying Decoction and Xi Jiao Di Huang Decoction.

Modifications: For persistent high fever, add Gypsum Fibrosum (Shi Gao) 30g and Rhizoma Anemarrhenae (Zhi Mu) 10g; for severe bleeding, add Radix Lithospermi seu Macrotomiae (Zi Cao) 9g, Rhizoma Imperatae Cylindricae (Bai Mao Gen) 20g, Herba Agrimoniae Pilosae (Xian He Cao) 12g, Herba seu Radix Cirsii Japonici (Da Ji) 12g and Herba Cephalanoploris (Xiao Ji) 15g.

3) Chronic Lymphocytic Leukemia (CLL)

Chronic lymphocytic leukemia (CLL) is a monoclonal disorder characterized by a progressive accumulation of functionally incompetent lymphocytes. It is the most common form of leukemia found in adults in Western countries. In the United States, more than 17,000 new cases are reported every year.

(1) Stagnation of Phlegm and Blood Stasis

Symptoms: Dim complexion, enlarged lymph nodes in the neck, axillae and groins (lymphadenopathy), localized or movable abdominal mass that is hard in texture (hepatomegaly or splenomegaly), low-grade fever, fatigue, cutaneous ecchymosis, or epistaxis, dark purple tongue with ecchymoses or petechiae, thick and greasy tongue coating, and deep, thready and rough pulse.

Therapeutic Principle: To resolve phlegm, remove stagnation and disperse mass.

Prescription: Modified Tao Hong Si Wu Decoction and Chai Hu Shu Gan Powder.

Modifications: For remarkable lymphadenopathy and organomegaly, add Pseudobulbus Cremastrae seu Pleiones (Shan Ci Gu) 5g, Herba Hedyotis Diffusae (Bai Hua She She Cao) 30g, Spica Prunellae Vulgaris (Xia Ku Cao) 12g, Concha Ostreae (Mu Li) 20g, Herba Sargassi (Hai Zao) 12g and Carapax Trionycis (Bie Jia) 20g.

(2) Deficiency of Both Qi and Yin

Symptoms: Low-grade fever, fatigue, shortness of breath, indolence of speaking, lusterless complexion, feverish sensation in palms and soles, cutaneous ecchymosis and petechiae, sore and weak loins and knees, anorexia, dry mouth, pale tongue, and deep and thready pulse.

Therapeutic Principle: To replenish qi and nourish yin.

Prescription: Modified Si Jun Zi Decoction and Sha Shen Mai Dong Decoction.

Modifications: For severe deficiency of yin, add Fructus Ligustri Lucidi (Nu Zhen Zi) 12g and Herba Ecliptae Prostratae (Han Lian Cao) 15g; for severe fever and remarkable lymphadenopathy, add Herba Hedyotis Diffusae (Bai Hua She She Cao) 30g, Herba Scutellaria Barbatae (Ban Zhi Lian) 20g and Herba Taraxaci Mongolici (Pu Gong Ying) 20g; for severe deficiency of qi, add Radix Astragali (Huang Qi) 10g, Rhizoma Polygonati (Huang Jing) 10g and Rhizoma Dioscoreae (Shan Yao) 20g.

What Kinds of Chinese Patent Drugs are Available to Treat Leukemia?

1) Acute Leukemia
   (1) Liu Shen Pill: 20 pill each time, thrice daily.
   (2) Xi Huang Pill: 1 pill each time, thrice daily.
   (3) Zhen Qi Fu Zheng Capsule: 3 capsules each time, thrice daily.
2) Chronic Myelogenous Leukemia (CML)
   (1) Dang Gui Long Hui Pill: 6g each time, thrice daily.
   (2) Liu Shen Pill: 30-40 pills each time, thrice daily.
3) Chronic Lymphocytic Leukemia (CLL)
   (1) Xi Huang Pill: 1 pill each time, twice daily.
   (2) Xiao Jin Pill: 1 pill each time, twice daily.

3. Lymphoma

Lymphoma is a cancer of a part of the immune system called the lymphatic system. There are many types of lymphoma. One type is called Hodgkin's disease. The rest are called non-Hodgkin's lymphoma.

1) Non-Hodgkin's Lymphoma (NHL)

Non-Hodgkin's lymphoma is a heterogeneous group of cancers of lymphocytes. Non-Hodgkin's lymphoma causes the cells in the lymphatic system to abnormally reproduce, eventually causing tumors to grow. Non-Hodgkin's disease cells can also spread to other organs and tissues in the body.

In the United States in 2004, there were about 54,320 new cases of non-Hodgkin's lymphoma. Non-Hodgkin's lymphoma has been one of the most rapidly increasing types of cancer in the United States, having more than doubled in incidence since the 1970s. Non-Hodgkin's lymphoma affects males more often than females.

Staging and classification of non-Hodgkin's lymphoma is based on the extent of the disease and the specific cells involved. There are three subtypes of non-Hodgkin's lymphoma: lymphoblastic non-Hodgkin's lymphoma, Burkitt's or non-Burkitt's lymphoma, large cell or diffuse histiocytic non-Hodgkin's lymphoma.

The specific cause of non-Hodgkin's lymphoma is unclear. It is possible that genetics and exposure to viral infections may increase the risk for developing this malignancy. Non-Hodgkin's lymphoma has also been linked to chemotherapy and radiation therapy. Non-Hodgkin's may be a second malignancy as a result of the treatment for certain cancers. The following are the most common symptoms of non-Hodgkin's lymphoma. However, each individual may experience the symptoms

differently. Symptoms may include:
- Painless swelling of the lymph nodes in neck, chest, abdomen, armpit, or groin
- Fever
- Sore throat
- Bone and joint pain
- Drenching night sweats
- Fatigue
- Weight loss
- Decreased appetite
- Coughing, trouble breathing or chest pain
- Pruritus
- Recurring infections
- Abdominal pain or swelling

How is NHL Diagnosed by Conventional Western Medicine?

In addition to a complete medical history and physical examination, diagnostic procedures for non-Hodgkin's lymphoma may include blood and urine tests, chest x rays, CT scan of the abdomen, chest, and pelvis, positron emission tomography (PET) scan, lymph node biopsy, lymphangiogram, bone marrow aspiration and/or biopsy, and lumbar puncture.

How is NHL Treated by Conventional Western Medicine?

Treatment may include (alone or in combination):
- Chemotherapy
- Radiation therapy
- Stem-cell transplantation
- Observation
- Biologic therapy, such as Rituximab (Rituxan)
- Radioimmunotherapy

2) Hodgkin's Disease (HD)

Hodgkin's disease is a group of cancers characterized by Reed-Sternberg cells in an appropriate reactive cellular background. Hodgkin's disease causes the cells in the lymphatic system to abnormally reproduce, eventually making the body less able to fight infection and cause swelling in the lymph nodes. Hodgkin's disease cells can also metastasize to other organs and tissue.

Hodgkin's disease most commonly affects people between the ages of 15 and 40 and people older than age 55. In the United States in 2004, there were about 7,880 new cases of Hodgkin's disease. The disease affects males more often than females.

The specific cause of Hodgkin's disease is unknown. It is possible that a genetic predisposition and exposure to viral infections may increase the risk for developing Hodgkin's lymphoma. The following are the most common symptoms of Hodgkin's disease. However, each individual may experience symptoms differently. Symptoms may include:

- Painless swelling of the lymph nodes in neck, underarm, groin, and chest
- Dyspnea
- Fever, chills
- Drenching night sweats
- Fatigue
- Weight loss
- Decreased appetite
- Pruritus
- Frequent viral infections

How is Hodgkin's Disease Diagnosed by Conventional Western Medicine?

In addition to a complete medical history and physical examination, diagnostic procedures for Hodgkin's lymphoma may include blood and urine tests, chest x rays, CT scan of the abdomen, chest, and pelvis, positron emission tomography (PET) scan, lymph node biopsy, lymphangiogram, bone marrow aspiration and/or biopsy.

How is Hodgkin's Disease Treated by Conventional Western Medicine?

Treatment may include (alone or in combination):

- Chemotherapy. Drug regimens include ABVD, BEACOPP, COPP/ABVD, Stanford V, and MOPP
- Radiation
- Bone marrow transplant
- Supportive care

What Causes Lymphoma According to Traditional Chinese Medicine?

1) Retention of Cold-Phlegm
2) Stagnation of Qi and Phlegm

3) Yin Deficiency of the Liver and Kidney

How is Lymphoma Differentiated and Treated by Traditional Chinese Medicine?

1) <u>Retention of Cold-Phlegm</u>

Symptoms: Non-painful and non-itching multiple enlarged lymph nodes, which are hard in texture (lymphadenopathy), in the neck and axillae; pale complexion, spiritlessness, fatigue, cold limbs, anorexia, loose stools, pale tongue, and thready and weak pulse.

Therapeutic Principle: To warm and resolve cold-phlegm, diminish stagnation and mass.

Prescription: Modified Yang He Decoction.

Modifications: For remarkable spiritlessness and fatigue, add Radix Codonopsitis Pilosulae (Dang Shen) 9g and Rhizoma Atractylodis Macrocephalae (Bai Zhu) 10g; for remarkable cold limbs, add Radix Aconiti Lateralis Praeparatae (Fu Zi) 10g, Ramulus Cinnamomi Cassiae (Gui Zhi) 9g and Radix Astragali (Huang Qi) 12g.

2) <u>Stagnation of Qi and Phlegm</u>

Symptoms: Non-painful and non-itching and localized multiple enlarged lymph nodes in the neck and axillae (lymphadenopathy), aversion to cold, fever, bitter taste in the mouth, dry throat, vertigo, tinnitus, irritability, constipation, yellow urine, red tongue with slight yellow coating, and taut and rapid pulse.

Therapeutic Principle: To soothe the liver, dismiss stagnation, resolve phlegm and disperse mass.

Prescription: Modified Chai Hu Shu Gan Powder.

Modifications: For constipation, add Radix et Rhizoma Rhei (Da Huang) 6g; for flushed face and irritability, add Radix Gentianae (Long Dan Cao) 5g, Cortex Moutan Radicis (Mu Dan Pi) 10g and Fructus Gardeniae Jasminoidis (Zhi Zi) 9g.

3) <u>Liver Fire Attacking the Lung</u>

Symptoms: Pain in the chest and hypochondrium, cough, belching, sensation of stuffiness in the chest, shortness of breath, irritability, palpitation, dyspnea, bitter taste in the mouth, dry throat, vertigo, fatigue, red tongue with thin and white or slight yellow coating, taut and rapid pulse.

Therapeutic Principle: To clear away liver fire, purge the lung and resolve stagnation.

Prescription: Modified Dai Ge Powder and Xie Bai Powder.

Modifications: For stuffiness in the chest, add Fructus Trichosanthis (Gua Lou) 15g and Rhizoma Coptidis (Huang Lian) 9g; for adverse flow of qi and cough, add Flos Inulae (Xuan Fu Hua) 9g and Ochra Haematitum (Dai Zhe Shi) 20g.

4) <u>Yin Deficiency of the Liver and Kidney</u>

Symptoms: Vertigo, tinnitus, hypochondriac pain, multiple enlarged lymph nodes, which are hard in texture (lymphadenopathy), in the neck; dry mouth and throat, dysphoria with feverish sensation in the chest, palms and soles, sore and weak loins and knees, seminal emission, or abnormal menstruation, red tongue with little coating, and thready and rapid pulse.

Therapeutic Principle: To nourish the liver and kidney, resolve stagnation and diminish mass.

Prescription: Modified Qi Ju Di Huang Pill.

Modifications: For fire hyperactivity and yin deficiency with feverish sensation in palms and soles, add Rhizoma Anemarrhenae (Zhi Mu) 10g and Cortex Phellodendri (Huang Bai) 10g; for severe night sweats, add Concha Ostreae (Mu Li) 20g and Fructus Tritici Aestivi Levis (Fu Xiao Mai) 20g.

5) <u>Stagnation of Blood Stasis</u>

Symptoms: Weight loss, abdominal distention, enlarged lymph nodes in the neck and axillae (lymphadenopathy), or abdominal mass, abdominal pain, anorexia, or cough and belching, nausea, vomiting, sensation of stuffiness in the chest, hectic fever in the afternoon, constipation or tarry stools, dark tongue with ecchymosis, and deep and taut pulse.

Therapeutic Principle: To promote circulation of blood and remove blood stasis, diminish stagnation and disperse mass.

Prescription: Modified Bie Jia Jian Pill and San Leng Decoction.

Modifications: For severe abdominal pain, add Radix Paeoniae Alba (Bai Shao Yao) 10g and Radix Glycyrrhizae Uralensis (Gan Cao) 6g; for vomiting, add Rhizoma Pinelliae Ternatae (Ban Xia) 10g and Caulis Bambusae in Taeniam (Zhu Ru) 10g.

6) <u>Deficiency of Both Qi and Blood</u>

Symptoms: Vertigo, blurred vision, palpitation, insomnia, pale complexion, shortness of breath, fatigue, multiple enlarged lymph nodes, which are hard in texture (lymphadenopathy), in the neck and axillae; or abdominal mass, anorexia, pale lips, pale tongue with thin and white coating, and thready and weak pulse.

Therapeutic Principle: To replenish qi and nourish blood.

Prescription: Modified Ba Zhen Decoction.

Modifications: For remarkable anemia, add Gelatinum Corii Asini (E Jiao) 10g and Radix et Caulis Jixueteng (Ji Xue Teng) 12g; for palpitation and insomnia, add Semen Ziziphi Spinosae (Suan Zao Ren) 15g, Mastodi Ossis Fossilia (Long Gu) 20g and Concha Ostreae (Mu Li) 20g; for anorexia, ad Fructus Crataegi (Shan Zha) 12g, Massa Medicata Fermentata (Shen Qu) 10g, Fructus Hordei Germinatus (Mai Ya) 12g and Pericarpium Citri Reticulatae (Chen Pi) 9g.

What Kinds of Chinese Patent Drugs are Available to Treat Lymphoma?

1) Xia Ku Cao Ointment: 15g each time, twice daily.
2) Xiao Jin Pill: 0.6g each time, twice daily.
3) Bie Jia Jian Pill: 6-9g each time, twice daily.
4) Xi Huang Pill: 3g each time, twice daily.

4. Allergic Purpura (Henoch-Schönlein Purpura)

Allergic purpura (AP) is also called Henoch-Schonlein purpura (HSP), named after the two German physicians who first recognized and described it in the 1880s. AP is also referred to as anaphylactoid purpura or vascular purpura.

Henoch-Schönlein purpura (HSP) is a form of vasculitis, a condition that involves inflammation of the small blood vessels in the skin, kidneys, and intestinal tract. Symptoms include a purple spotted skin rash, abdominal pain, gastrointestinal upsets, and joint inflammation, swelling, and pain. Although the exact cause of the disease is unknown, it often develops following a recent viral or bacterial infection of the respiratory tract and is possibly an allergic reaction of the immune system.

HSP is the most common acute vasculitis affecting children. In the United States, the prevalence of HSP is approximately 14 to 15 cases per 100,000 populations. Approximately 75 percent of cases occur in children between the ages of two and 11, and occurs more frequently in boys. A family connection has been noted with HSP. The following are the most common symptoms of Henoch-Schönlein purpura. However, each individual may experience symptoms differently. Symptoms may include:

- Purpura
- Arthralgia
- Swollen, sore joints (arthritis)
- Abdominal pain
- Gastrointestinal bleeding
- Nephritis
- Subcutaneous edema
- Encephalopathy
- Orchitis

How is Allergic Purpura Diagnosed by Conventional Western Medicine?

Diagnosis is based on the symptoms and their development, a careful medical history, and blood and urine tests. X rays or CT scans may be performed to assess complications in the bowel or other internal organs. In some cases a renal biopsy or skin biopsy may be ordered.

How is Allergic Purpura Treated by Conventional Western Medicine?

Treatments for HSP may include:

- Adequate hydration, or fluid intake
- Careful attention to nutrition
- Pain control with medications such as acetaminophen
- Nonsteroidal anti-inflammatory drugs (NSAIDs) to ease joint pain and swelling
- Glucocorticoids

What Causes Allergic Purpura According to Traditional Chinese Medicine?

1) Internal Retention of Pathogenic Factors
2) Deficiency of Yin and Interior-Heat
3) Dysfunction of the Spleen and Stomach
4) Blood Stasis

How is Allergic Purpura Differentiated and Treated by Traditional Chinese Medicine?

1) <u>Hyperactivity of Toxic Heat</u>

Symptoms: Abrupt onset, bluish purple petechiae, or red or reddish purple purpura of the skin, cutaneous pruritus that is more common in the lower extremities, fever, flushed face, swollen and sore throat, dry mouth, thirst, dark urine; or hematuria, abdominal pain, hematochezia, swollen and painful joints; red tongue with thin and yellow coating, and taut and rapid or slippery and rapid pulse.

Therapeutic Principle: To clear away heat, remove toxic substance, cool blood and stop hemorrhage.

Prescription: Modified Xi Jiao Di Huang Decoction and Qing Ying Decoction.

Modifications: For swollen and sore throat, remarkable dry mouth and thirst, add Herba seu Radix Cirsii Japonici (Da Ji) 10g, Herba Cephalanoploris (Xiao Ji) 20g and Rhizoma Imperatae Cylindricae (Bai Mao Gen) 20g; for widespread hemorrhage, constipation, add Gypsum Fibrosum (Shi Gao) 30g and Radix et Rhizoma Rhei (Da Huang) 6g; for abdominal pain, add Rhizoma Corydalis (Yan Hu Suo) 10g, Fructus Meliae Toosendan (Chuan Lian Zi) 10g and Radix Paeoniae Rubra (Chi Shao) 10g; for swollen and sore joints, add Lonicerae Caulis et Folium (Ren Dong Teng) 20g, Rhizoma Anemarrhenae (Zhi Mu) 10g, Cortex Fraxini (Qin Pi) 10g and Radix Gentianae Macrophyllae (Qin Jiao) 9g.

2) <u>Deficiency of Yin and Hyperactivity of Fire</u>

Symptoms: Recurrent and fluctuated bluish purple petechiae or reddish purple purpura, flushed cheeks, vexation, insomnia, feverish sensation in palms and soles, or hectic fever, night sweating, red tongue with little coating, and thready and rapid pulse.

Therapeutic Principle: To nourish yin, purge fire, calm collaterals and stop hemorrhage.

Prescription: Modified Qian Gen Powder.

Modifications: For remarkable purpura, add Cortex Moutan Radicis (Mu Dan Pi) 10g and Radix Lithospermi seu Macrotomiae (Zi Cao) 10g; for remarkable deficiency of yin, add Radix Scrophulariae Ningpoensis (Xuan Shen) 10g, Carapax et Plastrum Testudinis (Gui Ban) 15g, Fructus Ligustri Lucidi (Nu Zhen Zi) 10g and Herba Ecliptae Prostratae (Han Lian Cao) 15g; for sore lumbar region and weak knees, vertigo, fatigue, use Zhi Bai Di Huang Pill supplemented with Radix Lithospermi seu Macrotomiae (Zi Cao) 10g and Radix Rubiae Cordifoliae (Qian Cao) 12g.

3) Retention of Damp-Heat

Symptoms: Fluctuated purpura of the skin, which is more common in the lower extremities and buttocks; lassitude, sensation of stuffiness in the epigastrium, anorexia, dark urine or hematuria, edema, red tongue with yellow and greasy coating, and soft and rapid pulse.

Therapeutic Principle: To clear away heat, resolve dampness, cool blood and stop hemorrhage.

Prescription: Modified Xiao Ji Decoction.

Modifications: For epigastric stuffiness and anorexia, add Rhizoma Atractylodis (Cang Zhu) 10g, Semen Alpiniae Katsumadai (Cao Dou Kou) 5g and Herba Eupatorii (Pei Lan) 10g; for hematochezia, add Rhizoma Coptidis (Huang Lian) 10g and Radix Sanguisorbae Officinalis (Di Yu) 12g; for abdominal pain, add Rhizoma Corydalis (Yan Hu Suo) 10g and Fructus Meliae Toosendan (Chuan Lian Zi) 10g, for recurrent purpura, add Radix Salviae Miltiorrhizae (Dan Shen) 10g, Herba Leonuri Heterophylii (Yi Mu Cao) 10g and Radix Notoginseng (San Qi) 9g.

4) Inability of Qi to Arrest Blood

Symptoms: Lingering, recurrent and scattered light colored cutaneous purpura that is aggravated on exertion, palpitation, shortness of breath, fatigue, sallow complexion, pale tongue with thin and white coating, and thready and weak pulse.

Therapeutic Principle: To strengthen the spleen, replenish qi and arrest blood.

Prescription: Modified Gui Pi Decoction.

Modifications: For pruritus of the skin, add Periostracum Cicadae (Chan Tui) 9g and Cortex Dictamni Radicis (Bai Xian Pi) 10g; for lingering purpura, add Radix Salviae Miltiorrhizae (Dan Shen) 10g, Lumbricus (Di Long) 12g, Herba Leonuri Heterophylii (Yi Mu Cao) 12g and Pollen Typhae (Pu

Huang) 9g; for hematuria, add Gelatinum Corii Asini (E Jiao) 10g and Rhizoma Imperatae Cylindricae (Bai Mao Gen) 20g.

5) Obstruction of Collaterals by Blood Stasis

Symptoms: Chronic bluish purpura of the skin, dark black complexion, bluish purple lower eyelids, squamous and dry skin, joint pain, abdominal pain, or thirst without desire to drink, dark purple tongue with ecchymoses or petechiae, and rough pulse.

Therapeutic Principle: To promote qi circulation, remove blood stasis, regulate collaterals and stop hemorrhage.

Prescription: Modified Xue Fu Zhu Yu Decoction.

Modifications: For heat-blood, add Cortex Moutan Radicis (Mu Dan Pi) 10g, Cacumen Biotae Orientalis (Ce Bai Ye) 12g and Radix Rubiae Cordifoliae (Qian Cao) 12g; for swollen and painful joints, add Lonicerae Caulis et Folium (Ren Dong Teng) 15g, Fructus Chaenomelis (Mu Gua) 12g and Ramulus Mori (Sang Zhi) 20g.

What Kinds of Chinese Patent Drugs are Available to Treat Allergic Purpura?

1) San Qi Zong Gan Tablet: 5 tablets each time, thrice daily.
2) Lei Gong Teng Duo Gan Tablet: 1.0-1.5mg/kg/day, thrice daily.
3) Jin Lian Qing Re Granule: 1 bag each time, 4 times each day.
4) Xin Xue Pill: 1 little bottle each time, twice daily.

5. Idiopathic Thrombocytopenia Purpura (ITP)

Idiopathic thrombocytopenic purpura (ITP) is a blood disorder characterized by an abnormal decrease in the number of platelets in the blood. A decrease in platelets can result in easy bruising, bleeding gums, and internal bleeding. Normal platelet count is in the range of 150,000 to 450,000. With ITP, the platelet count is less than 100,000.

ITP is often divided into two categories: acute and chronic. Acute ITP is the most common form and occurs most frequently in children, typically after a viral infection. It usually goes away on its own within six months. Chronic ITP lasts longer than six months and is more common in adults.

Both children and adults can develop ITP. Children usually get the acute type of ITP. Adults tend to get the chronic type of ITP, rarely the acute type of ITP. Women are two to three times more likely than men to get chronic ITP.

In most cases, the cause of ITP is unknown. It is not contagious. ITP is largely an autoimmune disease. The decrease in platelets occurs because the immune system attacks and destroys the body's own platelets, for an unknown reason. Because "idiopathic" means "of unknown cause," a better name for most cases of ITP is immune thrombocytopenic purpura. Signs that typically indicate a low platelet count and possibly ITP include:

- Easy or excessive bruising (purpura)
- Petechiae
- Prolonged bleeding from cuts
- Spontaneous bleeding from the gums or nose
- Hematuria, hematemesis or hematochezia
- Unusually heavy menstrual flows
- Profuse bleeding during surgery

Serious or widespread bleeding indicates an emergency and requires immediate care.

How is ITP Diagnosed by Conventional Western Medicine?

In addition to a complete medical history and physical examination, diagnostic procedures for ITP may include complete blood count (CBC), blood smear, and bone marrow aspiration.

How is ITP Treated by Conventional Western Medicine?

Whether to treat ITP is based on the bleeding symptoms and platelet count. When treatment is needed, medicines are often used, at least at first. Treatments for ITP may include:

- Corticosteroids
- Immunoglobulin and anti-(Rh) D immunoglobulin
- Splenectomy
- Platelet transfusions
- Treating infections
- Stopping medicines that can lower the number of platelets or cause bleeding
- Hormone therapy

What Causes ITP According to Traditional Chinese Medicine?

1) Hyperactivity of Toxic Heat Forcing the Blood to Move Recklessly
2) Hyperactivity of Fire due to Deficiency of Yin
3) Failure of Qi to Control Blood
4) Obstruction and Stagnation of Blood Stasis

How is ITP Differentiated and Treated by Traditional Chinese Medicine?

1) <u>Hyperactivity of Heat Attacking Blood</u>

Symptoms: Abrupt onset with cutaneous purpura and petechiae, which are more common in the lower extremities; fever, thirst, constipation, dark urine, often accompanied with epistaxis, gingival bleeding, hematuria, hematochezia, or abdominal pain, red tongue with thin and yellow coating, and taut and rapid or slippery and rapid pulse.

Therapeutic Principle: To clear away heat, cool blood and stop bleeding.

Prescription: Modified Xi Jiao Di Huang Decoction.

Modifications: For severe hemorrhage, add Nodus Nelumbinis Nuciferae Rhizomatis (Ou Jie) 12g, Radix Sanguisorbae Officinalis (Di Yu) 12g and Herba Agrimoniae Pilosae (Xian He Cao) 12g; for hyperactive toxic heat with fever, thirst with a desire to drink, dysphoria, dense and wide-spread purple ecchymoses, add Gypsum Fibrosum (Shi Gao) 30g, Radix Gentianae (Long Dan Cao) 5g and Zi Xue Pill; for hematochezia, add Flos Sophorae Japonicae (Huai Hua) 12g and Radix Sanguisorbae Officinalis (Di Yu) 12g; for severe bleeding with thready and rapid pulse, pale complexion, cold limbs and drenching sweats, use Du Shen Decoction for emergency treatment.

2) Hyperactivity of Fire due to Deficiency of Yin

Symptoms: Multiple intermittent reddish purple ecchymoses, which are severer in the lower extremities; vertigo, tinnitus, low-grade fever, flushed cheeks, dysphoria, night sweats, epistaxis, gingival bleeding, menorrhagia, red tongue with little coating, and thready and rapid pulse.

Therapeutic Principle: To nourish yin, purge fire, clear away heat and stop bleeding.

Prescription: Modified Qian Gen Powder or Yu Nu Decoction.

Modifications: For remarkable deficiency of stomach yin with thirst, red tongue and little tongue coating, add Herba Dendrobii (Shi Hu) 10g and Rhizoma Polygonati Odorati (Yu Zhu) 12g; for deficiency of kidney yin with sore lumbar region, weak knees, vertigo, fatigue, feverish sensation in palms and soles, red tongue with little coating, deep, thready and rapid pulse, use Zhi Bai Di Huang Decoction supplemented with Radix Rubiae Cordifoliae (Qian Cao) 10g and Radix Lithospermi seu Macrotomiae (Zi Cao) 9g.

3) Failure of Qi to Control Blood

Symptoms: Scattered dull-colored intermittent purpura that is aggravated on exertion, spiritlessness, palpitation, shortness of breath, vertigo, anorexia, pale or sallow complexion, pale tongue with white coating, and weak pulse.

Therapeutic Principle: To replenish qi, arrest blood, strengthen the spleen and nourish blood.

Prescription: Modified Gui Pi Decoction.

Modifications: For yang deficiency with cold limbs, diarrhea, pale and chubby tongue with white and slippery coating, add Bao Yuan Decoction; for deficiency of kidney qi with sore and weak loins and knees, add Fructus Corni Officinalis (Shan Zhu Yu) 10g, Semen Cuscutae Chinensis (Tu Si Zi) 12g and Radix Dipsaci Asperi (Xu Duan) 15g.

4) Internal Obstruction of Blood Stasis

Symptoms: Bluish purple ecchymoses, muscular hemorrhage, epistaxis, hematemesis and hematochezia with dark purple colored blood, menses with clot, dry and lusterless hair, dark bluish complexion, dark purple tongue with ecchymoses or petechiae, thready and rough or taut pulse.

Therapeutic Principle: To promote circulation of blood, remove blood stasis and stop bleeding.

Prescription: Modified Tao Hong Si Wu Decoction.

Modifications: For remarkable deficiency of qi with spiritlessness, fatigue, shortness of breath, indolence of speaking, add Radix Astragali (Huang Qi) 12g and Radix Codonopsitis Pilosulae (Dang Shen) 9g; for yang deficiency of the spleen and kidney with cold limbs, aversion to cold, abdominal distention, diarrhea, soreness in lumbar region, chubby tongue, deep and slow pulse, add Radix Aconiti Lateralis Praeparatae (Fu Zi) 10g, Cortex Cinnamomi Cassiae (Rou Gui) 3g and Semen Cuscutae Chinensis (Tu Si Zi) 12g.

What Kinds of Chinese Patent Drugs are Available to Treat ITP?

1) Zi Dian Qing Tablet: 5-6 tablets each time, thrice daily.
2) Ren Shen Gui Pi Pill: 1 pill each time, thrice daily.

6. Leukopenia

Leukopenia (or leukocytopenia, or leucopenia) is a decrease in the number of circulating white blood cells (leukocytes) in the blood. As the principal function of white cells is to combat infection, a decrease in the number of these cells can place patients at increased risk for infection.

Granulocytopenia is defined as a reduced number of blood granulocytes, namely neutrophils, eosinophils, and basophils. Agranulocytosis refers to a complete absence of neutrophils in peripheral blood. Neutropenia is a decrease in the number of circulating neutrophil granulocytes, the most abundant white blood cells. The terms leukopenia and neutropenia may occasionally be used interchangeably. However, neutropenia is more properly considered a subset of leukopenia as a whole. Neutropenia can be caused by insufficient or injured bone marrow stem cells, shifts in neutrophils from the circulating pool to the marginal blood or tissue pools, increased destruction in the circulation, or a combination of these mechanisms.

A normal white blood cell count ranges from 4,500 to 10,000 cells per microliter of blood. A mild decrease in white blood cells below 4,500 cells per microliter doesn't necessarily indicate a serious illness. However, a dangerously low white blood cell count, i.e., below 2,500 cells per microliter, increases the risk of serious infection.

Low white cell counts are associated with chemotherapy, radiation therapy, leukemia, myelofibrosis and aplastic anemia. In addition, many common medications can cause leukopenia. Other causes of low white blood cell count include: influenza, systemic lupus erythematosus, typhus, malaria, HIV, tuberculosis, dengue, Rickettsial infections, splenomegaly, folate deficiencies and sepsis. Many other causes exist. Symptoms of leucopenia may include:

- Fever and chills
- Sweating
- Rash
- Diarrhea
- Signs of infection (anywhere in the body)

How is Leukopenia Diagnosed by Conventional Western Medicine?

Leukopenia can be identified with a complete blood count.

How is Leukopenia Treated by Conventional Western Medicine?

Treatment of leukopenia mostly is supportive and is based on the etiology, severity, and duration of leukopenia.

- Removal of any offending drugs or agents
- Correct nutritional deficiency
- Careful oral hygiene to prevent infections of the mucosa and teeth
- Avoidance of rectal temperature measurements and rectal examinations
- Administration of stool softeners for constipation
- Good skin care for wounds and abrasions
- Treat the fever as an infection
- Myeloid growth factors, granulocyte colony-stimulating factors (GCSFs), and granulocyte-macrophage colony-stimulating factor (GM-CSFs)
- Splenectomy
- Removal of indwelling central venous catheters

What Causes Leukopenia According to Traditional Chinese Medicine?

1) Congenial Insufficiency
2) Improper Diet
3) Exposure to Toxicants

How is Leukopenia Differentiated and Treated by Traditional Chinese Medicine?

1) Deficiency of Both Qi and Blood

Symptoms: Sallow complexion, vertigo, lassitude, insomnia, dreamfulness, palpitation, anorexia, abdominal distention, loose stools, pale tongue with thin and white coating, and thready and weak pulse.

Therapeutic Principle: To replenish qi and nourish blood.

Prescription: Modified Gui Pi Decoction.

Modifications: For deficiency of the spleen with remarkable anorexia, add Rhizoma Dioscoreae (Shan Yao) 20g and Fructus Hordei Germinatus (Mai Ya) 12g; for dark purple with petechiae or ecchymoses, add Radix Salviae Miltiorrhizae (Dan Shen) 10g, Herba Leonuri Heterophylii (Yi Mu Cao) 12g and Radix Paeoniae Rubra (Chi Shao) 10g.

2) Deficiency of the Spleen and Kidney

Symptoms: Spiritlessness, lassitude, weak and sore loins and knees, anorexia, loose stools, pale complexion, aversion to cold, cold limbs, polyuria with clear urine, pale and chubby tongue with teeth marks and white coating, deep and thready or deep and slow pulse.

Therapeutic Principle: To warm and nourish the spleen and kidney.

Prescription: Modified Huang Qi Jian Zhong Decoction and You Gui Pill.

Modifications: For cold-dampness with abdominal distention, nausea and vomiting, add Fructus Amomi Villosi (Sha Ren) 5g, Rhizoma Pinelliae Ternatae (Ban Xia) 9g and Pericarpium Citri Reticulatae (Chen Pi) 9g; for deficiency of kidney with seminal emission, add Fructus Rosae Laevigatae (Jin Ying Zi) 15g and Ootheca Mantidis (Sang Piao Xiao) 9g; for internal retention of dampness with edema and oliguria, add Sclerotium Polypori Umbellati (Zhu Ling) 10g, Rhizoma Alismatis Orientalis (Ze Xie) 10g and Sclerotium Poriae Cocos (Fu Ling) 12g.

3) Deficiency of Both Qi and Yin

Symptoms: Lusterless complexion, lassitude, vertigo, dysphoria with feverish sensation in the chest, palms and soles, insomnia, night sweating, or spontaneous sweating, red tongue with peeled coating, and thready and weak pulse.

Therapeutic Principle: To replenish qi and nourish yin.

Prescription: Modified Sheng Mai Powder.

Modifications: For sensation of stuffiness in the chest and palpitation, add Radix Salviae Miltiorrhizae (Dan Shen) 10g, Rhizoma Cyperi Rotundi (Xiang Fu) 10g and Semen Ziziphi Spinosae (Suan Zao Ren) 15g; for remarkable fatigue, shortness of breath and indolence of speaking, add Radix Astragali (Huang Qi) 12g and Fructus Corni Officinalis (Shan Zhu Yu) 10g.

4) Yin Deficiency of the Liver and Kidney

Symptoms: Sore and weak loins and knees, vertigo, dysphoria with feverish sensation in the chest, palms and soles, insomnia, dreamful sleep, seminal emission, low-grade fever, dry mouth and throat, red tongue with little coating, and thready and rapid pulse.

Therapeutic Principle: To nourish the liver and kidney.

Prescription: Modified Liu Wei Di Huang Pill.

Modifications: For constipation, add Semen Biotae Orientalis (Bai Zi Ren) 15g and Semen Cannabis Sativae (Huo Ma Ren) 12g; for insomnia and dreamful sleep, add Semen Ziziphi Spinosae (Suan Zao Ren) 15g and Mastodi Dentis Fossilia (Long Chi) 20g; for anorexia, add Fructus Crataegi (Shan Zha) 12g, Fructus Amomi Villosi (Sha Ren) 5g and Pericarpium Citri Reticulatae (Chen Pi) 9g.

5) Affected by Exogenous Pathogenic Heat

Symptoms: Persistent fever, thirst with a desire to drink, flushed face, sore throat, vertigo, fatigue, crimson tongue with yellow coating, slippery and rapid or thready and rapid pulse.

Therapeutic Principle: To clear sway heat, remove toxic substance, nourish yin and cool blood.

Prescription: Modified Xi Jiao Di Huang Decoction and Yu Nu Decoction.

Modifications: For sustained fever, add Gypsum Fibrosum (Shi Gao) 30g and Rhizoma Anemarrhenae (Zhi Mu) 10g; for aversion to cold and fever, add Herba Schizonepetae (Jing Jie) 10g, Radix Saposhnikoviae Divaricatae (Fang Feng) 10g and Flos Lonicerae (Jin Yin Hua) 15g; for lassitude and spontaneous sweating, add Fructus Schisandrae Chinensis (Wu Wei Zi) 5g and Radix Panacis Quinquefolii (Xi Yang Shen) 5g.

What Kinds of Chinese Patent Drugs are Available to Treat Leukopenia?

1) Sheng Bai Ning Granule: 15-30g each time, thrice daily.
2) Sheng Bai Kang Oral Liquid: 10ml each time, thrice daily.
3) Zhen Qi Fu Zheng Granule: 15g each time, thrice daily.
4) Feng Ling Capsule: 4-6 capsules each time, thrice daily.

7. Disseminated Intravascular Coagulation (DIC)

Disseminated intravascular coagulation (DIC) is an acquired syndrome characterized by the intravascular activation of coagulation with loss of localization arising from different causes. It can originate from and cause damage to the microvasculature, which if sufficiently severe, can produce organ dysfunction

DIC is associated with a number of well-defined clinical situations, including sepsis, major trauma, and placental abruption (abruptio placentae), and with laboratory evidence of procoagulant activation, fibrinolytic activation, inhibitor consumption and biochemical evidence of end-organ damage or failure.

Acute DIC is characterized by generalized bleeding. This leads to hypoperfusion, infarction, and end-organ damage. In severe cases, patients may develop fever and a shock-like picture with tachycardia, tachypnea, and hypotension. Chronic DIC is characterized by subacute bleeding and diffuse thrombosis. Localized DIC is characterized by bleeding or thrombosis confined to a specific anatomic location. It has been associated with aortic aneurysms, giant hemangiomas, and hyperacute renal allograft rejection. Bleeding from at least 3 unrelated sites is particularly suggestive of DIC. Risk factors for DIC include:

- Blood transfusion reaction
- Cancer, including leukemia
- Infections
- Pregnancy complications
- Recent surgery or anesthesia
- Sepsis
- Severe liver disease
- Severe tissue injury (as in burns and head injury)
- Liver disease
- Prosthetic devices, shunts (Denver, LeVeen), or ventricular assist devices
- Vascular conditions

Symptoms of DIC include:

- Bleeding, possibly from multiple sites in the body
- Cough
- Dyspnea
- Confusion, disorientation
- Blood clots

- Sudden bruising

How is DIC Diagnosed by Conventional Western Medicine?

Diagnosis is made based on medical history, physical exam, lab studies and other tests, including serum fibrinogen (low), prothrombin time (PT) (high), partial thromboplastin time (PTT) (high), and platelet count.

How is DIC Treated by Conventional Western Medicine?

The goal of management is to determine and treat the underlying disorder. The following supportive measures are essential:

- Monitor vital signs, assess and document extent of hemorrhage and thrombosis, correct hypovolemia, and administer basic hemostatic procedures when indicated
- Attend to life-threatening issues such as airway compromise or severe hemorrhage
- Determine the underlying cause of the patient's DIC and initiate therapy. Obtain appropriate imaging studies if necessary
- Draw specimens for appropriate coagulation studies and other diagnostic laboratory tests
- Begin anticoagulant therapy if indicated
- RBC transfusion, platelet concentrates, fresh frozen plasma (FFP) and cryoprecipitate as indicated
- Antithrombin III concentrate

What Causes DIC According to Traditional Chinese Medicine?

1) Affected by Exogenous Pathogenic Factors
2) Injury
3) Chronic Diseases or After Febrile Diseases

How is DIC Differentiated and Treated by Traditional Chinese Medicine?

1) <u>Heat invading Nutritive Division/Level (Ying fen) and Blood Division/Level (Xue fen)</u>

Symptoms: Fever aggravated at night, dysphoria, insomnia, or cloudy consciousness, thirst without much desire for drinks, vague rash and ecchymosis, or even hematemesis, epistaxis, hematochezia, yellow urine, constipation, crimson tongue, and thready, slippery and rapid pulse.

Therapeutic Principle: To clear away heat, cool blood and remove blood stasis.

Prescription: Modified Xi Jiao Di Huang Decoction.

Modifications: For hyperactive toxic heat with fever and widespread bleeding, add Radix Lithospermi seu Macrotomiae (Zi Cao) 10g, Radix Gentianae (Long Dan Cao) 5g and Gypsum Fibrosum (Shi Gao) 30g, and take Zi Xue Pill after mixing it with water; for constipation, abdominal distention and fullness, and excess pulse, add Radix et Rhizoma Rhei (Da Huang) 6g and Natrii Sulfas (Mang Xiao) 12g.

2) <u>Stagnation of Blood Stasis in Vessels and Collaterals</u>

Symptoms: Ecchymosis and purpura in the extremities, purplish lips, vertigo, headache, dark tongue with ecchymosis or petechiae, and rough pulse.

Therapeutic Principle: To promote circulation of qi, remove blood stasis and activate collaterals.

Prescription: Modified Xue Fu Zhu Yu Decoction.

3) <u>Qi Deficiency and Blood Stasis</u>

Symptoms: Light colored ecchymosis in the skin, or accompanied with epistaxis, gingival bleeding, hematemesis with dark colored blood, listlessness, fatigue, shortness of breath, indolence of speaking, dark purple tongue with ecchymosis or petechiae, and deficiency and rough pulse.

Therapeutic Principle: To promote circulation of qi and blood, and remove blood stasis.

Prescription: Modified Bu Yang Huan Wu Decoction.

Modifications: For palpitation and insomnia, add Radix Polygalae Tenuifoliae (Yuan Zhi) 10g and Semen Ziziphi Spinosae (Suan Zao Ren) 15g.

4) <u>Yin Deficiency Accompanied by Blood Stasis</u>

Symptoms: Local or general pricking pain, dark ecchymosis in the skin, or hematuria, epistaxis, feverish sensation in palms and soles, low-grade fever, vertigo, dry mouth, pale tongue with petechiae or ecchymosis, and thready and rough pulse.

Therapeutic Principle: To nourish yin and remove blood stasis.

Prescription: Modified Sheng Yu Decoction.

Modifications: For remarkable bleeding, add Herba Cephalanoploris (Xiao Ji) 20g, Radix Lithospermi seu Macrotomiae (Zi Cao) 10g and Radix Rubiae Cordifoliae (Qian Cao) 12g.

5) <u>Yang Deficiency and Blood Stasis</u>

Symptoms: Ecchymosis in the skin, or accompanied by epistaxis, hematochezia, lassitude, aversion to cold, cold limbs, shortness of breath, spontaneous sweating, feeble voice, dark purple tongue with ecchymosis, tinny and extremely faint pulse.

Therapeutic Principle: To warm yang and remove blood stasis.

Prescription: Modified Hui Yang Jiu Ji Decoction supplemented with Moschus (She Xiang) 0.06g.

Modifications: For severe bleeding, add Radix Notoginseng (San Qi) 10g, Radix Lithospermi seu Macrotomiae (Zi Cao) 10g and Radix Salviae Miltiorrhizae (Dan Shen) 10g; for cloudy consciousness, add Su He Xiang Pill.

What Kinds of Chinese Patent Drugs are Available to Treat DIC?

1) Qing Kai Ling Injection: 30-40ml each time, once daily.
2) Sheng Mai Injection: 30-50ml each time, once daily.
3) Fu Fang Dan Shen Injection: 10-20ml each time, once daily.

Chapter 6: Endocrinology and Metabolism

1. Diabetes Insipidus (DI)

Diabetes insipidus is a condition characterized by an increase in thirst and the passage of large quantities of urine of low specific gravity. It is caused by a deficiency of or resistance to antidiuretic hormone (ADH), also called vasopressin. Normally, ADH is secreted by the hypothalamus, stored in the pituitary gland and then released into the bloodstream. ADH is secreted to decrease the amount of urine output so that dehydration does not occur. Diabetes insipidus occurs when this system is disrupted and the body can't regulate how it handles fluids. Diabetes insipidus is categorized into three groups: central diabetes insipidus, nephrogenic diabetes insipidus and gestational diabetes insipidus. Diabetes insipidus can be caused by several conditions, including the following:

- Malfunctioning hypothalamus
- Malfunctioning pituitary gland
- Damage to hypothalamus or pituitary gland
- Brain injury
- Tumor
- Tuberculosis
- Blockage in the arteries leading to the brain
- Encephalitis
- Meningitis
- Sarcoidosis
- Family heredity

The following are the most common symptoms of diabetes insipidus. However, each individual may experience symptoms differently. Symptoms may include:

- Excessive thirst
- Excretion of an excessive volume of diluted urine

- Nocturia and bed-wetting
- Dehydration, hypovolemia

Infants and young children with diabetes insipidus may have the following symptoms:

- Unexplained fussiness or inconsolable crying
- Unusually wet diapers
- Fever, vomiting or diarrhea
- Dry skin with cool extremities
- Poor feeding

How is Diabetes Insipidus Diagnosed by Conventional Western Medicine?

In addition to a complete medical and family history and physical examination, diagnostic procedures for diabetes insipidus may include urinalysis, blood tests, water deprivation test, and magnetic resonance imaging (MRI).

How is Diabetes Insipidus Treated by Conventional Western Medicine?

Treatment for diabetes insipidus depends on the underlying causes of the disease. Treating the cause usually treats the diabetes insipidus. Treatment may include modified antidiuretic hormone medications, or medications that stimulate the production of the antidiuretic hormone (desmopressin). In addition, people with diabetes insipidus must maintain adequate fluid intake to compensate for the excessive urinary output, and eat a low-sodium diet. Reduction of aggravating factors, such as glucocorticoids, will improve polyuria. Hydrochlorothiazide, used alone or with other medications, may improve symptoms. Psychotherapy is required for patients with compulsive water drinking.

What Causes Diabetes Insipidus According to Traditional Chinese Medicine?

1) Congenital Insufficiency
2) Emotional Disturbance
3) Improper Diet
4) Injury
5) Invasion of Exogenous Heat Pathogenic Factors

How is Diabetes Insipidus Differentiated and Treated by Traditional Chinese Medicine?

1) <u>Yin Deficiency of the Lung and Stomach</u>

Symptoms: Polydipsia (intense thirst), urinary frequency, polyuria, dry mouth and throat, vexation, insomnia, dizziness, shortness of breath, low voice, timidity, fatigue, weight loss, red tongue with little coating and moisture, thready and rapid pulse.

Therapeutic Principle: To clear away lung heat, nourish the stomach, produce saliva and slake thirst.

Prescription: Modified Bai Hu Jia Ren Shen Decoction.

Modifications: For remarkable deficiency of qi, add Radix Panacis Quinquefolii (Xi Yang Shen) 5g; for remarkable stomach heat, add Radix Scrophulariae Ningpoensis (Xuan Shen) 10g and Rhizoma Coptidis (Huang Lian) 9g.

2) <u>Yin Deficiency of the Lung and Kidney</u>

Symptoms: Polydipsia, polyuria, urinary frequency, anorexia, dry mouth and tongue, vertigo, fatigue, insomnia, distending pain in the lumbar region, constipation, red tongue with dry and yellow coating, and thready and rapid pulse.

Therapeutic Principle: To nourish yin, clear away heat, produce saliva and slake thirst.

Prescription: Modified Sha Shen Mai Dong Decoction.

Modifications: For remarkable thirst, add Herba Dendrobii (Shi Hu) 12g, Schisandrae Fructus (Wu Wei Zi) 5g and Rhizoma Phragmitis Communis (Lu Gen) 20g; for remarkable yin deficiency and interior-heat, add Cortex Phellodendri (Huang Bai) 10g and Rhizoma Anemarrhenae (Zhi Mu) 10g.

3) <u>Deficiency of Both Yin an Yang</u>

Symptoms: Polydipsia, polyuria, urinary frequency, dry mouth and tongue, sore and weak loins and knees, aversion to cold, impotence, vertigo, fatigue, dysphoria with feverish sensation in the chest, palms and soles, emaciation, diarrhea or constipation, red tongue with thin coating, and thready and rapid pulse.

Therapeutic Principle: To nourish yin and yang, replenish qi and induce astringency.

Prescription: Modified Jin Gui Shen Qi Pill.

Modifications: For this syndrome, usually add Ootheca Mantidis (Sang Piao Xiao) 9g and Fructus Rubi Chingii (Fu Pen Zi) 10g to the above prescription; for chief deficiency of kidney yang, replace the prescription with You Gui Pill.

What Kinds of Chinese Patent Drugs are Available to Treat Diabetes Insipidus?

Suo Chuan Pill: 20g each time, 2-3 times each day.

2. Hyperthyroidism (Thyrotoxicosis)

Hyperthyroidism means overactivity of the thyroid gland, resulting in too much thyroid hormone in the bloodstream. The term "thyrotoxicosis" denotes a series of clinical disorders associated with increased circulating levels of free thyroxine or triiodothyronine. The over-secretion of thyroid hormones leads to overactivity of the body's metabolism, causing sudden weight loss, a rapid or irregular heartbeat, sweating, and nervousness or irritability.

The various causes of hyperthyroidism include Graves' disease, hyperfunctioning thyroid nodules (toxic adenoma, toxic multinodular goiter, Plummer's disease), and thyroiditis. The following are the most common symptoms of hyperthyroidism. However, each individual may experience symptoms differently. Symptoms may include:

- Sudden weight loss, even when the appetite and food intake remain normal or increase
- Tachycardia, arrhythmia or palpitations
- Nervousness, anxiety or anxiety attacks, irritability
- Tremor — usually a fine trembling in the hands and fingers
- Sweating
- Changes in menstrual patterns
- Increased sensitivity to heat
- Changes in bowel patterns, especially more frequent bowel movements
- An enlarged thyroid gland (goiter)
- Fatigue, muscle weakness
- High blood pressure
- Bulging eyes
- Difficulty sleeping

How is Hyperthyroidism Diagnosed by Conventional Western Medicine?

In addition to a complete medical history and physical examination, the diagnosis can be confirmed with blood tests that measure the levels of thyroxine and TSH. Other tests may include radioactive iodine uptake test and thyroid scan.

How is Hyperthyroidism Treated by Conventional Western Medicine?

Several treatments for hyperthyroidism exist. Specific treatment for hypothyroidism depends on the age and physical condition of a patient, and the severity of the disorder. Treatment may include radioactive iodine, anti-thyroid medications, beta blockers and surgery (thyroidectomy).

Treatment for Graves' ophthalmopathy may include avoiding wind and bright lights, artificial tears and lubricating gels, corticosteroids, orbital decompression surgery, or eye muscle surgery.

What Causes Hyperthyroidism According to Traditional Chinese Medicine?

1) Emotional Disturbance

2) Weak Constitution

How is Hyperthyroidism Differentiated and Treated by Traditional Chinese Medicine?

1) <u>Stagnation of Qi and Phlegm</u>

Symptoms: Goiter (enlargement of the thyroid), restlessness, irritability, sensation of stuffiness in the chest, distention and fullness in the hypochondrium, frequent sighing, insomnia, menstrual irregularities, abdominal distention, loose stools, slight red tongue with white and greasy coating, and taut or taut and slippery pulse.

Therapeutic Principle: To soothe the liver, regulate qi, resolve phlegm and disperse mass.

Prescription: Modified Xiao Yao Powder and Er Chen Decoction.

Modifications: For remarkable goiter, stuffy sensation in the chest and severe hypochondriac pain, add Fructus Meliae Toosendan (Chuan Lian Zi) 10g, Fructus Citri Aurantii (Zhi Ke) 10g, Concha Ostreae (Mu Li) 20g and Fructus Trichosanthis (Gua Lou) 15g; for menstrual irregularities, add Rhizoma Cyperi Rotundi (Xiang Fu) 10g, Radix Curcumae (Yu Jin) 10g and Herba Leonuri Heterophylii (Yi Mu Cao) 12g; for nausea, add Caulis Bambusae in Taeniam (Zhu Ru) 10g and Rhizoma Zingiberis Recens (Sheng Jiang) 10g; for abdominal distention and loose stools, add Pericarpium Citri Reticulatae (Chen Pi) 9g, Fructus Amomi Villosi (Sha Ren) 5g, Semen Coicis (Yi Yi Ren) 15g and Sclerotium Poriae Cocos (Fu Ling) 12g.

2) <u>Hyperactivity of Liver Fire</u>

Symptoms: Goiter, exophthalmos (bulging eyes), nervousness, restlessness, irritability, getting hungry easily, great appetite, fine resting finger tremors, heat intolerance, increased sweating, flushed and hot face, palpitation, insomnia, vertigo, bitter taste in the mouth, dry throat, constipation, menstrual irregularities, red tongue with yellow coating, and taut and rapid pulse.

Therapeutic Principle: To clear away liver heat, purge fire and disperse mass.

Prescription: Modified Long Dan Xie Gan Decoction.

Modifications: For getting hungry easily and intake of large amount of food, add Gypsum Fibrosum (Shi Gao) 30g, Rhizoma Anemarrhenae (Zhi Mu) 10g and Rhizoma Polygonati Odorati (Yu Zhu) 12g; for restlessness, irritability, vertigo, flushed and hot face, add Spica Prunellae Vulgaris (Xia Ku Cao) 12g, Tribulus Terrestris Fructus (Bai Ji Li) 10g and Flos Chrysanthemi Morifolii (Ju Hua) 12g; for finger tremors, add Ramulus Uncariae cum Uncis (Gou Teng) 12g, Concha Haliotidis (Shi Jue Ming) 20g and Concha Margaritiferae (Zhen Zhu Mu) 20g.

3) <u>Fire Hyperactivity due to Yin Deficiency</u>

Symptoms: Goiter, exophthalmos (bulging eyes), palpitation, increased sweating, finger tremors, polyorexia (getting hungry easily and increased appetite with intake of large amount of food), weight loss, dry mouth and throat, dysphoria with feverish sensation in the chest, palms and soles, restlessness, irritability, insomnia, dreamful sleep, menstrual irregularities, red tongue with little coating, and thready and rapid pulse.

Therapeutic Principle: To nourish yin, purge fire and disperse mass.

Prescription: Modified Tian Wang Bu Xin Pill.

Modifications: For remarkable deficiency of yin with dry mouth and throat, add Fructus Lycii (Gou Qi Zi) 10g, Radix Polygoni Multiflori (He Shou Wu) 20g and Carapax et Plastrum Testudinis (Gui Ban) 20g; for bulging eyes and finger tremors, add Radix Paeoniae Alba (Bai Shao Yao) 10g, Ramulus Uncariae cum Uncis (Gou Teng) 10g and Tribulus Terrestris Fructus (Bai Ji Li) 9g; for polydipsia (excessive thirst) and increased sweating, add Cortex Moutan Radicis (Mu Dan Pi) 10g, Fructus Tritici Aestivi Levis (Fu Xiao Mai) 15g and Fructus Schisandrae Chinensis (Wu Wei Zi) 5g; for menstrual irregularities, add Radix Scrophulariae Ningpoensis (Xuan Shen) 10g, Gelatinum Corii Asini (E Jiao) 10g and Herba Leonuri Heterophylii (Yi Mu Cao) 10g.

4) <u>Deficiency of Both Qi and Yin</u>

Symptoms: Goiter, exophthalmos (bulging eyes), palpitation, insomnia, finger tremors, weight loss, spiritlessness, fatigue, weakness, shortness of breath, increased sweating, dry mouth and throat, feverish sensation in palms and soles, anorexia, loose stools, red or slight red tongue with little coating, and thready or thready, rapid and forceless pulse.

Therapeutic Principle: To replenish qi, nourish yin and remove the goiter.

Prescription: Modified Sheng Mai Powder.

Modifications: For remarkable shortness of breath, fatigue and increased sweating, add Radix Astragali (Huang Qi) 12g, Radix Codonopsitis Pilosulae (Dang Shen) 9g, Rhizoma Atractylodis Macrocephalae (Bai Zhu) 10g and Fructus Tritici Aestivi Levis (Fu Xiao Mai) 15g; for remarkable yin deficiency with dry mouth and throat, feverish sensation in palms and soles, add Radix Scrophulariae Ningpoensis (Xuan Shen) 10g, Carapax et Plastrum Testudinis (Gui Ban) 20g, Fructus Ligustri Lucidi (Nu Zhen Zi) 12g and Cortex Lycii Radicis (Di Gu Pi) 12g; for chronic diseases accompanied by blood stasis, add Radix Salviae Miltiorrhizae (Dan Shen) 10g, Semen Pruni Persicae (Tao Ren) 10g, Flos Carthami Tinctorii (Hong Hua) 10g and Radix Notoginseng (San Qi) 9g.

What Kinds of Chinese Patent Drugs are Available to Treat Hyperthyroidism?

1) Jia Kang Ling Tablet: 7 tablets each time, thrice daily.

2) Yi Kang Pill: 1 pill each time, twice daily.

3. Hypothyroidism and Myxedema

Hypothyroidism is the condition in which the thyroid is underactive and is producing an insufficient amount of thyroid hormones. Thyroid hormone deficiency may affect virtually all body functions. The degree of severity ranges from mild and unrecognized hypothyroid states to striking myxedema. Hypothyroidism may be due to a number of different factors, including:

- Autoimmune disease (Hashimoto's thyroiditis)
- Treatment for hyperthyroidism
- Radiation therapy
- Thyroid surgery
- Medications, such as lithium
- Congenital disease
- Pituitary disorder
- Pregnancy
- Iodine deficiency

Women, especially those older than 50, are more likely to have hypothyroidism than men are. Hypothyroidism seldom causes symptoms in the early stages, but untreated hypothyroidism can lead to a number of health problems, including goiter, heart problems, mental health issues, myxedema (its symptoms include intense cold intolerance and drowsiness followed by profound lethargy, unconsciousness and myxedema coma), and birth defects.

The signs and symptoms of hypothyroidism vary widely, depending on the severity of the hormone deficiency. Symptoms may include:

- Increased sensitivity to cold
- Constipation
- Dry skin, carotenemic skin color
- Sparse, course and dry hair
- Slow speech
- Puffiness of the face and eyelids
- Thinning of the outer halves of the eyebrows
- Hoarse voice

- An elevated blood cholesterol level
- Unexplained weight gain
- Muscle aches, tenderness, stiffness and weakness
- Joint pain, stiffness or swelling
- Thin, brittle nails
- Menorrhagia or amenorrhea
- Depression
- Anemia, hyponatremia
- Bradycardia, delayed return of deep tendon reflexes

How is Hypothyroidism Diagnosed by Conventional Western Medicine?

Congenital hypothyroidism is usually detected during the routine newborn screening. Blood tests will reveal abnormal levels of thyroxine (T4) and thyroid-stimulating hormone (TSH). Further diagnosis may include a scan of the thyroid gland to check for abnormalities.

How is Hypothyroidism Treated by Conventional Western Medicine?

The goal of treatment is to restore the thyroid gland to normal function, producing normal levels of thyroid hormones. Standard treatment for hypothyroidism involves daily use of the synthetic thyroid hormone levothyroxine (Levothroid, Levoxyl, Synthroid, and Unithroid), and regular monitoring of the thyroid hormone levels during the course of treatment.

What Causes Hypothyroidism According to Traditional Chinese Medicine?

1) Congenital Insufficiency and Weak Constitution
2) Improper Diet and Emotional Disturbance
3) Chronic Disease Impairing the Kidney

How is Hypothyroidism Differentiated and Treated by Traditional Chinese Medicine?

1) <u>Deficiency of Spleen Qi</u>

Symptoms: Spiritlessness, fatigue, shortness of breath, indolence of speaking, lethargy, anorexia, abdominal distention, constipation or loose stools, cold limbs, sallow or pale complexion, dry skin, pale tongue with thin and white coating, and thready and weak pulse.

Therapeutic Principle: To strengthen the spleen and replenish qi.

Prescription: Modified Si Jun Zi Decoction.

Modifications: For severe abdominal distention, add Radix Aucklandiae Lappae (Mu Xiang) 10g and Pericarpium Citri Reticulatae (Chen Pi) 9g; for accompanied deficiency of yang, add Cortex Cinnamomi Cassiae (Rou Gui) 3g and Rhizoma Zingiberis Praeparatae (Pao Jiang) 10g; for deficiency of heart blood, add Sclerotium Poriae Circum Radicem Pini (Fu Shen) 12g, Radix Polygalae (Yun Zhi) 9g and Radix Angelicae Sinensis (Dang Gui) 10g; for blood stasis, add Radix Salviae Miltiorrhizae (Dan Shen) 10g and Radix Achyranthis Bidentatae (Niu Xi) 12g.

2) <u>Yang Deficiency of the Spleen and Kidney</u>

Symptoms: Spiritlessness, lethargy, shortness of breath, indolence of speaking, pallor, anorexia, abdominal distention, cold intolerance, cold limbs, sore and weak loins and knees, decreased libido, impotence, or amenorrhea, or infertility, or retarded development and intellectual impairment of a baby who was born from a woman with hypothyroidism; pale and chubby tongue with white and greasy coating, and deep, thready and slow pulse.

Therapeutic Principle: To strengthen the spleen, replenish qi, warm the kidney and nourish yang.

Prescription: Modified Ji Sheng Shen Qi Pill and Si Jun Zi Decoction.

Modifications: For severe deficiency of yang, add Rhizoma Curculiginis Orchioidis (Xian Mao) 10g and Herba Epimedii (Yin Yang Huo) 12g; for qi stagnation accompanied by dampness, remove Radix Rehmanniae Praeparatae (Shu Di Huang), and add Fructus Amomi Villosi (Sha Ren) 5g and Radix Aucklandiae Lappae (Mu Xiang) 10g; for intellectual impairment or dementia, add Gelatinum Cornu Cervi (Lu Jiao Jiao) 10g, Semen Cuscutae Chinensis (Tu Si Zi) 12g and Radix Morindae officinalis (Ba Ji Tian) 10g; for blood stasis, add Rhizoma Ligustici Chuanxiong (Chuan Xiong) 10g and Radix Salviae Miltiorrhizae (Dan Shen) 10g.

3) <u>Yang Deficiency of the Heart and Kidney</u>

Symptoms: Spiritlessness, lassitude, cold intolerance, cold limbs, puffiness of the face and eyelids, peripheral edema, palpitation, shortness of breath, sensation of stuffiness in the chest, sore and weak loins and knees, impotence, or amenorrhea, pale and chubby tongue with slippery and greasy coating, and slow pulse.

Therapeutic Principle: To warm and nourish the heart and kidney, promote qi circulation and induce diuresis.

Prescription: Modified Ji Sheng Shen Qi Pill and Bao Yuan Decoction.

Modifications: For severe stuffy sensation in the chest, or even chest pain, add Radix Curcumae (Yu Jin) 10g, Rhizoma Ligustici Chuanxiong (Chuan Xiong) 10g and Fructus Citri Aurantii (Zhi Ke) 10g; for remarkable cold intolerance and cold limbs, add Rhizoma Curculiginis Orchioidis (Xian Mao) 10g and Cornu Cervi Pantotrichum (Lu Rong) 1.5g; for dyspnea and shortness of breath aggravated by exertion, add Fructus Schisandrae Chinensis (Wu Wei Zi) 5g and Gecko (Ge Jie) 5g.

4) **Deficiency of Both Yang and Qi**

Symptoms: Lethargy, deep stupor or even coma, general coldness, weak knees, feeble respiration, pale tongue, and slow, tinny and weak or tinny and extremely faint pulse.

Therapeutic Principle: To replenish qi and restore yang from collapse.

Prescription: Modified Ren Shen Si Ni Decoction.

Modifications: May combine with large dosage of Shen Fu Injection.

What Kinds of Chinese Patent Drugs are Available to Treat Hypothyroidism?

1) Quan Lu Pill: 2-3g each time, 2-3 times each day.

2) You Gui Pill: 3-6g each time, 1-2 times each day.

4. Subacute Thyroiditis

Subacute thyroiditis, also called viral, de Quervain's, Giant Cell, or Granulomatous thyroiditis, is an inflammation of the thyroid gland probably caused by a viral infection. There is characteristic giant cell infiltration, PMNs, and follicular disruption in hypothyroidism. Subacute thyroiditis is a self-limited thyroid condition associated with a triphasic clinical course of hyperthyroidism, hypothyroidism, and return to normal thyroid function.

Initially, a person with subacute thyroiditis has signs and symptoms of hyperthyroidism. It results from excess thyroid hormone released from damaged thyroid cells. As the thyroid heals, thyroid hormone is eventually depleted and the patient may become hypothyroid. Often the hypothyroidism is mild, and no thyroid hormone therapy is required unless the patient has signs or symptoms of hypothyroidism. The hypothyroid phase may last up to 2 months. Symptoms may include:

- Acute and painful enlargement of the thyroid gland, which the pain may radiate to the ears
- Dysphagia
- Fever
- Fatigue, malaise
- Muscle and joint aches
- Initially, symptoms of hyperthyroidism
- Eventually, symptoms of hypothyroidism

How is Subacute Thyroiditis Diagnosed by Conventional Western Medicine?

Diagnosis is clinical and with thyroid function tests.

How is Subacute Thyroiditis Treated by Conventional Western Medicine?

Treatment of subacute thyroiditis may include:

- Pain relievers, such as high doses of NSAIDs
- Corticosteroids, such as prednisone
- During the hyperthyroid phase of the disease, beta blockers to block the effects of excess thyroid hormone
- Thyroid function typically returns to normal with no further problems. Rarely, hypothyroidism persists and requires treatment.

What Causes Subacute Thyroiditis According to Traditional Chinese Medicine?

1) Affected by Six Exogenous Pathogenic Factors
2) Internal Injury by Seven Emotions

How is Subacute Thyroiditis Differentiated and Treated by Traditional Chinese Medicine?

1) <u>Accumulation of Heat in the Liver and Gallbladder</u>

Symptoms: Distention and pain in the front neck (painful enlargement of the thyroid gland), fever, bitter taste in the mouth, dry throat, or palpitation, irritability, increased sweating, thirst, flushed face, oliguria with dark urine, constipation, red tongue with thin and yellow coating, and floating and rapid or taut and rapid pulse.

Therapeutic Principle: To clear away heat the liver and gallbladder, diminish mass and relieve pain.

Prescription: Modified Long Dan Xie Gan Decoction.

Modifications: For remarkable fever and cold intolerance, add Flos Lonicerae (Jin Yin Hua) 15g and Fructus Forsythiae Suspensae (Lian Qiao) 10g; for severe pain, add Rhizoma Corydalis (Yan Hu Suo) 10g and Fructus Meliae Toosendan (Chuan Lian Zi) 10g.

2) <u>Hyperactivity of Fire due to Deficiency of Yin</u>

Symptoms: Painful mass in the front neck (painful enlargement of the thyroid gland), which is pliable but strong in texture; dry mouth and throat, hectic fever, night sweating, palpitation, insomnia, dreamful sleep, red tongue with little or no coating, and thready and rapid pulse.

Therapeutic Principle: To nourish yin, clear away heat and eliminate mass.

Prescription: Modified Qing Gu Powder.

Modifications: For insomnia and dreamful sleep, add Semen Ziziphi Spinosae (Suan Zao Ren) 15g and Radix Ophiopogonis Japonici (Mai Dong) 12g; for severe pain, add Rhizoma Corydalis (Yan Hu Suo) 10g and Concha Ostreae (Mu Li) 20g.

3) <u>Stagnation of Phlegm and Blood Stasis</u>

Symptoms: Localized painful and hard mass in the front neck (painful enlargement of the thyroid gland), which is aggravated at night; depression, dry mouth without desire to drink, dark purple tongue with ecchymosis or petechiae, and thready and rough pulse.

Therapeutic Principle: To regulate qi, promote circulation of blood, resolve phlegm and eliminate mass.

Prescription: Modified Hai Zao Yu Hu Decoction.

4) Deficiency of Spleen Yang

Symptoms: Extreme painful mass in the front neck (painful enlargement of the thyroid gland), lusterless complexion, fatigue, weakness, dizziness, dreamfulness, cold intolerance, cold limbs, anorexia, abdominal distention, loose stools, pale tongue with white and greasy coating, and deep and thready pulse.

Therapeutic Principle: To warm yang, strengthen the spleen, promote qi circulation and induce diuresis.

Prescription: Modified Shi Pi Decoction.

What Kinds of Chinese Patent Drugs are Available to Treat Subacute Thyroiditis?

Liu Shen Pill: 10 pills each time, thrice daily.

5. Hashimoto's Thyroiditis (Chronic Lymphocytic Thyroiditis)

Hashimoto's thyroiditis (HT), also known as chronic lymphocytic thyroiditis, is an autoimmune disorder in which the immune system inappropriately attacks the thyroid gland. It is characterized by the destruction of thyroid cells by various cell- and antibody-mediated immune processes. Thyroid-stimulating hormone (TSH) receptor-blocking antibodies may also contribute to further impairment in thyroid function. The thyroid gland is typically goitrous but may be atrophic or normal in size.

The inflammation caused by Hashimoto's thyroiditis often leads to hypothyroidism, although it may cause transient hyperthyroidism during the initial destructive phase. Hashimoto's thyroiditis is the most common cause of hypothyroidism in the United States. It is most common in middle-aged women and tends to run in families

What causes the immune system to attack the thyroid gland is unknown. A virus or bacterium infection might trigger the response. Most likely, a combination of factors, including heredity, sex, and age, may determine the likelihood of developing the disorder. The signs and symptoms, if any, are those of an underactive thyroid gland (hypothyroidism), including:

- Increased sensitivity to cold
- Constipation
- Pale, dry skin

- A puffy face
- Hoarse voice
- An elevated blood cholesterol level
- Unexplained weight gain
- Muscle aches, tenderness and stiffness
- Joint pain, stiffness and swelling
- Muscle weakness
- Menorrhagia
- Depression
- Goiter

How is Hashimoto's Thyroiditis Diagnosed by Conventional Western Medicine?

Diagnosis is based on the signs and symptoms and the results of blood tests that measure levels of thyroid hormone, thyroid-stimulating hormone (TSH), and antithyroid antibodies.

How is Hashimoto's Thyroiditis Treated by Conventional Western Medicine?

Standard treatment for hypothyroidism involves observation, daily use of the synthetic thyroid hormone levothyroxine (Levothroid, Levoxyl, Synthroid), and regular monitoring of the thyroid hormone levels during the course of treatment.

What Causes Hashimoto's Thyroiditis According to Traditional Chinese Medicine?

1) Weak Constitution
2) Internal Injury by Emotional Disturbance
3) Improper Diet and Natural Environment (Water and Soil)

How is Hashimoto's Thyroiditis Differentiated and Treated by Traditional Chinese Medicine?

1) <u>Stagnation of Phlegm and Blood Stasis</u>

Symptoms: Enlargement of thyroid gland that is firm in texture and not tender to palpation, fatigue, weakness, anorexia, nausea, dark tongue with ecchymosis or petechiae, white and greasy tongue coating, and thready and rough pulse.

Therapeutic Principle: To promote circulation of qi and blood, remove blood stasis and eliminate mass.

Prescription: Modified Er Chen Decoction and Tao Hong Si Wu Decoction.

2) <u>Stagnation of Liver Qi and Deficiency of the Spleen</u>

Symptoms: Enlargement or atrophy of thyroid gland, sensation of stuffiness in the chest and hypochondrium, frequent sighing, anorexia, loose stools, dark and pale tongue with white and greasy coating, and taut and slippery pulse.

Therapeutic Principle: To soothe the liver, strengthen the spleen, promote qi circulation and resolve phlegm.

Prescription: Modified Xiao Yao Powder.

3) <u>Deficiency of Liver Yin and Kidney Yin</u>

Symptoms: Insidious onset of enlargement of thyroid gland that is firm in texture and not tender to palpation, flushed face in the afternoon, bitter taste in the mouth, dry throat, spiritlessness, fatigue, palpitation, insomnia, sore and weak loins and knees, vertigo, red tongue with little coating, and thready and rapid pulse.

Therapeutic Principle: To nourish the liver and kidney, and disperse mass.

Prescription: Modified Qi Ju Di Huang Pill.

Modifications: For accompanied deficiency of qi, add Radix Codonopsitis Pilosulae (Dang Shen) 10g and Radix Astragali (Huang Qi) 12g; for enlargement of thyroid gland, add Radix Scrophulariae Ningpoensis (Xuan Shen) 10g and Concha Ostreae (Mu Li) 20g.

4) <u>Deficiency of Spleen Yang and Kidney Yang</u>

Symptoms: Insidious onset of enlargement of thyroid gland that is firm in texture and not tender to palpation, pale complexion, spiritlessness, lethargy, anorexia, loose stools, cold intolerance, cold limbs, edema of the extremities, sore and weak loins and knees, impotence, or amenorrhea, pale and chubby tongue with white and greasy coating, and deep and weak or deep and slow pulse.

Therapeutic Principle: To warm and nourish the spleen and kidney, promote qi circulation and induce diuresis.

Prescription: Modified Si Ni Decoction and Wu Ling Powder.

Modifications: For impotence, add Cornu Cervi Pantotrichum (Lu Rong) 2g and Fructus Corni Officinalis (Shan Zhu Yu) 10g; for amenorrhea, add Radix Angelicae Sinensis (Dang Gui) 10g and Radix Dipsaci Asperi (Xu Duan) 15.

What Kinds of Chinese Patent Drugs are Available to Treat Hashimoto's Thyroiditis?

Xiao Yao Pill: 9g each time, twice daily.

6. Pheochromocytoma

A pheochromocytoma is an adrenal gland tumor that secretes epinephrine and norepinephrine hormones, resulting in high blood pressure and increased heart rate. A pheochromocytoma may be life-threatening if unrecognized or untreated.

A pheochromocytoma can develop at any age, but most commonly occurs in people between ages 30 and 60.

Many factors contribute to the cause of pheochromocytoma. In most cases, both genetic and environmental factors play a role. The condition can occur alone or in combination with other disorders. The following are the most common disorders associated with pheochromocytoma:

- Neurofibromatosis 1 (NF1)
- Von Hippel-Lindau disease
- Multiple endocrine neoplasia, type II (MEN II)
- Tuberous sclerosis
- Sturge-Weber syndrome
- Ataxia-telangiectasia

An attack of high blood pressure (hypertensive crisis) may be brought on by emotional distress or anxiety, by surgical anesthesia, or by physical activities. Symptoms of pheochromocytoma may include:

- High blood pressure
- Rapid heart rate
- Forceful heartbeat
- Dizziness
- Profound sweating
- Chest pain
- Upper abdominal pain
- Severe brief headaches of sudden onset
- Tremors of the hands
- Anxiety, extreme fright
- Nausea, vomiting
- Pale, clammy skin

How is Pheochromocytoma Diagnosed by Conventional Western Medicine?

In addition to a complete medical history and physical examination, diagnostic procedures for pheochromocytoma may include blood and urine tests, CT scan, and radioisotope scan.

How is Pheochromocytoma Treated by Conventional Western Medicine?

Treatment for pheochromocytoma usually includes surgery and medications, such as alpha blockers and beta blockers. The best treatment for most pheochromocytomas is surgery to remove the tumor. Continuous medical follow-up may be required to monitor the development of future tumors.

What Causes Pheochromocytoma According to Traditional Chinese Medicine?

1) Congenital Insufficiency
2) Acquired Malnutrition
3) Chronic Diseases

How is Pheochromocytoma Differentiated and Treated by Traditional Chinese Medicine?

1) <u>Flaring-up of Liver Yang</u>

Symptoms: Distending pain of the head, vertigo, tinnitus, restlessness, irritability, insomnia, dreamful sleep, flushed face, conjunctival congestion, bitter taste in the mouth, constipation, dark urine, red tongue with thin and yellow coating, and taut and rapid or taut and slippery coating.

Therapeutic Principle: To soothe the liver, suppress hyperactive yang, clear away heat and purge fire.

Prescription: Modified Tian Ma Gou Teng Decoction.

Modifications: For concurrent turbid phlegm, add Er Chen Decoction.

2) <u>Deficiency of Liver Yin and Kidney Yin</u>

Symptoms: Vertigo, blurred vision, dry and discomfort eyes, tinnitus, fatigue, sore loins and weak knees, heel pain, red or crimson tongue with no or little coating, and taut, thready and weak pulse.

Therapeutic Principle: To nourish the liver and kidney.

Prescription: Modified Yi Guan Decoction.

Modifications: For numbness of the extremities, add Radix et Caulis Jixueteng (Ji Xue Teng) 12g and Herba Taxilli (Sang Ji Sheng) 15g; for concurrent blood stasis, add Semen Pruni Persicae (Tao Ren) 10g, Flos Carthami Tinctorii (Hong Hua) 10g and Radix Salviae Miltiorrhizae (Dan Shen) 10g.

3) <u>Obstruction of Middle Warmer by Turbid Phlegm</u>

Symptoms: Vertigo, headache, sensation of heaviness in the head, restlessness, stuffy sensation in the chest, anorexia, lethargy, nausea, vomiting, distention and fullness in the abdomen, pale tongue with white and greasy coating, or slight red tongue with yellow and greasy coating, and taut and slippery pulse.

Therapeutic Principle: To resolve phlegm and lower adverse flow of qi.

Prescription: Modified Ban Xia Bai Zhu Tian Ma Decoction.

Modifications: For damp-heat, add Caulis Bambusae in Taeniam (Zhu Ru) 10g and Radix Scutellariae Baicalensis (Huang Qin) 9g; for remarkable nausea, add Caulis Perillae (Su Geng) 10g and Rhizoma Zingiberis Recens (Sheng Jiang) 10g.

4) Deficiency of Both Yin and Yang

Symptoms: Vertigo, blurred vision, tinnitus, fatigue, sore loins and weak knees, palpitation, shortness of breath, numbness of the extremities, abdominal distention, diarrhea, pale tongue with white or little coating, and deep and thready pulse.

Therapeutic Principle: To nourish yin and yang.

Prescription: Modified Er Xian Decoction.

Modifications: For remarkable sore loins and weak knees, add Cortex Eucommiae Ulmoidis (Du Zhong) 12g and Radix Dipsaci Asperi (Xu Duan) 15g; for remarkable vertigo and headache, add Rhizoma Ligustici Chuanxiong (Chuan Xiong) 10g.

7. Cushing's Syndrome (Hypercortisolism)

Cushing's syndrome is a condition that occurs when the body is exposed to high levels of the hormone cortisol for a prolonged period of time. The most common cause of Cushing's syndrome is the use of oral corticosteroid medication. The condition may also be caused by the body's own overproduction of cortisol (endogenous Cushing's syndrome) due to a pituitary gland tumor, an ectopic ACTH-secreting tumor and a primary adrenal gland disease.

Common signs and symptoms of Cushing's syndrome include:

- Weight gain, particularly around the midsection and upper back
- Fatigue
- Muscle weakness
- Round or moon face
- Facial flushing
- Fatty pad or hump between the shoulders (buffalo hump)
- Pink or purple stretch marks (striae) on the skin of the abdomen, thighs, breasts and arms
- Thin and fragile skin that bruises easily
- Slow healing of cuts, insect bites and infections
- Depression, anxiety and irritability
- Thicker or more visible body and facial hair (hirsutism)

- Acne
- Irregular or absent menstrual periods
- Impotence, infertility, reduce libido
- High blood pressure
- Darkened pigmentation of the skin

How is Cushing's Syndrome Diagnosed by Conventional Western Medicine?

In addition to a complete medical history and physical examination, diagnostic procedures for Cushing's syndrome may include blood tests, saliva test, x ray, 24-hour urinary test, CT scan, MRI, dexamethasone suppression test, and corticotropin-releasing hormone (CRH) stimulation test.

How is Cushing's Syndrome Treated by Conventional Western Medicine?

Treatments for Cushing's syndrome are designed to lower the high level of cortisol in the body. The best treatment depends on the cause of the syndrome. Surgery may be needed to remove tumors of the adrenal glands. Treatment options include:

- Reducing corticosteroid use
- Surgery
- Radiation therapy
- Medical therapy, such as ketoconazole (Nizoral), mitotane (Lysodren) and metyrapone (Metopirone)

What Causes Cushing's Syndrome According to Traditional Chinese Medicine?

1) Emotional Disturbance
2) Congenital Insufficiency and Sex Indulgence
3) Deficiency of Both Yin and Yang

How is Cushing's Syndrome Differentiated and Treated by Traditional Chinese Medicine?

1) <u>Flaring-up of Liver Fire</u>

Symptoms: Flushed face, conjunctival congestion, vertigo, tinnitus, restlessness, irritability, dry mouth with bitter taste, menstrual irregularities, abundant and yellow vaginal discharge (leukorrhea), vulvar pruritus, red tongue with yellow coating, and taut, slippery and forceful pulse.

Therapeutic Principle: To clear away liver heat and purge fire.

Prescription: Modified Long Dan Xie Gan Decoction.

2) <u>Damp-Heat in Middle Warmer</u>

Symptoms: Nausea, vomiting, stuffiness in the chest, abdominal distention, insipid mouth or sweat taste in the mouth, discomfort sensation in the epigastric area, lassitude and preference to lie down, heavy sensation in the head, red tongue with yellow and greasy or thick and greasy coating, and soft and rapid pulse.

Therapeutic Principle: To resolve dampness, clear away heat and strengthen the spleen.

Prescription: Modified Huo Po Xia Ling Decoction.

Modifications: For sustained fever, sweating without relieving fever and constipation, replace the prescription with Da Cheng Qi Decoction.

3) Deficiency of Liver Yin and Kidney Yin

Symptoms: "Moon face", flushed face in the afternoon, dry throat and bitter taste in the mouth aggravated at night, dysphoria with feverish sensation in the chest, palms and soles, vertigo, tinnitus, sore loins and weak knees, oligomenorrhea, or amenorrhea, red tongue with little dry coating, and thready and rapid or taut and thready pulse.

Therapeutic Principle: To nourish the liver and kidney, replenish yin and clear away heat.

Prescription: Modified Zi Shui Qing Gan Decoction.

Modifications: For insomnia, add Radix Polygalae Tenuifoliae (Yuan Zhi) 10g and Semen Ziziphi Spinosae (Suan Zao Ren) 15g; for headache and distending sensation of the eyes, add Concha Haliotidis (Shi Jue Ming) 20g, Herba Apocyni Veneti (Luo Bu Ma) 9g, Mastodi Ossis Fossilia (Long Gu) 20g and Concha Ostreae (Mu Li) 20g; for severe bitter taste in the mouth and dry throat, add Herba Dendrobii (Shi Hu) 12g and Radix Scutellariae Baicalensis (Huang Qin) 9g; for purple striae or ecchymosis of the skin, add Flos Carthami Tinctorii (Hong Hua) 10g and Semen Pruni Persicae (Tao Ren) 10g.

4) Deficiency of Spleen Yang and Kidney Yang

Symptoms: Spiritlessness, fatigue, dyspnea on exertion, dry mouth without desire for drinks, tinnitus, deafness, sore loins and weak knees, cold intolerance, cold limbs, amenorrhea, infertility, or impotence, seminal emission, chubby and tender tongue with thin coating, and deep, thready and weak pulse.

Therapeutic Principle: To warm and nourish the spleen and kidney.

Prescription: Modified You Gui Pill.

Modifications: For decreased sex function, add Radix Morindae officinalis (Ba Ji Tian) 12g and Herba Epimedii (Yin Yang Huo) 12g; for constipation, add Herba Cistanches (Rou Cong Rong) 15g and Rhizoma Polygonati (Huang Jing) 12g.

What Kinds of Chinese Patent Drugs are Available to Treat Cushing's Syndrome?

1) Qi Ju Di Huang Pill: 9g each time, twice daily.
2) Jin Gui Shen Qi Pill: 9g each time, twice daily.

8. Addison's Disease (Chronic Adrenocortical Hypofunction)

Addison's disease is a disorder caused by destruction of the adrenal cortices. An underactive adrenal gland produces insufficient amounts of cortisol, aldolsterone and adrenal androgens. One in every 100,000 people has Addison's disease. Onset of the disease may occur at any age, but is most common in people ages 30 to 50.

The cause of Addison's disease is unknown. The failure of the adrenal glands to produce adrenocortical hormones is most commonly the result of autoimmune process. About one-third of Addison's disease cases are caused by the actual destruction of the adrenal glands through cancer, infection, an autoimmune process, or other diseases. Other causes may include the following:

- Use of corticosteroids as a treatment
- Certain medications
- Tuberculosis
- Bleeding into the adrenal glands
- Rarely, Addison's disease is inherited as an X-linked trait

Lack of adrenal hormones may cause elevated levels of potassium, extreme sensitivity to insulin (may lead to low blood sugar levels), and increased risk during stressful periods. Corticosteroids play an important role in helping the body fight infection and promote health during physical stress. The following are the most common symptoms of Addison's disease. However, each individual may experience symptoms differently. Symptoms may include:

- Muscle weakness and fatigue
- Weight loss and anorexia
- Darkening of the skin (hyperpigmentation) especially prominent over the knuckles, elbows, knees, posterior neck, and nipples, and in palmar creases and nail beds
- Black freckles
- Hypotension, even fainting
- Salt craving
- Hypoglycemia

- Nausea, diarrhea or vomiting
- Abdominal pain
- Amenorrhea
- Irritability
- Depression
- Dizziness
- Scant axillary and pubic hair

In acute adrenal failure (addisonian crisis), the signs and symptoms may also include pain in the lower back, abdomen or legs, severe vomiting and diarrhea that may lead to dehydration, low blood pressure and loss of consciousness.

How is Addison's Disease Diagnosed by Conventional Western Medicine?

In addition to a complete medical history and physical examination, diagnostic procedures for Addison's disease may include blood tests to measure corticosteroid hormone levels, ACTH stimulation test, insulin-induced hypoglycemia test, and CT scan.

How is Addison's Disease Treated by Conventional Western Medicine?

The goal of treatment is to restore the adrenal glands to normal function. Since Addison's disease can be life threatening, treatment often begins with administration of corticosteroids. Treatment may also include restoring the body's level of sodium and potassium. Androgen replacement therapy may improve overall sense of well-being, libido and sexual satisfaction.

An addisonian crisis is a life-threatening situation that results in low blood pressure, hypoglycemia and high blood levels of potassium. Immediate medical treatment typically includes intravenous injections of hydrocortisone, saline solution and dextrose.

What Causes Addison's Disease According to Traditional Chinese Medicine?

1) Weak Constitution
2) Overstrain, Improper Diet and Sex Indulgence
3) Chronic Diseases

How is Addison's Disease Differentiated and Treated by Traditional Chinese Medicine?

1) Deficiency of Qi and Blood Stasis

Symptoms: Dim complexion, increased skin pigmentation, spiritlessness, fatigue, shortness of breath, indolence of speaking, anorexia, pale and red tongue with ecchymosis and petechiae, and slow or rough pulse.

Therapeutic Principle: To replenish kidney qi and remove blood stasis.

Prescription: Modified Shi Quan Da Bu Decoction.

Modifications: For abdominal distention, add Cortex Magnoliae Officinalis (Hou Po) 10g, Rhizoma Pinelliae Ternatae (Ban Xia) 10g and Fructus Amomi Villosi (Sha Ren) 5g; for loose stools, remove Radix Rehmanniae Praeparata, and add Rhizoma Dioscoreae (Shan Yao) 20g and Semen Euryales Ferocis (Qian Shi) 12g; for palpitation and insomnia, add Semen Ziziphi Spinosae (Suan Zao Ren) 15g, Mastodi Dentis Fossilia (Long Chi) 20g and Rhizoma Coptidis (Huang Lian) 9g; for depression, add Rhizoma Cyperi Rotundi (Xiang Fu) 10g, Cortex Albizziae Julibrissin (He Huan Pi) 12g and Radix Curcumae (Yu Jin) 10g.

2) Yang Deficiency of the Spleen and Kidney

Symptoms: Increased skin pigmentation, especially over palmar creases, pressure areas and nipples; lumbago, cold intolerance, cold limbs, general edema, sparse axillary and pubic hair, decreased libido, pale, chubby and tender tongue with white, moist and slippery coating, and deep, thready and slow or soft and weak pulse.

Therapeutic Principle: To nourish the heart, warm the kidney and strengthen the spleen.

Prescription: Modified You Gui Pill.

Modifications: For diarrhea, add Semen Myristicae Fragrantis (Rou Dou Kou) 9g and Fructus Psoraleae Corylifoliae (Bu Gu Zhi) 9g; for anorexia and abdominal distention, add Fructus Amomi Villosi (Sha Ren) 5g, Radix Aucklandiae Lappae (Mu Xiang) 10g and Pericarpium Citri Reticulatae (Chen Pi) 9g; for spiritlessness and fatigue, add Radix Astragali (Huang Qi) 12g, and replace Radix Codonopsitis Pilosulae with Radix Ginseng (Ren Shen) 9g; for abdominal cold pain, add Rhizoma Alpiniae Officinarum (Gao Liang Jiang) 10g, Rhizoma Cyperi Rotundi (Xiang Fu) 10g and Fructus Evodiae Rutaecarpae (Wu Zhu Yu) 3g; for remarkable blood stasis, add Flos Carthami Tinctorii (Hong Hua) 10g and Radix Salviae Miltiorrhizae (Dan Shen) 10g.

3) Yin Deficiency of the Liver and Kidney

Symptoms: Increased skin pigmentation, especially over palmar creases, pressure areas and nipples; vertigo, tinnitus, sore loins and weak knees, feverish sensation in palms and soles, or low-grade fever, seminal emission, or menstrual irregularities, or amenorrhea, red tongue with little moisture and thin coating, and taut and thready or thready and rapid pulse.

Therapeutic Principle: To nourish the liver and kidney, nourish blood and remove blood stasis.

Prescription: Modified Liu Wei Di Huang Pill and Si Wu Decoction.

Modifications: For persistent low-grade fever, add Herba Artemisiae Apiaceae seu Annuae (Qing Hao) 10g, Carapax Trionycis (Bie Jia) 20g and Cortex Lycii Radicis (Di Gu Pi) 10g; for anorexia, add

Fructus Crataegi (Shan Zha) 12g and Fructus Amomi Cardamomi (Bai Kou Ren) 5g; for night sweating, add Fructus Tritici Aestivi Levis (Fu Xiao Mai) 20g and Concha Ostreae (Mu Li) 20g; for seminal emission, add Jin Suo Gu Jing Pill.

4) Prostration of Yin and Yang

Symptoms: Shriveled skin, sunken eyes, sweating, fever, irritability, delirium, dry mouth and lips, dry and red tongue, and deficiency and rapid pulse (prostration of yin); extremely cold extremities, drenching oily sweats, feeble respiration, or even coma, pale tongue, and tinny and extremely faint pulse (prostration of yang).

Therapeutic Principle: To replenish qi and save yin, and restore yang from collapse.

Prescription: Modified Sheng Mai Powder for prostration of yin; modified Si Wei Hui Yang Di Huang Decoction for prostration of yang.

What Kinds of Chinese Patent Drugs are Available to Treat Addison's Disease?

Shi Quan Da Bu Oral Liquid: 10ml, thrice daily.

9. Diabetes Mellitus (DM)

Diabetes mellitus represents a syndrome with disordered metabolism and inappropriate hyperglycemia due to either an absolute deficiency of insulin secretion or a reduction in its biologic effectiveness or both. There are three basic types of diabetes including:

Type I diabetes: Type I diabetes, also called insulin dependent diabetes mellitus (IDDM), is an autoimmune disorder in which the body's immune system destroys, or attempts to destroy, the cells in the pancreas that produce insulin. Type I diabetes usually develops in children or young adults, but can start at any age. Type I diabetes accounts for 5 to 10 percent of all diagnosed cases of diabetes in the US. Type I diabetes may cause hypoglycemia, hyperglycemia, and ketoacidosis. Complications include heart disease, kidney disease, eye problems, neuropathy, and foot problems.

Type II diabetes: Type II diabetes, also called non-insulin-dependent diabetes mellitus (NIDDM), is a metabolic disorder resulting from the body's inability to produce enough, or to properly use, insulin. It usually develops after age 45 and is a chronic disease with no known cure. The exact cause of type II diabetes is unknown; however, heredity and obesity play a major role. Type II diabetes is the most common type of diabetes, accounting for 90 to 95 percent of diabetes cases. Risk factors for type II diabetes include age, family history of diabetes, overweight, not exercising regularly, certain racial and ethnic groups(such as African-Americans, Hispanic Americans, and Native Americans), a low level HDL, and a high triglyceride level.

Gestational diabetes: Gestational diabetes is a condition in which the blood glucose level is elevated and other diabetic symptoms appear during pregnancy in a woman who has not previously been diagnosed with diabetes. Unlike other types of diabetes, gestational diabetes is not caused by a lack of insulin, but by blocking effects of other hormones on the insulin that is produced, a condition referred to as insulin resistance.

There are 20.8 million children and adults in the United States, or 7% of the population, who have diabetes. Diabetes is a serious disease, which, if not controlled, can be life threatening. It is often associated with long-term complications that can affect every system and part of the body.

Type I diabetes often appears suddenly. The symptoms may include:

- High levels of plasma glucose
- High levels of glucosuria
- Polydipsia, polyuria
- Frequent urination
- Extreme hunger but rapid weight loss
- Blurred vision
- Nausea and vomiting
- Abdominal pain
- Extreme weakness and fatigue
- Irritability and mood changes
- Ketonemia, ketonuria

The symptoms of type II diabetes may include:

- Frequent infections that are not easily healed
- Candidal vaginitis
- Frequent urination
- Extreme hunger
- Polydipsia, polyuria
- Blurred vision
- Extreme weakness and fatigue
- Irritability and mood changes
- Nausea and vomiting

- High levels of plasma glucose
- High levels of glucosuria
- Dry, itchy skin
- Tingling or loss of feeling in the hands or feet
- Hypertension, hyperlipidemia, and atherosclerosis
- Ketonuria and weight loss generally are not common at time of diagnosis

How is Diabetes Mellitus Diagnosed by Conventional Western Medicine?

Diagnosis is made based on family and medical history, physical examination and diagnostic tests including urinalysis (for glucosuria and ketonuria), random blood sugar test, fasting blood glucose test, glucose challenge test, and glycated hemoglobin (A1C) test.

How is Diabetes Mellitus Treated by Conventional Western Medicine?

The goal of treatment is to keep blood glucose levels as close to normal as possible. Emphasis is on control of blood glucose by monitoring the levels, regular physical activity, meal planning, and routine healthcare. Treatment may include:

- Healthy diet with controlled amounts of carbohydrate
- Dietary fiber
- An appropriate exercise program
- Healthy weight
- Proper hygiene
- Daily blood glucose monitoring
- Regular blood testing
- Regular urine testing
- Insulin (for either type I or type II diabetes)
- Oral medications to keep glucose levels low (for type II diabetes)
- Transplantation, such as pancreas transplant and islet cell transplantation
- Special fetal testing and monitoring may be needed for pregnant diabetics, especially those who are taking insulin. These tests can include fetal movement counting, ultrasound, nonstress testing, biophysical profile, and Doppler flow studies.

What Causes Diabetes Mellitus According to Traditional Chinese Medicine?

1) Congenital Insufficiency
2) Improper Diet

3) Emotional Disorders

4) Overstrain and Excessive Sexual Activities

How is Diabetes Mellitus Differentiated and Treated by Traditional Chinese Medicine?

1) Asymptomatic Stage

Symptoms: Absence of remarkable clinical symptoms, increased appetite, fatigue, slightly increased blood glucose, absence of glucosuria; however, increased blood glucose and glucosuria on exertion.

Therapeutic Principle: To nourish kidney yin.

Prescription: Modified Mai Wei Di Huang Pill.

Modifications: For yin deficiency and hyperactive liver fire, add Si Ni Powder supplemented with Radix Scutellariae Baicalensis (Huang Qin) 9g, Fructus Gardeniae Jasminoidis (Zhi Zi) 9g and Flos Chrysanthemi Morifolii (Ju Hua) 12g; for yin deficiency and hyperactive yang with vertigo, add Concha Haliotidis (Shi Jue Ming) 20g.

2) Symptomatic Stage

(1) Fluid Consumption due to Lung Heat

Symptoms: Polydipsia with intake of large amount of fluid, dry mouth and tongue, frequent urination, polyuria, increased sweating, red tongue tip and margin, thin and yellow tongue coating, and full and rapid pulse.

Therapeutic Principle: To clear away heat, moisten the lung and promote fluid production to quench thirst.

Prescription: Modified Xiao Ke Formula and Er Dong Decoction.

Modifications: For extreme thirst, add Herba Dendrobii (Shi Hu) 10g; for constipation, add Semen Cassiae (Jue Ming Zi) 15g; for polydipsia with a desire to drink, dry and yellow tongue coating, and full and large pulse, add Radix Pseudostellariae Heterophyllae (Tai Zi Shen) 10g and Gypsum Fibrosum (Shi Gao) 30g.

(2) Excessive Heat in the Stomach

Symptoms: Polyorexia (polyphagia and easily getting hungry), thirst, polyuria, emaciation, dry mouth, constipation, red tongue with dry and yellow coating, and slippery, excess and forceful pulse.

Therapeutic Principle: To clear away stomach heat, purge fire, nourish yin and produce fluid.

Prescription: Modified Yu Nu Decoction.

Modifications: For constipation and difficult defecation, use Zeng Yie Cheng Qi Decoction.

(3) Deficiency of Kidney Yin

Symptoms: Frequent urination, polyuria with cloudy and sweet urine, sore loins and weak knees, fatigue, vertigo, tinnitus, dry mouth, lips and skin, pruritus, red tongue with little coating, thready and rapid pulse.

Therapeutic Principle: To nourish yin and strengthen the kidney.

Prescription: Modified Liu Wei Di Huang Pill.

Modifications: For ployuria with cloudy urine, add Fructus Alpinae Oxyphyllae (Yi Zhi Ren) 10g, Ootheca Mantidis (Sang Piao Xiao) 9g and Fructus Schisandrae Chinensis (Wu Wei Zi) 5g; for deficiency of both qi and yin, add Radix Codonopsitis Pilosulae (Dang Shen) 9g and Radix Astragali (Huang Qi) 12g, or add Sheng Mai Powder.

(4) Deficiency of Both Qi and Yin

Symptoms: Thirst with a desire to drink, polyphagia accompanied by loose stools, or decreased appetite, listlessness, weakness of extremities, emaciation, pale and red tongue with dry and white coating, and weak pulse.

Therapeutic Principle: To replenish qi, strengthen the spleen, and promote fluid production to quench thirst.

Prescription: Modified Qi Wei Bai Zhu Powder and Sheng Mai Powder.

Modifications: For dry-heat in the lung, add Cortex Lycii Radicis (Di Gu Pi) 10g, Rhizoma Anemarrhenae (Zhi Mu) 10g and Radix Scutellariae Baicalensis (Huang Qin) 9g; for remarkable thirst, add Radix Trichosanthis (Tian Hua Fen) 12g and Radix Rehmanniae (Di Huang) 15g; for increased sweating, add Fructus Schisandrae Chinensis (Wu Wei Zi) 5g and Fructus Corni Officinalis (Shan Zhu Yu) 10g.

(5) Deficiency of Both Yin and Yang

Symptoms: Frequent urination with cloudy urine (as frequent as once after each drink), dark complexion, dry ears, sore loins and weak knees, general coldness, aversion to cold, impotence, pale tongue with white coating, and deep, thready and forceless pulse.

Therapeutic Principle: To nourish yin, warm yang, tonify the kidney and induce astringency.

Prescription: Modified Jin Gui Shen Qi Pill.

Modifications: Add Fructus Rubi Chingii (Fu Pen Zi) 10g, Ootheca Mantidis (Sang Piao Xiao) 9g and Fructus Rosae Laevigatae (Jin Ying Zi) 10g to nourish the kidney and induce astringency; for polydipsia, headache, red lips, dry tongue, deep and rapid respiration, use Sheng Mai Powder supplemented with Tuber Asparagi Cochinchinensis (Tian Dong) 10g, Carapax Trionycis (Bie Jia) 20g and

Carapax et Plastrum Testudinis (Gui Ban) 20g; for coma, convulsion, tinny and thready pulse, add Shen Fu Long Mu Decoction.

(6) <u>Deficiency of Both Qi and Blood</u>

Symptoms: Chronic course of illness, spiritlessness, drowsiness, lassitude, shortness of breath, hypologia (indolence of speaking), pale lips and nails, lusterless hair, dry mouth, thirst, cloudy and sweat urine, good appetite with weight loss, or anorexia with abdominal distention, physical inactivity, palpitation, insomnia, white and dry tongue coating with little saliva, thready and weak pulse.

Therapeutic Principle: To nourish blood, replenish qi, moisten dryness and promote fluid production.

Prescription: Modified Gui Pi Decoction and Sheng Yu Decoction.

Modifications: For severe deficiency of blood, add Gelatinum Corii Asini (E Jiao) 10g and Placenta Hominis (Zi He Che) 3g, and increase the dosage of Radix Codonopsitis Pilosulae (Dang Shen) and Radix Astragali (Huang Qi); for anorexia and loose stools, remove Radix Angelicae Sinensis and add Semen Coicis (Yi Yi Ren) 15g, Radix Aucklandiae Lappae (Mu Xiang) 10g and Rhizoma Alismatis Orientalis (Ze Xie) 15g.

(7) <u>Phlegm Stagnation and Blood Stasis</u>

Symptoms: Obesity, distending sensation in the chest, epigastric distention, muscle soreness with distending sensation, sensation of heaviness and stabbing pain of the extremities, dark tongue with ecchymosis, thick and greasy tongue coating, and slippery pulse.

Therapeutic Principle: To promote circulation of blood, remove blood stasis and resolve phlegm.

Prescription: Modified Ping Wei Powder and Tao Hong Si Wu Decoction.

Modifications: Add Radix Salviae Miltiorrhizae (Dan Shen) 10g and Lumbricus (Di Long) 10g to promote blood circulation and remove blood stasis; add Radix Astragali (Huang Qi) 12g to replenish qi and nourish blood; add Radix Puerariae (Ge Gen) 15g for producing fluid production to quench thirst; add Fructus Trichosanthis (Gua Lou) 15g and Fructus Citri Aurantii (Zhi Ke) 10g to promote qi circulation and eliminate stagnation.

(8) <u>Obstruction of Vessels and Collaterals by Blood Stasis</u>

Symptoms: Dim complexion, emaciation, fatigue, stuffy sensation and pain in the chest, numbness or stabbing pain of the extremities, which is aggravated at night; purple lips, dark tongue with ecchymosis or with dark purple sublingual venous distention, little or thin and white tongue coating, and taut or deep and rough pulse.

Therapeutic Principle: To promote circulation of blood and activate collaterals.

Prescription: Modified Xue Fu Zhu Yu Decoction.

Modifications: For severe stuffy sensation and pain in the chest, add Lignum Santali Albi (Tan Xiang) 2g, Fructus Amomi Villosi (Sha Ren) 5g and Bulbus Allii Macrostemonis (Xie Bai) 10g; for severe pain of the extremities, add Buthus Martensi (Quan Xie) 3g and Zaocys Dhumnades (Wu Shao She) 9g.

3) Complications

(1) Blisters, Ulceration and Gangrene

Symptoms: Recurrent or lingering ulceration and gangrene, high fever and cloudy consciousness in severe cases, red tongue with yellow coating, and rapid pulse.

Therapeutic Principle: To clear away heat and remove toxic substance.

Prescription: Modified Wu Wei Xiao Du Decoction and Huang Qi Liu Yi Powder.

Modifications: For cloudy consciousness and delirium, add An Gong Niu Huang Pill.

(2) Diabetic Cataracts, Retinopathy and Deafness

Symptoms: From blurred vision to blindness; or normal vision during the day, but blindness at night; or progressive tinnitus and deafness.

Therapeutic Principle: To nourish the liver and kidney, and replenish essence and blood.

Prescription: Modified Qi Ju Di Huang Pill, Yang Gan Pill, or Ci Zhu Pill.

What Kinds of Chinese Patent Drugs are Available to Treat Diabetes Mellitus?

1) Xiao Ke Pill: 5-10 pills each time, thrice daily.
2) Jin Qi Jiang Tang Tablet: 7-10 tablets each time, thrice daily.

10. Hyperlipoproteinemia

Hyperlipoproteinemia is a metabolic disorder characterized by abnormally elevated concentrations of specific lipoprotein particles in the plasma. Hyperlipidemia, elevated plasma cholesterol (hypercholesterolemia) or triglyceride (hypertriglyceridemia) levels or both, is present in all hyperlipoproteinemias.

Levels of lipoproteins (and therefore lipids, particularly LDL cholesterol) increase slightly as people age. Levels are normally slightly higher in men than in women, but levels increase in women after menopause. The increase in levels of lipoproteins can result in hyperlipoproteinemia and increase the risk of atherosclerosis. Hyperlipoproteinemia has a high frequency in developed countries.

Causes or risk factors for hyperlipidemia include:

- Physical inactivity, obesity
- Heredity, age

- Eating excess calories or unhealthy foods
- Excessive consumption of alcohol
- Some hereditary disorders, such as hereditary hyperlipoproteinemias
- Diabetes, high blood pressure, kidney failure, obstructive liver disease, hypothyroidism, family history of heart disease
- Drugs such as estrogens, oral contraceptives, corticosteroids, and thiazide diuretics

The risk of developing atherosclerosis, heart attack or stroke increases as the total cholesterol level increases. For adults, a total cholesterol level of less than 200 mg/dL and triglyceride level of less than 150 mg/dL are desirable, and an LDL cholesterol level of less than 100 mg/dL is optimal. When the total cholesterol level approaches 300 mg/dL, the risk of a heart attack doubles. A high level of LDL (bad) cholesterol increases the risk. A high level of HDL (good) cholesterol decreases the risk, and a low level of HDL cholesterol (defined as less than 40 mg/dL) increases the risk.

High lipid levels in the blood usually cause no symptoms. Clinical manifestations of the hyperlipoproteinemias are caused by deposition of lipids in the vascular system and the eye. Occasionally, when levels are particularly high, fat is deposited in the skin and tendons and forms bumps called xanthomas. Very high triglyceride levels can cause the liver or spleen to enlarge and may increase the risk of developing pancreatitis.

How is Hyperlipoproteinemia Diagnosed by Conventional Western Medicine?

Blood tests, such as lipid panel or lipid profile, are the only way to measure plasma lipid and lipoprotein levels.

How is Hyperlipoproteinemia Treated by Conventional Western Medicine?

Usually, the best treatment for people who have high cholesterol or triglyceride levels is to lose weight if they are overweight, stop smoking, decrease the total amount of fat and cholesterol in their diet, increase physical activity, and, if necessary, take a lipid-lowering drug. These drugs include:

- Statins
- Bile-acid-binding resins.
- Cholesterol absorption inhibitors
- Combination cholesterol absorption inhibitor and statin
- Fibrates
- Niacin

What Causes Hyperlipoproteinemia According to Traditional Chinese Medicine?

1) Congenital Defect
2) Improper Diet
3) Seven Emotional Disorders
4) Debility after Chronic Illness
5) Overstrain

How is Hyperlipoproteinemia Differentiated and Treated by Traditional Chinese Medicine?

1) <u>Stagnation of Turbid Phlegm</u>

Symptoms: Weak extremities, sensation of stuffiness and fullness in the chest and abdomen, loose stools, obesity, palpitation, vertigo, chubby tongue with teeth marks on the margin, greasy tongue coating, and slippery pulse.

Therapeutic Principle: To resolve phlegm and eliminate turbidity.

Prescription: Modified Dao Tan Decoction.

Modifications: Add Rhizoma Atractylodis Macrocephalae (Bai Zhu) 10g, Rhizoma Alismatis Orientalis (Ze Xie) 10g and Semen Cassiae (Jue Ming Zi) 10g to strengthen the spleen, resolve dampness and promote laxation; for cough with abundant sputum, add Fructus Trichosanthis (Gua Lou) 15g, Rhizoma Arisaematis cum Bile (Dan Nan Xing) 3g and Caulis Bambusae in Taeniam (Zhu Ru) 10g.

2) <u>Stagnation of Liver Qi and Deficiency of the Spleen</u>

Symptoms: Depression or vexation and irritability, weak extremities, fatigue; distention, fullness and roving pain in the hypochondrium, menstrual irregularities, dry mouth, no desire for food, abdominal distention, anorexia, white tongue coating, taut and thready pulse.

Therapeutic Principle: To soothe the liver, relieve stagnation, strengthen the spleen and regulate the stomach.

Prescription: Modified Xiao Yao Powder.

Modifications: For shortness of breath and fatigue, add Radix Astragali (Huang Qi) 12g and Radix Pseudostellariae Heterophyllae (Tai Zi Shen) 20g; for severe distending pain in the chest and hypochondrium, Pericarpium Citri Reticulatae Viride (Qing Pi) 10g and Radix Salviae Miltiorrhizae (Dan Shen) 10g; for vertigo, Flos Chrysanthemi Morifolii (Ju Hua) 12g and Ochra Haematitum (Dai Zhe Shi) 20g.

3) <u>Accumulation of Heat in the Stomach and Spleen</u>

Symptoms: Polyphagia, polyorexia, obesity, distention and fullness in the abdomen, flushed and moist face, dry mouth with bitter taste, restlessness, dizziness, red tongue with yellow and greasy coating, and taut and slippery pulse.

Therapeutic Principle: To clear away stomach heat and purge fire.

Prescription: Modified Bao He Pill and Xiao Chen Qi Decoction.

Modifications: For severe stomach heat and abdominal distention, add Gypsum Fibrosum (Shi Gao) 30g and Fructus Citri Aurantii (Zhi Ke) 10g; for distention and fullness in the abdomen, and constipation, add Radix Scutellariae Baicalensis (Huang Qin) 10g, Rhizoma Coptidis (Huang Lian) 9g and Rhizoma Anemarrhenae (Zhi Mu) 10g.

4) <u>Deficiency of Liver Yin and Kidney Yin</u>

Symptoms: Vertigo, sore loins and weak knees, insomnia, dreamfulness, tinnitus, dementia, dry mouth and throat, feverish sensation in the chest, palms and soles, hypochondriac pain, flushed cheeks, night sweating, red tongue with little coating, thready and rapid pulse.

Therapeutic Principle: To nourish the liver and kidney.

Prescription: Modified Qi Ju Di Huang Decoction.

Modifications: Add Rhizoma Polygonati (Huang Jing) 10g, Radix Polygoni Multiflori (He Shou Wu) 15g, Semen Cuscutae Chinensis (Tu Si Zi) 12g, Radix Ophiopogonis Japonici (Mai Dong) 12g and Radix Adenophorae (Sha Shen) 12g to nourish yin, induce fluid production, and nourish the liver and kidney; for yin deficiency and interior-heat with insomnia and night sweats, add Rhizoma Anemarrhenae (Zhi Mu) 10g and Cortex Phellodendri (Huang Bai) 10g; for severe vertigo, add Herba Taxilli (Sang Ji Sheng) 15g and Ochra Haematitum (Dai Zhe Shi) 20g.

5) <u>Deficiency of Spleen Yang and Kidney Yang</u>

Symptoms: Cold intolerance, cold limbs, sore loins and weak knees, pale complexion, loose stools, abdominal distention and discomfort, anorexia, tinnitus, blurred vision, pale and chubby tongue with white and slippery coating, deep and thready pulse.

Therapeutic Principle: To warm and nourish the spleen and kidney.

Prescription: Modified Fu Zi Li Zhong Decoction.

Modifications: For cold intolerance and cold limbs, add Fructus Psoraleae Corylifoliae (Bu Gu Zhi) 10g, Rhizoma Curculiginis Orchioidis (Xian Mao) 10g and Fructus Alpinae Oxyphyllae (Yi Zhi Ren) 10g; for abdominal distention and loose stools, add Cortex Magnoliae Officinalis (Hou Po) 10g, Pericarpium Citri Reticulatae (Chen Pi) 9g, Rhizoma Atractylodis (Cang Zhu) 10g and Semen Raphani Sativi (Lai Fu Zi) 10g; for shortness of breath and spontaneous sweating, add Radix Ginseng (Ren Shen) 9g and Radix Astragali (Huang Qi) 12g.

6) <u>Qi Stagnation and Blood Stasis</u>

Symptoms: Sensation of stuffiness and distention in the chest and hypochondrium, tender hypochondriac lump with pricking pain, restlessness, irritability, anxiety, insomnia, dark purple tongue with ecchymosis, deep and rough pulse.

Therapeutic Principle: To promote circulation of blood and qi, remove blood stasis and relieve pain.

Prescription: Modified Xue Fu Zhu Yu Decoction and Shi Xiao Powder.

Modifications: For restlessness, irritability, dry mouth with bitter taste, and constipation, add Herba Artemisiae Scopariae (Yin Chen Hao) 20g, Fructus Gardeniae Jasminoidis (Zhi Zi) 10g, Radix et Rhizoma Rhei (Da Huang) 9g and Radix Scutellariae Baicalensis (Huang Qin) 9g; for irascible temperament, add Radix Scutellariae Baicalensis (Huang Qin) 10g and Radix Curcumae (Yu Jin) 10g; for severe chest pain, add Bulbus Allii Macrostemonis (Xie Bai) 10g and Fructus Trichosanthis (Gua Lou) 15g.

What Kinds of Chinese Patent Drugs are Available to Treat Hyperlipoproteinemia?

1) Zhi Bi Tuo Capsule: 1 capsule each time, thrice daily.
2) Shan Zha Jiang Zhi Tablet: 1-2 tablets each time, thrice daily.

11. Obesity

Obesity, in simple terms, is having a high proportion of body fat. Overweight and obesity together represent the second leading preventable cause of death in the United States.

The causes or risk factors for obesity can be a complex combination of genetics, socioeconomic factors, metabolic factors, and lifestyle choices, as well as other factors. Some endocrine disorders, diseases, and medications may also exert a powerful influence on an individual's weight. Although there are genetic and hormonal influences on body weight, ultimately excess weight is a result of an imbalance of calories consumed versus calories burned through physical activity. If a person consumes more calories than he or she expends through exercise and daily activities, the person gain weight. The following factors can contribute to weight gain and obesity:

- Diet
- Inactivity
- Quitting smoking
- Pregnancy
- Certain medications, such as corticosteroids, tricyclic antidepressants, some high blood pressure and antipsychotic medications

- Medical problems
- Genetics, family history
- Age, sex

In the United States in 2004, the prevalence of obesity in adults aged 20–74 is 32.9%, children aged 2–5 years 13.9%, those aged 6–11 years 18.8%, and those aged 12–19 years 17.4%. In another word, about one in three American adults is considered to be obese. Being overweight or obese increases the risk of many diseases and health conditions, including the following:

- Hypertension
- Dyslipidemia (for example, high total cholesterol or high levels of triglycerides)
- Type 2 diabetes
- Coronary heart disease
- Stroke
- Gallbladder disease
- Osteoarthritis
- Sleep apnea and respiratory problems
- Some cancers (endometrial, breast, and colon)

The following are the most common symptoms that indicate an adolescent is obese:

- Facial features often appear disproportionate
- Adiposity in the breast region in boys
- Large abdomen (white or purple marks are sometimes present)
- In males, external genitals may appear disproportionately small
- Puberty may occur early
- Increased adiposity in the upper arms and thighs
- Genu valgum (knock kneed) is common

People who are obese often experience significant social pressure, stress, and difficulties. Psychologic disturbances are also very common.

How is Obesity Diagnosed by Conventional Western Medicine?

Obesity is diagnosed by a physician. The body mass index (BMI) and waist circumference are usually used to define obesity.

How is Obesity Treated by Conventional Western Medicine?

The goal of obesity treatment is to achieve and maintain a healthier weight. Treatment goals should be realistic, focused on modest reduction of intake, changes in eating habits, and the incorporation of a healthy exercise-oriented lifestyle. Treatment for obesity may include the following:

- Dietary changes
- Increased physical activity
- Behavior modification
- Individual or group therapy
- Support and encouragement
- Prescription weight-loss medication
- Weight-loss surgery

What Causes Obesity According to Traditional Chinese Medicine?

1) Old Age and Weak Constitution
2) Over-Intake of Greasy Food
3) Physical Inactivity
4) Deficiency of Healthy Qi due to Chronic Illness
5) Seven Emotional Disorders

How is Obesity Differentiated and Treated by Traditional Chinese Medicine?

1) <u>Accumulation of Heat in the Stomach and Spleen</u>

Symptoms: Polyphagia, obesity, abdominal distention and fullness, flushed and moist face, dry mouth with bitter taste, restlessness, dizziness, burning pain and discomfort in the stomach, which is relieved after meals; red tongue with yellow and greasy coating, taut and slippery pulse.

Therapeutic Principle: To clear away stomach heat, purge fire and promote digestion.

Prescription: Modified Xiao Cheng Qi Decoction and Bao He Pill.

Modifications: For severe stomach heat, add Rhizoma Coptidis (Huang Lian) 6g and Fructus Gardeniae Jasminoidis (Zhi Zi) 10g; for severe dry mouth with bitter taste, add Rhizoma Anemarrhenae (Zhi Mu) 10g and Gypsum Fibrosum (Shi Gao) 30g.

2) <u>Dysfunction of the Spleen in Transportation</u>

Symptoms: Obesity, listlessness, fatigue, general heavy sensation, chest stuffy sensation and abdominal distention, slight edema of extremities, which is aggravated at night and by exertion; and alleviated in the morning; normal or slightly impaired appetite with history of ingestion of large quantities of food and drink, pale and chubby tongue with teeth marks on its margin, thin and white or white and greasy tongue coating, soft and slow pulse.

Therapeutic Principle: To strengthen the spleen, replenish qi, promote diuresis and eliminate dampness.

Prescription: Modified Shen Ling Bai Zhu Powder and Fang Ji Huang Qi Decoction.

Modifications: For severe edema of the limbs, add Pericarpium Areca Catechu (Da Fu Pi) 10g and Cortex Mori Alba Radicis (Sang Bai Pi) 12g; for abdominal distention and loose stools, add Pericarpium Citri Reticulatae (Chen Pi) 9g and Semen Raphani Sativi (Lai Fu Zi) 10g; for shortness of breath, cold intolerance and cold limbs, add Cortex Cinnamomi Cassiae (Rou Gui) 3g and increase the dosage of Radix Ginseng and Radix Astragali (Huang Qi).

3) Internal Retention of Phlegm

Symptoms: Obesity, general heavy sensation, weak limbs, thoracic lump and fullness, copious amounts of sputum and saliva, vertigo, vomiting and lack of appetite, dry mouth without desire for drinks, preference for greasy food and liquor, listlessness, somnolence, white and greasy tongue coating, and slippery pulse.

Therapeutic Principle: To dry dampness, resolve phlegm, regulate qi and eliminate mass.

Prescription: Modified Dao Tan Decoction.

Modifications: Add Rhizoma Atractylodis Macrocephalae (Bai Zhu) 10g, Rhizoma Alismatis Orientalis (Ze Xie) 10g and Semen Cassiae (Jue Ming Zi) 12g to strengthen the spleen, eliminate dampness and promote defecation; for phlegm-heat, add Semen Trichosanthis (Gua Lou Zi) 12g and Caulis Bambusae in Taeniam (Zhu Ru) 10.

4) Deficiency of Spleen Yang and Kidney Yang

Symptoms: Obesity, facial edema, listlessness, somnolence, shortness of breath, fatigue, abdominal distention, loose stools, spontaneous sweating and dyspnea aggravated on exertion, cold intolerance, cold limbs, edema of lower extremities, pale and chubby tongue with thin and white coating, deep and thready pulse.

Therapeutic Principle: To warm and nourish the spleen and kidney, induce diuresis and resolve fluid retention.

Prescription: Modified Zhen Wu Decoction and Ling Gui Zhu Gan Decoction.

Modifications: For shortness of breath and spontaneous sweats, add Radix Ginseng (Ren Shen) 6g and Radix Astragali (Huang Qi) 12g; for oliguria and edema of the extremities, add Rhizoma Alismatis Orientalis (Ze Xie) 10g, Sclerotium Polypori Umbellati (Zhu Ling) 10g and Pericarpium Areca Catechu (Da Fu Pi) 10g; for cold intolerance and cold limbs, add Fructus Psoraleae Corylifoliae (Bu Gu Zhi) 10g, Rhizoma Curculiginis Orchioidis (Xian Mao) 10g, Herba Epimedii (Yin Yang Huo) 12g and Fructus Alpinae Oxyphyllae (Yi Zhi Ren) 10g.

5) Qi Stagnation and Blood Stasis

Symptoms: Obesity, reddish purple or crimson complexion, stuffy sensation in the chest and hypochondriac distention, restlessness, irritability, insomnia, or restless sleep, constipation, dark red tongue with ecchymosis or petechiae, or engorged sublingual veins, deep and taut or rough pulse.

Therapeutic Principle: To promote circulation of blood and qi, remove blood stasis and relieve stagnation.

Prescription: Modified Xue Fu Zhu Yu Decoction and Tao Hong Si Wu Decoction.

Modifications: For stagnated heat in the body with restlessness, irritability, dry mouth with bitter taste, and constipation, add Herba Artemisiae Scopariae (Yin Chen Hao) 10g, Fructus Gardeniae Jasminoidis (Zhi Zi) 10g, Radix et Rhizoma Rhei Praeparatae (Zhi Da Huang) 6g and Radix Scutellariae Baicalensis (Huang Qin) 10; for stagnation of qi with chest distress, shortness of breath, abdominal distention and fullness, add Radix Curcumae (Yu Jin) 10g, Cortex Magnoliae Officinalis (Hou Po) 10g, Pericarpium Citri Reticulatae (Chen Pi) 9g and Semen Raphani Sativi (Lai Fu Zi) 10g.

What Kinds of Chinese Patent Drugs are Available to Treat Obesity?

1) Jian Fei Bolus: 1 bolus each time, 2-3 times each day.
2) Bai Jin Pill: 6g each time, thrice daily.
3) Fang Feng Tong Sheng Pill: 6g each time, thrice daily.

12. Gout

Gout is one of the most painful forms of arthritis. It can cause pain, swelling, redness, heat, and stiffness in joints. It occurs when too much uric acid builds up in the body. The buildup of uric acid can lead to:

- Sharp uric acid crystal deposits in joints, often in the big toe
- Deposits of uric acid (tophi) under the skin
- Kidney stones from uric acid crystals in the kidneys

Uric acid comes from the breakdown of substances called purines. Purines are found in all of the body's tissues. They are also in many foods, such as liver, dried beans and peas, and anchovies. Normally, uric acid dissolves in the blood. It passes through the kidneys and out of the body in urine. But uric acid can build up in the blood when the body increases the production of uric acid, or the kidneys do not get rid of enough uric acid, or person eats too many foods high in purines.

Most people with hyperuricemia do not develop gout. But if excess uric acid crystals form in the

body, gout can develop. The risk factors for gout include:
- Genetics
- Male, age
- Overweight
- Excess alcohol
- Medical conditions, such as hypertension, diabetes, hyperlipidemia, and arteriosclerosis
- Excess foods rich in purines
- An enzyme defect that makes it hard for the body to break down purines
- Exposure to lead in the environment
- Have had an organ transplant
- Medicines such as diuretics, aspirin, cyclosporine, or levodopa
- Vitamin niacin

For many people, the first attack of gout occurs in the big toe. Often, the attack wakes a person from sleep. The toe is very sore, red, warm, and swollen. Gout can also attack insteps, ankles, heels, knees, wrists, fingers and elbows. Gout almost always occurs suddenly, often at night, and without any warning. Signs and symptoms of gout may include:

- Hyperuricemia
- Uric acid crystals in joint fluid
- More than one attack of acute arthritis
- Arthritis that develops in 1 day, producing a tender, swollen, red, and warm joint
- Attack of arthritis in only one joint, usually the toe, ankle, or knee

How is Gout Diagnosed by Conventional Western Medicine?
Diagnosis is made based on the symptoms, medical history, and family history of gout.

To confirm a diagnosis of gout, a sample of fluid from an inflamed joint may be drawn to look for crystals of uric acid. Other tests may include blood test and urine test.

How is Gout Treated by Conventional Western Medicine?
Treatment of gout includes: Nonsteroidal anti-inflammatory drugs (NSAIDs), Corticosteroids, such as prednisone, and Colchicine.

What Causes Gout According to Traditional Chinese Medicine?
1) Invasion of Exogenous Pathogenic Wind, Cold, Dampness and Heat
2) Congenital Insufficiency and Deficiency of Healthy Qi

3) Stagnation of Phlegm and Blood Stasis

4) Blockage of Channels and Collaterals

How is Gout Differentiated and Treated by Traditional Chinese Medicine?

1) <u>Retention of Wind, Cold and Dampness</u>

Symptoms: Painful and stiff joints with limited flexibility or roving pain or localized intense pain; or swollen and painful joints with heavy sensation, numbness of muscle and skin, which is aggravated in cloudy and raining days; thin and white tongue coating, taut and tense or soft and slow pulse.

Therapeutic Principle: To expel wind, eliminate cold, remove dampness and activate the collaterals.

Prescription: Modified Juan Bi Decoction.

Modifications: For excessive pathogenic wind with wandering pain, add Radix Saposhnikoviae Divaricatae (Fang Feng) 10g, Radix Angelicae Pubescentis (Du Huo) 10g and increase the dosage of Rhizoma et Radix Notopterygii (Qiang Huo); for excessive pathogenic cold with intense pain, add Radix Aconiti Lateralis Praeparatae (Fu Zi) 10g, Herba cum Radice Asari (Xi Xin) 3g and Cortex Cinnamomi Cassiae (Rou Gui) 5g; for excessive dampness with numbness of the limbs and joints, add Radix Stephaniae Tetrandrae (Fang Ji) 10g and Semen Coicis (Yi Yi Ren) 20g.

2) <u>Stagnation of Wind, Dampness and Heat</u>

Symptoms: Swollen, red, warm, painful and exquisitely tender joints, which are aggravated by warmth and alleviated by coldness; sudden onset, fever, thirst, restlessness, sweating without relieving fever, red tongue with yellow or yellow and greasy coating, slippery and rapid pulse.

Therapeutic Principle: To clear away heat, remove dampness, expel wind and activate the collaterals.

Prescription: Modified Bai Hu Jia Gui Zhi Decoction.

Modifications: For severe heat, add Lonicerae Caulis et Folium (Ren Dong Teng) 20g, Fructus Forsythiae Suspensae (Lian Qiao) 10g and Cortex Phellodendri (Huang Bai) 10g; for swollen joints, add Ramulus Mori (Sang Zhi) 20g, Radix Stephaniae Tetrandrae (Fang Ji) 10g, Rhizoma Curcumae Longae (Jiang Huang) 10g and Radix Clematidis (Wei Ling Xian) 10g; for ecchymosis of the skin, add Radix Paeoniae Rubra (Chi Shao) 10g, Cortex Moutan Radicis (Mu Dan Pi) 10g and Radix Rehmanniae (Di Huang) 15g; for remarkable deficiency of yin, add Radix Gentianae Macrophyllae (Qin Jiao) 10g, Herba Artemisiae Apiaceae seu Annuae (Qing Hao) 10g and Folium Mahoniae (Shi Da Gong Lao) 12g.

3) <u>Phlegm Stagnation and Blood Stasis Blocking the Channels and Collaterals</u>

Symptoms: Recurrent, swollen and painful joints (pain fluctuates in severity), or even swollen and stiff joints with limited flexibility and deformities, or ruptured subcutaneous nodules, dark purple tongue with petechiae or ecchymosis, white and greasy or thick and greasy tongue coating, thready and rough pulse.

Therapeutic Principle: To resolve phlegm, remove blood stasis, activate the collaterals and relieve pain.

Prescription: Modified Tao Hong Decoction.

Modifications: For severe phlegm and blood stasis, add Zaocys Dhumnades (Wu Shao She) 9g, Squama Manitis Pentadactylae (Chuan Shan Jia) 9g, Buthus Martensi (Quan Xie) 3g and Lumbricus (Di Long) 10g; for subcutaneous nodules, add Semen Sinapis Albae (Bai Jie Zi) 10g and Bombyx Batryticatus (Jiang Can) 10g.

4) <u>Deficiency of the Liver and kidney</u>

Symptoms: Recurrent, lingering, swollen and painful joints, or roving joint pain, or heavy sensation, numbness, stiffness and deformities of the joints with limited flexibility, sore loins and weak knees, listlessness, fatigue, pale tongue with white coating, and thready or thready and weak pulse.

Therapeutic Principle: To nourish the liver and kidney, expel wind and activate collaterals.

Prescription: Modified Du Huo Ji Sheng Decoction.

Modifications: For severe sore loins and weak knees, add Radix Astragali (Huang Qi) 12g, Radix Dipsaci Asperi (Xu Duan) 15g and Fructus Psoraleae Corylifoliae (Bu Gu Zhi) 10g; for remarkable cold pain in the joints, add Radix Aconiti Lateralis Praeparatae (Fu Zi) 10g and Cortex Cinnamomi Cassiae (Rou Gui) 3g; for numbness, add Caulis Trachelospermi Jasminoidis (Luo Shi Teng) 10g and Radix et Caulis Jixueteng (Ji Xue Teng) 12g.

What Kinds of Chinese Patent Drugs are Available to Treat Gout?

1) Wang Bi Granule: 1 bag each time, 2-3 times daily.

2) Yi She Juan Bi Granule: 1 bag each time, 2-3 times, daily.

3) Shu Jin Huo Xue Tablet: 5 tablets each time, thrice daily.

Chapter 7: Disorders of Connective Tissue and Joints

1. Rheumatoid Arthritis (RA)

Rheumatoid arthritis is a chronic systemic inflammatory disease of unknown cause, chiefly affecting synovial membranes of multiple joints, causing synovitis. This inflammation results in the release of proteins that, over months or years, cause thickening of the synovium. These proteins can also damage cartilage, bone, tendons and ligaments. Gradually, the joint loses its shape and alignment. Eventually, it may be destroyed. Rheumatoid arthritis is probably an autoimmune disease.

Rheumatoid arthritis is the most crippling form of arthritis and affects approximately 2.1 million Americans. Two to three times more women are affected than men. The average onset for rheumatoid arthritis is between the ages of 30 and 50 years old. But rheumatoid arthritis can also affect young children and adults older than age 50. The risk factors for rheumatoid arthritis may include age, sex, infection (possibly a virus or bacterium), inheriting specific genes, and smoking.

Rheumatoid arthritis usually causes problems in several joints at the same time. Early in rheumatoid arthritis, the joints in the wrists, hands, feet and knees are most affected. As the disease progresses, the shoulders, elbows, hips, jaw and neck can become involved. It generally affects both sides of the body at the same time. Rheumatoid arthritis can also cause inflammation of tear glands, salivary glands, the linings of the heart and lungs, lungs themselves and, in rare cases, blood vessels.

The signs and symptoms of rheumatoid arthritis may come and go over time. Each individual may experience symptoms differently. They include:

- Painful and swollen joints, especially in the smaller joints of the hands and feet
- Generalized aching or stiffness of the joints and muscles, especially in the morning, after sleep or after periods of rest
- Loss of motion of the affected joints
- Loss of strength in muscles attached to the affected joints
- Fatigue, which can be severe during a flare-up
- Low-grade fever

- Deformity of the joints over time
- Malaise
- Subcutaneous rheumatoid nodules

How is Rheumatoid Arthritis Diagnosed by Conventional Western Medicine?

In addition to a complete medical history and physical examination, the following tests may be recommended: blood tests and other laboratory tests (antinuclear antibody (ANA), arthrocentesis, complement, complete blood count, creatinine, erythrocyte sedimentation rate (ESR or sed rate), hematocrit, rheumatoid factor (RF), urinalysis, and white blood cell count), x ray, CT scan, MRI, and bone scan.

How is Rheumatoid Arthritis Treated by Conventional Western Medicine?

Most treatments involve basic nonpharmacologic management and medications. But in some cases, surgical or other procedures, such as joint replacement surgery, may be necessary. Medications include:

- Nonsteroidal anti-inflammatory drugs (NSAIDs).
- COX-2 inhibitors, such as celecoxib (Celebrex)
- Corticosteroids
- Disease-modifying antirheumatic drugs (DMARDs), such as hydroxychloroquine (Plaquenil), the gold compound auranofin (Ridaura), sulfasalazine (Azulfidine), minocycline (Dynacin, Minocin) and methotrexate (Rheumatrex)
- Immunosuppressants, such as leflunomide (Arava), azathioprine (Imuran), cyclosporine (Neoral, Sandimmune) and cyclophosphamide (Cytoxan)
- TNF blockers
- Interleukin-1 receptor antagonist (IL-1Ra)
- Abatacept (Orencia)
- Rituximab (Rituxan)
- Antidepressant drugs

What Causes Rheumatoid Arthritis According to Traditional Chinese Medicine?

1) Congenital Insufficiency and Deficiency of Kidney Essence
2) Exogenous Cold-Damp Obstructing Channels and Collaterals
3) Accumulation of Pathogenic Wind, Cold and Dampness
4) Damp-Heat Impairing Yin and Toxic Heat Impairing the Blood

5) Internal Retention of Damp-Heat, Phlegm Stagnation and Blood Stasis

How is Rheumatoid Arthritis Differentiated and Treated by Traditional Chinese Medicine?

1) <u>Accumulation of Pathogenic Wind, Cold and Dampness</u>

Symptoms: Wandering pain of joints with localized swelling, heavy sensation and numbness; or localized cold pain of joints, which is aggravated in cloudy and raining days, and is worsened by cold and is alleviated by warmth; stiffness of the joints, which is prominent in the morning and subsides during the day; limited flexibility, aversion to wind and cold, dark and pale tongue with thin and white or greasy and white coating, floating and tense or deep and tense or soft and slow pulse.

Therapeutic Principle: To expel wind, eliminate cold, remove dampness and activate collaterals.

Prescription: Modified Yi Yi Ren Decoction and Wu Tou Decoction.

Modifications: For remarkable wandering pain, add Radix Saposhnikoviae Divaricatae (Fang Feng) 9g, Radix Angelicae Dahuricae (Bai Zhi) 9g and Rhizoma seu Herba Aristolochiae Mollissimae (Xun Gu Feng) 10g; for severe swollen joints, add Radix Stephaniae Tetrandrae (Fang Ji) 10g, Diosceae Hypoglaucae Rhizoma (Bi Xie) 10g and Bombycis Mori Excrementum (Can Sha) 10g; for severe pain, add Radix Aconiti Lateralis Praeparatae (Fu Pian) 10g, Ramulus Cinnamomi Cassiae (Gui Zhi) 10g and Herba cum Radice Asari (Xi Xin) 3g.

2) <u>Retention of Wind, Heat and Dampness</u>

Symptoms: Red and swollen joints with associated stiffness, warmth, tenderness and pain, rigidity, or subcutaneous nodules, low-grade fever, flushed face, polydipsia with a desire to drink, sore throat, oliguria with dark urine, red tongue with thin and yellow or yellow and greasy coating, slippery and rapid or taut and rapid pulse.

Therapeutic Principle: To clear away heat, activate collaterals, expel wind and remove dampness.

Prescription: Modified Bai Hu Jia Gui Zhi Decoction and Si Miao Pill.

Modifications: For persistent high fever and polydipsia with a desire to drink, add Fructus Forsythiae Suspensae (Lian Qiao) 10g, Fructus Gardeniae Jasminoidis (Zhi Zi) 10g and Herba Hedyotis Diffusae (Bai Hua She She Cao) 20g; for warmth and pain of the lower extremities, difficult urination with dark urine, add Radix Achyranthis Bidentatae (Niu Xi) 10g and Cortex Erythrinae (Hai Tong Pi) 10g; for persistent low-grade fever or afternoon hectic fever, red tongue with little coating, thready and rapid pulse, add Carapax et Plastrum Testudinis (Gui Ban) 15g, Radix Rehmanniae Praeparatae (Shu Di Huang) 12g, Radix Angelicae Sinensis (Dang Gui) 10g, Radix Paeoniae Alba (Bai Shao Yao) 10g, Radix Gentianae Macrophyllae (Qin Jiao) 10g and Herba Artemisiae Apiaceae seu Annuae (Qing

Hao) 10g; for subcutaneous nodules, add Rhizoma Polygoni Cuspidati (Hu Zhang) 15g, Semen Sinapis Albae (Bai Jie Zi) 6g and Thallus Laminariae (Kun Bu) 10g.

3) Yin Deficiency and Interior-Heat

Symptoms: Afternoon fever or night fever, night sweating, or spontaneous sweating, dry mouth and throat, feverish sensation in palms and soles, swollen and painful joints, difficult urination with dark yellow urine, constipation, red and dry tongue with little coating, thready and rapid pulse.

Therapeutic Principle: To nourish yin, clear away heat, expel wind and activate collaterals.

Prescription: Modified Ding Shi Qing Luo Decoction.

Modifications: For concurrent damp-heat, add Cortex Phellodendri (Huang Bai) 10g, Rhizoma Atractylodis (Cang Zhu) 10g and Radix Achyranthis Bidentatae (Niu Xi) 10g.

4) Concurrence of Cold and Heat

Symptoms: Low-grade fever, burning sensation, warmth and pain of the joints, or with redness and swelling (joint pain is aggravated in cloudy and raining days, and is relieved by warmth), general coldness and cold limbs, red tongue with white coating, taut and thready or rapid pulse.

Therapeutic Principle: To expel wind, eliminate cold, clear away heat and remove dampness.

Prescription: Modified Gui Zhi Shao Yao Zhi Mu Decoction.

Modifications: For severe redness, swelling, warmth and pain of joints, add Flos Lonicerae (Jin Yin Hua) 12g, Herba Taraxaci Mongolici (Pu Gong Ying) 12g and Radix Isatidis seu Baphicacanthi (Ban Lan Gen) 10g; for severe cold intolerance, add Radix Astragali (Huang Qi) 12g and Radix Aconiti (Wu Tou) 3g.

5) Phlegm Stagnation and Blood Stasis

Symptoms: Swollen and painful joints with deformities and limited flexibility, or localized muscular stabbing pain, elasticity loss of skin with stiffness to palpation, dark purple skin and complexion, or subcutaneous nodules, numbness of the limbs, crimson tongue with petechiae or ecchymosis, thin and white tongue coating, taut and rough pulse.

Therapeutic Principle: To promote blood circulation, remove blood stasis, resolve phlegm and activate collaterals.

Prescription: Modified Shen Tong Zhu Yu Decoction and Zhi Mi Fu Ling Pill.

Modifications: For concurrent vasculitis, add Si Miao Yong An Decoction; for severe pain, add Gummi Olibanum (Ru Xiang) 10g, Rhizoma Corydalis (Yan Hu Suo) 10g and Eupolyphagae seu Opisthoplatia (Di Bie Chong) 9g.

6) Deficiency of the Liver and Kidney

Symptoms: Emaciation, joint deformities, atrophy of muscles, excessive pain and stiffness of joints with limited flexibility, muscle cramps or tremors, sore loins and weak knees, vertigo, palpitation, shortness of breath, pale nails, pale tongue with thin coating, thready and weak pulse.

Therapeutic Principle: To nourish the kidney and liver, replenish qi and blood, eliminate rheumatism and activate collaterals.

Prescription: Modified Du Huo Ji Sheng Decoction.

Modifications: For vertigo and tinnitus, insomnia, dreamfulness, night sweats, dysphoria with feverish sensation, and flushed cheeks, add Zuo Gui Pill; for pale complexion, edema, cold intolerance and cold limbs, add You Gui Pill; for severe swelling, add Semen Sinapis Albae (Bai Jie Zi) 9g and Fructus Gleditsiae Sinensis (Zao Jia) 3g; for severe joint pain, add Lonicerae Caulis et Folium (Ren Dong Teng) 15g, Rhizoma Polygoni Cuspidati (Hu Zhang) 15g and Herba Erodii seu Geranii (Lao Guan Cao) 15g; for chronic syndromes, add Zaocys Dhumnades (Wu Shao She) 6g, Agkistrodon seu Bungarus (Bai Hua She) 6g and Agkistrodon (Qi She) 6g.

What Kinds of Chinese Patent Drugs are Available to Treat Rheumatoid Arthritis?

1) Lei Gong Teng Duo Gan Tablet: 1-1.5mg/kg/day, thrice daily.
2) Huo Ba Hua Gen Tablet: 3-5 tablets each time, 2-3 times each day.

2. Systemic Lupus Erythematosus (SLE)

Systemic lupus erythematosus, also known as SLE, or simply lupus, is an inflammatory autoimmune disorder that may affect multiple organ systems. It is characterized by periodic episodes of inflammation of and damage to the joints, tendons, other connective tissues, and organs, including the heart, lungs, blood vessels, brain, kidneys, and skin. The heart, lungs, kidneys, and brain are the organs most affected. SLE affects each individual differently and the effects of the illness range from mild to severe.

SLE is considered to be a multifactorial condition. The factors are usually both genetic and environmental. Many of its clinical manifestations are secondary to the trapping of antigen-antibody complexes in capillaries of visceral structures or to autoantibody-mediated destruction of host cells. SLE may be triggered by many factors, such as infection, certain prescription medications, sunlight, hormones, stress, certain foods, the artificial sweetener aspartame, silicone breast implants, mercury dental fillings, hair dye, pesticides and other toxic chemicals. Although anyone can develop lupus at any age, common risk factors include sex, age, race, family history, infection with the Epstein-Barr virus, and pregnancy.

The disease is known to have periods of flare-ups and periods of remission. Women account for the vast majority of lupus cases and are approximately nine times as likely to develop the disease as men are. The following are the most common symptoms of SLE. However, each individual may experience symptoms differently. Symptoms may include:

- Malar rash, discoid rash
- Fever
- Arthritis
- Sunlight sensitivity
- Hair loss
- Mucosal ulcers
- Hear problems, lung problems
- Blood vessel disorders
- Digestive problems
- Swelling
- Kidney problems
- Low white blood cell or low platelet count
- Raynaud's phenomenon
- Weight loss, fatigue
- Dysfunction of brain or central nervous system
- Anemia, thrombocytopenia, or leukopenia

How is SLE Diagnosed by Conventional Western Medicine?

The American College of Rheumatology has developed clinical and laboratory criteria to help physicians diagnose and classify lupus. A patient is classified as have SLE if any 4 or more of 11 criteria are met (the 11 criteria will not be listed here). In addition to using the clinical history and a physical examination to check for the classification criteria, the following laboratory tests may be ordered:

- Complete blood count
- Erythrocyte sedimentation rate
- Kidney and liver assessment
- Urinalysis
- Antinuclear antibody (ANA) test

- Complement test
- Chest X-ray
- ECG
- Syphilis test

How is SLE Treated by Conventional Western Medicine?

The treatments for SLE can be varied and individual and may change over time. But rest, protection from sunlight, exercise, not smoking, stress reduction and a healthy diet are important for everyone with SLE. Treatments of SLE may include:

- Nonsteroidal anti-inflammatory drugs (NSAIDs)
- Antimalarial drugs
- Corticosteroids
- Immunosuppressive medications
- Immediate treatment of infections
- Kidney dialysis or kidney transplantation, if kidney failure is permanent
- New treatments are under investigation

What Causes SLE According to Traditional Chinese Medicine?

1) Congenital Insufficiency
2) Invasion of Six Exogenous Pathogenic Factors
3) Blood Stasis Blocking Collaterals

How is SLE Differentiated and Treated by Traditional Chinese Medicine?

1) <u>Hyperactive Heat Invading Qi Level (qi fen) and Nutritive Level (ying fen)</u>

Symptoms: High fever, not aversion to cold, flushed face, bright red erythema of the skin, dry throat, thirst with a desire for cold drinks, oliguria with dark yellow urine, joint pain, crimson tongue with yellow coating, slippery and rapid or full and rapid pulse.

Therapeutic Principle: To clear away heat, remove toxic substance, cool blood and resolve erythema.

Prescription: Modified Qing Wen Bai Du Decoction.

Modifications: For persistent high fever, add Calculus Bovis Powder (Niu Huang Powder), Cornu Saigae Tataricae Powder (Ling Yang Jiao Powder) or Zi Xue Powder; for joint pain, add Lonicerae Caulis et Folium (Ren Dong Teng) 15g and Ramulus Mori (Sang Zhi) 15g; for epistaxis and hematuria, add Nodus Nelumbinis Nuciferae Rhizomatis (Ou Jie) 12g and Rhizoma Imperatae Cylindricae

(Bai Mao Gen) 20g and Cornu Bubali (Shui Niu Jiao) 10g; for toxic heat with headache, vomiting, chill, thick and yellow tongue coating, increase the dosage of Rhizoma Coptidis and add Cortex Phellodendri (Huang Bai) 10g, Radix et Rhizoma Rhei (Da Huang) 9g, Rhizoma Guanzhong (Guan Zhong) 15g and Radix Isatidis seu Baphicacanthi (Ban Lan Gen) 15g; for cloudy consciousness, add An Gong Niu Huang Pill.

2) <u>Yin Deficiency Generating Interior-Heat</u>

Symptoms: Chronic low-grade fever, feverish sensation in palms and soles, afternoon flushed face with dark purple erythematous plaque, dry mouth, sore throat, thirst with desire for cold drinks, conjunctivitis, gingival bleeding, swollen and painful joints, dysphoria, insomnia, red tongue with little or thin and yellow coating, thready and rapid pulse.

Therapeutic Principle: To nourish yin and clear away heat.

Prescription: Modified Yu Nu Decoction and Zeng Ye Decoction.

Modifications: For joint pain, add Caulis Piperis Kadsurae (Hai Feng Teng) 9g and Rhizoma Polygoni Cuspidati (Hu Zhang) 15g; for low-grade fever, add Herba Artemisiae Apiaceae seu Annuae (Qing Hao) 9g and Cortex Lycii Radicis (Di Gu Pi) 10g; for dry mouth, add Herba Dendrobii (Shi Hu) 10g and Rhizoma Phragmitis Communis (Lu Gen) 15g; for alopecia, add Radix Polygoni Multiflori (He Shou Wu) 15g and Radix Rehmanniae Praeparatae (Shu Di Huang) 15.

3) <u>Heat Stagnation and Fluid Retention</u>

Symptoms: Stuffy sensation and pain in the chest, palpitation, occasional low-grade fever, dry throat, thirst, irritability, anxiety, skin rash and erythema, red tongue with thick and greasy coating, slippery and rapid, soft and rapid or occasional knot and intermittent pulse.

Therapeutic Principle: To clear away heat and induce diuresis.

Prescription: Modified Ting Li Da Zao Xie Fei Decoction and Xie Bai Powder.

Modifications: For fever, add Gypsum Fibrosum (Shi Gao) 30g; for cold intolerance or abundant white sputum, add Ramulus Cinnamomi Cassiae (Gui Zhi) 10g and Semen Sinapis Albae (Bai Jie Zi) 10g; for palpitation, knot and intermittent pulse, add Radix Glycyrrhizae Uralensis (Gan Cao) 6g, Fructus Schisandrae Chinensis (Wu Wei Zi) 5g, Radix Salviae Miltiorrhizae (Dan Shen) 10g and Mastodi Dentis Fossilia (Long Chi) 15g; for cough with sputum, add Bulbus Fritillariae Cirrhosae (Bei Mu) 10g and Radix Stemonae (Bai Bu) 9g; for dyspnea and stuffy sensation in the chest, add Fructus Perillae (Su Zi) 9g, Pericarpium Trichosanthis (Gua Lou Pi) 9g and Cortex Magnoliae Officinalis (Hou Po) 9g.

4) <u>Blood Stasis Blocking Vessels and Collaterals</u>

Symptoms: Petechiae, rash and erythema over the hands, feet and legs, nail fold infarcts, splinter hemorrhages, mucous membrane lesions, alopecia, aphtha, epistaxis, muscular hemorrhage, joint swelling and pain, menstrual irregularities, oliguria with dark yellow urine, proteinuria, hematuria, low-grade fever or general hot sensation, restlessness, irritability, red and smooth tongue with thin coating or prickles or ecchymosis on its margin, thready and taut or rough and rapid pulse.

Therapeutic Principle: To clear away heat, cool blood, promote blood circulation and remove blood stasis.

Prescription: Modified Xi Jiao Di Huang Decoction.

Modifications: For muscular hemorrhage, epistaxis and thrombocytopenia, add Radix Polygoni Multiflori (He Shou Wu) 20g, Radix Rubiae Cordifoliae (Qian Cao) 12g, Nodus Nelumbinis Nuciferae Rhizomatis (Ou Jie) 12g, Radix Sanguisorbae Officinalis (Di Yu) 12g and Cornu Bubali (Shui Niu Jiao) 10g; for concurrence of heat and cold with severe Raynaud's syndrome, add Ramulus Cinnamomi Cassiae (Gui Zhi) 10g and Flos Carthami Tinctorii (Hong Hua) 10g; for amenorrhea, add Radix Angelicae Sinensis (Dang Gui) 10g and Herba Leonuri Heterophylii (Yi Mu Cao) 12g.

5) <u>Deficiency of the Spleen and Kidney</u>

Symptoms: Lusterless complexion, occasional flushed face, pale fingers, listlessness, fatigue, cold intolerance, cold limbs, occasional hectic fever in the afternoon, dry mouth, oliguria, edema of the extremities, progressive edema in the lumbar region, abdominal enlargement, chubby and slight red or chubby and pale tongue with thin and white or thin and greasy coating, taut and thready, thready and rapid or thready and weak pulse.

Therapeutic Principle: To nourish the kidney essence, strengthen the spleen and induce diuresis.

Prescription: Modified Ji Sheng Shen Qi Pill.

Modifications: For lusterless complexion, anemia and leukopenia, add Radix Astragali (Huang Qi) 12g, Fructus Ligustri Lucidi (Nu Zhen Zi) 12g and Radix Polygoni Multiflori (He Shou Wu) 15g; for sore loins and knees, add Cortex Eucommiae Ulmoidis (Du Zhong) 12g, Radix Dipsaci Asperi (Xu Duan) 15g and Herba Taxilli (Sang Ji Sheng) 15g; for flushed face, add Rhizoma Anemarrhenae (Zhi Mu) 10g and Radix Scutellariae Baicalensis (Huang Qin) 9g; for cold intolerance, pale tongue and proteinuria, add Rhizoma Smilacis Glabrae (Tu Fu Ling) 30g and Folium Mori Alba (Sang Ye) 10g; for anorexia and loose stools, add Semen Euryales Ferocis (Qian Shi) 10g, Endothelium Corneum Gigeriae Galli (Ji Nei Jin) 10g and Fructus Crataegi (Shan Zha) 12g; for vertigo, headache and hypertension, add Flos Chrysanthemi Morifolii (Ju Hua) 12g, Ramulus Uncariae cum Uncis (Gou Teng) 12g, Tribulus Terrestris Fructus (Bai Ji Li) 9g and Rhizoma Gastrodiae Elatae (Tian Ma) 9g; for nausea, vomiting, oliguria and constipation, add Radix et Rhizoma Rhei (Da Huang) 6g, Natrii Sulfas (Mang Xiao) 10g, Radix Aucklandiae Lappae (Mu Xiang) 9g and Cortex Magnoliae Officinalis (Hou Po) 10g.

6) <u>Deficiency of Both Qi and Blood</u>

Symptoms: Palpitation, amnesia, insomnia, dreamfulness, lusterless complexion, numbness of the extremities, pale tongue with thin and white, thready and slow pulse.

Therapeutic Principle: To replenish qi and nourish blood.

Prescription: Modified Ba Zhen Decoction.

Modifications: For epistaxis, add Gelatinum Corii Asini (E Jiao) 9g, Fructus Citri Aurantii (Zhi Ke) 9g and Herba Ecliptae Prostratae (Han Lian Cao) 15g; for anemia, add Gelatinum Corii Asini (E Jiao) 10g and Cornu Cervi (Lu Jiao) 10g; for thrombocytopenia, add Radix Boehmeriae (Zhu Ma Gen) 15g and Radix Sanguisorbae Officinalis (Di Yu) 12g; for leukopenia, add Radix Astragali (Huang Qi) 12g, Rhizoma Atractylodis Macrocephalae (Bai Zhu) 10g and Fructus Ligustri Lucidi (Nu Zhen Zi) 12g.

7) <u>Stagnant Heat Invading the Mind</u>

Symptoms: Burning sensation over the body, fever, convulsion, cloudy consciousness, delirium, or muddleheadedness, or seizures, or strokes, or copious amount of sputum and dyspnea, bright crimson tongue, thready and rapid pulse.

Therapeutic Principle: To clear away heart fire and cause resuscitation.

Prescription: Modified Qing Gong Decoction, An Gong Niu Huang Pill, or Zhi Bao Pill.

Modifications: For severe headache, add Buthus Martensi (Quan Xie) 3g, Scolopendra Subspinipes (Wu Gong) 2g and Tribulus Terrestris Fructus (Bai Ji Li) 9g; for seizures, add Ramulus Uncariae cum Uncis (Gou Teng) 12g, Rhizoma Arisaematis (Tian Nan Xing) 10g and Rhizoma Acori Tatarinowii (Shi Chang Pu) 10g.

8) <u>Stagnant Heat Impairing the Liver</u>

Symptoms: Lingering low-grade fever, bitter taste in the mouth, anorexia, distending pain in the hypochondrium, menstrual irregularities with dark purplish blood and clot, restlessness, irritability, or jaundice, splenomegaly, hepatomegaly, erythema and ecchymosis of the skin, dark purple tongue with ecchymosis, and taut pulse.

Therapeutic Principle: To soothe the liver, clear away heat, cool blood and promote blood circulation.

Prescription: Modified Yin Chen Hao Decoction and Chai Hu Shu Gan Powder.

Modifications: For constipation, add Radix et Rhizoma Rhei (Da Huang) 6g; for ascites, add Herba Leonuri Heterophylii (Yi Mu Cao) 12g and Herba Verbenae (Ma Bian Cao) 20g.

What Kinds of Chinese Patent Drugs are Available to Treat SLE?

1) Lei Gong Teng Duo Gan Tablet: 1-1.5mg/kg/day, thrice daily.
2) Huo Ba Hua Gen Tablet: 3-5 tablets each time, 2-3 times each day.

3. Sjögren's Syndrome

Sjögren's syndrome, an autoimmune disorder, is the result of chronic dysfunction of exocrine glands in many areas of the body. It is characterized by dryness of the mouth, eyes, and other areas covered by mucous membranes. Sjögren's syndrome is frequently associated with other autoimmune disorders, such as rheumatoid arthritis, lupus and others. Most people with Sjögren's syndrome are older than 40. Nine of 10 are women.

Sjögren's syndrome is probably caused by a combination of genetic and environmental factors. A viral or bacterial infection may trigger the attack. In Sjögren's syndrome, the immune system attacks healthy tissue. The mucous membranes and moisture-secreting glands of the eyes and mouth are usually affected first, resulting in decreased production of tears and saliva. This can lead to difficulty swallowing, dental cavities, light-sensitive eyes, corneal ulcers and other problems. It may also affect joints, lungs, kidneys, blood vessels, digestive organs and nerves. Typical signs and symptoms of Sjögren's syndrome:

- Dry eyes and mouth (sicca components)
- Burning, itching, rosy secretions, and impaired tear production of the eyes
- Dental cavities
- Fatigue
- Fever
- Enlarged parotid glands
- Difficulty swallowing, chewing or speaking
- Loss of taste and smell
- Hoarseness
- Oral yeast infections, such as candidiasis
- Irritation and mild bleeding in the nose
- Skin rashes or dry skin
- Vaginal dryness
- Dry cough

- Joint pain, swelling and stiffness

How is Sjögren's Syndrome Diagnosed by Conventional Western Medicine?

In addition to medical history, and physical examination, the following tests may be recommended: blood test, tear test, and imaging tests such as sialogram, salivary scintigraphy and chest x ray. Sometimes biopsy, urine sample and slit-lamp exam may be helpful.

How is Sjögren's Syndrome Treated by Conventional Western Medicine?

Treatment can vary from person to person, depending on what parts of the body are affected. But in all cases, the doctor will help relieve the symptoms, especially dryness. The following medications and procedures may also be prescribed to help ease certain symptoms:

- Nonsteroidal anti-inflammatory drugs (NSAIDs)
- Corticosteroids
- Hydroxychloroquine (Plaquenil)
- Pilocarpine (Salagen)
- Cevimeline (Evoxac)
- Cyclosporine
- Immunosuppressants
- Surgery

What Causes Sjögren's Syndrome According to Traditional Chinese Medicine?

1) Congenital Insufficiency and Imbalance between Yin and Yang
2) Emotional Disturbance, Overstrain, Malnutrition due to Chronic Illness and Senility
3) Six Pathogenic Factors

How is Sjögren's Syndrome Differentiated and Treated by Traditional Chinese Medicine?

1) <u>Pathogenic Dryness Attacking the Lung</u>

Symptoms: Dry mouth and nose, dry cough without sputum or with little thick and sticky sputum that is difficult to be expectorated, chest pain, fever, headache, malaise, red tongue with dry, thin and yellow coating, thready and rapid pulse.

Therapeutic Principle: To clear away lung heat, moisten dryness and relieve cough.

Prescription: Modified Qing Zao Jiu Fei Decoction.

Modifications: For exterior wind-heat syndrome, use Sang Xing Decoction.

2) <u>Deficiency of Spleen Yin and Stomach Yin</u>

Symptoms: Dry mouth and tongue, belching, non-productive vomiting, hunger without desire to eat, epigastric dull pain, constipation, red tongue with little moisture, thready and slightly rapid pulse.

Therapeutic Principle: To strengthen the spleen, regulate the stomach, nourish yin and promote fluid production.

Prescription: Modified Yi Wei Decoction and Yu Nu Decoction.

Modifications: For difficult defecation, add Ma Zi Ren Pill.

3) Deficiency of Lung Yin and Kidney Yin

Symptoms: Dry mouth and throat, hoarse voice, cough with little sputum, vexation, restlessness, insomnia, hectic fever, warm sensation in the bones, sore loins and weak knees, red tongue with little coating, thready and rapid pulse.

Therapeutic Principle: To clear away lung heat, tonify the kidney, nourish yin and promote fluid production.

Prescription: Modified Bai He Gu Jin Decoction.

Modifications: For shortness of breath aggravated by exertion, add Radix Astragali (Huang Qi) 12g and Rhizoma Polygonati (Huang Jing) 12g; for severe dry mouth and throat, add Rhizoma Phragmitis Communis (Lu Gen) 20g and Fructus Pruni Mume (Wu Mei) 20g; for internal heat due to yin deficiency, add Cortex Lycii Radicis (Di Gu Pi) 10g, Radix Cynanchi Atrati (Bai Wei) 10g and Carapax Trionycis (Bie Jia) 15g.

4) Qi Deficiency and Blood Stasis

Symptoms: Dry mouth and throat, dryness of eyes with burning and discomfort sensation, shortness of breath and fatigue aggravated by exertion, vertigo, coarse skin with ecchymosis, joint pain with limited flexibility, dark tongue with little moisture, or bluish and purplish tongue with petechiae, thready and rough pulse.

Therapeutic Principle: To replenish qi, promote blood circulation and remove blood stasis.

Prescription: Modified Bu Yang Huan Wu Decoction.

Modifications: For joint deformity, coarse skin with ecchymosis, add Radix Salviae Miltiorrhizae (Dan Shen) 10g and Hirudo seu Whitmania (Shui Zhi) 5g.

What Kinds of Chinese Patent Drugs are Available to Treat Sjögren's Syndrome?

Lei Gong Teng Duo Gan Tablet: 1-1.5mg/kg/day, thrice daily.

4. Osteoarthritis

Osteoarthritis, sometimes called degenerative joint disease or osteoarthrosis, is the most common form of arthritis. Osteoarthritis is characterized by the breakdown of joint cartilage and may affect any joint in the body, including those in the fingers, hips, knees, lower back and feet. Initially osteoarthritis may strike only one joint. Over time multiple joints may become arthritic.

The exact cause of osteoarthritis isn't known. It's probably a combination of factors, including being overweight, the aging process, joint injury or stress, heredity, and muscle weakness. The cartilage damage may be due to a mechanical stress that results in an imbalance of enzymes released from the cells that synthesize the components of cartilage, such as collagen and proteoglycans. Too much of the enzymes can cause the joint cartilage to break down faster than it's rebuilt. The following factors may increase the risk of getting osteoarthritis:

- Age, sex
- Having certain hereditary conditions, including defective cartilage and malformed joints
- Having joint injuries
- Being obese
- Having diseases, such as rheumatoid arthritis, hemochromatosis, gout or pseudogout
- Having weak thigh muscles

Osteoarthritis affects most people to some degree by age 70. Before the age of 40, men develop osteoarthritis more often than do women, because of injury. From age 40 to 70, women develop the disorder more often than do men. After age 70, the disorder develops in both sexes equally. There's no cure for osteoarthritis, but available treatments can relieve pain and help remain active.

Osteoarthritis often develops slowly, and some people may not experience any signs or symptoms. However, osteoarthritis can cause the following signs and symptoms:

- Articular swelling and stiffness
- Pain on motion worsened by activity or weight bearing and relieved by rest
- Discomfort in a joint before or during a change in the weather
- Deformity
- Bony lumps on the middle or end joints of the fingers or the base of the thumb
- Loss of joint flexibility

Areas osteoarthritis typically affects include fingers, spine and weight bearing joints. It's uncommon for osteoarthritis to affect the jaw, shoulder, elbows, wrists or ankles unless they are injured or bear unusual stress.

How is Osteoarthritis Diagnosed by Conventional Western Medicine?

No single test can diagnose osteoarthritis. Diagnosis is based on medical history, physical examination, and the following tests: blood tests, joint aspiration tests, x rays, bone scans, computerized tomography (CT) scans, magnetic resonance imaging (MRI) scans and arthrography.

How is Osteoarthritis Treated by Conventional Western Medicine?

The goals of osteoarthritis treatment are to control pain, improve joint function, maintain normal body weight, and achieve a healthy lifestyle. Treatments include:

- Exercise
- Weight control
- Rest and relief from stress on joints
- Nondrug pain relief techniques
- Medications to control pain, including topical pain relievers, acetaminophen, NSAIDs, COX-2 inhibitors, tramadol, antidepressants, and injections of pain relievers
- Surgery and other procedures, including joint replacement, arthroscopic lavage and debridement, repositioning bones (osteotomy), and fusing bones
- Complementary and alternative therapies

What Causes Osteoarthritis According to Traditional Chinese Medicine?

1) Senility and Deficiency of the Kidney
2) Invasion of Exogenous Pathogenic Factors
3) Overstrain
4) Joint Injury
5) Damp-Heat Blocking the Channels and Collaterals

How is Osteoarthritis Differentiated and Treated by Traditional Chinese Medicine?

1) <u>Invasion of Pathogenic Wind, Cold and Dampness</u>

Symptoms: Joint pain alleviated by warmth and rest, and aggravated by cold, activity or weight bearing; absence of warmth and redness in the overlying skin of the joints; articular stiffness, thin and white or white and slippery tongue coating, taut and tense or rough pulse.

Therapeutic Principle: To dispel wind, eliminate cold, remove dampness and activate collaterals.

Prescription: Modified Wu Tou Decoction.

Modifications: For numbness or pain of upper extremities, add Rhizoma et Radix Notopterygii (Qing Huo) 10g and Ramulus Cinnamomi Cassiae (Gui Zhi) 10g; for numbness or pain of the lower extremities, add Radix Stephaniae Tetrandrae (Fang Ji) 10g and Radix Achyranthis Bidentatae (Niu

Xi) 15g; for severe damp-heat, add Cortex Phellodendri (Huang Bai) 10g, Rhizoma Arisaematis cum Bile (Dan Nan Xing) 3g and Rhizoma Smilacis Glabrae (Tu Fu Ling) 30g.

2) <u>Blood Stasis Blocking the Collaterals</u>

Symptoms: Chronic, recurrent and localized joint stabbing pain, or joint pain with numbness, articular stiffness, deformity, dark purplish skin overlying the joints, dark purple tongue with petechiae or ecchymosis, thready and rough pulse.

Therapeutic Principle: To promote blood circulation, remove blood stasis, activate collaterals and relieve pain.

Prescription: Modified Shen Tong Zhu Yu Decoction.

Modifications: For pain in the lower back region and extremities, remove Rhizoma et Radix Notopterygii (Qiang Huo) and add Radix Angelicae Pubescentis (Du Huo) 10g and Zaocys Dhumnades (Wu Shao She) 6g; for pain in the upper back region, remove Radix Achyranthis Bidentatae (Niu Xi) and add Caulis Sinomenii (Qing Feng Teng) 10g.

3) <u>Deficiency of the Kidney</u>

Symptoms: Chronic and intermittent joint pain, or tendon spasm aggravated by flexibility of the joints, or articular deformity, atrophy of muscle and tendon, sore loins and weak knees, general coldness, cold limbs, polyuria, loose stools, palpitation, shortness of breath, anorexia, fatigue, sallow complexion, or vertigo, tinnitus, dysphoria with feverish sensation, night sweating, pale and white tongue, or red tongue with little moisture, thready and deep or deep, thready and rapid pulse.

Therapeutic Principle: To nourish blood and yin, warm yang, replenish qi, promote blood circulation, activate collaterals and relieve pain.

Prescription: Modified San Bi Decoction.

Modifications: For excessive coldness, add Cortex Cinnamomi Cassiae (Rou Gui) 3g and Radix Aconiti Lateralis Praeparatae (Fu Zi) 10g; for severe lower backache, add Cortex Eucommiae Ulmoidis (Du Zhong) 12g, Rhizoma Cibotii Barometz (Gou Ji) 12g, Radix Dipsaci Asperi (Xu Duan) 15g, Radix Morindae officinalis (Ba Ji Tian) 12g and Radix Angelicae Pubescentis (Du Huo) 9g; for severe pain of the knees, add Herba Taxilli (Sang Ji Sheng) 15g, Radix et Caulis Jixueteng (Ji Xue Teng) 12g, Herba Artemisiae Anomalae (Liu Ji Nu) 9g and Herba Speranskiae seu Impatientis (Tou Gu Cao) 12g; for severe heel pain, add Gummi Olibanum (Ru Xiang) 10g and Myrrha (Mo Yao) 10g.

4) <u>Pathogenic Damp-Heat Blocking Channels and Collaterals</u>

Symptoms: Swollen joints and joint effusion with pain and burning sensation (the knees and ankles are more remarkable), general weakness, lassitude, heavy and sore sensation of lower extremities, red and chubby tongue with teeth marks on its margin, yellow and greasy tongue coating, slippery and rapid pulse.

Therapeutic Principle: To clear away heat, remove toxic substance, eliminate dampness and activate collaterals.

Prescription: Modified Si Miao Pill.

Modifications: For remarkable red, swollen, warm and painful joints, add Flos Lonicerae (Jin Yin Hua) 15g, Herba Taraxaci Mongolici (Pu Gong Ying) 15g, Radix Isatidis seu Baphicacanthi (Ban Lan Gen) 12g and Rhizoma Polygoni Cuspidati (Hu Zhang) 15g.

What Kinds of Chinese Patent Drugs are Available to Treat Osteoarthritis?

1) Tian Ma Pill: 10 pills each time, thrice daily.
2) Shu Jin Huo Luo Pill: 6g each time, thrice daily.
3) Kang Gu Zhi Zeng Sheng Pill: 6g each time, twice daily.

Chapter 8: Neurological Disorders

1. Trigeminal Neuralgia (tic douloureux)

Trigeminal neuralgia (TN), also called tic douloureux, is a chronic pain condition that causes extreme, sporadic, sudden burning or shock-like face pain that lasts anywhere from a few seconds to as long as two minutes per episode. The intensity of pain can be physically and mentally incapacitating. TN pain is typically felt on one side of the jaw or cheek. Episodes can last for days, weeks, or months at a time and then disappear for months or years. In the days before an episode begins, some patients may experience a tingling or numbing sensation or a somewhat constant and aching pain. The attacks often worsen over time, with fewer and shorter pain-free periods before they recur. The intense flashes of pain can be triggered by vibration or contact with the cheek (such as when shaving, washing the face, stroking the face or applying makeup), brushing teeth, eating, drinking, talking, smiling or encountering a breeze.

The pain of trigeminal neuralgia is due to a disturbance in the function of the trigeminal nerve. The presumed cause is a blood vessel pressing on the trigeminal nerve in the head as it exits the brainstem. Other less frequent sources of pain to the trigeminal nerve may include compression by a tumor, multiple sclerosis and stroke.

TN occurs most often in people over age 50, but it can occur at any age, and is more common in women than in men. About 5 percent of people with trigeminal neuralgia have other family members with the disorder (perhaps because of an inherited pattern of blood vessel formation), which suggests a possible genetic cause in some cases.

The pain of trigeminal neuralgia is described as "lightning-like or electric-shock-like", "shooting", "jabbing", or "like having live wires in the face" by patients. Trigeminal neuralgia usually affects just one side of the face. Rarely, trigeminal neuralgia can affect both sides, but not at the same time.

How is Trigeminal Neuralgia Diagnosed by Conventional Western Medicine?

Diagnosis is made based on medical history, physical examination, and a magnetic resonance imaging (MRI) scan of the head, and by excluding other possible conditions.

How is Trigeminal Neuralgia Treated by Conventional Western Medicine?

It is important to find the cause of the pain because the treatments for different types of pain may differ. Treatment options include medicines (anticonvulsants and tricyclic antidepressants), surgery (alcohol injection, glycerol injection, balloon compression, percutaneous stereotactic radiofrequency thermal rhizotomy (PSRTR), microvascular decompression (MVD), severing the nerve, and gamma-knife radiosurgery (GKR)), and complementary approaches (acupuncture, biofeedback, vitamin therapy, nutritional therapy, and electrical stimulation of the nerves).

What Causes Trigeminal Neuralgia According to Traditional Chinese Medicine?

1) Exogenous Pathogenic Factors: Wind, Cold and Heat
2) Obstruction of Wind and Phlegm due to Improper Diet and Pathogenic Wind
3) Fire Attacking Upwards
4) Yin Deficiency and Yang Hyperactivity
5) Blood Stasis Blocking Collaterals

How is Trigeminal Neuralgia Differentiated and Treated by Traditional Chinese Medicine?

1) <u>Wind-Cold Attacking Collaterals</u>

Symptoms: Momentary episodes of sudden severe lancinating facial pain, which is triggered or aggravated by coldness and alleviated by warmth; sensation of facial tightness during episodes, aversion to cold and wind, absence of thirst, thin and white tongue coating, floating and tense pulse.

Therapeutic Principle: To disperse wind, expel cold, activate collaterals and relieve pain.

Prescription: Modified Chuan Xiong Cha Tiao Powder.

Modifications: For severe aversion to cold, add Herba Ephedrae (Ma Huang) 6g and Folium Perillae Frutescentis (Su Ye) 10g; for facial muscle spasm, add Scolopendra Subspinipes (Wu Gong) 2g and Lumbricus (Di Long) 10g; for severe general aching and headache, increase the dosage of Rhizoma et Radix Notopterygii (Qiang Huo) and Herba cum Radice Asari (Xi Xin); for cold stagnation with severe pain, add Rhizoma Zingiberis Recens (Sheng Jiang) 9g and Rhizoma Ligustici (Gao Ben) 9g; for nasal stuffiness and running nose, add Fructus Xanthii Sibirici (Cang Er Zi) 9g and Flos Magnoliae (Xin Yi Hua) 9g; for chronic stagnation of wind and cold that generates heat, add Flos Chrysanthemi Morifolii (Ju Hua) 12g and Fructus Viticis (Man Jing Zi) 10g.

2) <u>Wind-Heat Impairing Collaterals</u>

Symptoms: Momentary episodes of sudden burning or lancinating facial pain, which is aggravated by warmth and slightly alleviated by coldness; flushed face and perspiration during episodes; fever, aversion to wind, dry mouth, sore throat, red tongue tip and margin, thin and yellow tongue coating, floating and rapid pulse.

Therapeutic Principle: To disperse wind, clear away heat, activate collaterals and relieve pain.

Prescription: Modified Xiong Zhi Shi Gao Decoction.

Modifications: For severe wind-heat syndrome, add Flos Lonicerae (Jin Yin Hua) 15g and Fructus Forsythiae Suspensae (Lian Qiao) 10g; for constipation, add Radix et Rhizoma Rhei (Da Huang) 6g and Natrii Sulfas (Mang Xiao) 10g; for oliguria with dark yellow urine, add Herba Lophatheri Gracilis (Dan Zhu Ye) 10g, Plumula Nelumbinis Nuciferae (Lian Zi Xin) 2g and Caulis Akebiae (Mu Tong) 5g; for severe sore throat, add Fructus Arctii Lappae (Niu Bang Zi) 10g, Semen Sterculiae Scaphigerae (Pang Da Hai) 3 pieces and Radix Scrophulariae Ningpoensis (Xuan Shen) 10g; for severe thirst, add Radix Trichosanthis (Tian Hua Fen) 10g and Rhizoma Phragmitis Communis (Lu Gen) 15g.

3) <u>Wind-Phlegm Blocking Collaterals</u>

Symptoms: Facial spasm, numbness and pain, vertigo, distending sensation in the chest and abdomen, vomiting, copious amounts of saliva, obesity, white and greasy tongue coating, taut and slippery pulse.

Therapeutic Principle: To disperse wind, resolve phlegm, eliminate spasm and relieve pain.

Prescription: Modified Xiong Xin Dao Tan Decoction.

Modifications: For facial numbness, add Radix et Caulis Jixueteng (Ji Xue Teng) 12g and Scolopendra Subspinipes (Wu Gong) 2g; for cold intolerance and cold limbs, remove fresh Rhizoma Zingiberis Recens (Sheng Jiang) and add dried Rhizoma Zingiberis Officinalis (Gan Jiang) 10g and Fructus Evodiae Rutaecarpae (Wu Zhu Yu) 3g; for turbid phlegm generating heat, remove Herba cum Radice Asari (Xi Xin) and Rhizoma Arisaematis (Tian Nan Xing), and add Rhizoma Arisaematis cum Bile (Dan Nan Xing) 3g and Succus Bambosae (Zhu Li) 30g; for feeling of oppression in the chest and anorexia, add Rhizoma Atractylodis (Cang Zhu) 9g and Cortex Magnoliae Officinalis (Hou Po) 9g.

4) <u>Stomach Fire Attacking Upwards</u>

Symptoms: Episodes of paroxysmal severe facial burning pain, distending pain in the forehead, flushed face, conjunctival congestion, foul odor in the mouth, dry throat, gingival swelling and pain, preference to cold drinks, constipation, dark urine, red tongue with yellow coating, slippery and rapid pulse.

Therapeutic Principle: To clear away stomach heat and purge fire.

Prescription: Modified Qing Wei Powder.

Modifications: For severe stomach heat consuming fluid, add Rhizoma Anemarrhenae (Zhi Mu) 10g and Radix Ophiopogonis Japonici (Mai Dong) 12g; for constipation, add Natrii Sulfas (Mang Xiao) 10g and Radix et Rhizoma Rhei (Da Huang) 6g; for gingival swelling and pain, and epistaxis, add Radix Cyathulae Officinalis (Chuan Niu Xi) 12g and Rhizoma Imperatae Cylindricae (Bai Mao Gen) 20g; for restlessness and insomnia, add Fructus Gardeniae Jasminoidis (Zhi Zi) 9g, Caulis Polygoni Multiflori (Ye Jiao Teng) 20g and Plumula Nelumbinis Nuciferae (Lian Zi Xin) 2g; for facial spasm, add Ramulus Uncariae cum Uncis (Gou Teng) 10g, Bombyx Batryticatus (Jiang Can) 9g and Buthus Martensi (Quan Xie) 3g.

5) Hyperactivity of Liver Fire and Gallbladder Fire

Symptoms: Episodes of paroxysmal severe facial shocking pain, hot and flushed face, vertigo, conjunctival congestion, restlessness, irritability, bitter taste in the mouth, dry throat, sensation of stuffiness and fullness in the chest and hypochondrium, constipation, dark yellow urine, red tongue with dry and yellow coating, taut and rapid pulse.

Therapeutic Principle: To clear away liver heat, purge fire and relieve pain.

Prescription: Modified Long Dan Xie Gan Decoction.

Modifications: For vertigo, add Flos Chrysanthemi Morifolii (Ju Hua) 12g, Ramulus Uncariae cum Uncis (Gou Teng) 12g and Radix Paeoniae Alba (Bai Shao Yao) 10g; for restlessness and insomnia, add Semen Ziziphi Spinosae (Suan Zao Ren) 15g and Cortex Albizziae Julibrissin (He Huan Pi) 12g; for facial spasm, add Buthus Martensi (Quan Xie) 3g, Scolopendra Subspinipes (Wu Gong) 2g and Rhizoma Gastrodiae Elatae (Tian Ma) 9g; for feeling of oppression in the chest and hypochondriac pain, add Radix Curcumae (Yu Jin) 10g, Fructus Meliae Toosendan (Chuan Lian Zi) 9g and Rhizoma Corydalis (Yan Hu Suo) 9g; for constipation, add Semen Cassiae Torae (Cao Jue Ming) 12g and Radix et Rhizoma Rhei (Da Huang) 6g; for thirst with a desire to drink, add Radix Trichosanthis (Tian Hua Fen) 10g and Radix Ophiopogonis Japonici (Mai Dong) 12g.

6) Deficiency of Yin and Hyperactivity of Yang

Symptoms: Episodes of paroxysmal severe facial spasmodical pain, dizziness, distending sensation in the eyes, insomnia, restlessness, irritability, bitter taste in the mouth, dry throat, sore loins and weak knees, red tongue with little moisture, and taut, thready and rapid pulse.

Therapeutic Principle: To nourish yin, suppress yang, calm wind and activate collaterals.

Prescription: Modified Zhen Gan Xi Feng Decoction.

Modifications: For facial spasm, add Scolopendra Subspinipes (Wu Gong) 2g and Lumbricus (Di Long) 10g; for restlessness and insomnia, remove Ochra Haematitum (Dai Zhe Shi) and add Caulis

Polygoni Multiflori (Ye Jiao Teng) 20g, Radix Polygalae Tenuifoliae (Yuan Zhi) 9g and Semen Ziziphi Spinosae (Suan Zao Ren) 12g; for severe headache, add Rhizoma Ligustici Chuanxiong (Chuan Xiong) 9g and increase the dosage of Radix Paeoniae Alba (Bai Shao Yao); for sore loins and weak knees, add Cortex Eucommiae Ulmoidis (Du Zhong) 12g and Radix Dipsaci Asperi (Xu Duan) 12g; for constipation, add Semen Cannabis Sativae (Huo Ma Ren) 12g; for accompanied phlegm, add Rhizoma Arisaematis cum Bile (Dan Nan Xing) 3g and Bulbus Fritillariae Cirrhosae (Bei Mu) 9g.

7) <u>Blood Stasis Blocking Collaterals</u>

Symptoms: Recurrent lancinating facial pain, dim complexion, coarse skin, dark purple tongue with ecchymosis, taut and rough or thready and rough pulse.

Therapeutic Principle: To promote blood circulation, remove blood stasis, activate collaterals and relieve pain.

Prescription: Modified Tong Qiao Huo Xue Decoction.

Modifications: For severe facial pain, add Buthus Martensi (Quan Xie) 3g and Scolopendra Subspinipes (Wu Gong) 2g, for accompanied qi stagnation, add Fructus Meliae Toosendan (Chuan Lian Zi) 9g and Pericarpium Citri Reticulatae Viride (Qing Pi) 9g; for accompanied deficiency of blood, add Radix Rehmanniae Praeparatae (Shu Di Huang) 15g and Radix Angelicae Sinensis (Dang Gui) 10g; for deficiency of qi, use Bu Yang Huan Wu Decoction.

What Kinds of Chinese Patent Drugs are Available to Treat Trigeminal Neuralgia?

1) Qi Ye Lian Tablet: 4 tablets each time, thrice daily.
2) Yan Hu Suo Tablet: 3 tablets each time, thrice daily.

2. Bell's Palsy (Idiopathic Facial Palsy)

Bell's palsy is a form of temporary facial paralysis resulting from damage or trauma to one of the two facial nerves. It is the most common cause of facial paralysis. Generally, Bell's palsy affects only one of the paired facial nerves and one side of the face, however, in rare cases, it can affect both sides. Most scientists believe that a viral infection such as viral meningitis or the common cold sore virus-herpes simplex-causes the disorder when the facial nerve swells and becomes inflamed in reaction to the infection.

The prognosis for individuals with Bell's palsy is generally very good. The extent of nerve damage determines the extent of recovery. With or without treatment, most individuals begin to get better within 2 weeks after the initial onset of symptoms and recover completely within 3 to 6 months.

Symptoms of Bell's palsy usually begin suddenly and reach their peak within 48 hours. Symptoms range in severity from mild weakness to total paralysis and may include twitching, weakness, or paralysis, drooping eyelid or corner of the mouth, drooling, dry eye or mouth, impairment of taste, and excessive tearing in the eye. Bell's palsy often causes significant facial distortion.

How is Bell's Palsy Diagnosed by Conventional Western Medicine?

Diagnosis is made based on medical history, physical examination, and tests such as electromyography (EMG), MRI or CT scan.

How is Bell's Palsy Treated by Conventional Western Medicine?

There is no cure or standard course of treatment for Bell's palsy. The most important factor in treatment is to eliminate the source of the nerve damage. Some cases are mild and do not require treatment since the symptoms usually subside on their own within 2 weeks. For others, treatment may include medications such as acyclovir (Zovirax) or famciclovir (Famvir) (used to fight viral infections) combined with an anti-inflammatory drug such as the steroid prednisone (used to reduce inflammation and swelling). Massage and analgesics such as aspirin, acetaminophen, or ibuprofen may relieve pain. In general, decompression surgery for Bell's palsy to relieve pressure on the nerve is controversial and is seldom recommended.

What Causes Bell's Palsy According to Traditional Chinese Medicine?

1) Insufficiency of Healthy Qi and Invasion of Pathogenic Wind
2) Internal Generation of Damp-Phlegm and Obstruction of Channels and Collaterals
3) Qi Deficiency and Blood Stagnation Resulting in Malnourishment of Channels and Collaterals

How is Bell's Palsy Differentiated and Treated by Traditional Chinese Medicine?

1) <u>Wind-Cold Attacking Collaterals</u>

Symptoms: Abrupt onset of facial paresis with deviation of the eyes and mouth, restriction of eye closure, or saliva drooling from one corner of the mouth, spilling tears, aversion to wind and cold, headache, nasal stuffiness, stiff facial muscles, soreness of extremities, thin and white tongue coating, floating and tense pulse.

Therapeutic Principle: To disperse wind, expel cold, warm channels and activate collaterals.

Prescription: Modified Xiao Xu Ming Decoction.

Modifications: For spontaneous sweating, remove Herba Ephedrae (Ma Huang) and add Radix Astragali (Huang Qi) 12g and Rhizoma Atractylodis Macrocephalae (Bai Zhu) 10g; for headache, add Radix Angelicae Dahuricae (Bai Zhi) 9g and Rhizoma et Radix Notopterygii (Qiang Huo) 9g; for facial spasm, add Rhizoma Gastrodiae Elatae (Tian Ma) 9g, Scolopendra Subspinipes (Wu Gong) 2g and Buthus Martensi (Quan Xie) 3g; for angular salivation, add Bombyx Batryticatus (Bai Jiang Can) 9g.

2) <u>Wind-Heat Blocking Collaterals</u>

Symptoms: Abrupt onset of deviation of the eyes and mouth, restriction of eye closure, headache, hot face, or fever, wind intolerance, restlessness, thirst, pain behind the ear, red tongue with thin and yellow coating, floating and rapid pulse.

Therapeutic Principle: To disperse wind, clear away heat, activate channels and collaterals.

Prescription: Modified Yin Qiao Powder.

Modifications: For bitter taste in the mouth, add Radix Bupleuri (Chai Hu) 9g and Gypsum Fibrosum (Shi Gao) 30g; for dizziness and conjunctival congestion, add Flos Chrysanthemi Morifolii (Ju Hua) 12g and Ramulus Uncariae cum Uncis (Gou Teng) 12g.

3) <u>Wind-Phlegm Blocking Collaterals</u>

Symptoms: Abrupt onset of deviation of the eyes and mouth, facial muscle spasm or numbness, distending sensation of the face, or saliva drooling from one corner of the mouth, sensation of heaviness and tightness in the head, thoracic stuffiness and fullness, vomiting, copious amounts of saliva, chubby tongue with white and greasy coating, taut and slippery pulse.

Therapeutic Principle: To disperse wind, resolve phlegm, activate collaterals and eliminate spasm.

Prescription: Modified Qian Zheng Powder and Dao Tan Decoction.

Modifications: For frequent facial spasm, add Scolopendra Subspinipes (Wu Gong) 2g and Zaocys Dhumnades (Wu Shao She) 9g; for turbid phlegm generating heat, add Radix Scutellariae Baicalensis (Huang Qin) 9g and Caulis Bambusae in Taeniam (Zhu Ru) 9g; for thoracic fullness and stuffiness, add Fructus Citri Sarcodactyli (Fo Shou) 9g and Rhizoma Atractylodis (Cang Zhu) 9g.

4) <u>Qi Deficiency and Blood Stasis</u>

Symptoms: Chronic deviation of the eyes and mouth, occasional facial spasm, pale complexion, shortness of breath, spiritlessness, fatigue, dark purple tongue with thin and white coating, thready and rough or taut and rough pulse.

Therapeutic Principle: To replenish qi, promote blood circulation and activate collaterals.

Prescription: Modified Bu Yang Huan Wu Decoction.

Modifications: For persistent syndrome, add Radix Notoginseng (San Qi) 9g, Squama Manitis Pentadactylae (Chuan Shan Jia) 9g and Ramulus Euonymi (Gui Jian Yu) 9g; for facial spasm, add Scolopendra Subspinipes (Wu Gong) 2g and Buthus Martensi (Quan Xie) 3g; for concurrent deficiency of blood, add Radix Rehmanniae Praeparatae (Shu Di Huang) 15g and Radix Paeoniae Alba

(Bai Shao Yao) 9g; for deficiency of yin fluid, add Radix Scrophulariae Ningpoensis (Xuan Shen) 12g and Radix Ophiopogonis Japonici (Mai Dong) 12g.

C What Kinds of Chinese Patent Drugs are Available to Treat Bell's Palsy?

Da Huo Luo Pill: 1 pill each time, twice daily.

3. Acute Idiopathic Polyneuropathy (AIDP, Guillain-Barré Syndrome)

Guillain-Barré syndrome (GBS) is an inflammatory disorder in which the immune system attacks the peripheral nerves and, rarely, parts of the brain itself. Severe weakness and numbness in the legs and arms characterize GBS. Paresthesias, dysesthersias and paralysis may occur in the legs, arms, upper body and face. The exact cause of Guillain-Barré syndrome is unknown. GBS is probably an autoimmune disorder that can occur after a viral infection, surgery, trauma, or reaction to an immunization. Immune system may destroy the myelin sheath of the peripheral nerves, which disables the nerves from transmitting signals to the muscles.

GBS affects an estimated one to three in every 100,000 persons annually in the United States. It can strike any race at any age, but its incidence increases with age. Most people with GBS return to normal within months. In its most severe form, GBS is a medical emergency and may require hospitalization. Severe GBS may result in total paralysis, potentially dangerous fluctuations in heart rate and blood pressure, and inability to breathe without respiratory assistance. People with severe GBS often need long-term rehabilitation to regain normal independence, and as many as 15 percent experience lasting physical impairment. In some cases, GBS can be fatal.

The following are the most common symptoms of Guillain-Barré syndrome. However, each individual may experience symptoms differently.

- Weakness, tingling or loss of sensation that often begins in the feet and legs and spreads to the upper body and arms
- Moderate pain throughout the body
- Difficulty breathing
- Paralysis of the legs, arms, respiratory muscles and face
- Difficulty with eye movement, facial movement, speaking, chewing or swallowing
- Very slow heart rate or low blood pressure
- Difficulty with bladder control or intestinal functions

GBS usually appear rapidly over the course of a single day and progresses quickly, with most people experiencing the most significant weakness in the legs, arms, chest and other areas within three weeks of the start of this disorder. In some cases, the signs and symptoms of GBS may progress very rapidly with complete paralysis of legs, arms and breathing muscles over the course of a few hours.

How is Guillain-Barré Syndrome Diagnosed by Conventional Western Medicine?

The diagnosis is made based on medical and family history, physical examination and diagnostic tests such as blood tests, urine tests, lumbar puncture (spinal tap) and electromyogram (EMG).

How is Guillain-Barré Syndrome Treated by Conventional Western Medicine?

There is no cure for Guillain-Barré syndrome. The goal of treatment is to prevent breathing problems and provide supportive care to help with activities of daily living. Early detection is the key to medically managing GBS. Treating GBS early, within two to four weeks after signs and symptoms first appear, may speed recovery time. The options of treatment may include:

- Plasmapheresis
- Immunoglobulin
- Pain medications including acetaminophen and nonsteroidal anti-inflammatory drugs, possibly in combination with narcotic painkillers
- Physical therapy
- Whirlpool therapy (hydrotherapy)
- Rehabilitation
- Adaptive devices such as a wheelchair or braces

What Causes Guillain-Barré Syndrome According to Traditional Chinese Medicine?

1) Hyperactive Heat Impairing Fluid
2) Internal Hyperactivity of Damp-Heat
3) Deficiency of the Spleen and Stomach
4) Deficiency of the Liver and Kidney

How is Guillain-Barré Syndrome Differentiated and Treated by Traditional Chinese Medicine?

1) <u>Hyperactive Heat Impairing Fluid</u>

Symptoms: Early stage of onset, fever, sore throat, irritating cough, dry mouth and tongue, paralysis of extremities, oliguria with dark yellow urine, constipation, red tongue with little coating, thready and rapid pulse.

Therapeutic Principle: To clear away heat, moisten dryness, nourish yin and promote fluid production.

Prescription: Modified Qing Zao Jiu Fei Decoction.

Modifications: For high fever, thirst and abundant sweats, add Flos Lonicerae (Jin Yin Hua) 15g and Fructus Forsythiae Suspensae (Lian Qiao) 10g; for dry throat and thirst, add Rhizoma Phragmitis Communis (Lu Gen) 20g and Radix Trichosanthis (Tian Hua Fen) 12g.

2) <u>Stagnation of Damp-Heat</u>

Symptoms: Weakness, heaviness, numbness and slightly swelling of extremities, thirst without desire to drink, sensation of distention and fullness in the chest and abdomen, oliguria with dark urine, red tongue with yellow and greasy coating, slippery and rapid pulse.

Therapeutic Principle: To clear away heat and eliminate dampness.

Prescription: Modified Si Miao Pill.

Modifications: For feeling of oppression and fullness in the chest, add Cortex Magnoliae Officinalis (Hou Po) 9g and Herba Agastache seu Pogostemonis (Huo Xiang) 9g; for severe heat, add Gypsum Fibrosum (Shi Gao) 30g and Fructus Gardeniae Jasminoidis (Zhi Zi) 9g.

3) <u>Deficiency of the Spleen and Stomach</u>

Symptoms: Weakness of extremities, anorexia, loose stools, lusterless complexion or facial edema, spiritlessness, lassitude, thin and white tongue coating, thready and weak pulse.

Therapeutic Principle: To strengthen the spleen and replenish qi.

Prescription: Modified Shen Ling Bai Zhu Powder.

Modifications: For swollen hands and feet, add Fructus Chaenomelis (Mu Gua) 10g and Caulis Trachelospermi Jasminoidis (Luo Shi Teng) 10g; for remarkable anorexia, add Endothelium Corneum Gigeriae Galli (Ji Nei Jin) 9g and Fructus Crataegi (Shan Zha) 12g.

4) <u>Deficiency of the Liver and Kidney</u>

Symptoms: Weakness, paralysis, paresthesias and dysesthesias of extremities, sore loins and weak knees, vertigo, dry mouth and tongue, red tongue with little coating, thready and rapid pulse.

Therapeutic Principle: To nourish yin, the kidney and liver.

Prescription: Modified Liu Wei Di Huang Pill.

Modifications: For remarkable dizziness, add Fructus Lycii (Gou Qi Zi) 10g and Flos Chrysanthemi Morifolii (Ju Hua) 12g; for hyperactivity of deficient fire, add Rhizoma Anemarrhenae (Zhi Mu) 10g and Cortex Phellodendri (Huang Bai) 9g; for deficiency of both yin and yang, use Hu Qian Pill.

4. Transient Ischemic Attacks (TIA)

A transient ischemic attack (TIA) is a transient stroke that lasts only a few minutes. It occurs when the blood supply to part of the brain is briefly interrupted. TIA symptoms, which usually occur suddenly, are similar to those of stroke but do not last as long. Most symptoms of a TIA disappear within an hour, although they may persist for up to 24 hours.

Risk factors for TIA include family history, age, sex, race, high blood pressure, cardiovascular disease, cigarette smoking, diabetes, undesirable levels of blood cholesterol, elevated homocysteine level, blood disorders such as sickle cell anemia, sleep apnea, migraine, sedentary lifestyle, obesity, carotid artery disease, peripheral artery disease, and heavy drinking.

TIAs are often warning signs that a person is at risk for a more serious and debilitating stroke. About one-third of those who have a TIA will have an acute stroke some time in the future. Many strokes can be prevented by heeding the warning signs of TIAs and treating underlying risk factors.

Transient ischemic attacks usually last for a few minutes. Most signs and symptoms disappear within an hour, and, by definition, all effects disappear within 24 hours. The signs and symptoms of TIA resemble those found early in a stroke and may include:

- Sudden weakness, numbness or paralysis in the face, arm or leg, typically on one side of the body
- Slurred or garbled speech
- Sudden blindness in one or both eyes or diplopia
- Vertigo, ataxia, slowness of movement

How is TIA Diagnosed by Conventional Western Medicine?

Diagnosis is made based on medical history, physical examination and tests such as carotid ultrasonography, CT scan, computerized tomography angiography (CTA) scanning, MRI, magnetic resonance angiography (MRA), transesophageal echocardiography (TEE), and arteriography.

How is TIA Treated by Conventional Western Medicine?

The goal of treatment is to correct the underlying causes and prevent a stroke. Treatments may include medications such as antiplatelet agents or anticoagulants to reduce the tendency for blood to clot, surgery such as endarterectomy, or carotid angioplasty.

What Causes TIA According to Traditional Chinese Medicine?

1) Hyperactivity of Liver Yang
2) Internal Generation of Turbid Phlegm
3) Blood Stasis

How is TIA Differentiated and Treated by Traditional Chinese Medicine?

1) <u>Yin Deficiency of the Liver and Kidney, and Upward Disturbance of Wind and Yang</u>

Symptoms: Vertigo, or even drop attacks due to bilateral leg weakness, distending sensation of the eyes, tinnitus, dysphoria with feverish sensation in the chest, dreamfulness, amnesia, numbness of the extremities, or abrupt onset of hemiplegia and dysphasia that recover rapidly; red tongue with little or thin and white coating, and taut or thready and rapid pulse.

Therapeutic Principle: To soothe the liver, calm wind, nourish yin and suppress yang.

Prescription: Modified Zhen Gan Xi Feng Decoction.

Modifications: For headache and distending sensation of the eyes, add Spica Prunellae Vulgaris (Xia Ku Cao) 12g and Flos Chrysanthemi Morifolii (Ju Hua) 12g; for dysphasia, add Radix Polygalae Tenuifoliae (Yuan Zhi) 9g and Rhizoma Acori Tatarinowii (Shi Chang Pu) 9g; for sore loins and weak knees, red tongue, thready and rapid pulse, add Radix Rehmanniae Praeparatae (Shu Di Huang) 20g, Fructus Corni Officinalis (Shan Zhu Yu) 10g and Radix Polygoni Multiflori (He Shou Wu) 20g; for facial flushing, conjunctival congestion, bitter taste in the mouth and dysphoria, add Spica Prunellae Vulgaris (Xia Ku Cao) 12g and Radix Gentianae (Long Dan Cao) 5g.

2) <u>Obstruction of Vessels and Collaterals due to Qi Deficiency and Blood Stasis</u>

Symptoms: Vertigo aggravated on exertion, dysphasia, or weakness or paralysis of the extremities in one side of the body, occasional convulsive jerking of limbs, saliva drooling from the mouth, dark pale tongue with petechiae and white coating, and deep, thready and forceless or rough pulse.

Therapeutic Principle: To replenish qi, nourish blood, promote blood circulation and activate collaterals.

Prescription: Modified Bu Yang Huan Wu Decoction.

Modifications: For paralysis of upper extremities, add Ramulus Cinnamomi Cassiae (Gui Zhi) 9g and Ramulus Mori (Sang Zhi) 15g; for paralysis of lower extremities, add Radix Dipsaci Asperi (Xu Duan) 15g and Radix Achyranthis Bidentatae (Niu Xi) 12g; for stiff tongue or dysphasia, add Radix Polygalae Tenuifoliae (Yuan Zhi) 9g and Rhizoma Acori Tatarinowii (Shi Chang Pu) 9g.

3) <u>Obstruction of Vessels and Collaterals due to Phlegm Stagnation and Blood Stasis</u>

Symptoms: Vertigo, sensation of heaviness and tightness in the head, numbness of limbs, distending sensation in the chest and abdomen, or abrupt onset of hemiplegia that recovers rapidly, dark tongue with white and greasy or yellow, thick and greasy coating, slippery and rapid or rough pulse.

Therapeutic Principle: To resolve phlegm, remove blood stasis, activate channels and collaterals.

Prescription: Modified Huang Lian Wen Dan Decoction and Tao Hong Si Wu Decoction.

Modifications: For severe turbid phlegm, add Rhizoma Arisaematis (Tian Nan Xing) 12g; for distending sensation in the chest and abdomen, add Cortex Magnoliae Officinalis (Hou Po) 9g and Fructus Citri Aurantii Immaturus (Zhi Shi) 9g.

What Kinds of Chinese Patent Drugs are Available to Treat TIA?

1) Nao Xue Shuan Tablet: 4 tablets each time, thrice daily.
2) Xuan Yun Ning Granule: 1 bag each time, thrice daily.
3) Fu Fang Dan Shen Injection: 20ml each time, once daily.
4) Chuan Xiong Qin Injection: 80-160ml each time, once daily.

5. Stroke (thrombotic Infarct, embolic Infarct and Hemorrhage)

Stroke, also called brain attack, occurs when blood flow to the brain is disrupted. Disruption in blood flow is caused when either a blood clot or piece of plaque blocks one of the vital blood vessels in the brain, or when a blood vessel in the brain bursts, spilling blood into surrounding tissues. Strokes can be classified into two main categories: about 80% are ischemic strokes - strokes caused by blockage of an artery; about 20% are hemorrhagic strokes - strokes caused by bleeding.

An ischemic stroke occurs when a blood vessel that supplies the brain becomes blocked or "clogged", leading to impairment of blood flow to part of the brain. Ischemic strokes are further divided into two groups: thrombotic strokes - caused by a blood clot that develops in the blood vessels inside the brain, and embolic strokes - caused by a blood clot or plaque debris that develops elsewhere in the body and then travels to one of the blood vessels in the brain via the bloodstream.

Hemorrhagic strokes occur when a blood vessel that supplies the brain ruptures and bleeds. Hemorrhagic strokes are divided into two main categories: intracerebral hemorrhage - bleeding from the blood vessels within the brain, and subarachnoid hemorrhage - bleeding in the subarachnoid space.

Many factors can increase the risk of a stroke. A number of these factors can also increase the chances of having a heart attack. They include family history, high blood pressure, diabetes mellitus, heart disease, cigarette smoking, history of transient ischemic attacks (TIAs) or prior stroke, high red blood cell count, elevated homocysteine level, high blood cholesterol and lipids, physical inactivity, obesity, excessive alcohol use, drug abuse, use of birth control pills and hormone therapy, abnormal heart rhythm, cardiac structural abnormalities, age, race, where a person lives, temperature, season, and climate, and socioeconomic factors.

Recovery from stroke and the specific ability affected depends on the size and location of the stroke. A small stroke may result in only minor problems such as weakness in an arm or leg. Larger strokes may cause paralysis, loss of speech, or even death. The signs and symptoms of stroke usually occur suddenly; frequently there's more than one. Signs and symptoms include:

- Sudden numbness, weakness, or paralysis of the face, arm or leg, usually on one side of the body
- Sudden difficulty speaking or understanding speech (aphasia)
- Sudden blurred, double or decreased vision
- Sudden dizziness, loss of balance or loss of coordination
- A sudden, severe headache or an unusual headache, which may be accompanied by a stiff neck, facial pain, pain between the eyes, vomiting or altered consciousness
- Confusion or problems with memory, spatial orientation or perception
- Sudden nausea, vomiting, or fever not caused by a viral illness
- Transient ischemic attack (TIA)

How is Stroke Diagnosed by Conventional Western Medicine?

In addition to a complete medical history and physical examination, diagnostic procedures for stroke may include CT scan, MRI, radionuclide angiography, computed tomographic angiography (CTA), and tests that evaluate the brain's electrical activity such as electroencephalogram (EEG), evoked potentials, carotid phonoangiography, Doppler sonography, ocular plethysmography, cerebral blood flow test (inhalation method) and digital subtraction angiography (DSA).

How is Stroke Treated by Conventional Western Medicine?

Getting prompt medical treatment for stroke is of utmost importance. Treatment itself depends on the type of stroke.

1) Ischemic stroke

To treat an ischemic stroke, any obstruction must be removed and blood flow to the brain must be restored.

- Emergency treatment. Therapy with clot busters (thrombolytics or fibrinolytics) such as a tissue plasminogen activator (TPA) must start within three hours. Quick treatment not only improves the chances of survival, but may also reduce the amount of disability resulting from the stroke. Currently, though, only a small proportion of Americans who have had a stroke receive thrombolytic therapy. Reasons for this include a limited time window and a limited group of people who benefit from this therapy.

- Surgical and other procedures may include carotid endarterectomy, angioplasty, and other techniques such as catheter embolectomy.
- Preventive medications may include anti-platelet drugs such as aspirin, Aggrenox, clopidogrel (Plavix) or ticlopidine (Ticlid), and anticoagulants such as heparin and warfarin (Coumadin).
- Medications to treat existing medical conditions such as diabetes, heart, or blood pressure problems
- Life support measures including such treatments as ventilators, IV fluids, adequate nutrition, blood pressure control, and prevention of complications
- Rehabilitation

2) Hemorrhagic stroke

- Medications and therapy such as corticosteroids and special types of intravenous (IV) fluids to reduce or control brain swelling
- Life support measures including such treatments as ventilators, IV fluids, adequate nutrition, blood pressure control, and prevention of complications
- Surgery may include aneurysm clipping, coiling (aneurysm embolization), and surgical AVM removal.
- Rehabilitation

What Causes Stroke According to Traditional Chinese Medicine?

1) Emotional Disorders, Hyperactivity of Liver Yang and Upward Disturbance of Wind and Fire
2) Overstrain, Senility, Generation of Internal Wind, Phlegm and Blood Stasis, and Blockage of Vessels and Collaterals
3) Improper Diet, Stagnation of Phlegm, Heat and Fu Organ Qi, Generation of Toxic Turbidity, Blockage of Heart Orifice
4) Congenital Insufficiency, Deficiency of Healthy Qi, Blood Stasis, Obstruction of Vessels and Collaterals

How is Stroke Differentiated and Treated by Traditional Chinese Medicine?

1) <u>Hyperactivity of Liver Yang and Upward Disturbance of Wind and Fire</u>

Symptoms: Dizziness, tinnitus, vertigo, abrupt onset of deviation of the eyes and mouth, stiff tongue, dysphasia, or heaviness and numbness of the hands and feet, or even hemiplegia, red tongue with yellow coating, and taut pulse.

Therapeutic Principle: To soothe the liver, suppress yang, promote blood circulation and activate collaterals.

Prescription: Modified Tian Ma Gou Teng Decoction.

Modifications: For accompanied turbid phlegm with feeling of oppression in the chest, nausea and greasy tongue coating, add Rhizoma Arisaematis cum Bile (Dan Nan Xing) 3g and Radix Curcumae (Yu Jin) 10g; for severe headache, add Cornu Saigae Tataricae (Ling Yang Jiao) 2g and Spica Prunellae Vulgaris (Xia Ku Cao) 12g; for heaviness and numbness of lower extremities, add Cortex Eucommiae Ulmoidis (Du Zhong) 12g and Herba Taxilli (Sang Ji Sheng) 15g.

2) Wind, Phlegm and Blood Stasis Blocking Vessels and Collaterals

Symptoms: Dysesthesias of muscles and skin, numbness of hands and feet, abrupt onset of deviation of the eyes and mouth, stiff tongue and dysphasia, saliva drooling from one corner of the mouth, hemiplegia, or spasm of the hands and feet, joint pain, cold intolerance, fever, thin and white tongue coating, floating and rapid pulse.

Therapeutic Principle: To disperse wind, resolve phlegm and activate collaterals.

Prescription: Modified Zhen Fang Bai Pill.

Modifications: For slurred speech, add Rhizoma Acori Tatarinowii (Shi Chang Pu) 9g and Radix Polygalae Tenuifoliae (Yuan Zhi) 9g; for stagnation of phlegm and blood stasis, dark purple tongue with petechiae or ecchymosis, thready and rough pulse, add Radix Salviae Miltiorrhizae (Dan Shen) 10g, Semen Pruni Persicae (Tao Ren) 9g, Flos Carthami Tinctorii (Hong Hua) 9g, Lumbricus (Di Long) 10g and Radix Paeoniae Rubra (Chi Shao) 10g.

3) Qi Stagnation of Fu Organ due to Phlegm and Heat

Symptoms: Hemiplegia, stiff tongue, dysphasia, or aphasia, deviation of the eyes and mouth, numbness in one side of the body, sticky sensation in the mouth, abundant sputum, abdominal distention, constipation, vertigo, red tongue with yellow and greasy or thick, dry and yellow coating, taut and slippery pulse.

Therapeutic Principle: To remove obstructions from fu organs, purge heat, resolve phlegm and regulate qi.

Prescription: Modified Xing Lou Cheng Qi Decoction.

Modifications: For remarkable heat syndrome, add Radix Scutellariae Baicalensis (Huang Qin) 9g and Fructus Gardeniae Jasminoidis (Zhi Zi) 9g; for little saliva, add Radix Rehmanniae (Di Huang) 15g and Radix Ophiopogonis Japonici (Mai Dong) 12g; for dysphasia, add Rhizoma Acori Tatarinowii (Shi Chang Pu) 9g and Radix Curcumae (Yu Jin) 10g.

4) Qi Deficiency and Blood Stasis

Symptoms: Paralysis and weakness of the extremities, obesity, shortness of breath, weak voice, sallow complexion, pale or dark tongue with ecchymosis, thin or thick tongue coating, thready and weak or deep and weak pulse.

Therapeutic Principle: To replenish qi, nourish blood, remove blood stasis and activate collaterals.

Prescription: Modified Bu Yang Huan Wu Decoction.

Modifications: For severe deficiency of blood, add Fructus Lycii (Gou Qi Zi) 10g and Radix Polygoni Multiflori (He Shou Wu) 15g; for cold limbs, add Ramulus Cinnamomi Cassiae (Gui Zhi) 9g; for sore loins and weak knees, add Herba Taxilli (Sang Ji Sheng) 15g, Cortex Eucommiae Ulmoidis (Du Zhong) 12g and Radix Dipsaci Asperi (Xu Duan) 12g.

5) Yin Deficiency of the Liver and Kidney and Stirring-Up of Internal Wind

Symptoms: Abrupt onset of deviation of the eyes and mouth, stiff tongue and dysphasia, hemiplegia, vertigo, headache, tinnitus, sore loins and weak knees, red tongue with yellow coating, and taut, thready and rapid or taut and slippery pulse.

Therapeutic Principle: To nourish yin, suppress yang, tranquilize the liver and calm wind.

Prescription: Modified Zhen Gan Xi Feng Decoction.

Modifications: For flushed face, dry mouth, red tongue with little coating, add Radix Rehmanniae (Di Huang) 15g, Radix Rehmanniae Praeparatae (Shu Di Huang) 15g, Radix Polygoni Multiflori (He Shou Wu) 15g and Fructus Lycii (Gou Qi Zi) 10g; for vertigo, add Concha Margaritiferae (Zhen Zhu Mu) 20g and Spica Prunellae Vulgaris (Xia Ku Cao) 12g; for severe feverish sensation in the chest, add Gypsum Fibrosum (Shi Gao) 30g; for abundant sputum, add Rhizoma Arisaematis cum Bile (Dan Nan Xing) 3g; for loose stools, remove Carapax et Plastrum Testudinis (Gui Ban) and Ochra Haematitum (Dai Zhe Shi), and add Halloysitum Rubrum (Chi Shi Zhi) 15g.

6) Invasion of Vessels and Collaterals by Pathogenic Wind

Symptoms: Numbness of the hands and feet, dysesthesias of the muscles and skin, or abrupt onset of deviation of the eyes and mouth, dysphasia, saliva drooling from one corner of the mouth, hemiplegia; or cold intolerance, fever, spasm, joint soreness, thin and white tongue coating, floating and taut or taut and thready pulse.

Therapeutic Principle: To disperse wind, activate collaterals, nourish blood and enforce nutrition.

Prescription: Modified Da Qin Jiao Decoction.

Modifications: For deviation of the eyes and mouth without hemiplegia, use Qian Zheng Powder supplemented with Herba Schizonepetae (Jing Jie) 9g, Radix Saposhnikoviae Divaricatae (Fang Feng)

9g and Radix Angelicae Dahuricae (Bai Zhi) 9g; for accompanied exterior-heat syndrome, add Flos Lonicerae (Jin Yin Hua) 12g, Fructus Forsythiae Suspensae (Lian Qiao) 10g and Herba Menthae Haplocalycis (Bo He) 9g.

7) Phlegm Heat Blocking the Heart Orifice

Symptoms: Sudden onset of coma followed by trip and fall, unconsciousness, trismus, tightly closed mouth difficult to be opened, coarse breathing sound, or firmly clenched hands, or restlessness, deviation of the eyes and mouth, hemiplegia, flushed face, constipation, red tongue with yellow and greasy coating, and taut, slippery and rapid pulse.

Therapeutic Principle: To clear away heat, resolve phlegm and restore consciousness.

Prescription: Forced feeding or nasal feeding of Zhi Bao Pill or An Gong Niu Huang Pill, followed by modified Ling Yang Jiao Decoction.

Modifications: For constipation, add Radix et Rhizoma Rhei (Da Huang) 6g; for profuse sputum, add Succus Bambosae (Zhu Li) 30g and Rhizoma Arisaematis cum Bile (Dan Nan Xing) 3g; for severe heat syndrome, add Radix Scutellariae Baicalensis (Huang Qin) 9g and Fructus Gardeniae Jasminoidis (Zhi Zi) 9g; for coma, add Radix Curcumae (Yu Jin) 10g.

8) Phlegm Dampness Blocking the Heart Orifice

Symptoms: Sudden onset of coma followed by trip and fall, unconsciousness, trismus, tightly closed mouth difficult to be opened, copious amounts of sputum and saliva, quietness without agitation, or even cold limbs, pale tongue with white, slippery and greasy coating, and deep pulse.

Therapeutic Principle: To open heart orifice (restore consciousness) with pungent and warm drugs, resolve phlegm and calm wind.

Prescription: Emergency forced feeding or nasal feeding of Su He Xiang Pill, followed by modified Di Tan Decoction.

Modifications: For copious amounts of saliva and sputum, add Vesica Fellea (Zhu Dan Zhi) 9g, Pericarpium Citri Reticulatae (Chen Pi) 6g and Fructus Gleditsiae Sinensis (Zao Jia) 3g; for excessive wind manifestations, add Rhizoma Gastrodiae Elatae (Tian Ma) 9g, Ramulus Uncariae cum Uncis (Gou Teng) 12g and Bombyx Batryticatus (Jiang Can) 9g.

9) Exhaustion of Primordial Qi

Symptoms: Sudden onset of coma followed by trip and fall, unconsciousness, closed eyes and opened mouth, feeble breathing, cold limbs with hands stretching out, profuse sweating, incontinence of urine and stools, flaccid paralysis of extremities, lingual atrophy, tinny and extremely faint pulse.

Therapeutic Principle: To replenish qi and restore yang from collapse.

Prescription: Modified Shen Fu Decoction and Sheng Mai Decoction.

Modifications: For persistent sweating, add Radix Astragali (Huang Qi) 12g, Mastodi Ossis Fossilia (Long Gu) 20g, Concha Ostreae (Mu Li) 20g and Fructus Corni Officinalis (Shan Zhu Yu) 10g.

What Kinds of Chinese Patent Drugs are Available to Treat Stroke?

1) Yin Xing Ye Tablet: 2 tablets each time, thrice daily.
2) Hua Tuo Zai Zao Pill: 8g each time, twice daily.
3) Ren Shen Zai Zao Pill: 1 pill each time, twice daily.

6. Parkinson's Disease (Paralysis Agitans)

Parkinson's disease (PD), also called paralysis agitans or shaking palsy, is a progressive loss of nerve cell function in the part of the brain that controls muscle movement. People with Parkinson's disease often experience trembling, muscle rigidity, difficulty walking, problems with balance and slowed movements. These symptoms usually develop after age 60, but it can start earlier.

The signs and symptoms of Parkinson's disease develop when certain neurons in the substantia nigra are damaged or destroyed. Normally, these nerve cells release dopamine, a chemical that transmits signals between the substantia nigra and the corpus striatum. These signals cause the muscles to make smooth, controlled movements. Parkinson's disease may result from a combination of genetic and environmental factors. Certain drugs, diseases and toxins also may cause symptoms similar to those of Parkinson's disease.

Risk factors for Parkinson's disease include heredity, age, sex, exposure to pesticides and herbicides, and reduced estrogen levels. Typical signs and symptoms of Parkinson's disease may include:

- Tremor of hands, arms, legs, jaw and face
- Slowed motion (bradykinesia)
- Rigid muscles
- Impaired balance
- Loss of automatic movements
- Impaired speech
- Difficulty swallowing
- Dementia

How is Parkinson's Disease Diagnosed by Conventional Western Medicine?

A diagnosis is based on the medical and family history, observations of the signs and a neurological examination. No diagnostic tests are available for Parkinson's disease. If symptoms go away or get better when a person takes levodopa, it's fairly certain that he or she has Parkinson's disease.

How is Parkinson's Disease Treated by Conventional Western Medicine?

For many people with Parkinson's, the initial response to treatment can be dramatic. Over time, however, the benefits of drugs frequently diminish or become less consistent, although symptoms can usually still be fairly well controlled. Treatment may include:

- Lifestyle changes, such as physical therapy, a healthy diet and exercise
- Medications, including levodopa and carbidopa, dopamine agonists such as bromocriptine (Parlodel), apomorphine (Apokyn), pramipexole (Mirapex) and ropinirole (Requip), selegiline (Eldepryl), catechol-O-methyltransferase (COMT) inhibitors such as tolcapone (Tasmar) and Entacapone, anticholinergics such as trihexyphenidyl and benztropine (Cogentin), amantadine, and coenzyme Q10
- Surgery, such as thalamotomy, pallidotomy, deep brain stimulation

What Causes Parkinson's Disease According to Traditional Chinese Medicine?

1) Senility and Overstrain
2) Emotional Disorders
3) Improper Diet
4) Congenital Insufficiency

How is Parkinson's Disease Differentiated and Treated by Traditional Chinese Medicine?

1) <u>Deficiency of Both Qi and Blood</u>

Symptoms: Chronic and severe tremor of limbs, rigidity of the neck, or spasm of the limbs, reduction in automatic movements, unsteadiness on turning and walking, shortness of breath, fatigue, vertigo, spontaneous sweating, saliva drooling from the mouth, pale and chubby tongue with teeth marks, thin and white or white and greasy tongue coating, thready and forceless pulse.

Therapeutic Principle: To replenish qi, nourish blood, calm wind and activate collaterals.

Prescription: Modified Ba Zhen Decoction and Tian Ma Gou Teng Decoction.

Modifications: For palpitation and insomnia, add Semen Ziziphi Spinosae (Suan Zao Ren) 15g and Radix Polygalae Tenuifoliae (Yuan Zhi) 9g; for constipation, add Semen Cannabis Sativae (Huo Ma Ren) 12g, Semen Armeniacae Amarum (Xing Ren) 9g and Fructus Citri Aurantii (Zhi Ke) 9g.

2) <u>Deficiency of Liver Yin and Kidney Yin</u>

Symptoms: Immobile face and fixity of facial expression, severe tremor of the limbs, bradykinesia (slowness of voluntary movement and reduction in automatic movements), rigidity in the limbs, clumsiness in movement, vertigo, tinnitus, amnesia, irritability, dreamfulness, lumbar soreness and knee weakness, red and small tongue with little coating, and taut, thready and rapid pulse.

Therapeutic Principle: To tonify the kidney, nourish yin, soothe the liver and calm wind.

Prescription: Modified Da Ding Feng Pill.

Modifications: For severe tremor, add Concha Margaritiferae (Zhen Zhu Mu) 20g and Rhizoma Gastrodiae Elatae (Tian Ma) 9g; for severe rigidity of the limbs, add Lumbricus (Di Long) 12g and Buthus Martensi (Quan Xie) 3g; for remarkable fire hyperactivity due to yin deficiency, add Rhizoma Anemarrhenae (Zhi Mu) 10g and Cortex Phellodendri (Huang Bai) 9g.

3) <u>Wind and Phlegm Blocking Collaterals</u>

Symptoms: Tremor and rigidity of the limbs, clumsiness in movement, bradykinesia, feeling of oppression and fullness in the chest and hypochondrium, excessive saliva and sputum, pale and chubby tongue with white and greasy coating, taut and slippery pulse.

Therapeutic Principle: To promote qi circulation, resolve phlegm, calm wind and activate collaterals.

Prescription: Modified Dao Tan Decoction.

Modifications: For heat manifestation, add Cortex Phellodendri (Huang Bai) 9g and Spica Prunellae Vulgaris (Xia Ku Cao) 12g; for severe tremor, add Mastodi Ossis Fossilia (Long Gu) 20g, Concha Ostreae (Mu Li) 20g and Lumbricus (Di Long) 10g; for spiritlessness, abdominal lump and distention, add Rhizoma Arisaematis cum Bile (Dan Nan Xing) 3g and Radix Curcumae (Yu Jin) 10g.

4) <u>Blood Stasis and Stirring-Up of Wind</u>

Symptoms: Immobile face and fixity of facial expression, dim complexion, rigidity of the limbs, bradykinesia, severe tremor, pain in the shoulders and back, stiff tongue and dysphasia, dark purple tongue with ecchymosis, taut and rough pulse.

Therapeutic Principle: To promote blood circulation, remove blood stasis, calm wind and activate collaterals.

Prescription: Modified Bu Yang Huan Wu Decoction.

Modifications: For dysphasia, add Radix Curcumae (Yu Jin) 10g, Radix Polygalae Tenuifoliae (Yuan Zhi) 9g and Rhizoma Acori Tatarinowii (Shi Chang Pu) 9g; for constipation, add Radix et Rhizoma Rhei (Da Huang) 6g, Semen Trichosanthis (Gua Lou Zi) 12g and Semen Cannabis Sativae (Huo Ma Ren) 12g; for excessive phlegm, add Succus Bambosae (Zhu Li) 30g, Concretio Silicea Bambusae (Tian Zhu Huang) 5g and Rhizoma Arisaematis (Tian Nan Xing) 10g; for restlessness and insomnia, add Fructus Gardeniae Jasminoidis (Zhi Zi) 9g, Caulis Polygoni Multiflori (Ye Jiao Teng) 20g and Semen Ziziphi Spinosae (Suan Zao Ren) 15g.

5) Deficiency of Both Yin and Yang

Symptoms: Chronic tremor, immobile face and fixity of facial expression, rigidity of the limbs, bradykinesia, dysphasia, postural instability, lusterless complexion, spiritlessness, lassitude, spontaneous sweating, cold intolerance, anorexia, insomnia, pale tongue, and deep, thready and weak pulse.

Therapeutic Principle: To nourish yin and yang, and calm wind.

Prescription: Modified Di Huang Decoction.

Modifications: For vexation and insomnia, add Semen Ziziphi Spinosae (Suan Zao Ren) 15g; for dementia, add Rhizoma Acori Tatarinowii (Shi Chang Pu) 9g and Radix Polygalae Tenuifoliae (Yuan Zhi) 10g; for severe tremor, add Mastodi Ossis Fossilia (Long Gu) 20g, Concha Ostreae (Mu Li) 20g, Concha Margaritiferae (Zhen Zhu Mu) 20g, Buthus Martensi (Quan Xie) 3g and Rhizoma Gastrodiae Elatae (Tian Ma) 9g; for clumsiness in movement and bradykinesia, add Radix Paeoniae Alba (Bai Shao Yao) 9g and Radix Dipsaci Asperi (Xu Duan) 15g.

What Kinds of Chinese Patent Drugs are Available to Treat Parkinson's Disease?

1) Liu Wei Di Huang Pill: 8g each time, twice daily.
2) Tian Ma Pill: 3-6g each time, thrice daily.

7. Epilepsy

Epilepsy is a disorder characterized by recurrent seizure due to an abnormal transmission of electrical signals inside the brain. About one in 100 people in the United States has experienced an unprovoked seizure at some point in life, however at least two unprovoked seizures are required for a diagnosis of epilepsy. The onset of epilepsy is most common during childhood and after age 65, but the condition can occur at any age.

Epilepsy has many possible causes, including defective genes, genetic inheritance, an accident, disease, metabolic disorder, medical trauma, brain tumor and abnormal brain development. However, epilepsy has no identifiable cause in about half of all affected people. Risk factors for epilepsy include a family history of epilepsy, head injuries, stroke and other vascular diseases, degenerative disorder, brain infections, and prolonged seizures in childhood due to high fevers.

Seizures are divided into partial seizures such as simple partial seizures and complex partial seizures, and generalized seizures such as absence (petit mal) seizures, atypical absences, myoclonic seizures, tonic-clonic (grand mal) seizures and atonic seizures. Symptoms vary depending on the type of seizure.

Partial seizures

Simple partial seizures: These seizures don't result in loss of consciousness. They may alter emotions or change the way things look, smell, feel, taste or sound.

Complex partial seizures: These seizures alter consciousness, causing loss of awareness for a period of time. Complex partial seizures often result in staring and nonpurposeful movements such as hand rubbing, lip smacking, arm positioning, vocalization or swallowing.

Generalized seizures

Absence seizures (petit mal): These seizures are characterized by staring, subtle body movement and brief lapses of awareness.

Atypical absences: Changes in tone may be more remarkable, or attacks may have a more gradual onset and termination than in typical absences.

Myoclonic seizures: These seizures usually appear as sudden jerks of the arms and legs.

Atonic seizures: Also known as drop attacks, these seizures cause sudden collapse or fall down.

Tonic-clonic seizures (grand mal): The most intense of all types of seizures, these are characterized by a loss of consciousness, body stiffening and shaking, and sometimes tongue biting or loss of bladder control.

How is Epilepsy Diagnosed by Conventional Western Medicine?

Diagnosis is made based on medical and family history, physical examination and tests such as blood tests, electroencephalogram (EEG), CT scan, magnetic resonance imaging (MRI), positron emission tomography (PET), and single-photon emission computerized tomography (SPECT).

How is Epilepsy Treated by Conventional Western Medicine?

Most people with epilepsy can become seizure-free by using a single anti-epileptic drug. Others can decrease the frequency and intensity of their seizures with medication. More than half the children with medication-controlled epilepsy can eventually stop medications and live a seizure-free life. Many adults also can discontinue medication after two or more years without seizures.

If anti-epileptic medications don't provide satisfactory results, other treatment options such as surgery, vagus nerve stimulation or a ketogenic diet may be suggested.

What Causes Epilepsy According to Traditional Chinese Medicine?

1) Congenital Insufficiency

2) Emotional Disorders (Fear and Fright) Impairing visceral organs, resulting in generation of internal heat and wind and accumulation of turbid phlegm

3) High Fever, Trauma and toxicosis

How is Epilepsy Differentiated and Treated by Traditional Chinese Medicine?

1) Upward Disturbance of Wind and Phlegm

Symptoms: Sudden onset of trip and fall, upward deviation of eyes, white and foamy saliva drooling from the mouth, convulsive jerking of the hands and feet, wheezing sound in the throat, white and greasy tongue coating, taut and slippery pulse.

Therapeutic Principle: To resolve phlegm, calm wind, cause resuscitation and relieve epilepsy.

Prescription: Modified Ding Xian Pill.

Modifications: For persistent jerking, add Ling Yang Jiao Power and Bai Shao Powder (mix with water and drink); for sticky sputum difficult to be expectorated, add Fructus Trichosanthis (Gua Lou) 15g; for abdominal distention, add Pericarpium Citri Reticulatae Viride (Qing Pi) 9g and Fructus Citri Aurantii (Zhi Ke) 9g.

2) Internal Disturbance of Phlegm-Heat

Symptoms: Sudden onset of trip and fall during the seizures, sudden loss of consciousness, myoclonic and tonic jerking of the limbs, uttering during attacks, white and foamy saliva drooling from the mouth, irritability, panting and coarse breathing sound, wheezing sound in the throat, foul odor in the mouth, constipation, dark red tongue with yellow and greasy coating, taut and slippery pulse.

Therapeutic Principle: To clear away heat, resolve phlegm, calm wind and stop epilepsy.

Prescription: Modified Huang Lian Wen Dan Decoction.

Modifications: For coma and severe seizure, add Rhizoma Gastrodiae Elatae (Tian Ma) 9g, Buthus Martensi (Quan Xie) 3g, Bombyx Batryticatus (Jiang Can) 9g and Lumbricus (Di Long) 12g; and also oral intake or nasal feeding of Zi Yue Powder and Zhi Bao Pill. For constipation, add Radix et Rhizoma Rhei (Da Huang) 6g; for accumulation of phlegm and coarse breathing, add Rhizoma Arisaematis cum Bile (Dan Nan Xing) 3g, Concretio Silicea Bambusae (Tian Zhu Huang) 5g and Chloriti Lapis (Qing Meng Shi) 8g.

3) Stagnation of the Liver and Phlegm-Fire

Symptoms: Irascible temperament, vexation, insomnia, bitter taste in the mouth, dry throat, occasional spitting of sputum and saliva, constipation; sudden onset of coma with trip and fall, myoclonic or tonic jerking and foamy saliva drooling during seizure; red tongue with yellow coating, and taut, slippery and rapid pulse.

Therapeutic Principle: To clear away liver heat, purge fire, resolve phlegm and calm wind.

Prescription: Modified Long Dan Xie Gan Decoction and Di Tan Decoction.

Modifications: For remarkable spasm, add Rhizoma Gastrodiae Elatae (Tian Ma) 9g, Lumbricus (Di Long) 12g and Ramulus Uncariae cum Uncis (Gou Teng) 12g, and oral intake (with water) of Ling Yang Jiao Powder; for constipation, add Radix et Rhizoma Rhei (Da Huang) 6g; for abundant and sticky sputum, add Succus Bambosae (Zhu Li) 30g.

4) <u>Blood Stasis Blocking the Heart Orifice</u>

Symptoms: Sudden onset of coma with trip and fall during seizures, myoclonic or tonic jerking; or jerking in the mouth, eyelids and limbs, which is the only manifestation; bluish and purplish complexion and lips, dark purple tongue with ecchymosis, and rough or deep and taut pulse.

Therapeutic Principle: To promote blood circulation, remove blood stasis, activate collaterals and calm wind.

Prescription: Modified Tong Qiao Huo Xue Decoction.

Modifications: Could add Rhizoma Gastrodiae Elatae (Tian Ma) 9g, Buthus Martensi (Quan Xie) 3g, Lumbricus (Di Long) 12g and Radix Salviae Miltiorrhizae (Dan Shen) 10g to the prescription. For abundant sputum, add Rhizoma Pinelliae Ternatae (Ban Xia) 9g and Caulis Bambusae in Taeniam (Zhu Ru) 9g; for concurrent deficiency of qi, add Radix Astragali (Huang Qi) 12g and Radix Pseudostellariae Heterophyllae (Tai Zi Shen) 15g.

5) <u>Deficiency of the Spleen and Phlegm-Dampness</u>

Symptoms: Chronic epilepsy, listlessness, fatigue, recurrent vertigo, lusterless complexion, feeling of oppression in the chest, abundant sputum, or nausea, anorexia, loose stools, pale and chubby tongue with white and greasy coating, soft and weak pulse.

Therapeutic Principle: To strengthen the spleen, regulate the stomach, resolve phlegm and calm wind.

Prescription: Modified Xing Pi Decoction.

Modifications: For nausea and vomiting, add Caulis Bambusae in Taeniam (Zhu Ru) 9g and Flos Inulae (Xuan Fu Hua) 9g; for anorexia, add Fructus Hordei Germinatus (Mai Ya) 12g, Fructus Crataegi (Shan Zha) 12g and Massa Medicata Fermentata (Shen Qu) 12g; for abdominal distention, add Fructus Citri Aurantii (Zhi Ke) 9g and Pericarpium Areca Catechu (Da Fu Pi) 9g.

6) <u>Deficiency of Liver Yin and Kidney Yin</u>

Symptoms: Severe epilepsy, vertigo, dry and discomfort eyes, vexation, insomnia, lumbar soreness, weak knees, red tongue with little coating, thready and rapid pulse.

Therapeutic Principle: To nourish the liver and kidney, replenish yin and calm wind.

Prescription: Modified Zuo Gui Pill.

Modifications: Could add Radix Paeoniae Alba (Bai Shao Yao) 9g, Carapax Trionycis (Bie Jia) 15g, Concha Ostreae (Mu Li) 20g and Mastodi Dentis Fossilia (Long Chi) 20g to the prescription. For sore loins and weak knees, add Cortex Eucommiae Ulmoidis (Du Zhong) 12g, Radix Dipsaci Asperi (Xu Duan) 15g; for somnolence, add Concha Ostreae (Mu Li) 20g, Semen Biotae Orientalis (Bai Zi Ren) 15g and Magnetitum (Ci Shi) 12g; for concurrent phlegm-heat, add Concretio Silicea Bambusae (Tian Zhu Huang) 5g and Caulis Bambusae in Taeniam (Zhu Ru) 9g; for restlessness and irritability, add Fructus Gardeniae Jasminoidis (Zhi Zi) 9g and Plumula Nelumbinis Nuciferae (Lian Zi Xin) 2g.

What Kinds of Chinese Patent Drugs are Available to Treat Epilepsy?

1) Meng Shi Guen Tan Pill: 1-3g each time, twice daily.
2) Niu Huang Qing Xin Pill: 6g each time, twice daily.

8. Vascular Dementia (Multi-Infarct Dementia or Atherosclerotic Dementia)

Vascular dementia (VD) is a disorder characterized by impairments in cognitive function caused by problems in the blood vessels that feed the brain. It is most often caused by either a narrowing or a complete blockage of one or more blood vessels in the brain. The complete blockage of an artery in the brain usually causes a stroke (infarction), but some blockages don't produce stroke symptoms. These "silent brain infarctions" increase a person's risk of vascular dementia. The risk increases with the number of infarctions experienced over time. Vascular dementia also can occur when blood vessels in the brain narrow, reducing the amount of blood flow to those sections of the brain. Vascular dementia can also be caused by profoundly low blood pressure, brain damage caused by brain hemorrhage, blood vessel damage from such disorders as lupus erythematosus or temporal arteritis.

The prevalence of vascular dementia ranges from 1 percent to 4 percent in people over the age of 65. The risk increases dramatically with age. Most people with vascular dementia also have some Alzheimer's disease. One difference between vascular dementia and Alzheimer's disease is that memory loss is one of the first symptoms of Alzheimer's; however in vascular dementia, memory problems typically occur much later in the disease process.

Increasing age is one of the biggest risk factors for vascular dementia. Other risk factors include history of stroke, high blood pressure and diabetes. Vascular dementia symptoms can vary, depending on the part of the brain that's affected. Symptoms may include:

- Confusion and agitation

- Problems with language and memory
- Unsteady gait, causing falls
- Urinary frequency, urgency or incontinence
- Personality and mood changes

Vascular dementia symptoms often begin suddenly and may worsen gradually, following a series of strokes or mini-strokes.

How is Vascular Dementia Diagnosed by Conventional Western Medicine?

Diagnosis is made based on medical history, physical examination and tests such as CT scan, MRI, MR angiogram, Doppler ultrasound or neuropsychological tests.

How is Vascular Dementia Treated by Conventional Western Medicine?

There is no cure for vascular dementia. Treatment focuses on preventing future strokes by controlling or avoiding the diseases and medical conditions that put people at high risk for stroke. The best treatment is prevention early in life, including eating a healthy diet, exercising, not smoking, moderately using alcohol, and maintaining a healthy weight.

Medications designed to treat the symptoms of Alzheimer's disease, such as donepezil (Aricept), galantamine (Razadyne), rivastigmine (Exelon), and memantine (Namenda), also appear to help people with vascular dementia.

What Causes Vascular Dementia According to Traditional Chinese Medicine?

1) Senility and Physical Weakness with Deficiency of the Kidney
2) Chronic Illness with Impaired Function of the Kidney, Spleen and Stomach
3) Internal Injury of Seven Emotions with Impaired Function of the Liver

How is Vascular Dementia Differentiated and Treated by Traditional Chinese Medicine?

1) <u>Insufficiency of Brain (Sea of Marrow)</u>

Symptoms: Impaired intellectual function, stiff and dull expression, amnesia, impairment of computational ability, listlessness, somnolence, dry hair and teeth, lumbar soreness, weak knees, dizziness, tinnitus, slight red and small tongue, and deep, thready and weak pulse.

Therapeutic Principle: To replenish marrow and essence, and tranquilize the mind.

Prescription: Modified Qi Fu Decoction.

Modifications: Could add Placenta Hominis (Zi He Che) 2g and Gelatinum Cornu Cervi (Lu Jiao Jiao) 9g. For remarkable lumbar soreness and weakness, add Radix Dipsaci Asperi (Xu Duan) 15g and Cortex Eucommiae Ulmoidis (Du Zhong) 12g.

2) *Deficiency of the Spleen and Kidney*

Symptoms: Dull expression, slowness of movement, forgetfulness, loss of computational ability, cognitive impairment, slurred speech, lumbar soreness and knee weakness, anorexia, indolence of speaking, saliva drooling from the mouth, pale and chubby tongue with white coating, deep and weak pulse.

Therapeutic Principle: To warm and nourish the spleen and kidney.

Prescription: Modified Huan Shao Pill.

Modifications: For remarkable yang deficiency of the spleen and kidney, use Jin Gui Shen Qi Pill or You Gui pill; for cold intolerance and cold limbs, add Radix Morindae officinalis (Ba Ji Tian) 12g and Radix Dipsaci Asperi (Xu Duan) 15g; for severe shortness of breath and fatigue, add Radix Astragali (Huang Qi) 12g and Placenta Hominis (Zi He Che) 2g.

3) *Deficiency of Liver Yin and Kidney Yin*

Symptoms: Reticence in temperament, dementia, vertigo, tinnitus, lumbar soreness and weak knees, dysphoria with feverish sensation in the chest, palms and soles, dry mouth, red tongue with little coating, thready and rapid pulse.

Therapeutic Principle: To nourish the liver and kidney.

Prescription: Modified Zhi Bai Di Huang Pill.

Modifications: For remarkable deficiency of kidney yin, add Zuo Gui Pill; for remarkable fire hyperactivity due to yin deficiency, add Cortex Moutan Radicis (Mu Dan Pi) 10g and Cortex Lycii Radicis (Di Gu Pi) 10g; for stirring-up of internal wind, add Concha Ostreae (Mu Li) 20g, Rhizoma Gastrodiae Elatae (Tian Ma) 9g, Ramulus Uncariae cum Uncis (Gou Teng) 12g and Mastodi Ossis Fossilia (Long Gu) 20g.

4) *Turbid Phlegm Blocking Heart Orifice*

Symptoms: Dull expression, impaired intellectual function, reticence, or crying and laughing for no particular reason, anorexia, dizziness, heaviness of the head, abdominal distention and fullness, excessive saliva and sputum, shortness of breath, fatigue, pale tongue with greasy coating, and slippery or soft pulse.

Therapeutic Principle: To strengthen the spleen, replenish qi, resolve phlegm and cause resuscitation.

Prescription: Modified Xi Xin Decoction.

Modifications: For remarkable deficiency of the spleen, add Sclerotium Poriae Cocos (Fu Ling) 12g and Radix Codonopsitis Pilosulae (Dang Shen) 9g; for hyperactive turbid phlegm, add Herba Eupatorii (Pei Lan) 9g and Pericarpium Trichosanthis (Gua Lou Pi) 9g, and increase the dosage of Pericarpium Citri Reticulatae (Chen Pi) and Rhizoma Pinelliae Ternatae (Ban Xia); for heat due to stagnant phlegm, add Radix Scutellariae Baicalensis (Huang Qin) 9g and Caulis Bambusae in Taeniam (Zhu Ru) 9g.

5) <u>Internal Obstruction of Blood Stasis</u>

Symptoms: Dull expression, dysphasia, or odd thinking, or eccentric conduct, forgetfulness, panic, scaly dry skin, dry mouth without desire to drink, dark tongue with ecchymosis,

Therapeutic Principle: To promote blood circulation, remove blood stasis, tranquilize the mind and cause resuscitation.

Prescription: Modified Tong Qiao Huo Xue Decoction.

Modifications: For concurrent deficiency of yin blood, add Radix Polygoni Multiflori (He Shou Wu) 15g, Radix Angelicae Sinensis (Dang Gui) 10g and Fructus Lycii (Gou Qi Zi) 10g; for concurrent deficiency of qi, add Radix Astragali (Huang Qi) 12g and Rhizoma Atractylodis Macrocephalae (Bai Zhu) 10g.

What Kinds of Chinese Patent Drugs are Available to Treat Vascular Dementia?

1) Xue Shuan Xin Mai Ning Pill: 4 pills each time, thrice daily.
2) Hua Bao Tong Yin Xing Ye Tablet: 2 tablets each time, thrice daily.
3) Chuan Xiong Qin Injection: 40-80ml each time, once daily.

9. Alzheimer's Disease (AD)

Dementia is a brain disorder with loss of intellectual and social abilities that seriously affects a person's ability to carry out daily activity. The most common form of dementia among older people is Alzheimer's disease (AD), which initially involves the parts of the brain that control thought, memory, and language.

About 4.5 million older Americans have Alzheimer's disease, a disorder that usually develops in people age 65 or older. About 5 percent of men and women ages 65 to 74 have Alzheimer's disease, and nearly half of those age 85 and older may have the disease.

Alzheimer's disease is named after Dr. Alois Alzheimer, a German neurologist. In 1906, he examined the brain of a woman who had died after years of progressive dementia. Her brain tissue showed abnormal clumps (now called amyloid plaques) and tangled bundles of fibers (now called neurofibrillary tangles). Today, these plaques and tangles are considered hallmarks of Alzheimer's disease.

The causes of Alzheimer's disease are poorly understood. Alzheimer's disease is a complex disease probably caused by a combination of factors such as infection or reduced circulation, and genetic susceptibility. Risk factors for this disease include age, heredity, sex, lifestyle, education levels, toxicity, head injury, and hormone replacement therapy. Alzheimer's disease is a slow disease, starting with mild memory problems and ending with severe brain damage. The course the disease takes and how fast changes occur vary from person to person. On average, patients with Alzheimer's disease live from 8 to 10 years after they are diagnosed, though some people may live with this disease for as many as 20 years.

Alzheimer's disease may start with slight memory loss and confusion, but it eventually leads to irreversible mental impairment that destroys a person's ability to remember, reason, learn and imagine. Symptoms of Alzheimer's disease may include:

- Increasing and persistent forgetfulness
- Difficulties with abstract thinking
- Difficulty finding the right word
- Disorientation
- Loss of judgment
- Difficulty performing familiar tasks
- Personality changes

How is Alzheimer's Disease Diagnosed by Conventional Western Medicine?

There's no single test to diagnose Alzheimer's disease. Typically, the diagnostic process is started by ruling out other diseases and conditions that also can cause memory loss. The diagnostic methods include:

- Medical history
- Basic medical tests, such as tests of blood, urine, or spinal fluid
- Mental status evaluation
- Neuropsychological testing
- Brain scans, including CT scan, MRI and a positron emission tomography (PET) scan

Alzheimer's can be diagnosed with complete accuracy only after death, using a microscopic examination of brain tissue, which checks for plaques and tangles.

How is Alzheimer's Disease Treated by Conventional Western Medicine?

Currently, there's no cure for Alzheimer's disease. Sometimes drugs are prescribed to improve symptoms that often accompany Alzheimer's disease, including sleeplessness, wandering, anxiety, agitation and depression. But only two varieties of medications have been proved to slow the cognitive decline associated with Alzheimer's disease. These include cholinesterase inhibitors such as donepezil (Aricept), rivastigmine (Exelon) and galantamine (Reminyl), and memantine (Namenda).

What Causes Alzheimer's Disease According to Traditional Chinese Medicine?

1) Phlegm Blocking the Orifice to the Brain due to Impaired Function of the Spleen in Transportation and Transformation
2) Emptiness of Marrow and Brain due to Congenital Insufficiency and Deficiency of Liver Yin and Kidney Yin
3) Deficiency of Qi and Blood Leading to the Malnourished Brain
4) Emotional Injury Resulting in Internal Stagnation of Qi
5) Obstruction of the Orifice to the Brain due to Qi Stagnation and Blood Stasis

How is Alzheimer's Disease Differentiated and Treated by Traditional Chinese Medicine?

1) <u>Emptiness of Marrow and Brain (Sea of Marrow)</u>

Symptoms: Failing memory, impairment of expressive and comprehensive language, slowness of movement, or childish deeds, dull facial expression, social withdrawal, shaking of the head and tremor of the limbs, vertigo, tinnitus, impaired hearing, scanty hair and teeth, pale complexion, red tongue with little coating, or smooth tongue with no coating, deep, thready and forceless pulse.

Therapeutic Principle: To nourish the liver and kidney, replenish marrow and brains.

Prescription: Modified Qi Fu Decoction.

Modifications: Add Gelatinum Cornu Cervi (Lu Jiao Jiao) 9g, Colla Testudinis Plastri (Gui Ban Jiao) 9g, Gelatinum Corii Asini (E Jiao) 9g and Placenta Hominis (Zi He Che) 2g.

2) <u>Deficiency of Qi and Blood</u>

Symptoms: Dull facial expression, amnesia, cognitive impairment, loss of computational ability, somnolence, lassitude, lusterless complexion, shortness of breath, no desire to speak, palpitation, insomnia, anorexia, loose stools, pale and chubby tongue with teeth marks on its margin, thin and white tongue coating, thready and weak pulse.

Therapeutic Principle: To replenish qi, nourish blood, and tranquilize the mind.

Prescription: Modified Ba Zhen Decoction.

Modifications: Add Radix Polygalae Tenuifoliae (Yuan Zhi) 9g and Semen Ziziphi Spinosae (Suan Zao Ren) 15g.

3) <u>Liver Qi Stagnation with Hyperactivity of Fire</u>

Symptoms: Impaired memory, frequent sighing, irritability, suspiciousness, misgivings, childish words and deeds, headache, vertigo, restlessness, insomnia, flushed face, conjunctival congestion, dry mouth, dry and red tongue with yellow coating, taut and rapid pulse.

Therapeutic Principle: To soothe the live, disperse stagnant liver qi, reduce fire and tranquilize the mind.

Prescription: Dan Zhi Xiao Yao Powder.

4) <u>Phlegm Disturbing the Mind</u>

Symptoms: Heaviness of the head, sallow complexion, fatigue, lassitude, lethargy, depression, wheezing sound in the throat, dull facial expression, reticence, impaired intellectual function (difficulty with problem-solving and ordinary activities), disorientation, cognitive impairment, impairment of expressive and comprehensive language, crying and laughing for no particular reason, no judgment about good and bad, lost interest in human appearances, social withdrawal, excessive saliva and sputum, saliva drooling from the mouth, abdominal distention, pale and chubby tongue with teeth marks and greasy coating, and slippery pulse.

Therapeutic Principle: To invigorate the spleen, resolve phlegm, open the orifices and induce resuscitation.

Prescription: Modified Zhi Mi Decoction supplemented with Add Radix Bupleuri (Chai Hu) 9g, Radix Paeoniae Alba (Bai Shao Yao) 9g, Semen Ziziphi Spinosae (Suan Zao Ren) 15g, Semen Biotae Orientalis (Bai Zi Ren) 15g, and Radix Polygalae Tenuifoliae (Yuan Zhi) 9g. Or use modified Xi Xin Decoction.

Modifications: For excessive saliva drooling from the mouth, add Bulbus Fritillariae Thunbergii (Zhe Bei Mu) 9g.

5) <u>Blood Stasis Obstructing the Orifice to the Brain</u>

Symptoms: Dull facial expression, slurred speech, cognitive impairment, slowness of response, amnesia, irritability, or delusions and insomnia, stare, black complexion, dark purple lips and nails, scaly dry skin, dark eyes, dark purple tongue with ecchymosis and petechiae, or varicosity under the tongue, and thready, rough or slow pulse.

Therapeutic Principle: To promote blood circulation, remove blood stasis, open the orifices and tranquilize the mind.

Prescription: Modified Tong Qiao Huo Xue Decoction.

Modifications: Add Rhizoma Acori Tatarinowii (Shi Chang Pu) 9g, Radix Curcumae (Yu Jin) 10g, Radix et Caulis Jixueteng (Ji Xue Teng) 12g, Gelatinum Corii Asini (E Jiao) 9g, Carapax Trionycis (Bie Jia) 20g, and Radix Polygoni Multiflori (He Shou Wu) 15g.

6) Stagnation of Liver Qi

Symptoms: Vexation, irritability, depression, no desire to speak, hypochondriac distention and pain, dark tongue with ecchymosis and sticky coating, taut and slippery pulse.

Therapeutic Principle: To soothe the liver, promote qi and blood circulation, and resolve phlegm.

Prescription: Modified Chai Hu Shu Gan Powder and Tao Hong Si Wu Decoction.

Modifications: For dampness and phlegm, add Rhizoma Pinelliae Ternatae (Ban Xia) 9g and Rhizoma Acori Tatarinowii (Shi Chang Pu) 9g; for deficiency of the spleen, add Rhizoma Atractylodis Macrocephalae (Bai Zhu) 10g and Sclerotium Poriae Cocos (Fu Ling) 12g.

7) Deficiency of Liver Yin and Kidney Yin

Symptoms: Vertigo, tinnitus, numbness and tingling or trembling of the hands and feet, impaired intellectual function and coordination, amnesia, spiritlessness of the eyes, dull facial expression, malar flushing, night sweats, scaly dry skin, irritability, lumbar soreness and weak knees, dysphoria with feverish sensation in the chest, palms and soles, dry mouth, red tongue with little coating, thready and rapid pulse.

Therapeutic Principle: To nourish the liver and kidney, promote blood circulation and resolve phlegm.

Prescription: Modified Liu Wei Di Huang Pill.

Modifications: For concurrent deficiency of the spleen, add Rhizoma Pinelliae Ternatae (Ban Xia) 9g, Rhizoma Dioscoreae (Shan Yao) 15g and Pericarpium Citri Reticulatae (Chen Pi) 6g; for fire hyperactivity due to yin deficiency, add Rhizoma Anemarrhenae (Zhi Mu) 10g, Cortex Phellodendri (Huang Bai) 9g, Cortex Moutan Radicis (Mu Dan Pi) 10g and Cortex Lycii Radicis (Di Gu Pi) 10g; for vertigo, add Magnetitum (Ci Shi) 12g, Rhizoma Gastrodiae Elatae (Tian Ma) 9g, Ramulus Uncariae cum Uncis (Gou Teng) 12g and Fructus Ligustri Lucidi (Nu Zhen Zi) 12g; for dry mouth and constipation, add Fructus Mori Alba (Sang Shen) 12g, Semen Biotae Orientalis (Bai Zi Ren) 12g and Radix Trichosanthis (Tian Hua Fen) 12g; for irritability and a stiff tongue, add Concha Margaritiferae (Zhen Zhu Mu) 20g and Bulbus Lilii (Bai He) 12g; for remarkable deficiency of kidney yin, add Zuo Gui Pill

8) Deficiency of Spleen Yang and Kidney Yang

Symptoms: Slowness of movement, dull facial expression, slurred speech, or even aphasia, problems with word finding and concentration, amnesia, numbness of the limbs, loss of mental and physical sharpness and coordination, cold limbs, pale complexion, lumbar soreness, weak knees, cold pain in the lower abdomen, polyuria with clear urine, pale and chubby tongue with teeth marks on its margin, and deep, slow and forceless pulse.

Therapeutic Principle: To warm and nourish the spleen and kidney.

Prescription: Modified Shi Pi Decoction and Jin Gui Shen Qi Pill.

Modifications: For dizziness and tinnitus, add Herba Taxilli (Sang Ji Sheng) 12g, Fructus Lycii (Gou Qi Zi) 10g, Rhizoma Gastrodiae Elatae (Tian Ma) 9g and Radix Dipsaci Asperi (Xu Duan) 12g; for cold intolerance and cold limbs, add Radix Morindae officinalis (Ba Ji Tian) 12g and Radix Dipsaci Asperi (Xu Duan) 15g; for severe shortness of breath and fatigue, add Radix Astragali (Huang Qi) 12g and Placenta Hominis (Zi He Che) 2g.

9) <u>Deficiency of the Heart and Spleen</u>

Symptoms: Disorientation, thought disorder, melancholy, excessive stillness, scanty speech, slowness of movement, social withdrawal, spiritlessness, amnesia, spontaneous perspiration, lassitude, weight loss, palpitations, panic, shortness of breath on exertion, decreased sense of smell and taste, pale and large tongue with thin coating, and thready and weak pulse.

Therapeutic Principle: To nourish the heart, invigorate the spleen and tranquilize the mind.

Prescription: Modified Yang Xin Decoction.

Modifications: For severe blood deficiency, add Radix Rehmanniae Praeparatae (Shu Di Huang) 10g, Radix Paeoniae Alba (Bai Shao Yao) 10g and Gelatinum Corii Asini (E Jiao) 10g; for severe insomnia, add Cortex Albizziae Julibrissin (He Huan Pi) 12g and Caulis Polygoni Multiflori (Ye Jiao Teng) 20g; for abdominal distention, anorexia and greasy tongue coating, add Pericarpium Citri Reticulatae (Chen Pi) 6g and Cortex Magnoliae Officinalis (Hou Po) 9g.

10) <u>Hyperactivity of Liver Yang</u>

Symptoms: Headache, dizziness, flushed face and red eyes, irritability, restless, personality changes (usually paranoid), insomnia, dreamfulness, stiff tongue with slurred speech, numbness and tingling of the limbs, or deviation of the mouth and eyes, hemiplegia, red tongue with yellow coating, taut and slippery or taut and rapid pulse.

Therapeutic Principle: To soothe the liver, subdue yang and cause resuscitation.

Prescription: Modified Tian Ma Gou Teng Decoction.

Modifications: For constipation, add Radix et Rhizoma Rhei (Da Huang) 6g; for hypochondriac distention and pain, add Pericarpium Citri Reticulatae Viride (Qing Pi) 9g and Rhizoma Corydalis (Yan Hu Suo) 9g; for restlessness and irritability, add Concha Ostreae (Mu Li) 12g and Mastodi Ossis Fossilia (Long Gu) 15g.

11) Hyperactivity of Heart Fire

Symptoms: Headache, vexation, anxiety, red face and lips, insomnia, dreamfulness, impairment of expressive and comprehensive language, eccentric laughing and crying, thought disorder, rash behavior, frequent urination with dark urine, constipation, red tongue tip, thin and yellow tongue coating, taut and rapid pulse.

Therapeutic Principle: To clear away heart fire and tranquilize the mind.

Prescription: Modified Xie Xin Decoction and Dao Chi Powder.

Modifications: For dry mouth and throat, add Radix Ophiopogonis Japonici (Mai Dong) 12g, Tuber Asparagi Cochinchinensis (Tian Dong) 12g, Bulbus Lilii (Bai He) 12g and Herba Dendrobii (Shi Hu) 10g; for insomnia and dreamful sleep, add Semen Ziziphi Spinosae (Suan Zao Ren) 12g, Caulis Polygoni Multiflori (Ye Jiao Teng) 15g and Sclerotium Poriae Circum Radicem Pini (Fu Shen) 10g.

What Kinds of Chinese Patent Drugs are Available to Treat Alzheimer's Disease?

1) Xue Shuan Xin Mai Ning Pill: 4 pills each time, thrice daily.
2) Hua Bao Tong Yin Xing Ye Tablet: 2 tablets each time, thrice daily.
3) Chuan Xiong Qin Injection: 40-80ml each time, once daily.

10. Myasthenia Gravis (MG)

Myasthenia gravis is a chronic autoimmune neuromuscular disease characterized by varying degrees of weakness of the skeletal (voluntary) muscles of the body. The hallmark of myasthenia gravis is muscle weakness that increases during periods of activity and improves after periods of rest. Certain muscles such as those of the face, eyes, arms and legs, and those involved in chewing, swallowing and talking are often involved in the disorder. The muscles that control breathing and neck and limb movements may also be affected.

Myasthenia gravis is caused by a defect in the transmission of nerve impulses to muscles. It occurs when normal communication between the nerve and muscle is interrupted at the neuromuscular junction. In myasthenia gravis, for unknown reasons, the immune system produces antibodies that block, alter, or destroy the receptors for acetylcholine at the neuromuscular junction, which prevents the muscle contraction from occurring.

The relationship between the thymus gland and myasthenia gravis is not yet fully understood. Sometimes myasthenia gravis is associated with lymphoid hyperplasia, thymomas or tumors of the thymus gland. Some factors can make myasthenia gravis worse, including fatigue, illness, stress, extreme heat, and some medications, such as beta blockers, calcium channel blockers, quinine and some antibiotics.

In the United States, myasthenia gravis affects about 14 people in 100,000. It is more common in women younger than 40 or older than 70, and in men older than 50. However, myasthenia gravis can occur at any age. Males are more often affected than females. Myasthenia gravis can affect any of voluntary muscles. Signs and symptoms may include:

- Facial muscle weakness, including drooping eyelids (ptosis)
- Double vision (diplopia)
- Difficulty in breathing, talking, chewing or swallowing
- Muscle weakness in the arms or legs
- Fatigue brought on by repetitive motions

How is Myasthenia Gravis Diagnosed by Conventional Western Medicine?

The first steps of diagnosing myasthenia gravis include a review of the individual's medical history, and physical and neurological examinations. Tests to confirm the diagnosis may include neurological examination, blood analysis, edrophonium test, nerve conduction studies and single-fiber electromyography.

How is Myasthenia Gravis Treated by Conventional Western Medicine?

There are several therapies available to help reduce and improve muscle weakness:

- Medications: Cholinesterase inhibitors, such as pyridostigmine (Mestinon) and neostigmine (Prostigmin); Corticosteroids; other medications that alter the immune system, such as azathioprine (Imuran), mycophenolate mofetil (CellCept), cyclophosphamide (Cytoxan) or cyclosporine (Sandimmune, Neoral)
- Surgery: Thymectomy
- Plasmapheresis
- Intravenous immune globulin
- Physical therapy and occupational therapy

Myasthenia crisis is a condition of extreme muscle weakness, particularly of the diaphragm and chest muscles that support breathing. In severe crisis, a person may have to be placed on a ventilator to assist breathing until muscle strength returns with treatment.

What Causes Myasthenia Gravis According to Traditional Chinese Medicine?

1) Pathogenic Dampness or Improper Diet, with Damp-Heat Invading Channels
2) Congenital Insufficiency
3) Chronic Illness or Overstrain

How is Myasthenia Gravis Differentiated and Treated by Traditional Chinese Medicine?

1) <u>Deficiency of Spleen Qi</u>

Symptoms: Lassitude, weakness, ptosis, sallow complexion, feeble voice, anorexia, abdominal distention that is alleviated by pressing, loose stools, pale, chubby and tender tongue with thin and white coating, thready and weak pulse.

Therapeutic Principle: To strengthen the spleen and replenish qi.

Prescription: Modified Bu Zhong Yi Qi Decoction.

Modifications: For abundant sputum, feeling of oppression in the chest, general heaviness and sensation of heaviness in the head, add Rhizoma Pinelliae Ternatae (Ban Xia) 9g and Folium Perillae Frutescentis (Su Ye) 9g; for spleen deficiency generating dampness, add Fructus Amomi Villosi (Sha Ren) 5g and Semen Coicis (Yi Yi Ren) 15g; for anorexia, add Fructus Hordei Germinatus (Mai Ya) 12g and Fructus Germinatus Oryzae Sativae (Gu Ya) 12g; for excessive sweats, add Radix Saposhnikoviae Divaricatae (Fang Feng) 9g and Radix Oryzae Glutinosae (Nuo Dao Gen Xu) 20g; for sore throat and cough, add Radix Scrophulariae Ningpoensis (Xuan Shen) 12g, Radix Platycodi Grandiflori (Jie Geng) 6g and Bulbus Fritillariae Thunbergii (Zhe Bei Mu) 9g.

2) <u>Deficiency of Spleen Yang and Kidney Yang</u>

Symptoms: Lassitude and weakness of limbs, difficulty in raising head, coldness of the body and limbs, pale complexion, puffy face, lumbar soreness, weak knees, cold pain in the lower abdomen, undigested food in the stools, polyuria with clear urine, pale and chubby tongue with teeth marks on its margin, and deep, slow and forceless pulse.

Therapeutic Principle: To warm and nourish the spleen and kidney.

Prescription: Modified You Gui Decoction.

Modifications: For vertigo and tinnitus, add Carapax Trionycis (Bie Jia) 20g, Carapax et Plastrum Testudinis (Gui Ban) 20g and Radix Polygoni Multiflori (He Shou Wu) 15g; for remarkable yang deficiency with cold body and cold limbs, add Cornu Cervi Degelatinatum (Lu Jiao Shuang) 12g, Herba Epimedii (Yin Yang Huo) 12g and Radix Morindae officinalis (Ba Ji Tian) 12g; for undigested food in the stools, add Fructus Psoraleae Corylifoliae (Bu Gu Zhi) 9g and Semen Myristicae Fragrantis (Rou Dou Kou) 9g.

3) Deficiency of Both Qi and Blood

Symptoms: Stare, strabismus and difficulty in opening eyes (weakness of extraocular muscles), atrophy of muscles, lusterless complexion and nails, dizziness, listlessness, lassitude, indolence of speaking, pale and small tongue with little or thin and white coating, thready and weak pulse.

Therapeutic Principle: To replenish qi and nourish blood.

Prescription: Modified Gui Pi Decoction.

Modifications: For insomnia and dreamfulness, add Radix Salviae Miltiorrhizae (Dan Shen) 10g, Flos Albizziae Julibrissin (He Huan Hua) 9g and Caulis Polygoni Multiflori (Ye Jiao Teng) 20g; for constipation, add Semen Cannabis Sativae (Huo Ma Ren) 12g and Radix Scrophulariae Ningpoensis (Xuan Shen) 12g.

4) Deficiency of Liver Yin and Kidney Yin

Symptoms: Lassitude, weakness, ptosis, diplopia, dry mouth, anorexia, lumbar soreness, weak knees, dizziness, tinnitus, insomnia, amnesia, constipation, slight red tongue with little or peeled coating, thready and weak or thready and rapid pulse.

Therapeutic Principle: To nourish the liver and kidney.

Prescription: Modified Yi Guan Decoction.

Modifications: For concurrent hyperactivity of yang, add Concha Haliotidis (Shi Jue Ming) 20g and Ramulus Uncariae cum Uncis (Gou Teng) 12g; for deficient heat or excessive sweats, add Cortex Moutan Radicis (Mu Dan Pi) 10g and Rhizoma Anemarrhenae (Zhi Mu) 10g; for leg weakness, add Radix Achyranthis Bidentatae (Niu Xi) 12g.

5) Qi Deficiency and Blood Stasis

Symptoms: Weakness and numbness of the limbs with localized pricking pain and ecchymosis, listlessness, lassitude, dark purple tongue, deficiency and rough pulse.

Therapeutic Principle: To replenish qi and promote blood circulation.

Prescription: Modified Bu Yang Huan Wu Decoction.

Modifications: For remarkable deficiency of qi, add Radix Codonopsitis Pilosulae (Dang Shen) 9g and Rhizoma Atractylodis Macrocephalae (Bai Zhu) 10g; for concurrent yin deficiency, add Fructus Lycii (Gou Qi Zi) 10g and Radix Ophiopogonis Japonici (Mai Dong) 12g.

6) Damp-Heat Blocking Collaterals

Symptoms: Weakness, soreness and sensation of distention in the limbs; or ptosis, general heavy sensation, distending sensation in the chest and abdomen, yellow and greasy tongue coating, and slippery pulse.

Therapeutic Principle: To clear away heat, eliminate dampness and activate collaterals.

Prescription: Modified Jia Wei Er Miao Powder.

Modifications: For excessive heat, add Talcum (Hua Shi Fen) 10g and Radix Scutellariae Baicalensis (Huang Qin) 9g; for excessive dampness, add Fructus Amomi Kravanh (Bai Dou Kou) 5g and Herba Eupatorii (Pei Lan) 9g.

What Kinds of Chinese Patent Drugs are Available to Treat Myasthenia Gravis?

1) Bu Zhong Yi Chi Pill: 6g each time, twice daily.
2) Kun Ming Shan Hai Tang Tablet: 2 tablets each time, thrice daily.

Chapter 9: Psychiatric Disorders

1. Insomnia/Dyssomnias

A. Etiology and Pathogenesis

1) Improper Diet

2) Emotional Disorder

3) Overstrain or Too Much Leisure

4) Weak Constitution after Illness

5) Senility

6) Congenital Insufficiency

B. Syndrome Differentiation and Treatment

1) <u>Generation of Fire due to Liver Qi Stagnation</u>

Symptoms: Anxiety, irritability, dreamful sleep, insomnia or even inability to fall asleep all night, dizziness, distending sensation in the head, conjunctival congestion, tinnitus, dry mouth with bitter taste, anorexia, constipation, dark urine, red tongue with yellow coating, taut and rapid pulse.

Therapeutic Principle: To soothe the liver, purge fire, and tranquilize the mind.

Prescription: Modified Long Dan Xie Gan Decoction.

Modifications: For sensation of stuffiness in the chest, distention in hypochondriac region and frequent sighing, add Rhizoma Cyperi Rotundi (Xiang Fu) 10g, Radix Curcumae (Yu Jin) 10g and Fructus Citri Sarcodactyli (Fo Shou) 9g; for vertigo, splitting headache, constipation, irritability and anger, use Dang Gui Long Hui Pill.

2) <u>Internal Disturbance of Phlegm-Heat</u>

Symptoms: Vexation, insomnia, feeling of oppression in the chest, epigastric distention, nausea, belching, bitter taste in the mouth, heavy sensation in the head, vertigo, slight red tongue with yellow and greasy coating, slippery and rapid pulse.

Therapeutic Principle: To clear away heat, resolve phlegm, regulate the stomach and tranquilize the mind.

Prescription: Modified Huang Lian Wen Dan Decoction.

Modifications: For palpitation and fright, add Mastodi Dentis Fossilia (Long Chi) 20g, Concha Margaritiferae (Zhen Zhu Mu) 20g and Magnetitum (Ci Shi) 15g; for sensation of stuffiness in the chest, belching, abdominal distention and fullness, dyschezia, greasy tongue coating and slippery pulse, add Ban Xia Shu Mi Decoction; for retention of food, gastric discomfort, belching with rotten odor, acid regurgitation and distending pain in the abdomen, add Massa Medicata Fermentata (Shen Qu) 12g, Fructus Crataegi (Shan Zha) 12g and Semen Raphani Sativi (Lai Fu Zi) 9g; for insomnia and constipation, add Radix et Rhizoma Rhei Praeparatae (Zhi Da Huang) 9g.

3) <u>Hyperactivity of Heart Fire</u>

Symptoms: Vexation, insomnia, restlessness, anxiety, dry mouth and tongue, oliguria with dark urine, aphthous stomatitis, red tongue tip, thin and yellow tongue coating, and rapid pulse.

Therapeutic Principle: To clear away heart fire, soothe the heart and tranquilize the mind.

Prescription: Modified Zhu Sha An Shen Pill.

Modifications: Add Radix Scutellariae Baicalensis (Huang Qin) 9g and Fructus Gardeniae Jasminoidis (Zhi Zi) 9g to clear away heart fire and soothe the heart; for constipation and dark urine, add Herba Lophatheri Gracilis (Dan Zhu Ye) 10g, Radix et Rhizoma Rhei (Da Huang) 6g and Plumula Nelumbinis Nuciferae (Lian Zi Xin) 2g; for persistent insomnia, vexation, slight dark tongue with petechiae, use Xue Fu Zhu Yu Decoction.

4) <u>Hyperactivity of Fire due to Yin Deficiency</u>

Symptoms: Vexation, insomnia, difficulty in falling asleep, palpitation, dreamfulness, dizziness, tinnitus, lumbar soreness and weak knees, hectic fever, night sweats, dysphoria with feverish sensation in the chest, palms and soles, amnesia, dry throat and mouth, seminal emission, or menstrual irregularities, red tongue with little coating, thready and rapid pulse.

Therapeutic Principle: To nourish yin, purge fire, clear heart fire and tranquilize the mind.

Prescription: Modified Liu Wei Di Huang Pill and Huang Lian E Jiao Decoction.

Modifications: For vexation, insomnia with inability to fall asleep all night, add Mastodi Dentis Fossilia (Long Chi) 20g, Magnetitum (Ci Shi) 15g and Mastodi Ossis Fossilia (Long Gu) 20g.

5) <u>Deficiency of the Heart and Spleen</u>

Symptoms: Difficulty in falling asleep, dreamful and restless sleep, palpitation, amnesia, listlessness, anorexia, vertigo, lassitude of the limbs, abdominal distention, loose stools, lusterless complexion, pale tongue with thin coating, thready and forceless pulse.

Therapeutic Principle: To nourish the heart, invigorate the spleen and tranquilize the mind.

Prescription: Modified Gui Pi Decoction.

Modifications: For severe insomnia, add Fructus Schisandrae Chinensis (Wu Wei Zi) 5g, Caulis Polygoni Multiflori (Ye Jiao Teng) 20g, Flos Albizziae Julibrissin (He Huan Hua) 9g, Semen Biotae Orientalis (Bai Zi Ren) 15g, Mastodi Ossis Fossilia (Long Gu) 20g and Concha Ostreae (Mu Li) 20g; for severe blood deficiency, add Radix Rehmanniae Praeparatae (Shu Di Huang) 20g, Gelatinum Corii Asini (E Jiao) 9g and Radix Paeoniae Alba (Bai Shao Yao) 9g; for epigastric distention, anorexia, slippery and greasy tongue coating, add Rhizoma Pinelliae Ternatae (Ban Xia) 9g, Pericarpium Citri Reticulatae (Chen Pi) 6g, Sclerotium Poriae Cocos (Fu Ling) 12g and Cortex Magnoliae Officinalis (Hou Po) 9g.

6) <u>Deficiency of Heart Qi and Gallbladder Qi</u>

Symptoms: Vexation, restlessness, insomnia, dreamful and restless sleep, timidity, panic, palpitation, shortness of breath, spontaneous sweating, lassitude, pale tongue, taut and thready pulse.

Therapeutic Principle: To replenish qi, relieve panic and tranquilize the mind.

Prescription: Modified An Shen Ding Zhi Pill and Suan Zao Ren Decoction.

Modifications: For severe palpitation, panic and anxiety, add Mastodi Ossis Fossilia (Long Gu) 20g, Concha Ostreae (Mu Li) 20g and Cinnabaris (Zhu Sha) 0.5g; for blood deficiency of the liver and heart with panic, palpitation and sweating, add Radix Paeoniae Alba (Bai Shao Yao) 9g, Radix Angelicae Sinensis (Dan Gui) 10g and Radix Astragali (Huang Qi) 12g.

2. Mood Disorders (Depression and Mania)

A. Etiology and Pathogenesis

1) Smoldering Anger, with Stagnation of Liver Qi
2) Depression and Pensiveness, with Impaired Function of the Spleen in Transportation
3) Emotional Disturbance, with Malnourished Heart
4) Imbalance of Yin and Yang
5) Mental Confusion due to Phlegm
6) Pathogenic Fire Attacking the Heart
7) Stagnation of Qi and Blood Stasis

B. Syndrome Differentiation and Treatment

1) Depression

(1) <u>Stagnation of Liver Qi</u>

Symptoms: Mental depression, restlessness, fullness and stuffiness in the chest, distending and wandering pain in the hypochondrium, epigastric stuffiness, belching, anorexia, irregular bowel movement, slight red tongue with thin and greasy coating, and taut pulse.

Therapeutic Principle: To soothe the liver, relieve stagnation and regulate Middle Warmer Qi.

Prescription: Modified Chai Hu Shu Gan Powder.

Modifications: For frequent belching, epigastric stuffiness and discomfort, add Flos Inulae (Xuan Fu Hua) 9g, Ochra Haematitum (Dai Zhe Shi) 10g, Rhizoma Pinelliae Ternatae (Ban Xia) 9g and Pericarpium Citri Reticulatae (Chen Pi) 6g; for retention of food and abdominal distention, add Massa Medicata Fermentata (Shen Qu) 10g, Fructus Hordei Germinatus (Mai Ya) 12g, Fructus Crataegi (Shan Zha) 12g and Endothelium Corneum Gigeriae Galli (Ji Nei Jin) 9g; for blood stasis with pricking pain in the chest and hypochondrium, petechiae and ecchymosis on the tongue, add Radix Angelicae Sinensis (Dang Gui) 10g, Radix Salviae Miltiorrhizae (Dan Shen) 10g, Radix Curcumae (Yu Jin) 10g, Flos Carthami Tinctorii (Hong Hua) 9g and Rhizoma Corydalis (Yan Hu Suo) 9g.

(2) <u>Stagnation of Qi Transforming into Fire</u>

Symptoms: Irascible temperament, distention and fullness in the chest and hypochondrium, dry mouth with bitter taste, or headache, conjunctival congestion, tinnitus, or gastric discomfort, acid regurgitation, constipation, red tongue with yellow coating, taut and rapid pulse.

Therapeutic Principle: To soothe the liver, relieve stagnation and purge liver fire.

Prescription: Modified Dan Zhi Xiao Yao Powder.

Modifications: For liver fire attacking the stomach with hypochondriac pain, bitter taste in the mouth, gastric discomfort, acid regurgitation, belching and vomiting, add Rhizoma Coptidis (Huang Lian) 6g, Fructus Evodiae Rutaecarpae (Wu Zhu Yu) 3g, Concha Arcae (Wa Leng Zi) 12g and Concha Ostreae (Mu Li) 20g; for flaming-up of liver fire with headache, conjunctival congestion and tinnitus, add Flos Chrysanthemi Morifolii (Ju Hua) 12g, Ramulus Uncariae cum Uncis (Gou Teng) 12g and Fructus Tribuli (Ci Ji Li) 9g; for excessive heat impairing yin with red tongue with little coating, thready and rapid pulse, add Radix Rehmanniae (Di Huang) 12g, Radix Ophiopogonis Japonici (Mai Dong) 10g and Rhizoma Dioscoreae (Shan Yao) 15g.

(3) <u>Stagnation of Qi and Retention of Phlegm</u>

Symptoms: Mental depression, sensation of stuffiness in the chest, distention and fullness in the hypochondrium, feeling of a foreign body in the throat, which is difficult to swallow or spit out; white and greasy tongue coating, taut and slippery pulse.

Therapeutic Principle: To promote circulation of qi, alleviate depression, resolve phlegm and relieve stagnation.

Prescription: Modified Ban Xia Hou Po Decoction.

Modifications: For excessive retention of phlegm, add Concha Meretricis seu Cyclinae (Hai Ge Qiao) 10g, Radix Asteris Tatarici (Zi Wan) 9g, Bulbus Fritillariae Cirrhosae (Bei Mu) 9g and Pericarpium Citri Reticulatae (Chen Pi) 6g; for irritability, red tongue with yellow coating, add Caulis Bambusae in Taeniam (Zhu Ru) 9g, Fructus Trichosanthis (Gua Lou) 12g, Radix Scutellariae Baicalensis (Huang Qin) 9g and Rhizoma Coptidis (Huang Lian) 6g; for chronic illness with blood stasis, stabbing pain in the chest and hypochondrium, dark purple tongue with petechiae and ecchymosis, and rough pulse, add Radix Curcumae (Yu Jin) 10g, Radix Salviae Miltiorrhizae (Dan Shen) 10g, Lignum Dalbergiae Odoriferae (Jiang Xiang) 5g and Rhizoma Curcumae Longae (Jiang Huang) 6g.

(4) <u>Deficiency of Qi and Retention of Phlegm</u>

Symptoms: Apathetic and indifferent expression, reticence, stare, discouragement, confusion, feeling of guilt, sallow complexion, loose stools and clear urine, pale and chubby tongue with white and greasy coating, and slippery or weak and forceless pulse.

Therapeutic Principle: To replenish qi, strengthen the spleen, relieve phlegm and induce resuscitation.

Prescription: Modified Si Jun Zi Decoction and Di Tan Decoction.

Modifications: For severe confusion and dull facial expression, use Su He Xiang Pill.

(5) <u>Stagnation of Blood</u>

Symptoms: Mental depression, irritability, headache, insomnia, amnesia, or pain in the chest and hypochondrium, or cold or feverish sensation in certain part of the body, dark purple tongue with petechiae and ecchymosis, and taut or rough pulse.

Therapeutic Principle: To promote blood circulation, remove blood stasis, regulate qi and alleviate depression.

Prescription: Modified Xue Fu Zhu Yu Decoction.

Modifications: For concurrent deficiency of qi, add Radix Codonopsitis Pilosulae (Dang Shen) 9g, Radix Astragali (Huang Qi) 12g and Rhizoma Atractylodis Macrocephalae (Bai Zhu) 10g.

(6) <u>Mental Confusion due to Melancholy</u>

Symptoms: Trance, restlessness, suspiciousness, timidity, sentimentality, depression, or frequent stretching and yawning or unrestrained flourishing and shouting, pale tongue with thin and white coating, and taut pulse.

Therapeutic Principle: To relieve the acute case with sweat and lubricant herbs, nourish the heart and tranquilize the mind.

Prescription: Modified Gan Mai Da Zao Decoction.

Modifications: For pathogenic internal wind due to deficiency of blood with convulsion or tremor of the hands and feet, add Radix Angelicae Sinensis (Dang Gui) 10g, Radix Rehmanniae (Di Huang) 12g, Concha Margaritiferae (Zhen Zhu Mu) 20g and Ramulus Uncariae cum Uncis (Gou Teng) 12gp; for restlessness and insomnia, add Semen Ziziphi Spinosae (Suan Zao Ren) 12g, Semen Biotae Orientalis (Bai Zi Ren) 12g, Sclerotium Poriae Circum Radicem Pini (Fu Shen) 10g and Radix Polygoni Multiflori (He Shou Wu) 12g; for dyspnea and adverse flow of qi, add Wu Mo Yin Zi; for palpitation, insomnia and restlessness, use Ren Shen Hu Po Pill.

(7) <u>Deficiency of the Heart and Spleen</u>

Symptoms: Suspiciousness, dizziness, listlessness, palpitation, timidity, insomnia, amnesia, anorexia, lusterless complexion, pale tongue with thin and white coating, and thready pulse.

Therapeutic Principle: To invigorate the spleen, nourish the heart, and replenish qi and blood.

Prescription: Modified Gui Pi Decoction.

Modifications: For sensation of stuffiness in the chest and emotional upsets, add Radix Curcumae (Yu Jin) 10g and Fructus Citri Sarcodactyli (Fo Shou) 9g; for headache, add Rhizoma Ligustici Chuanxiong (Chuan Xiong) 9g and Tribulus Terrestris Fructus (Bai Ji Li) 9g.

(8) <u>Deficiency of Heart Yin and Kidney Yin</u>

Symptoms: Restlessness, palpitation, amnesia, insomnia, dreamfulness, dysphoria with feverish sensation in the chest, palms and soles, night sweating, dry mouth and throat, red tongue with little coating, thready and rapid pulse.

Therapeutic Principle: To nourish the heart and kidney, and tranquilize the mind.

Prescription: Modified Tian Wang Bu Xin Pill and Liu Wei Di Huang Pill.

Modifications: For incoordination between the heart and kidney with vexation, insomnia, dreamfulness and seminal emission, add Rhizoma Coptidis (Huang Lian) 5g and Cortex Cinnamomi Cassiae (Rou Gui) 3g; for frequent seminal emission, add Semen Euryales Ferocis (Qian Shi) 12g, Stamen Nelumbinis Nuciferae (Lian Xu) 3g and Fructus Rosae Laevigatae (Jin Ying Zi)10g.

2) Mania

(1) <u>Phlegm-Fire Disturbing the Heart</u>

Symptoms: Irascible temperament, headache, insomnia, angry stare, flushed face, conjunctival congestion; sudden onset of madness and violent rage, muddled speech, climbing walls and roofs, grandiosity, extraordinary strength, racket and scolding, not caring about relationship, or smashing things and hitting people, eccentric laugh and cry, thirst with preference to cold drinks, constipation, dark urine, refusing to eat and sleep, crimson tongue with yellow and greasy coating, taut and slippery or slippery, rapid and forceful pulse.

Therapeutic Principle: To purge fire, relieve phlegm and tranquilize the mind.

Prescription: Modified Xie Xin Decoction and Meng Shi Gun Tan Pill.

Modifications: For lingering phlegm-fire after treatment, with relatively clear consciousness, vexation, insomnia, abnormal laugh and cry, use Wen Dan Decoction and Zhu Sha An Shen Pill.

(2) Hyperactivity of Fire due to Yin Deficiency

Symptoms: Chronic manic psychosis that is gradually alleviated, listlessness, emotional instability, nervousness, anxiety, palpitation, panic, occasional mania, irritability, insomnia, feverish sensation in the chest, palms and soles, emaciation, oliguria with dark urine, constipation, red tongue with no or little coating, thready and rapid or thready, taut and rapid pulse.

Therapeutic Principle: To nourish yin, purge fire and tranquilize the mind.

Prescription: Modified Er Yin Decoction and Ding Zhi Pill.

Modifications: To clear away deficiency-heat, add Radix Cynanchi Atrati (Bai Wei) 9g and Cortex Lycii Radicis (Di Gu Pi) 10g; to tranquilize the mind, add Sclerotium Poriae Circum Radicem Pini (Fu Shen) 12g, Semen Ziziphi Spinosae (Suan Zao Ren) 12g and Radix Glycyrrhizae Uralensis (Gan Cao) 6g.

(3) Stagnation and Retention of Blood and Qi

Symptoms: Restlessness, anger, talkativeness, or grandiosity, auditory or visual hallucinations, or dull facial expression and reticence, mental confusion, dim complexion, distention, stuffiness and pricking pain in the chest and hypochondrium, palpitation, dysmenorrhea with dark purple blood and clot, headache or distending feeling in the head, dark purple tongue with ecchymosis, thin and white or thin and yellow tongue coating, taut and thready or deep and taut pulse.

Therapeutic Principle: To promote circulation of blood and qi, and remove blood stasis.

Prescription: Modified Dian Kuang Meng Xing Decoction, Xue Fu Zhu Yu Decoction, or Tao He Cheng Qi Decoction.

Modifications: For heat accumulation due to blood stasis, add Caulis Akebiae (Mu Tong) 3g and Radix Scutellariae Baicalensis (Huang Qin) 9g; for cold manifestation, add Rhizoma Zingiberis Officinalis (Gan Jiang) 9g and Radix Aconiti Lateralis Praeparatae (Fu Zi) 10g; for severe blood stasis, add Da Huang Zhe Chong Pill.

3. Schizophrenia

A. Etiology and Pathogenesis

1) Congenital Insufficiency
2) Anger, Fear and Fright
3) Alternate Grief and Joy
4) Excessive Anxiety
5) Disturbance of Turbid Phlegm in the Heart

B. Syndrome Differentiation and Treatment

1) <u>Stagnation of Phlegm Qi</u>

Symptoms: Depression, apathetic facial expression, reticence, dementia, incoherent speech or muttering to oneself, mood instability, no sense of hygiene, no desire for meals, red tongue with white and greasy coating, and taut and slippery pulse.

Therapeutic Principle: To regulate qi, relieve stagnation, resolve phlegm and restore consciousness.

Prescription: Modified Shun Qi Dao Tan Decoction.

Modifications: For frequent belching and sensation of stuffiness and fullness in the chest and epigastrium, add Flos Inulae (Xuan Fu Hua) 9g, Ochra Haematitum (Da Zhe Shi) 15g and Caulis Perillae (Zi Su Geng) 9g; for phlegm stagnation transforming into heat, with restlessness, yellow and greasy tongue coating, slippery and rapid pulse, add Rhizoma Coptidis (Huang Lian) 6g and Concretio Silicea Bambusae (Tian Zhu Huang) 6g.

2) <u>Deficiency of Both Heart and Spleen</u>

Symptoms: Trance, fantasy, palpitation, fright, grief, lassitude of the limbs, impaired appetite, pale tongue with greasy coating, and deep, thready and forceless pulse.

Therapeutic Principle: To invigorate the spleen, nourish the heart and regulate the functional activity of qi.

Prescription: Modified Yang Xin Decoction.

Modifications: For palpitation and fright, add Magnetitum (Ci Shi) 20g and Mastodi Dentis Fossilia (Long Chi) 20g; for consumption of heart qi with grief and sadness, add Radix Glycyrrhizae Uralensis (Gan Cao) 10g and Fructus Tritici Aestivi (Xiao Mai) 15g.

3) <u>Phlegm Fire Disturbing the Mind</u>

Symptoms: Irascible temperament, headache, insomnia, staring angrily, flushed face, conjunctival congestion, sudden onset of madness and violent rage, muddled speech, climbing walls and roofs, grandiosity, extraordinary energy, racket and scolding, not caring about relationship, or smashing things and harming people, eccentric laugh and cry, thirst with preference to cold drinks, constipation, dark urine, refusing to eat and sleep, crimson tongue with yellow and greasy or yellow, dry and dirty coating, and taut, slippery, large and rapid pulse.

Therapeutic Principle: To purge liver fire, resolve phlegm and induce resuscitation.

Prescription: Modified Sheng Tie Luo Decoction and Meng Shi Gun Tan Pill.

Modifications: For polydipsia with a desire to drink, add Gypsum Fibrosum (Shi Gao) 30g and Rhizoma Anemarrhenae (Zhi Mu) 10g; for restlessness and insomnia due to lingered phlegm-heat, add Rhizoma Coptidis (Huang Lian) 6g, Caulis Bambusae in Taeniam (Zhu Ru) 10g and Fructus Citri Aurantii Immaturus (Zhi Shi) 10g; for excessive Yang Ming fire with constipation, yellow and coarse tongue coating, excess and large pulse, add Natrii Sulfas (Mang Xiao) 5g.

4) <u>Excessive Fire Impairing Yin</u>

Symptoms: Prolonged manic state that is gradually alleviated and is controllable by persuasion; listlessness, lassitude, talkativeness, susceptibility to fright, occasional restlessness, emaciation, flushed face, red tongue with no or little coating, thready and rapid pulse.

Therapeutic Principle: To nourish yin, subdue fire, tranquilize mind and stabilize emotion.

Prescription: Modified Er Yin Decoction.

Modifications: For yellow and greasy tongue coating due to lingered phlegm-fire, add Rhizoma Arisaematis cum Bile (Dan Nan Xing) 5g and Caulis Bambusae in Taeniam (Zhu Ru) 9g; for amnesia, lumbar soreness and weak knees, add Carapax et Plastrum Testudinis (Gui Ban) 20g, Fructus Lycii (Gou Qi Zi) 10g and Gelatinum Corii Asini (E Jiao) 9g.

5) <u>Blood Stasis Blocking the Heart Orifice</u>

Symptoms: Insomnia, fright, suspiciousness, visual and auditory hallucination, incoherent speech, dim complexion, purple tongue with ecchymosis, thin and slippery tongue coating, small and taut or thready and rough pulse.

Therapeutic Principle: To remove blood stasis and induce resuscitation.

Prescription: Modified Dian Kuang Meng Xing Decoction.

Modifications: For dry mouth with bitter taste, yellow and greasy tongue coating, add Radix Astragali (Huang Qi) 12g; for cold intolerance and cold limbs, add Rhizoma Zingiberis Officinalis (Gan Jiang) 9g and Radix Aconiti Lateralis Praeparatae (Fu Zi) 10g; for dark purple tongue, add Radix Salviae Miltiorrhizae (Dan Shen) 12g and Flos Carthami Tinctorii (Hong Hua) 10g.

4. Autism

Autism is the most common condition in a group of developmental disorders known as the autism spectrum disorders (ASD). Autism is characterized by impairment in social interaction, problems with verbal and nonverbal communication, and restricted, unusual, repetitive, or stereotyped patterns of behavior. In addition, children with autism often have unusual responses to sensory experiences, such as certain sounds or the way objects look. Other ASD include Asperger syndrome, Rett syndrome, childhood disintegrative disorder, and pervasive developmental disorder not otherwise specified (PDD-NOS). Many children with ASD have some degree of mental impairment. 1/4 children with ASD develops seizures, often starting either in early childhood or adolescence. Fragile X syndrome affects about 2-5 percent of people with ASD. 1-4 percent of people with ASD also have tuberous sclerosis. A study of a U.S. metropolitan area estimated that 3.4 of every 1,000 children 3-10 years old had autism. In 2007, the Centers for Disease Control (CDC) found that the rate of autism is higher. The risk is 3-4 times higher in males than females. Autism is diagnosed by screening and comprehensive diagnostic evaluation. There is no single best treatment package for all children with autism. Early therapy and behavioral intervention have a dramatic impact on reducing symptoms and increasing a child's ability to grow and learn new skills.

A. Etiology and Pathogenesis

1) Congenital Insufficiency or Abnormality
2) Deficiency of the Liver and Kidney
3) Postnatal Pathogenic Factors or Malnourishment
4) Deficiency of Qi and Blood

B. Syndrome Differentiation and Treatment

1) <u>Deficiency of Kidney Essence</u>

Symptoms: Delayed closure of fontanels, sparse hair, dull spirit and expression, delays in the acquisition of language, poor sleep, fondness of sleeping curled up on one side, lusterless complexion, enuresis (bedwetting), unstable movements, pale tongue with white coating, thready and forceless pulse.

Therapeutic Principle: To replenish kidney essence.

Prescription: Modified Zuo Gui Pill.

Example Prescription: Radix Rehmanniae Praeparatae (Shu Di Huang), Fructus Corni Officinalis (Shan Zhu Yu), Rhizoma Dioscoreae (Shan Yao), Fructus Lycii (Gou Qi Zi), Semen Cuscutae Chinensis (Tu Si Zi), Gelatinum Cornu Cervi (Lu Jiao Jiao), Colla Testudinis Plastri (Gui Ban Jiao), and Radix Cyathulae Officinalis (Chuan Niu Xi).

2) Deficiency of the Heart and Spleen

Symptoms: Dull expression, low intelligence, delays in language, growth retardation, spiritlessness, weakness, impaired social interaction, impaired verbal communication, limited interests, pale or lusterless complexion, dull or chlorotic hair, dreamful sleep, poor appetite, loose stools, cold extremities, pale tongue with thin coating, thready and weak pulse.

Therapeutic Principle: To replenish qi, nourish blood, strengthen the spleen and nourish the heart.

Prescription: Modified Gui Pi Decoction, or Modified Gui Pi Decoction and Yang Xin Decoction.

Example Prescription: Radix Ginseng (Ren Shen), Rhizoma Atractylodis Macrocephalae (Bai Zhu), Sclerotium Poriae Circum Radicem Pini (Fu Shen), Semen Zizyphi Spinosae (Suan Zao Ren), Arillus Longanae Euphoriae (Long Yan Rou), Radix Astragali (Huang Qi), Radix Angelicae Sinensis (Dang Gui), Radix Polygalae Tenuifoliae (Yuan Zhi), Radix Aucklandiae Lappae (Mu Xiang), Radix Glycyrrhizae Praeparatae (Zhi Gan Cao), Rhizoma Zingiberis Recens (Sheng Jiang), and Fructus Zizyphi Jujubae (Da Zao).

Modifications: For severe insomnia, add Fructus Schisandrae Chinensis (Wu Wei Zi) and Semen Biotae Orientalis (Bai Zi Ren) to nourish the heart and calm spirit; or add Flos Albizziae Julibrissin (He Huan Hua), Caulis Polygoni Multiflori (Ye Jiao Teng), Mastodi Ossis Fossilia (Long Gu) and Concha Ostreae (Mu Li) to tranquilize the mind.

3) Deficiency of Liver Yin and Kidney Yin

Symptoms: Growth retardation, repetitive language, language imitation, deficits in social interaction, concentration difficulty or short attention span, absentmindedness, irritability, insomnia, dysphoria with feverish sensation in the chest, palms and soles, frequent urination, dark urine, or enuresis (bedwetting), spontaneous sweating, night sweats, red tongue with little coating, and thready or thready and rapid pulse.

Therapeutic Principle: To nourish the liver and kidney, tonify yin and blood.

Prescription: Modified Liu Wei Di Huang Pill supplemented with Radix Polygalae Tenuifoliae (Yuan Zhi) and Rhizoma Acori Tatarinowii (Shi Chang Pu), or Huang Lian E Jiao Decoction supplemented with Magnetitum (Ci Shi) and Cinnabaris (Zhu Sha).

Example Prescription: Radix Rehmanniae Praeparatae (Shu Di Huang), Fructus Corni Officinalis (Shan Zhu Yu), Rhizoma Dioscoreae (Shan Yao), Cortex Moutan Radicis (Mu Dan Pi), Sclerotium Poriae Cocos (Fu Ling), Rhizoma Alismatis Orientalis (Ze Xie), Radix Polygalae Tenuifoliae (Yuan Zhi), and Rhizoma Acori Tatarinowii (Shi Chang Pu).

5. Impotence/Erectile Dysfunction

A. Etiology and Pathogenesis

1) Excessive Sexual Activities and Masturbation
2) Frequent Seminal Emission, with Deficiency of Essence
3) Emotional Disturbance
4) Chronic Illness and Weak Constitution
5) Downward movement of Damp-Heat

B. Syndrome Differentiation and Treatment

1) <u>Decline of Fire of the Life Gate</u>

Symptoms: Inability to achieve or maintain erections, clear, thin and cold seminal fluid, dizziness, tinnitus, pale complexion, listlessness, lumbar soreness, weak knees, cold intolerance, cold limbs, pale tongue with white coating, deep and thready pulse.

Therapeutic Principle: To warm and nourish the kidney.

Prescription: Modified You Gui Pill and Zan Yu Pill.

Modifications: For marked sore and weak loins and knees, add Cortex Eucommiae Ulmoidis (Du Zhong) 12g and Radix Achyranthis Bidentatae (Niu Xi) 12g.

2) <u>Impairment of the Heart and Spleen</u>

Symptoms: Inability to achieve or maintain erections, listlessness, insomnia, anorexia, lusterless complexion, pale tongue with thin and greasy coating, and thready pulse.

Therapeutic Principle: To nourish the heart and spleen.

Prescription: Modified Gui Pi Decoction.

Modifications: For palpitation and insomnia, add Bulbus Lilii (Bai He) 12g and Cortex Albizziae Julibrissin (He Huan Pi) 12g.

3) <u>Impairment of the Kidney due to Fright</u>

Symptoms: Inability to achieve or maintain firm erections, timidity, suspiciousness, palpitation, panic, insomnia, thin and greasy tongue coating, taut and thready pulse.

Therapeutic Principle: To nourish the kidney and tranquilize the mind.

Prescription: Modified Da Bu Yuan Decoction.

Modifications: For restlessness, add Semen Ziziphi Spinosae (Suan Zao Ren) 12g and Radix Polygalae Tenuifoliae (Yuan Zhi) 9g; for descent of qi due to fright, add Rhizoma Cimicifugae (Sheng Ma) 6g and Radix Bupleuri (Chai Hu) 6g.

4) <u>Stagnation of Liver Qi</u>

Symptoms: Inability to achieve or maintain erections, depression or irritability, discomfort in the chest and epigastrium, distention and stuffiness in the hypochondrium, anorexia, loose stools, thin tongue coating, and taut pulse.

Therapeutic Principle: To soothe the liver and relieve depression.

Prescription: Modified Xiao Yao Powder.

Modifications: For qi stagnation transforming into fire, add Cortex Moutan Radicis (Mu Dan Pi) 10g and Fructus Gardeniae Jasminoidis (Zhi Zi) 10g; for yin impairment due to fire, add Radix Polygoni Multiflori (He Shou Wu) 12g, Fructus Lycii (Gou Qi Zi) 10g and Radix Rehmanniae Praeparatae (Shu Di Huang) 12g.

5) Downward Movement of Damp-Heat

Symptoms: Inability to achieve or maintain erections, damp and stinking scrotum, soreness of lower limbs, dark yellow urine, yellow and greasy tongue coating, soft and rapid pulse.

Therapeutic Principle: To clear away heat and remove dampness.

Prescription: Modified Long Dan Xie Gan Decoction.

Modifications: For impaired liver yin and kidney yin and disturbance of deficient fire with penis erection and seminal emission in the dream, night sweating, dysphoria with feverish sensation in the chest, palms and soles, lumbar soreness, weak knees, red tongue with little saliva, and taut, thready and rapid pulse, use Rhizoma Anemarrhenae (Zhi Mu) 10g, Cortex Phellodendri (Huang Bai) 9g, Radix Rehmanniae Praeparatae (Shu Di Huang) 12g, Rhizoma Dioscoreae (Shan Yao) 15g, Fructus Corni Officinalis (Shan Zhu Yu) 10g, Fructus Lycii (Gou Qi Zi) 10g, Sclerotium Poriae Cocos (Fu Ling) 12g, Cortex Moutan Radicis (Mu Dan Pi) 10g and Rhizoma Alismatis Orientalis (Ze Xie) 9g.

6. Frigidity and Disorders of Sexual Desire

A. Etiology and Pathogenesis

1) Emotional Disturbance
2) Dysfunction of the Kidney, Leading to Decline of Fire of the Life Gate and Inability of the Kidney to Arrest Essence
3) Dysfunction of the Liver, Leading to Qi Stagnation in the Liver
4) Dysfunction of the Spleen Impairs the Function of Transportation and Transformation of the Spleen, Resulting in Downward Movement of Damp-Heat

B. Syndrome Differentiation and Treatment

1) Deficiency of Kidney Qi

Symptoms: Diminished or absent libido, pale complexion, lumbar soreness and weak knees, cold intolerance, cold limbs, listlessness, lassitude, or impotence, pale and chubby tongue, deep, thready and weak pulse

Therapeutic Principle: To warm the kidney and strengthen Yang.

Prescription: Modified Wu Zi Yan Zong Pill.

Modifications: For restless and insomnia, add Caulis Polygoni Multiflori (Ye Jiao Teng) 20g and Ganoderma (Ling Zhi) 9g; for inability to achieve or maintain erections, add Actinolitum (Yang Qi Shi) 5g

2) <u>Deficiency of the Heart and Spleen</u>

Symptoms: Diminished or absent libido, sentimentality, palpitation, timidness, insomnia, amnesia, dizziness, spiritlessness, anorexia, lusterless complexion, pale tongue, and thready and weak pulse.

Therapeutic Principle: To nourish the heart and spleen.

Prescription: Modified Gui Pi Decoction.

Modifications: Add Herba Epimedii (Xian Ling Pi) 12g, Cervi Cornu Degelatinatum (Lu Jiao Shuang) 12g and Herba Cistanches (Rou Cong Rong) 12g to strengthen yang and increase libido.

3) <u>Stagnation of Liver Qi</u>

Symptoms: Diminished or absent libido, moodiness, frequent sighing, insomnia, discomfort in the chest and epigastrium, distention and stuffiness in the hypochondrium, pale tongue with thin coating, taut and thready pulse.

Therapeutic Principle: To soothe the liver and relieve stagnation.

Prescription: Modified Xiao Yao Powder.

Modifications: Add Fructus Lycii (Gou Qi Zi) 10g and Fructus Ligustri Lucidi (Nu Zhen Zi) 12g to nourish liver yin; add Herba Epimedii (Yin Yang Huo) 12g to strengthen yang.

7. Premature Ejaculation

A. Etiology and Pathogenesis

1) Emotional Disturbance
2) Dysfunction of the Kidney, Leading to Decline of Fire of the Life Gate and Inability of the Kidney to Arrest Essence
3) Dysfunction of the Liver, Leading to Qi Stagnation in the Liver
4) Dysfunction of the Spleen Impairs the Function of Transportation and Transformation of the Spleen, Resulting in Downward Movement of Damp-Heat

B. Syndrome Differentiation and Treatment

1) Yin Deficiency and Hyperactivity of Fire

Symptoms: Premature ejaculation, increased libido, dreamful sleep, nocturnal emission, dry mouth, dysphoria with feverish sensation in the heart, lumbar soreness and weak knees, vertigo, palpitation, insomnia, hectic fever, night sweats, red tongue, thin and yellow tongue coating or no coating, thready and rapid pulse.

Therapeutic Principle: To nourish yin, reduce fire, nourish the kidney and arrest semen.

Prescription: Modified Zhi Bai Di Huang Pill.

Modifications Add Fructus Lycii (Gou Qi Zi) 9g, Fructus Rosae Laevigatae (Jin Ying Zi) 9g, Fructus Schisandrae (Wu Wei Zi) 3g, Mastodi Ossis Fossilia (Long Gu) 20g, and Concha Ostreae (Mu Li) 20g to the prescription.

2) Damp-Heat in the Liver Channel

Symptoms: Premature ejaculation, increased libido, fidgety, irritability, hypochondriac pain, anorexia, genital pruritus, dysuria, bitter taste in the mouth, sticky and greasy mouth, dark yellow urine, dribbling after urination, red tongue with yellow and greasy coating, taut and rapid pulse.

Therapeutic Principle: To clear away damp-heat in the liver channel.

Prescription: Modified Long Dan Xie Gan Decoction.

Modifications: For red, hot, or swollen genitals, add Herba Taraxaci (Pu Gong Ying) 15g and Rhizoma Smilacis Glabrae (Tu Fu Ling) 30g; for distensible pain in the hypochondriac region, lower abdomen and testicles, add Fructus Meliae Toosendan (Chuan Lian Zi) 9g and Semen Citri Reticulatae (Ju He) 9g.

3) Deficiency of Kidney Qi

Symptoms: Premature ejaculation, diminished libido, tardy erection, lumbar soreness and weak knees, listlessness, nocturnal polyuria and urinary frequency, cold limbs, cold intolerance, lusterless complexion, pale and chubby tongue with thin and white coating, deep and weak pulse.

Therapeutic Principle: To warm and replenish kidney qi, arrest semen and stop premature ejaculation.

Prescription: Modified Zan Yu Pill.

Modifications: Add Fructus Rosae Laevigatae (Jin Ying Zi) 9g, Ootheca Mantidis (Sang Piao Xiao) 9g and Sclerotium Poriae Circum Radicem Pini (Fu Shen) 12g to the prescription.

4) Deficiency of the Heart and Spleen

Symptoms: Premature ejaculation, scanty seminal fluid, palpitation, insomnia, shortness of breath, spiritlessness, emaciation, anorexia, loose stools, dizziness, spontaneous sweating, lusterless complexion, pale tongue with thin and white coating, thready and weak pulse.

Therapeutic Principle: To nourish the heart and spleen, arrest semen and stop premature ejaculation.

Prescription: Modified Gui Pi Decoction.

Modifications: Add Semen Euryales (Qian Shi) 12g, Mastodi Ossis Fossilia (Long Gu) 20g and Concha Ostreae (Mu Li) 20g to the prescription.

Chapter 10: Environmental Hazards and Poisoning

1. Acute Carbon Monoxide Poisoning

Carbon monoxide (CO) is a colorless, odorless and tasteless gas. It can be created whenever a fuel (such as wood, gasoline, coal, natural gas, or kerosene) is burning. Carbon monoxide poisoning is caused by inhaling carbon monoxide fumes. Carbon monoxide replaces the oxygen in the hemoglobin of the red blood cells, keeping oxygen from reaching the tissues and organs. Carbon monoxide also causes harm to the central nervous system. People with existing health problems such as anemia, heart and lung disease are especially vulnerable, as are infants, children, pregnant women, the elderly, and people who are sleeping or intoxicated.

The majority of carbon monoxide exposures occur in the winter months. Various appliances fueled by wood, gas or coal produce carbon monoxide.

Carbon monoxide poisoning is dangerous. Depending on the degree and length of exposure, carbon monoxide poisoning can cause permanent brain damage, and it can damage the heart as well, possibly leading to life-threatening cardiac complications years after the poisoning. The following are the most common symptoms of carbon monoxide poisoning. However, each individual may experience symptoms differently. Symptoms may include:

- Headache, the most common early symptom
- Dizziness
- Nausea and vomiting
- Chest pain
- Confusion
- Irritability
- Weakness
- Rapid heartbeat
- Seizures
- Cardiac arrest

- Loss of hearing
- Blurry vision
- Respiratory failure
- Impaired judgment
- Loss of consciousness or coma

How is Acute Carbon Monoxide Poisoning Diagnosed by Conventional Western Medicine?

Diagnosis is made based on medical history and specific measurement of the arterial or venous carboxyhemoglobin saturation.

How is Acute Carbon Monoxide Poisoning Treated by Conventional Western Medicine?

The goal of treatment is to replace the carbon monoxide in the blood with oxygen. Treatments may include:

- Remove the victim from exposure
- Maintain a patent airway and assist ventilation
- Administer 100% oxygen through face mask
- Hyperbaric oxygen therapy
- Treat patients with coma, hypotension, or seizures

What Causes Acute Carbon Monoxide Poisoning According to Traditional Chinese Medicine?

1) Inhalation of Turbid Qi, with Pathogenic Fire and Phlegm Block the Pericardium
2) Hyperactive Fire Flaring up Internal Wind
3) Pathogenic Phlegm Blocking Heart Orifice
4) Pathogenic Heat and Fire Forcing the Blood not to Follow Its Vessels

How is Acute Carbon Monoxide Poisoning Differentiated and Treated by Traditional Chinese Medicine?

1) <u>Liver Fire and Turbid Phlegm</u>

Symptoms: Headache, dizziness, nausea, vomiting, abdominal pain, weakness of the limbs, blurred vision, or cherry-red lips, or syncope, or even coma and seizures, stare, bluish conjunctivae of the eyes, pale tongue with white and greasy coating, taut and slippery pulse.

Therapeutic Principle: To eliminate dampness with aromatic drugs, resolve phlegm, cause resuscitation, soothe the liver and calm the wind.

Prescription: Modified Di Tan Decoction.

Modifications: Forced feeding of Su He Xiang Pill for coma. For fever, red tongue with yellow and greasy coating, taut, slippery and rapid pulse, add An Gong Niu Huang Pill or Xing Nao Jing Injection; for hematemesis and tarry stools, add Radix et Rhizoma Rhei (Da Huang) 6g, Os Sepiae seu Sepiellae (Hai Piao Xiao) 10g and Rhizoma Bletillae Striatae (Bai Ji) 9g; for distending pain in the chest, add Radix Salviae Miltiorrhizae (Dan Shen) 12g and Bulbus Allii Macrostemonis (Xie Bai) 9g.

2) <u>Collapse of Yin and Yang</u>

Symptoms: Coma or muddleheadedness, fever, flushed face, drenching sweats, coarse breathing, dyspnea, red and dry tongue, rapid and forceless pulse (in first stage); pale complexion, bluish purple lips, extremely cold limbs, drenching sweats, shortness of breath, feeble respiration, tinny and extremely faint pulse (in second stage).

Therapeutic Principle: To replenish qi, and restore yin and yang from collapse.

Prescription: Sheng Mai Injection and Shen Fu Injection; or modified large dosage of Sheng Mai Powder and Shen Fu Decoction.

Modifications: For chest pain, add Fu Fang Dan Shen Injection.

3) <u>Retention of Turbid Phlegm</u>

Symptoms: Dementia, reticence, or slurred speech, disorientation, physical instability and unstable gait, dull facial complexion, stare, amnesia, insomnia, delusion, fear, or even delirium and coma, slight red tongue with white coating, deep and slippery or deep and floating pulse.

Therapeutic Principle: To strengthen the spleen, eliminate dampness, resolve phlegm and cause resuscitation.

Prescription: Modified Ban Xia Bai Zhu Tian Ma Decoction.

Modifications: For cloudy consciousness, add Su He Xiang Pill; for spasm or tremors of the head and limbs, add Concha Haliotidis (Shi Jue Ming) 20g, Tribulus Terrestris Fructus (Bai Ji Li) 9g, Ramulus Uncariae cum Uncis (Gou Teng) 12g and Buthus Martensi (Quan Xie) 3g; for rigidity of the limbs or paralysis, add Bombyx Batryticatus (Jiang Can) 9g and Hirudo seu Whitmania (Shui Zhi) 5g.

4) <u>Obstruction of Collaterals due to Qi Deficiency and Phlegm Stagnation</u>

Symptoms: Hemiplegia, slurred speech or aphasia, numbness of the limbs, pale complexion, shortness of breath, fatigue, saliva drooling from one corner of the mouth, swelling and distending sensation of the limbs, or blindness, dark and pale tongue with thin and white or white and greasy coating, thready and slow or taut and thready pulse.

Therapeutic Principle: To replenish qi, promote blood circulation, resolve phlegm and activate collaterals.

Prescription: Modified Bu Yang Huan Wu Decoction.

Modifications: For urinary incontinence, Ootheca Mantidis (Sang Piao Xiao) 9g, Fructus Alpinae Oxyphyllae (Yi Zhi Ren) 9g and Radix Linderae Strychnifoliae (Wu Yao) 9g; for severe blood stasis, add Hirudo seu Whitmania (Shui Zhi) 5g, Rhizoma Curcumae Ezhu (E Zhu) 9g, Radix et Caulis Jixueteng (Ji Xue Teng) 12g and Ramulus Euonymi (Gui Jian Yu) 9g; for severe numbness of the limbs, add Fructus Chaenomelis (Mu Gua) 10g and Herba Lycopodii (Shen Jin Cao) 10g.

What Kinds of Chinese Patent Drugs are Available to Treat Acute Carbon Monoxide Poisoning?

1) Su He Xiang Pill: 1 pill each time, 1-2 times daily.
2) An Gong Niu Huang Pill: 3g each time, 1-2 times daily.
3) Xing Nao Jing Injection: 10-40ml each time, once daily.
4) Qing Kai Ling Injection: 10ml each time, once daily.

2. Barbiturates Poisoning

Barbiturates are drugs that act as central nervous system (CNS) depressants; they are used mainly as anesthetics, as anticonvulsants, and in the resuscitation of patients with cerebral injuries. Barbiturates are also used commonly in combination with other substances for the treatment of gastrointestinal illness and migraine. The most common scenario for a massive barbiturate poisoning is an intentional overdose of barbiturate-based anticonvulsants or barbiturate-containing combination medications (e.g., Fiercest, Farina, and Don natal).

Barbiturates suppress the activity of all excitable tissue, including the CNS, the peripheral nervous system, and the cardiovascular system. They also depress gastrointestinal function and have a number of effects on hepatic function. Fatal poisonings have occurred with the ingestion of as little as 6 g of Phenobarbital and 2-3 g of short-acting barbiturates. The presence of co-ingestants (e.g., alcohol, tricyclic antidepressants) may increase the lethality of barbiturates. Signs and symptoms of barbiturate poisoning may include:

- Hypothermia
- Bradypnea, apnea, or rapid and shallow respirations
- Hypotension, bradycardia, pulmonary edema, cardiovascular collapse, shock, or occasional tachycardia
- Disorders of mentation, slurred speech, loss of coordination, ataxia, stupor, deeply comatose, hypotonia, and areflexia

- Nystagmus (rapid involuntary oscillation of the eyes) and a dysconjugate gaze
- Bowel distention, or bowel necrosis with decreased bowel sounds and abdominal distention
- Urinary retention, or acute tubular necrosis with azotemia, volume overload, hyperkalemia, and acidosis
- Tense, clear, bullous skin lesions

How is Barbiturates Poisoning Diagnosed by Conventional Western Medicine?

Diagnosis is made based on medical history, physical examination and tests such as blood tests, arterial blood gas tests, electrolytes and glucose tests, renal function tests, liver function tests, CBC count, toxicology, pregnancy test, chest x ray, CT scan, electrocardiogram or electroencephalogram.

How is Barbiturates Poisoning Treated by Conventional Western Medicine?

The treatment of barbiturate poisoning cases is supportive. Airway protection, cardiovascular support, and the immediate identification and treatment of correctable metabolic and structural abnormalities have a great impact on patient survival. Once the patient is stabilized, bowel decontamination, bowel and kidney elimination enhancement are performed.

Patients with delayed gastric emptying and ileus should receive nothing by mouth (NPO) until the gastrointestinal tract recovers. Patients with barbiturate toxicity should be monitored closely when out of bed.

What Causes Barbiturates Poisoning According to Traditional Chinese Medicine?

1) Taking Barbiturates by Accident or Overdose of Barbiturates
2) Internal Generation of Turbid Phlegm and Blood Stasis

How is Barbiturates Poisoning Differentiated and Treated by Traditional Chinese Medicine?

1) <u>Phlegm Blocking Heart Orifice</u>

Symptoms: Dizziness, headache, palpitation, lassitude, lethargy, nausea, vomiting, abdominal distention and fullness, or wheezing sound in the throat, spasm of limbs, white and greasy tongue coating, and slippery pulse.

Therapeutic Principle: To resolve phlegm, remove turbidity and cause resuscitation.

Prescription: Di Tan Decoction and Su He Xiang Pill.

Modifications: For spasm of limbs, add Ramulus Uncariae cum Uncis (Gou Teng) 12g, Rhizoma Gastrodiae Elatae (Tian Ma) 9g and Concha Haliotidis (Shi Jue Ming) 20g.

2) <u>Blood Stasis Blocking Heart Orifice</u>

Symptoms: Severe headache, palpitation, restlessness, anxiety, moist and cold skin, cyanosis of skin, dark tongue with ecchymosis or petechiae, thin and white tongue coating, and rough pulse.

Therapeutic Principle: To promote blood circulation, remove blood stasis and activate collaterals.

Prescription: Modified Tong Qiao Huo Xue Decoction.

Modifications: To activate collaterals, add Radix Curcumae (Yu Jin) 10g and Rhizoma Acori Tatarinowii (Shi Chang Pu) 9g; for palpitation and restlessness, add Mastodi Ossis Fossilia (Long Gu) 15g and Concha Ostreae (Mu Li) 20g.

3) <u>Deficiency of Both Qi and Blood</u>

Symptoms: Lusterless complexion, pale lips and nails, vertigo, palpitation, lassitude, listlessness, pale tongue with white coating, thready and weak pulse.

Therapeutic Principle: To replenish qi and nourish blood.

Prescription: Modified Ba Zhen Decoction.

What Kinds of Chinese Patent Drugs are Available to Treat Barbiturates Poisoning?

1) Qing Kai Ling Injection: 40ml each time, once daily.
2) Fu Fang Dan Shen Injection: 20ml each time, once daily.
3) Sheng Mai Injection: 40-100ml each time, once daily.

3. Alcohol (Ethanol) Poisoning

Alcohol poisoning is a serious, sometimes fatal, result of consuming dangerous amounts of alcohol. Overdose of alcohol can directly impact the central nervous system, slowing breathing, heart rate and gag reflex. This can lead to choking, coma and even death.

Alcohol poisoning most often occurs as a result of drinking too many alcoholic beverages over a short period of time. Binge drinking is a common cause of alcohol poisoning. Accidental ingestion is another one, particularly among children. Alcohol poisoning can also occur by drinking household products that contain ethyl alcohol (ethanol), or by ingesting isopropyl alcohol (isopropanol) or methyl alcohol (methanol).

The effects of ethanol on the body system depend on the blood alcohol concentration, or BAC. Factors that affect the blood alcohol concentration include how strong the alcohol is, how quickly and how much a person drinks it, and how empty the stomach is at the time a person drinks it. Signs and symptoms of alcohol poisoning may include:

- Confusion, stupor
- Vomiting
- Slurred speech, ataxia
- Seizures

- Slow or irregular breathing
- Blue-tinged skin or pale skin
- Hypothermia
- Unconsciousness

How is Alcohol Poisoning Diagnosed by Conventional Western Medicine?

Diagnosis is made based on medical history, and signs and symptoms of alcohol poisoning. Blood tests and urine tests may help to confirm a diagnosis of alcohol poisoning.

How is Alcohol Poisoning Treated by Conventional Western Medicine?

The management for alcohol poisoning usually is supportive. Treatment of alcohol poisoning consists of providing breathing support and intravenous fluids and vitamins until all of the alcohol is eliminated from the body. Treatment may include:

- Careful monitoring
- Airway protection to prevent breathing or choking problems
- Oxygen therapy
- Administration of fluids intravenously to prevent dehydration
- Kidney dialysis

What Causes Alcohol Poisoning According to Traditional Chinese Medicine?

1) Alcohol Indulgence and Overdose
2) Impairment of the Stomach, Brain, Spleen, Liver and Kidney
3) Obstruction of Middle Warmer by Dampness and Deficiency of Kidney Essence

How is Alcohol Poisoning Differentiated and Treated by Traditional Chinese Medicine?

1) <u>Retention of Damp-Heat</u>

Symptoms: Overdose of alcohol, muddleheadedness, or irritability, or aphasia, or vomiting with sputum and saliva, or dyspnea and fever, or cough and hematemesis, constipation, red tongue with yellow and greasy coating, and excess pulse.

Therapeutic Principle: To clear away heat and eliminate dampness.

Prescription: Modified Chou Xin Decoction.

Modifications: For remarkable muddleheadedness, add Radix Curcumae (Yu Jin) 10g, Rhizoma Acori Tatarinowii (Shi Chang Pu) 9g and Flos Puerariae (Ge Hua) 10g; for remarkable vomiting with sputum and saliva, add Rhizoma Pinelliae Ternatae (Ban Xia) 9g and Caulis Bambusae in Taeniam (Zhu Ru) 9g; for remarkable fever and dyspnea, add Rhizoma Coptidis (Huang Lian) 9g and Semen

Hoveniae (Zhi Ju Zi) 6g.

2) <u>Internal Accumulation of Alcohol Toxicity</u>

Symptoms: Overdose of alcohol, vomiting with sputum and saliva, headache, vexation, distending sensation in the chest and abdomen, tremors of the hands and feet, or cloudy consciousness, thick and greasy tongue coating, taut and slippery pulse.

Therapeutic Principle: To promote food digestion and remove toxic substance.

Prescription: Modified Ge Hua Jie Cheng Decoction.

Modifications: Remove Radix Ginseng (Ren Shen) and Rhizoma Zingiberis Officinalis (Gan Jiang), and add Rhizoma Coptidis (Huang Lian) 6g, Semen Hoveniae (Zhi Ju Zi) 6g and Rhizoma Acori Tatarinowii (Shi Chang Pu) 9g to the prescription.

3) <u>Deficiency of Kidney Essence</u>

Symptoms: Alcohol drinking for years, amnesia, dementia, decreased libido or impotence, pale tongue with white coating, deep and thready pulse.

Therapeutic Principle: To nourish the kidney and replenish essence.

Prescription: Modified Di Huang Decoction.

Modifications: For numbness in one side of the body or tremor, add Rhizoma Ligustici Chuanxiong (Chuan Xiong) 9g, Radix Salviae Miltiorrhizae (Dan Shen) 9g, Radix Curcumae (Yu Jin) 10g, Buthus Martensi (Quan Xie) 3g and Ramulus Uncariae cum Uncis (Gou Teng) 12g.

4) <u>Stagnation of the Liver and Deficiency of the Spleen</u>

Symptoms: Alcohol indulgence for years, dizziness, fatigue, sticky mouth without a desire to drink, anorexia, distention and fullness in the chest and hypochondrium, irritability, pale tongue with white and greasy coating, taut and thready pulse.

Therapeutic Principle: To soothe the liver and strengthen the spleen.

Prescription: Modified Xiao Yao Powder.

Modifications: For fatigue and remarkable anorexia, add Radix Codonopsitis Pilosulae (Dang Shen) 9g, Radix Astragali (Huang Qi) 12g and Fructus Hordei Germinatus (Mai Ya) 12g; for distention and fullness in the chest and hypochondrium, add irritability, add Radix Aucklandiae Lappae (Mu Xiang) 9g, Rhizoma Cyperi Rotundi (Xiang Fu) 10g and Radix Curcumae (Yu Jin) 10g; for yellow and greasy tongue coating, and concurrent damp-heat, add Caulis Bambusae in Taeniam (Zhu Ru) 9g and Radix Gentianae (Long Dan Cao) 3g.

4. Heat Disorders (Heat Syncope, Heat Cramps, Heat Exhaustion and Heat Stroke)

Heat disorders, also known as hyperthermia, are a group of illnesses caused by prolonged exposure to hot temperatures, restricted fluid intake, or failure of the body's ability to regulate its temperature. Sweat production and evaporation is a major mechanism of heat removal. Conduction (the direct transfer of heat from the skin to the surrounding air) also occurs. Heat disorders can affect people of all ages. But its effects are more serious with increasing age.

Risk factors for heat disorders include obesity, generalized skin diseases, diminished cutaneous blood flow, dehydration, malnutrition, hypotension, reduced cardiac output, some medications, alcohol, and illicit drugs. The four most common forms of heat disorders are heat stroke, heat exhaustion, heat cramps, and heat syncope.

Heat Syncope can result from cutaneous vasodilation with consequent systemic and cerebral hypotension. There is typically a history of vigorous physical activity for 2 hours or more just preceding the episode. Heat cramps can result from fluid and electrolyte depletion. There is almost always a history of vigorous activity just preceding the onset of symptoms. Heat exhaustion results from prolonged heavy activity with inadequate salt intake in a hot environment and is characterized by dehydration, sodium depletion, or isotonic fluid loss with accompanying cardiovascular changes. Heat stroke is a life-threatening medical emergency resulting from failure of the thermoregulatory mechanism.

Symptoms for the different types of heat disorders vary.

- Heat syncope: Sudden unconsciousness, hypotension, cool and moist skin, and weak pulse
- Heat Cramps: Slow, painful skeletal muscle contractions or even severe muscle spasms, muscle twitching, cool and moist skin, tender, hard and lumpy muscles, alertness, agitation, and normal or slightly increased body temperature
- Heat Exhaustion: Increased pulse rate, moist skin, thirst, weakness, headache, fatigue, anxiety, paresthesias, impaired judgment, hysteria, psychosis, respiratory alkalosis, and rectal temperature over 37.8ºC
- Heat Stroke: Cerebral dysfunction with impaired consciousness, high fever, and absence of sweating

How is Heat Disorders Diagnosed by Conventional Western Medicine?

The two key factors are the patient's visible symptoms and recent personal history. Testing temperature, heart rate, and other vital factors may confirm the diagnosis quickly. Blood and urine tests can also be used to confirm a diagnosis of heat disorders.

How is Heat Disorders Treated by Conventional Western Medicine?

Treatment of heat disorders may include:

- Moving the patient to a cooler location
- Providing the patient with cool water
- Giving the patient liquids that contain electrolytes such as salt water or a sports drink such as Gatorade
- Massage of leg muscles
- Making patients lie down with their feet elevated
- Placing ice packs around the neck, under the arms and knees, and in the groin
- Intravenous administration of fluids and electrolytes
- Bed rest
- Patients should be observed for renal failure, hypokalemia, cardiac arrhythmias, DIC, and hepatic failure

What Causes Heat Disorders According to Traditional Chinese Medicine?

1) Attack by Exogenous Pathogenic Summer Heat
2) Insufficiency of Healthy Qi due to Senility, Infancy, Under Age, Postpartum, Obesity, Hunger, Fatigue or Insufficient Sleep

How is Heat Disorders Differentiated and Treated by Traditional Chinese Medicine?

1) Yang Type Heat Disorder

Symptoms: High fever, or cold intolerance, sweating or no sweats, restlessness, thirst with a desire for excessive water, oliguria with dark urine, red tongue with little moisture, full and large pulse.

Therapeutic Principle: To clear away heat, remove summer heat and promote fluid production.

Prescription: Modified Bai Hu Decoction.

Modifications: For fever, thirst, excessive sweats, large and forceless pulse, add Radix Ginseng (Ren Shen) 6g; for fever, excessive sweats, hiccup, nausea, red tongue with little coating, deficiency and rapid pulse, use Zhu Ye Shi Gao Decoction; for fever, vexation, dark yellow urine, thirst, spontaneous sweating, listlessness, lassitude of the limbs, deficiency and forceless pulse, use Qing Shu Yi Qi Decoction; for concurrent dampness with cold intolerance, fever, irritability, thirst, loose stools, use Huang Lian Xiang Ru Decoction.

2) Yin Type Heat Disorder

Symptoms: Fever, sweating, listlessness, drowsiness, weakness of the limbs, fullness in the chest, shortness of breath, no desire for food, diarrhea, full and slow pulse (early stage with yin deficiency and excessive qi deficiency); extremely cold limbs, spontaneous cold sweats, pale complexion, irritability, progressive shallowness and shortness of breath, and tinny, thready and extremely faint pulse, or even coma, unconsciousness (prostration of qi and yin after persistent drenching sweats or persistent vomiting and diarrhea).

Therapeutic Principle: To replenish qi and restore yang from collapse.

Prescription: Sheng Mai Powder and Shen Fu Long Mu Decoction.

Modifications: For coma, use Su He Xiang Pill.

3) <u>Summer Heat Attacking the Heart</u>

Symptoms: High fever, irritability, sweating, feeling of oppression in the chest, abrupt onset of syncope, unconsciousness, crimson tongue, full and rapid pulse.

Therapeutic Principle: To clear away heart heat and induce resuscitation.

Prescription: An Gong Niu Huang Pill, Zhi Bao Pill or Zi Xue Pellet.

Modifications: Once unconsciousness is recovered, use Qing Gong Decoction or Qing Ying Decoction.

4) <u>Summer Heat Stirring up Internal Wind</u>

Symptoms: Persistent high fever, restlessness, or even unconsciousness, spasm of the limbs, trismus, flushed face, dyspnea, red tongue with yellow coating and little moisture, taut and rapid pulse.

Therapeutic Principle: To clear away heat, remove summer heat and calm wind.

Prescription: Ling Yang Jiao Decoction and Zi Xue Pellet.

Modifications: For unconsciousness, add An Gong Niu Huang Pill.

Chapter 11: Other Diseases

1. Headache

A. Etiology and Pathogenesis

1) Exogenous Pathogenic Factors (the chief factor is wind, which is accompanied with cold, heat and dampness)
2) Hyperactivity of Liver Yang
3) Deficiency of Kidney Essence
4) Deficiency of the Spleen and Stomach
5) Blood Stasis Blocking Collaterals

B. Syndrome Differentiation and Treatment

1) <u>Wind-Cold Headache</u>

Symptoms: Abrupt onset of headache, which radiates to the neck and the back, and is aggravated by exposure to wind; preference to warmth in the head, aversion to wind and cold, absence of thirst, or nasal congestion and watery rhinorrhea, thin and white tongue coating, and floating or floating and tense pulse.

Therapeutic Principle: To eliminate wind and disperse cold.

Prescription: Modified Chuan Xiong Cha Tiao Powder.

Modifications: For severe headache aggravated by coldness, absence of sweats, add Radix Aconiti Lateralis Praeparatae (Fu Pian) 9g and Herba Ephedrae (Ma Huang) 6g; for pathogenic cold invading Jue Yin Channel with headache in the vertex, retching, salivation, or even extremely cold limbs, white tongue coating and taut pulse, use Wu Zhu Yu Decoction supplemented with Rhizoma Pinelliae Ternatae (Ban Xia) 9g, Rhizoma Ligustici (Gao Ben) 9g and Rhizoma Ligustici Chuanxiong (Chuan Xiong) 9g.

2) <u>Wind-Heat Headache</u>

Symptoms: Distending or even splitting pain in the head, fever, wind intolerance, thirst with a desire to drink, flushed face, conjunctival congestion, constipation or dyschezia, dark yellow urine, red tongue with yellow coating, floating and rapid pulse.

Therapeutic Principle: To eliminate wind and clear away heat.

Prescription: Modified Xiong Zhi Shi Gao Decoction.

Modifications: For concurrent thirst, red tongue with little moisture, add Radix Trichosanthis (Tian Hua Fen) 12g, Herba Dendrobii (Shi Hu) 9g and Rhizoma Anemarrhenae (Zhi Mu) 10g; for constipation, add Huang Lian Shang Qing Pill.

3) <u>Wind-Dampness Headache</u>

Symptoms: Headache with a feeling that the head is tightly wrapped, heavy sensation of the limbs, feeling of oppression in the chest, anorexia, loose stools, difficult urination, white and greasy tongue coating, soft and slippery pulse.

Therapeutic Principle: To expel wind and eliminate dampness.

Prescription: Modified Qiang Huo Sheng Shi Decoction.

Modifications: For nausea and vomiting, add Rhizoma Pinelliae Ternatae (Ban Xia) 9g, Pericarpium Citri Reticulatae (Chen Pi) 6g and Caulis Bambusae in Taeniam (Zhu Ru) 9g; for chest discomfort, anorexia and loose stools, add Rhizoma Atractylodis (Cang Zhu) 9g, Cortex Magnoliae Officinalis (Hou Po) 9g and Pericarpium Citri Reticulatae (Chen Pi) 6g; for oliguria, add Semen Coicis (Yi Yi Ren) 15g and Herba Lophatheri Gracilis (Dan Zhu Ye) 10g; for distending pain of the head, fever, vexation, thirst, feeling of oppression in the chest, use Huang Lian Xiang Ru Decoction supplemented with Herba Agastache seu Pogostemonis (Huo Xiang) 9g, Herba Eupatorii (Pei Lan) 9g, Fructus Viticis (Man Jing Zi) 10g and Folium Nelumbinis Nuciferae (He Ye) 9g.

4) <u>Headache due to Hyperactivity of Liver Yang</u>

Symptoms: Distending pain in the head, dizziness, distending pain in the hypochondriac region, restlessness, irritability, insomnia, bitter taste in the mouth, flushed face, conjunctival congestion, red tongue with thin and yellow coating, taut and forceful or taut, thready and rapid pulse.

Therapeutic Principle: To calm the liver and suppress hyperactive yang.

Prescription: Modified Tian Ma Gou Teng Decoction.

Modifications: For insufficiency of liver yin, add Radix Paeoniae Alba (Bai Shao Yao) 9g, Fructus Ligustri Lucidi (Nu Zhen Zi) 12g and Herba Dendrobii (Shi Hu) 10g; for hyperactivity of liver fire with severe headache, hypochondriac pain, bitter taste in the mouth, flushed face, constipation, dark yellow urine, yellow tongue coating, taut and rapid pulse, add Radix Curcumae (Yu Jin) 10g, Radix Gentianae (Long Dan Cao) 5g and Spica Prunellae Vulgaris (Xia Ku Cao) 10g.

5) <u>Headache due to Kidney Deficiency</u>

Symptoms: Headache with and empty sensation, vertigo, lumbar soreness, weak knees, spiritlessness, lassitude, seminal emission, leukorrhea, tinnitus, insomnia, red tongue with little coating, thready and forceless pulse.

Therapeutic Principle: To replenish yin and nourish the kidney.

Prescription: Modified Da Bu Yuan Decoction.

Modifications: For severe seminal emission and leukorrhea, add Stamen Nelumbinis Nuciferae (Lian Xu) 3g, Semen Euryales Ferocis (Qian Shi) 12g and Fructus Rosae Laevigatae (Jin Ying Zi) 12g; and in normal times, take Liu Wei Di Huang Pill or Qi Ju Di Huang Pill. For deficiency of kidney yang with headache, cold intolerance, pale complexion, cold limbs, pale tongue, deep and thready pulse, add Cornu Cervi (Lu Jiao) 9g and Radix Aconiti Lateralis Praeparatae (Fu Zi) 10g, or use You Gui Pill, for concurrent attack by exogenous cold, use Ma Huang Fu Zi Xi Xin Decoction.

6) <u>Headache due to Blood Deficiency</u>

Symptoms: Headache, dizziness, palpitation, lusterless complexion, spiritlessness, lassitude, pale tongue with thin coating, and thready pulse.

Therapeutic Principle: To nourish blood and replenish yin.

Prescription: Modified Jia Wei Si Wu Decoction.

Modifications: For concurrent yin deficiency with tinnitus, vexation, insomnia and dizziness, add Radix Polygoni Multiflori (He Shou Wu) 15g, Fructus Lycii (Gou Qi Zi) 10g, Rhizoma Polygonati (Huang Jing) 12g and Semen Ziziphi Spinosae (Suan Zao Ren) 12g.

7) <u>Headache due to Qi Deficiency</u>

Symptoms: Lingering headache aggravated by overstrain, sallow complexion, emaciation, lassitude, insipid mouth, anorexia, loose stools, pale and chubby tongue with thin and white coating, and thready, weak and forceless pulse.

Therapeutic Principle: To strengthen the spleen, replenish qi, lift lucid yang.

Prescription: Modified Shun Qi He Zhong Decoction.

Modifications: Add Fructus Viticis (Man Jing Zi) 10g, Rhizoma Ligustici Chuanxiong (Chuan Xiong) 9g and Herba cum Radice Asari (Xi Xin) 3g to disperse wind and relieve pain; for concurrent blood deficiency, add Si Wu Decoction.

8) <u>Headache due to Turbid Phlegm</u>

Symptoms: Headache, dizziness, fullness and stuffiness in the chest and epigastrium, anorexia, nausea and vomiting, white and greasy tongue coating, slippery and rapid pulse or taut and slippery pulse.

Therapeutic Principle: To strengthen the spleen, resolve phlegm, descend the adverse flow of qi and relieve pain.

Prescription: Modified Ban Xia Bai Zhu Tian Ma Decoction.

Modifications: For stagnation of dampness and phlegm with stuffiness and fullness in the chest and epigastrium, and anorexia, add Fructus Citri Aurantii (Zhi Ke) 9g and Cortex Magnoliae Officinalis (Hou Po) 9g; for retention of turbid phlegm with bitter taste in the mouth, dyschezia, yellow and greasy tongue coating, slippery and rapid pulse, remove Rhizoma Atractylodis Macrocephalae (Bai Zhu) and add Rhizoma Coptidis (Huang Lian) 9g, Fructus Citri Aurantii (Zhi Ke) 9g and Caulis Bambusae in Taeniam (Zhu Ru) 9g.

9) Headache due to Blood Stasis

Symptoms: Localized persistent stabbing headache, or history of trauma in the head, purple tongue with ecchymosis and petechiae, thin and white tongue coating, deep and thready or rough pulse.

Therapeutic Principle: To remove blood stasis and dredge the orifices.

Prescription: Modified Tong Qiao Huo Xue Decoction.

Modifications: For severe headache, add Buthus Martensi (Quan Xie) 3g, Scolopendra Subspinipes (Wu Gong) 2g, Excrementum Trogopteri seu Pteromydis (Wu Ling Zhi) 9g and Lumbricus (Di Long) 10g; for concurrent pathogenic cold, add Ramulus Cinnamomi Cassiae (Gui Zhi) 9g and Herba cum Radice Asari (Xi Xin) 3g; for deficiency of qi and blood due to chronic illness, add Radix Astragali (Huang Qi) 12g and Radix Angelicae Sinensis (Dang Gui) 10g.

2. Chest Pain

A. Etiology and Pathogenesis

1) Invasion of Exogenous Pathogenic Factors
2) Improper Diet
3) Emotional Disturbance
4) Senility

B. Syndrome Differentiation and Treatment

1) Stagnation of Liver Qi

Symptoms: Wandering distending pain, which varies with emotional disturbance, in the chest; or stuffiness in the chest, anorexia, frequent belching, slight red tongue with thin and white or thin and yellow coating, and taut pulse.

Therapeutic Principle: To soothe the liver, regulate qi, promote qi circulation and relieve pain.

Prescription: Modified Chai Hu Shu Gan Powder.

Modifications: For qi stagnation and blood stasis with severe chest pain, add Shi Xiao Powder; for epigastric distention, belching and anorexia, add Xiao Yao Powder; for dry mouth, vexation, red tongue and yellow tongue coating, use Dan Zhi Xiao Yao Powder.

2) <u>Blood Stasis Blocking Vessels and Collaterals</u>

Symptoms: Localized pricking pain in the chest, which is aggravated at night; or intermittent and lingering sensation of stuffiness in the chest and palpitation, dark purple tongue with ecchymosis, rough or knot and intermittent pulse.

Therapeutic Principle: To promote blood circulation, remove blood stasis, activate collaterals and relieve pain.

Prescription: Modified Xue Fu Zhu Yu Decoction.

Modifications: For severe chest pain, add Rhizoma Corydalis (Yan Hu Suo) 9g, Radix et Caulis Jixueteng (Ji Xue Teng) 12g, Lignum Dalbergiae Odoriferae (Jiang Xiang) 5g and Radix Curcumae (Yu Jin) 10g; for cold limbs and bluish purple tongue, add Ramulus Cinnamomi Cassiae (Gui Zhi) 9g, Herba cum Radice Asari (Xi Xin) 3g, Rhizoma Alpiniae Officinarum (Gao Liang Jiang) 9g and Bulbus Allii Macrostemonis (Xie Bai) 9g; for phlegm stagnation and blood stasis with stuffiness in the chest, white and greasy tongue coating, add Di Tan Decoction; for yellow and greasy tongue coating, add Wen Dan Decoction or Xiao Xian Xiong Decoction; for qi deficiency and blood stasis with shortness of breath, fatigue, spontaneous sweating, thready and weak pulse, add Bao Yuan Decoction; for deficiency of yang and qi, add Radix Ginseng (Ren Shen) 6g and Radix Aconiti Lateralis Praeparatae (Fu Zi) 10g.

3) <u>Internal Obstruction of Turbid Phlegm</u>

Symptoms: Chest pain with feeling of oppression and stuffiness radiating to the shoulders and the back, or accompanied shortness of breath, dyspnea, heaviness of the limbs, obesity, abundant sputum, pale tongue with turbid and greasy coating, and slippery pulse.

Therapeutic Principle: To resolve phlegm, activate yang and relieve pain.

Prescription: Modified Gua Lou Xie Bai Ban Xia Decoction.

Modifications: For severe phlegm stagnation with epigastric stuffiness and anorexia, add Er Chen Decoction; for phlegm stagnation and blood stasis with dark and purple tongue, add Semen Pruni Persicae (Tao Ren) 9g, Flos Carthami Tinctorii (Hong Hua) 9g, Rhizoma Ligustici Chuanxiong (Chuang Xiong) 9g, Radix Salviae Miltiorrhizae (Dan Shen) 10g and Radix Curcumae (Yu Jin) 10g;

for red tongue with yellow and greasy coating, slippery and rapid pulse, add Huang Lian Wen Dan Decoction.

4) <u>Stagnation of Yin-Cold</u>

Symptoms: Chest Pain that radiates to the back and aggravated by exposure to cold; general coldness, cold limbs, feeling of oppression in the chest, shortness of breath, palpitation, pale complexion, white tongue coating, deep and thready or deep and tense pulse.

Therapeutic Principle: To activate yang with pungent and warm herbs, and expel cold.

Prescription: Modified Zhi Shi Xie Bai Gui Zhi Decoction and Dang Gui Si Ni Decoction.

Modifications: For chest pain radiating to the back, occasional angina pectoris, general coldness, cold limbs, dyspnea and inability to maintain recumbency, use Wu Tou Chi Shi Zhi Pill and Su He Xiang Pill.

5) <u>Retention of Phlegm-Heat in the Lung</u>

Symptoms: Chest pain, dyspnea, cough with yellow, thick and foul odor sputum, or hemoptysis, dysphoria, fever, red tongue with yellow and greasy coating, slippery and rapid pulse.

Therapeutic Principle: To clear away heat, resolve phlegm and relieve pain.

Prescription: Xiao Xian Xiong Decoction and Qian Jin Wei Jing Decoction.

Modifications: Add Flos Lonicerae (Jin Yin Hua) 15g, Fructus Forsythiae Suspensae (Lian Qiao) 10g and Herba cum Radice Houttuyniae Cordatae (Yu Xing Cao) 15g; for hemoptysis, add Fructus Gardeniae Jasminoidis (Zhi Zi) 9g, Radix Scutellariae Baicalensis (Huang Qin) 9g, Rhizoma Imperatae Cylindricae (Bai Mao Gen) 15g and Nodus Nelumbinis Nuciferae Rhizomatis (Ou Jie) 12g; for night sweats, dysphoria with feverish sensation in the chest, palms and soles, add Rhizoma Phragmitis Communis (Lu Gen) 12g, Radix Ophiopogonis Japonici (Mai Dong) 12g and Radix Adenophorae (Sha Shen) 12g.

6) <u>Deficiency of Heart Qi</u>

Symptoms: Intermittent and dull chest pain, chest discomfort and stuffiness, palpitation and shortness of breath aggravated by exertion, spontaneous sweating, lassitude, pale tongue, and thready or deficiency, large and forceless pulse.

Therapeutic Principle: To replenish qi, nourish the heart, warm yang and relieve pain.

Prescription: Modified Bao Yuan Decoction.

Modifications: For concurrent blood stasis with localized chest pain, pale and dark tongue, add Rhizoma Ligustici Chuanxiong (Chuan Xiong) 9g and Radix Paeoniae Rubra (Chi Shao) 10g; for concurrent blood deficiency with lusterless complexion, pale lips and tongue, and dizziness, add Radix Angelicae Sinensis (Dang Gui) 10g and Gelatinum Corii Asini (E Jiao) 9g.

7) Deficiency of Heart Yang

Symptoms: Chest pain with feeling of stuffiness, which is aggravated by exertion and exposure to cold; palpitation, shortness of breath, spiritlessness, cold intolerance, cold limbs, spontaneous sweating, pale and chubby tongue with teeth marks on its margin, white or greasy tongue coating, and deep, theady and slow pulse.

Therapeutic Principle: To replenish qi, warm and activate yang.

Prescription: Modified Ren Shen Decoction.

Modifications: For yang deficiency of the heart and kidney with lumbar soreness, cold limbs and edema, add Jin Gui Shen Qi Pill; for yang deficiency of the heart and kidney with dyspnea, inability to lie flat, edema of the face and limbs, add Zhen Wu Decoction.

8) Deficiency of Both Qi and Yin

Symptoms: Lingering, intermittent and dull chest pain, dizziness, palpitation, spiritlessness, lassitude, shortness of breath, no desire to speak, dysphoria with feverish sensation in the chest, palms and soles, dry mouth with little moisture, red tongue with little coating, and theady, weak and forceless pulse.

Therapeutic Principle: To replenish qi, nourish yin, promote blood circulation and activate collaterals.

Prescription: Modified Sheng Mai Powder and Zhi Gan Cao Decoction.

Modifications: For concurrent blood stasis, use Sheng Mai Powder and Dan Shen Decoction; for stagnation of phlegm and heat with chest stuffiness, abundant sputum, yellow and greasy tongue coating, use Sheng Mai Powder and Wen Dan Decoction.

3. Abdominal Pain

A. Etiology and Pathogenesis

1) Infection of Exogenous Pathogenic Factors
2) Improper Diet
3) Emotional Disturbance
4) Congenital Insufficiency of Yang

B. Syndrome Differentiation and Treatment

1) Internal Stagnation of Pathogenic Cold

Symptoms: Abrupt onset of severe abdominal pain that is aggravated by exposure to cold and alleviated by warmth; insipid mouth, absence of thirst, clear urine, loose stools, white and greasy tongue coating, deep and tense pulse.

Therapeutic Principle: To warm Middle Warmer and dispel cold.

Prescription: Modified Liang Fu Pill and Zheng Qi Tian Xiang Powder.

Modifications: For severe pain in the middle abdomen, which is alleviated by pressure and warmth; extremely cold limbs, tinny and extremely faint pulse, use Tong Mai Si Ni Decoction; for coldness and pain in the lower abdomen, white tongue coating, deep and tense pulse, use Nuan Gan Decoction; for coldness and pain in the abdomen, extremely cold limbs and general aching, use Wu Tou Gui Zhi Decoction; for loud borborygmi and cutting pain in the abdomen, sensation of fullness in the chest and hypochondrium, belching and vomiting, use Fu Zi Nuo Mi Decoction.

2) Retention of Damp-Heat

Symptoms: Abdominal pain aggravated by pressure, chest discomfort and stuffiness, constipation or dyschezia, polydipsia with a desire to drink, spontaneous sweating, oliguria with dark yellow urine, yellow and greasy tongue coating, soft and rapid pulse.

Therapeutic Principle: To purge heat and loosen the bowel.

Prescription: Modified Da Cheng Qi Decoction.

Modifications: For abdominal pain radiating to hypochondriac region, add Radix Bupleuri (Chai Hu) 9g and Radix Curcumae (Yu Jin) 10g.

3) Deficiency Cold of the Middle Warmer

Symptoms: Lingering and intermittent abdominal pain, which is aggravated by coldness, exertion and hunger, and alleviated by warmth, pressure, meals or rest; loose stools, spiritlessness, shortness of breath, cold intolerance, pale tongue with white coating, deep and thready pulse.

Therapeutic Principle: To warm the Middle Warmer and nourish deficiency.

Prescription: Xiao Jian Zhong Decoction.

Modifications: For deficiency cold with severe abdominal pain, vomiting, cold limbs and tinny pulse, use Da Jian Zhong Decoction; for yang deficiency of the spleen and kidney with abdominal pain, diarrhea, cold limbs, deep and slow pulse, use Fu Zi Li Zhong Decoction.

4) Food Retention

Symptoms: Abdominal distention and fullness, tenderness, anorexia, belching with rotten odor, acid regurgitation, or abdominal pain relieved after diarrhea; or constipation, greasy tongue coating, slippery and excess pulse.

Therapeutic Principle: To promote digestion and eliminate food retention.

Prescription: Modified Bao He Pill.

Modifications: For severe abdominal pain due to food retention, use Zhi Shi Dao Zhi Pill.

5) <u>Qi Stagnation and Blood Stasis</u>

Symptoms: Wandering abdominal stuffiness or distending pain radiating to the lower abdomen, which is alleviated by belching and passing flatus and aggravated by emotional disturbance; thin tongue coating, and taut pulse (qi stagnation); or severe localized abdominal pain, dark purple tongue, and taut or rough pulse (blood stasis).

Therapeutic Principle: To soothe the liver, regulate qi, promote blood circulation and remove blood stasis.

Prescription: Modified Chai Hu Shu Gan Powder to soothe the liver and regulate qi; Shao Fu Zhu Yu Decoction to promote blood circulation and remove blood stasis.

Modifications: For abdominal pain due to surgery, add Herba Lycopi Lucidi (Ze Lan) 12g and Flos Carthami Tinctorii (Hong Hua) 9g; for abdominal pain due to trauma, add Gummi Olibanum (Ru Xiang) 9g, Myrrha (Mo Yao) 9g and Semen Vaccariae Segetalis (Wang Bu Liu Xing) 9g.

4. Lumbar Pain

A. Etiology and Pathogenesis

1) Attack by Damp-Cold
2) Attack by Damp-Heat
3) Qi Stagnation and Blood Stasis
4) Deficiency of the Kidney due to Congenial Insufficiency. Overstrain, Chronic Illness, Senility or Sex Indulgence

B. Syndrome Differentiation and Treatment

1) <u>Lumbar Pain due to Damp-Cold</u>

Symptoms: Progressive coldness, heaviness and pain in the lumbar region, which is not alleviated by maintaining recumbency and is aggravated in cloudy weather or by exposure to cold; difficulty in turning round, pale tongue with white and greasy coating, deep and slow pulse.

Therapeutic Principle: To dispel cold, remove dampness, warm channels and activate collaterals.

Prescription: Modified Gan Jiang Ling Zhu Decoction.

Modifications: For pathogenic cold with lumbar coldness, discomfort and pain, add Radix Aconiti Lateralis Praeparatae (Fu Pian) 12g and Herba cum Radice Asari (Xi Xin) 3g; for pathogenic dampness with pain and heaviness, thick and greasy tongue coating, add Rhizoma Atractylodis (Cang Zhu) 9g and Semen Coicis (Yi Yi Ren) 15g; for concurrent pathogenic wind with wandering lumbar pain, add Ramulus Cinnamomi Cassiae (Gui Zhi) 9g, Radix Angelicae Pubescentis (Du Huo) 9g and Rhizoma et Radix Notopterygii (Qiang Huo) 9g; for senility and chronic ill with lumbar soreness and weak knees, deep and weak pulse, use Du Huo Ji Sheng Decoction.

2) Lumbar Pain due to Damp-Heat

Symptoms: Lumbar pain with feverish sensation, which is aggravated in cloudy, damp and raining weather, and is alleviated on motion; oliguria with dark yellow urine, yellow and greasy tongue coating, soft and rapid or taut and rapid pulse.

Therapeutic Principle: To clear away heat, eliminate dampness and relieve pain.

Prescription: Modified Si Miao Pill.

Modifications: For severe heat, polydipsia, oliguria with dark urine, red tongue, taut and rapid pulse, add Fructus Gardeniae Jasminoidis (Zhi Zi) 9g, Rhizoma Alismatis Orientalis (Ze Xie) 9g and Rhizoma Anemarrhenae (Zhi Mu) 10g; for lumbar pain, dry throat, feverish sensation in palms and soles, add Fructus Ligustri Lucidi (Nu Zhen Zi) 12g and Herba Ecliptae Prostratae (Han Lian Cao) 15g.

3) Lumbar Pain due to Blood Stasis

Symptoms: Localized pricking pain and tenderness in the lumbar region, which are relieved during the day and aggravated at night; inability to turn round, dark purple tongue with ecchymosis, and rough pulse.

Therapeutic Principle: To promote blood circulation, remove blood stasis, regulate qi and relieve pain.

Prescription: Modified Shen Tong Zhu Yu Decoction.

Modifications: For concurrent dampness and wind, add Radix Angelicae Pubescentis (Du Huo) 9g and Rhizoma Cibotii Barometz (Gou Ji) 12g; for concurrent kidney deficiency with lumbar soreness and weak knees, add Cortex Eucommiae Ulmoidis (Du Zhong) 12g, Radix Dipsaci Asperi (Xu Duan) 12g and Herba Taxilli or Ramulus Loranthi Seu Visci (Sang Ji Sheng) 12g; for severe blood stasis with lumbar pain aggravated at night, add Buthus Martensi (Quan Xie) 3g, Scolopendra Subspinipes (Wu Gong) 2g and Agkistrodon seu Bungarus (Bai Hua She) 9g.

4) Lumbar Pain due to Deficiency of Kidney Yang

Symptoms: Lingering and recurrent soreness and pain in the lumbar region, which are alleviated by pressing, massage and maintaining recumbency, and aggravated by exertion; weakness of lower extremities and knees; lower abdominal pain, pale complexion, cold limbs, aversion to cold, shortness of breath, fatigue, pale tongue, deep and thready pulse.

Therapeutic Principle: To warm kidney yang

Prescription: Modified You Gui Pill

Modifications: For chronic lumbar pain, use Qing E Pill.

5) <u>Lumbar Pain due to Deficiency of Kidney Yin</u>

Symptoms: Lingering and recurrent soreness and pain in the lumbar region, which are alleviated by pressing, massage and maintaining recumbency, and aggravated by exertion; vexation, insomnia, dry mouth and throat, flushed face, feverish sensation in palms and soles, red tongue with little coating, and taut, thready and rapid pulse.

Therapeutic Principle: To nourish kidney yin.

Prescription: Modified Zuo Gui Pill.

Modifications: For chronic lumbar pain, use Qing E Pill.

5. Vertigo/Dizziness

A. Etiology and Pathogenesis

1) Hyperactivity of Liver Yang
2) Deficiency of Qi and Blood
3) Insufficiency of Kidney Essence
4) Dampness and Phlegm Blocking Middle Warmer
5) Stagnation of Blood Stasis
6) Affection of Exogenous Pathogenic Factors

B. Syndrome Differentiation and Treatment

1) <u>Hyperactivity of Liver Yang</u>

Symptoms: Dizziness, tinnitus, distending pain in the head, irritability, insomnia, dreamfulness, and taut pulse; or accompanied flushed face, conjunctival congestion, bitter taste in the mouth, constipation, dark yellow urine, red tongue with yellow coating, taut and rapid pulse; or accompanied sore and weak loins and knees, amnesia, seminal emission, red tongue with little coating, and taut, thready and rapid pulse; or dizziness, posture instability, nausea, headache with distending sensation, numbness and tremor of the limbs, dysphasia and staggering movement.

Therapeutic Principle: To soothe the liver, suppress yang, remove fire and stop wind.

Prescription: Modified Tian Ma Gou Teng Decoction.

Modifications: For hyperactive liver fire, add Radix Gentianae (Long Dan Cao) 5g and Cortex Moutan Radicis (Mu Dan Pi) 10g; or use Long Dan Xie Gan Decoction supplemented with Concha Haliotidis (Shi Jue Ming) 20g and Ramulus Uncariae cum Uncis (Gou Teng) 12g. For constipation, add Radix et Rhizoma Rhei (Da Huang) 6g and Natrii Sulfas (Mang Xiao) 10g; for yin deficiency of the liver and kidney, add Concha Ostreae (Mu Li) 20g, Carapax et Plastrum Testudinis (Gui Ban) 20g, Carapax Trionycis (Bie Jia) 15g, Radix Polygoni Multiflori (He Shou Wu) 15g and Radix Rehmanniae (Di Huang) 15g; for internal wind due to extremely hyperactive liver yang, use modified Ling Yang Jiao Decoction.

2) Deficiency of Both Qi and Blood

Symptoms: Dizziness aggravated by exertion and overstrain, listlessness, indolence of speaking, shortness of breath, low voice, pale and lusterless complexion, palpitation, insomnia, anorexia, or postprandial bloating, loose stools, or cold intolerance, cold limbs, pale lips and nails, pale, tender and chubby tongue with teeth marks on its margin, little or thick tongue coating, and thready or deficiency and large pulse.

Therapeutic Principle: To replenish qi, nourish blood, invigorate the spleen and regulate the stomach.

Prescription: Modified Ba Zhen Decoction.

Modifications: For collapse of qi due to deficiency of the spleen, use Bu Zhong Yi Qi Decoction; for deficiency of spleen yang, use Li Zhong Decoction supplemented with Radix Polygoni Multiflori (He Shou Wu) 15g, Radix Angelicae Sinensis (Dang Gui) 10g, Rhizoma Ligustici Chuanxiong (Chuan Xiong) 9g and Cortex Cinnamomi Cassiae (Rou Gui) 3g; if main manifestation is palpitation, insomnia and amnesia, use Gui Pi Decoction; severe blood deficiency, add Gelatinum Corii Asini (E Jiao) 9g and Placenta Hominis (Zi He Che) 3g, and increase the dosage of Radix Astragali (Huang Qi).

3) Deficiency of Kidney Essence

Symptoms: Dizziness, spiritlessness, sore and weak loins and knees, or seminal emission, tinnitus, alopecia, loose teeth, insomnia, dreamfulness, amnesia, small and tender or red and tender tongue with no or little coating, taut and thready or weak or thready and rapid pulse.

Therapeutic Principle: To replenish kidney essence.

Prescription: Modified He Che Da Zao Pill.

Modifications: For severe dizziness, add Mastodi Ossis Fossilia (Long Gu) 20g, Concha Ostreae (Mu Li) 20g, Carapax Trionycis (Bie Jia) 15g, Magnetitum (Ci Shi) 15g and Concha Margaritiferae

(Zhen Zhu Mu) 20g; for frequent seminal emission, add Stamen Nelumbinis Nuciferae (Lian Xu) 3g, Semen Euryales Ferocis (Qian Shi) 12g, Ootheca Mantidis (Sang Piao Xiao) 9g, Semen Astragali Complanati (Sha Yuan Zi) 12g and Fructus Rubi Chingii (Fu Pen Zi) 9g; for yin deficiency with headache, flushed cheeks, sore throat, emaciation, feverish sensation in the chest, palms and soles, red and tender tongue with little or peeled coating, thready and rapid pulse, use Zuo Gui Pill supplemented with Rhizoma Anemarrhenae (Zhi Mu) 10g, Cortex Phellodendri (Huang Bai) 9g and Radix Salviae Miltiorrhizae (Dan Shen) 10g; for yang deficiency with pale or black complexion, emaciation, cold limbs, pale and tender tongue with white coating, and weak pulse, use You Gui Pill supplemented with Radix Morindae officinalis (Ba Ji Tian) 12g, Herba Epimedii (Yin Yang Huo) 12g, Rhizoma Curculiginis Orchioidis (Xian Mao) 12g and Herba Cistanches (Rou Cong Rong) 15g.

4) <u>Stagnation of Turbid Phlegm</u>

Symptoms: Dizziness, lassitude, or heaviness and tightness in the head, sensation of stuffiness in the chest, nausea, vomiting with sputum and saliva, anorexia, dreamful sleep, chubby tongue with white and greasy coating, taut and slippery pulse.

Therapeutic Principle: To dry up dampness, resolve phlegm, invigorate the spleen and regulate the stomach.

Prescription: Modified Ban Xia Bai Zhu Tian Ma Decoction.

Modifications: For severe dizziness and frequent vomiting, add Ochra Haematitum (Dai Zhe Shi) 15g, Flos Inulae (Xuan Fu Hua) 9g and Rhizoma Arisaematis cum Bile (Dan Nan Xing) 3g; for sensation of stuffiness in the chest, and anorexia, add Fructus Amomi Cardamomi (Bai Kou Ren) 3g and Fructus Amomi Villosi (Sha Ren) 5g; for tinnitus, add Bulbus Allii Fistulosi (Cong Bai) 9g, Radix Curcumae (Yu Jin) 10g and Rhizoma Acori Tatarinowii (Shi Chang Pu) 9g; for distending pain in the head and eyes, vexation, bitter taste in the mouth, thirst without desire to drink, yellow and greasy tongue coating, taut and slippery pulse, use Wen Dan Decoction supplemented with Rhizoma Coptidis (Huang Lian) 9g and Radix Scutellariae Baicalensis (Huang Qin) 9g.

5) <u>Blood Stasis Blocking Collaterals</u>

Symptoms: Dizziness due to trauma or lingering dizziness, recurrent and localized stabbing pain in the head, amnesia, insomnia, palpitation, listlessness, tinnitus, dark purple complexion and lips, dark purple tongue with ecchymosis or petechiae, taut and slippery or thready and rough pulse.

Therapeutic Principle: To remove blood stasis, activate collaterals and promote blood circulation.

Prescription: Modified Tong Qiao Huo Xue Decoction.

Modifications: For pain in the chest and hypochondrium, and frequent sighing, add Radix Bupleuri (Chai Hu) 9g, Fructus Citri Aurantii (Zhi Ke) 9g and Radix Curcumae (Yu Jin) 10g; for concurrent qi deficiency with lassitude, excessive sweats and aversion to wind, add Radix Astragali (Huang Qi) 12g and Radix Codonopsitis Pilosulae (Dang Shen) 9g; for concurrent yang deficiency with cold intolerance and cold limbs, add Radix Aconiti Lateralis Praeparatae (Fu Zi) 10g and Ramulus Cinnamomi Cassiae (Gui Zhi) 9g; for concurrent yin deficiency with hot sensation in the bones and scaly dry skin, add Cortex Moutan Radicis (Mu Dan Pi) 10g, Rhizoma Anemarrhenae (Zhi Mu) 10g, Cortex Phellodendri (Huang Bai) 9g and Radix Rehmanniae (Di Huang) 15g.

6. Diarrhea

A. Etiology and Pathogenesis

1) Affection by Exogenous Pathogenic Factors
2) Improper Diet
3) Emotional Disturbance and Chronic Illness
4) Stagnation of Liver Qi Attacking the Spleen
5) Weakness of the Spleen and Stomach
6) Deficiency of Kidney Yang

B. Syndrome Differentiation and Treatment

1) Fulminant Diarrhea

(1) <u>Cold-Damp Impairing the Spleen</u>

Symptoms: Diarrhea with clear and thin or even watery stools, epigastric distention, abdominal pain, loud borborygmi, anorexia, or cold intolerance, fever, soreness of the limbs, headache, white or white and greasy tongue coating, soft and slow pulse.

Therapeutic Principle: To dispel cold and remove dampness.

Prescription: Modified Huo Xiang Zheng Qi Powder.

Modifications: For severe exterior cold syndrome, add Herba Schizonepetae (Jing Jie) 9g and Radix Saposhnikoviae Divaricatae (Fang Feng) 9g; for excessive dampness with abdominal distention, loud borborygmi and difficult urination, use Wei Ling Decoction; for excessive cold syndrome with abdominal distention, coldness and pain, use Li Zhong Decoction.

(2) <u>Damp-Heat in the Bowels</u>

Symptoms: Sudden onset of acute diarrhea with yellow, brown and foul stools, abdominal pain, or discomfort after diarrhea, burning sensation in the anus, dysphoria with feverish sensation, thirst, oliguria with yellow urine, red tongue with yellow and greasy coating, soft and rapid or slippery and rapid pulse.

Therapeutic Principle: To clear away heat and eliminate dampness.

Prescription: Modified Ge Gen Qin Lian Decoction.

Modifications: For excessive dampness with stuffiness and fullness in the chest and abdomen, and absence of thirst, remove Radix Scutellariae Baicalensis (Huang Qin) and add Cortex Magnoliae Officinalis (Hou Po) 9g, Herba Agastache seu Pogostemonis (Huo Xiang) 9g and Rhizoma Atractylodis (Cang Zhu) 9g; for fever, headache and floating pulse, add Flos Lonicerae (Jin Yin Hua) 15g, Fructus Forsythiae Suspensae (Lian Qiao) 10g and Herba Menthae Haplocalycis (Bo He) 9g; for fever, headache, dysphoria with feverish sensation, spontaneous sweating, oliguria with dark urine, soft and rapid pulse during summer season, use Xin Jia Xiang Ru Decoction and Liu Yi Powder.

(3) Food Retention in the Stomach and Bowels

Symptoms: Abdominal pain that is relieved after diarrhea, loud borborygmi, diarrhea with foul stools, abdominal distention and fullness, belching with rotten odor, anorexia, thick and greasy tongue coating, and slippery pulse.

Therapeutic Principle: To promote digestion and remove food retention.

Prescription: Modified Bao He Pill.

Modifications: For yellow tongue coating and slippery pulse in patients with overeating of pungent, sweat and fried food, add Radix Scutellariae Baicalensis (Huang Qin) 9g and Rhizoma Coptidis (Huang Lian) 9g; for white tongue coating and slow pulse in patients with overeating of cold meals, add Ping Wei Powder; for severe food retention, abdominal distention and fullness, and dyschezia, use Zhi Shi Dao Zhi Pill.

2) Chronic Diarrhea

(1) Deficiency of Spleen Qi

Symptoms: Recurrent, lingering and chronic diarrhea with watery stools and undigested food, anorexia, postprandial epigastric discomfort and distention, increased defecation after intake of fatty and greasy meals, sallow complexion, listlessness, lassitude, pale tongue with thin and white coating, thready and weak pulse.

Therapeutic Principle: To invigorate the spleen, replenish qi, eliminate dampness and relieve diarrhea.

Prescription: Modified Shen Ling Bai Zhu Powder.

Modifications: For qi collapse of Middle Warmer with persistent and chronic diarrhea, shortness of breath and prolapse of anus, use Bu Zhong Yi Qi Decoction; for deficiency of spleen yang with cold limbs, abdominal coldness and pain alleviated by warmth and pressure, use Fu Zi Li Zhong Decoction.

(2) <u>Deficiency of Kidney Yang</u>

Symptoms: Middle abdominal pain before dawn, immediate diarrhea with undigested food after loud borborygmi, comfort after diarrhea, abdominal coldness and pain that are alleviated by warmth and pressure, general coldness, cold limbs, lumbar soreness and weak knees, pale tongue with white coating, deep and thready pulse.

Therapeutic Principle: To warm the kidney, strengthen the spleen and relieve diarrhea.

Prescription: Modified Si Shen Pill.

Modifications: For senility and qi collapse of the Middle Warmer with persistent and chronic diarrhea, and prolapse of anus, add Rhizoma Cimicifugae (Sheng Ma) 9g, Radix Bupleuri (Chai Hu) 9g, Radix Astragali (Huang Qi) 12g and Radix Codonopsitis Pilosulae (Dang Shen) 9g; for chronic diarrhea and fecal incontinence, add Limonitum (Yu Yu Liang) 15g, Fructus Terminaliae Chebulae (He Zi) 9g and Halloysitum Rubrum (Chi Shi Zhi) 15g, or add Zhen Ren Yang Zang Decoction.

(3) <u>Stagnation of Liver Qi</u>

Symptoms: Abdominal pain and diarrhea after emotional disturbance, slight relief of abdominal pain after diarrhea, passing flatus frequently, distention and stuffiness in the chest and hypochondrium, belching, anorexia, slight red tongue, and taut pulse.

Therapeutic Principle: To suppress the hyperactive liver qi and support the spleen.

Prescription: Modified Tong Xie Formula.

Modifications: For distention and fullness in the chest, hypochondrium and abdomen, and belching, add Radix Bupleuri (Chai Hu) 9g, Fructus Citri Aurantii (Zhi Ke) 9g, Radix Aucklandiae Lappae (Mu Xiang) 9g and Rhizoma Cyperi Rotundi (Xiang Fu) 10g; for persistent and chronic diarrhea, add Fructus Pruni Mume (Wu Mei) 20g, Galla Rhois Chinensis (Wu Bei Zi) 5g and Pericarpium Punicae Granati (Shi Liu Pi) 9g; for severe spleen deficiency with lassitude and anorexia, add Radix Codonopsitis Pilosulae (Dang Shen) 9g, Sclerotium Poriae Cocos (Fu Ling) 12g, Semen Dolichoris Lablab (Bian Dou) 15g and Rhizoma Dioscoreae (Shan Yao) 15g.

7. Constipation

A. Etiology and Pathogenesis

1) Improper Diet
2) Emotional Disorders
3) Affection by Exogenous Pathogenic Factors
4) Senility and Postpartum Weakness

B. Syndrome Differentiation and Treatment

1) <u>Heat Accumulation in the Stomach and Bowels</u>

Symptoms: Dry stools, distending pain in the abdomen, flushed face, fever, dry mouth with foul odor, or aphthous stomatitis, red tongue with dry and yellow coating, slippery and rapid pulse.

Therapeutic Principle: To clear away heat, relieve stagnation, moisten the bowels and promote defecation.

Prescription: Modified Ma Zi Ren Pill.

Modifications: For depletion of body fluid with thirst with a desire to drink, red tongue with little coating, add Radix Rehmanniae (Di Huang) 15g, Radix Ophiopogonis Japonici (Mai Dong) 12g and Radix Scrophulariae Ningpoensis (Xuan Shen) 12g; for irritability, conjunctival congestion, taut and rapid pulse, add Cortex Moutan Radicis (Mu Dan Pi) 10g and Fructus Gardeniae Jasminoidis (Zhi Zi) 10g.

2) <u>Qi Stagnation in the Bowels</u>

Symptoms: Dry or not very dry stools, urgency and difficulty in defecation, or discomfort after defecation, borborygmus, passing flatus, distending pain in the abdomen, fullness and stuffiness in the chest and hypochondrium, frequent belching, anorexia, thin and greasy tongue coating, and taut pulse.

Therapeutic Principle: To restore the free flow of qi and relieve stagnation.

Prescription: Modified Liu Mo Decoction.

Modifications: For emotional disturbance, depression and reticence, add Radix Bupleuri (Chai Hu) 9g, Radix Paeoniae Alba (Bai Shao Yao) 9g and Rhizoma Cyperi Rotundi (Xiang Fu) 10g; for qi stagnation turning into fire with bitter taste in the mouth, dry throat, red tongue with yellow coating, taut and rapid pulse, add Fructus Gardeniae Jasminoidis (Zhi Zi) 9g, Cortex Moutan Radicis (Mu Dan Pi) 10g and Radix Gentianae (Long Dan Cao) 5g.

3) <u>Retention of Yin Cold</u>

Symptoms: Dyschezia, abdominal pain and distention aggravated by pressure, hypochondriac pain, cold limbs, belching and vomiting, white and greasy tongue coaling, taut and tense pulse.

Therapeutic Principle: To warm the interior, expel cold, relieve stagnation and promote bowel movement.

Prescription: Modified Da Huang Fu Zi Decoction.

Modifications: For distending pain in the abdomen, add Cortex Magnoliae Officinalis (Hou Po) 9g and Fructus Citri Aurantii Immaturus (Zhi Shi) 9g; for cold limbs and cold pain in the abdomen, add Rhizoma Zingiberis Officinalis (Dan Jiang) 9g and Fructus Feoniculi (Xiao Hui Xiang) 9g.

4) Deficiency of Spleen Qi

Symptoms: Neither dry nor hard stools, urgency to defecate with difficult defecation, sweating, shortness of breath, fatigue after bowel movement, pale complexion, listlessness, lassitude, indolence of speaking, pale tongue with white coating, and weak pulse.

Therapeutic Principle: To replenish qi and lubricate the bowels.

Prescription: Modified Huang Qi Decoction.

Modifications: For severe qi deficiency with sweating and shortness of breath, add Radix Codonopsitis Pilosulae (Dang Shen) 9g and Fructus Schisandrae Chinensis (Wu Wei Zi) 5g; for sinking of qi with prolapse of anus, add Bu Zhong Yi Qi Decoction; for dizziness, pale finger and nails, add Radix Polygoni Multiflori (He Shou Wu) 15g and Radix Rehmanniae (Di Huang) 12g; for severe shortness of breath, add Ge Jie Powder; for anorexia, add Fructus Hordei Germinatus (Mai Ya) 15g.

5) Deficiency of Blood and Body Fluid

Symptoms: Dry stools, lusterless complexion, vertigo, palpitation, shortness of breath, insomnia, dreamfulness, amnesia, pale lips and nails, pale tongue with white coating, and thready or thready and weak pulse.

Therapeutic Principle: To nourish blood and moisten dryness.

Prescription: Modified Run Chang Pill.

Modifications: For concurrent qi deficiency with shortness of breath, listlessness, fatigue, add Radix Astragali (Huang Qi) 12ga and Radix Codonopsitis Pilosulae (Dang Shen) 9g; for dry stools after recovery of blood deficiency, add Wu Ren Pill; for blood deficiency and internal heat, add Rhizoma Picrorrhizae (Hu Huang Lian) 9g and Rhizoma Anemarrhenae (Zhi Mu) 10g.

6) Deficiency of Yin

Symptoms: Dry and hard stools, dizziness, tinnitus, emaciation, vexation, insomnia, flushed cheeks, or hectic fever, night sweats, lumbar soreness and weak knees, red tongue with no or little coating, thready and rapid pulse.

Therapeutic Principle: To nourish yin and promote bowel movement.

Prescription: Modified Zeng Ye Decoction.

Modifications: For constipation with dry and hard stools, add Semen Cannabis Sativae (Huo Ma Ren) 12g, Semen Biotae Orientalis (Bai Zi Ren) 12g and Semen Trichosanthis (Gua Lou Zi) 12g; for deficiency of stomach yin with dry mouth and thirst, use Yi Wei Decoction; for deficiency of kidney yin with lumbar soreness and weak knees, use Liu Wei Di Huang Pill.

7) <u>Deficiency of Spleen Yang and Kidney Yang</u>

Symptoms: Dry or not dry stools, dyschezia, polyuria with clear urine, pale complexion, cold limbs, cold pain in the abdomen relieved by warmth and pressure, soreness and coldness in the lumbar region and knees, pale tongue with white coating, deep and slow pulse.

Therapeutic Principle: To warm yang, lubricate bowels and promote bowel movement.

Prescription: Modified Ji Chuan Decoction.

Modifications: For senility with deficient-cold and constipation, use Ban Liu Pill; for stagnation of cold and qi with cold pain in the abdomen, add Rhizoma Zingiberis Officinalis (Gan Jiang) 10g and Radix Aucklandiae Lappae (Mu Xiang) 9g; for nocturnal polyuria, add Fructus Rosae Laevigatae (Jin Ying Zi) 15g, Radix Linderae Strychnifoliae (Wu Yao) 9g and Rhizoma Dioscoreae (Shan Yao) 15g.

8. Vomiting

A. Etiology and Pathogenesis

1) Exogenous Pathogenic Factors Attacking the Stomach
2) Improper Diet
3) Emotional Disturbance
4) Deficiency of the Spleen and Stomach

B. Syndrome Differentiation and Treatment

1) <u>Pathogenic Cold Attacking the Stomach</u>

Symptoms: Sudden onset of vomiting, fever, cold intolerance, headache, absence of sweats, abdominal distention and stuffiness, anorexia, thin and white tongue coating, floating and tense pulse.

Therapeutic Principle: To relieve exterior syndrome, dispel cold, regulate the stomach and lower the adverse flow of qi.

Prescription: Modified Huo Xiang Zheng Qi Powder.

Modifications: For food retention with vomiting of undigested food, abdominal distention and fullness, remove Rhizoma Atractylodis Macrocephalae (Bai Zhu) and Fructus Zizyphi Jujubae (Da Zao), and add Endothelium Corneum Gigeriae Galli (Ji Nei Jin) 9g and Fructus Hordei Germinatus (Mai

Ya) 12g; for excessive wind-cold, add Herba Schizonepetae (Jing Jie) 10g and Radix Saposhnikoviae Divaricatae (Fang Feng) 10g.

2) Retention of Food in the Stomach

Symptoms: Vomiting of undigested food aggravated by meals, comfort after vomiting, abdominal distention and fullness, eructation, anorexia, abdominal pain, thick and greasy tongue coating, and slippery pulse.

Therapeutic Principle: To promote digestion, relieve retention, regulate the stomach and lower adverse flow of qi.

Prescription: Modified Bao He Pill.

Modifications: For severe stomach heat, add Rhizoma Phragmitis Communis (Lu Gen) 15g and Rhizoma Coptidis (Huang Lian) 9g; for abdominal fullness and constipation, add Radix et Rhizoma Rhei (Da Huang) 6g and Fructus Citri Aurantii Immaturus (Zhi Shi) 10g; for chronic food retention turning into fire with abdominal distention and constipation, use Da Cheng Qi Decoction.

3) Retention of Phlegm and Fluid in the Body

Symptoms: Vomiting saliva, sputum and watery fluid, distention and stuffiness in the chest and epigastric area, anorexia, vertigo, palpitation, white and greasy tongue coating, and slippery pulse.

Therapeutic Principle: To warm and remove phlegm and fluid, regulate the stomach and lower adverse flow of qi.

Prescription: Modified Er Chen Decoction and Ling Gui Zhu Gan Decoction.

Modifications: For insufficiency of spleen qi with epigastric distention and anorexia, add Fructus Amomi Villosi (Sha Ren) 5g, Rhizoma Atractylodis (Cang Zhu) 9g and Herba Eupatorii (Pei Lan) 9g; for stagnation of Middle Warmer with bitter taste in the mouth, feeling of stuffiness in the chest, nausea, vomiting, yellow and greasy tongue coating, use Wen Dan Decoction.

4) Hyperactive Liver Qi Attacking the Stomach

Symptoms: Vomiting with acid regurgitation, which is aggravated by emotional disturbance; frequent belching, fullness and pain in the chest and hypochondrium, red tongue margin, thin tongue coating, and taut pulse.

Therapeutic Principle: To soothe the liver, regulate qi, regulate the stomach and lower the adverse flow of qi.

Prescription: Modified Ban Xia Hou Po Decoction.

Modifications: For qi stagnation turning into fire with dysphoria, discomfort, vomiting acid and watery fluid, use Si Ni Powder and Zuo Jin Pill; for constipation, add Radix et Rhizoma Rhei (Da

Huang) 6g and Natrii Sulfas (Mang Xiao) 10g; for qi stagnation and blood stasis with pricking pain in the chest and hypochondrium, use Ge Xia Zhu Yu Decoction.

5) Insufficiency of Spleen Yang

Symptoms: Intermittent vomiting after improper diet, anorexia, dry mouth without desire to drink, pale and lusterless complexion, fatigue, preference to warmth and aversion to cold, loose stools, pale tongue with thin coating, thready and weak pulse.

Therapeutic Principle: To warm the Middle Warmer, strengthen the spleen, regulate the stomach and lower the adverse flow of qi.

Prescription: Modified Li Zhong Decoction.

Modifications: For vomiting saliva, sputum and watery fluid, add Ramulus Cinnamomi Cassiae (Gui Zhi) 9g, Fructus Evodiae Rutaecarpae (Wu Zhu Yu) 3g and Rhizoma Zingiberis Recens (Sheng Jiang) 9g; for cold sensation in the epigastric area, cold limbs, sore and weak loins and knees, add Cortex Cinnamomi Cassiae (Rou Gui) 3g and Radix Aconiti Lateralis Praeparatae (Fu Zi) 10g.

6) Insufficiency of Stomach Yin

Symptoms: Recurrent vomiting without much contents, occasional retching, dry mouth and throat, hunger but anorexia, gastric discomfort, red tongue with little moisture and coating, thready and rapid pulse.

Therapeutic Principle: To nourish yin, moisten dryness, lower the adverse flow of qi and relieve vomiting.

Prescription: Modified Mai Men Dong Decoction.

Modifications: For frequent vomiting, add Caulis Bambusae in Taeniam (Zhu Ru) 9g and Pericarpium Citri Reticulatae (Ju Pi) 9g; for constipation, add Semen Cannabis Sativae (Huo Ma Ren) 12g and honey; for severe yin deficiency, decrease the dosage of Rhizoma Pinelliae Ternatae (Ban Xia) and add Herba Dendrobii (Shi Hu) 10g and Radix Trichosanthis (Tian Hua Fen) 12g.

9. Edema

A. Etiology and Pathogenesis

1) Invasion of Exogenous Pathogenic Wind, with Impairment of Lung Function in Regulation and Ventilation.
2) Retention of Water and Dampness, with Impaired Function of the Spleen in Transportation
3) Invasion of the Spleen and Lung by Damp-Heat and Sore Toxins
4) Improper Diet and Overstrain, with Impairment of the Spleen and Stomach

5) Congenital Insufficiency, Chronic Illness, Sexual Indulgence and Postpartum Weakness

B. Syndrome Differentiation and Treatment

1) <u>Invasion of Wind and Overflow of Water</u>

Symptoms: Acute onset of edema starting from the eyelids, followed by limbs and the whole body, aversion to cold, fever, soreness of the limbs and joints, difficult urination; swollen and sore throat, red tongue, floating, slippery and rapid pulse (predominant wind-heat); or aversion to cold, cough, dyspnea, thin and white tongue coating, floating and slippery or floating and tense pulse (predominant wind-cold).

Therapeutic Principle: To eliminate wind, disperse lung qi, promote water circulation and relieve edema.

Prescription: Modified Yue Bi Jia Zhu Decoction.

Modifications: Could add Herba Spirodelae (Fu Ping) 9g, Rhizoma Alismatis Orientalis (Ze Xie) 9g and Sclerotium Poriae Cocos (Fu Ling) 12g to the prescription. For swollen and sore throat, add Radix Isatidis seu Baphicacanthi (Ban Lan Gen) 12g, Radix Platycodi Grandiflori (Jie Geng) 9g, Fructus Forsythiae Suspensae (Lian Qiao) 10g and Rhizoma Phragmitis Communis (Lu Gen) 15g; for severe heat and oliguria, add Rhizoma Imperatae Cylindricae (Bai Mao Gen) 20g and Semen Phaseoli (Chi Xiao Dou) 15g; for excessive wind-cold syndrome, remove Gypsum Fibrosum (Shi Gao) and add Folium Perillae Frutescentis (Su Ye) 9g, Radix Saposhnikoviae Divaricatae (Fang Feng) 9g and Ramulus Cinnamomi Cassiae (Gui Zhi) 9g; for severe cough and dyspnea, add Radix Peucedani (Qian Hu) 9g and Semen Armeniacae Amarum (Xing Ren) 9g; for sweating, aversion to wind, general heavy sensation and edema, use Fang Ji Huang Qi Decoction.

2) <u>Invasion of Toxic Dampness</u>

Symptoms: Edema of the eyelids followed by generalized edema, shiny skin, oliguria with dark urine, pyogenic infection or even ulceration of skin, aversion to wind, fever, red tongue with thin and yellow coating, floating and rapid or slippery and rapid pulse.

Therapeutic Principle: To disperse lung qi, remove toxic substance, promote diuresis and relieve edema.

Prescription: Modified Ma Huang Lian Qiao Chi Xiao Dou Decoction and Wu Wei Xiao Du Decoction.

Modifications: For severe septic condition, increase the dosage of Herba Taraxaci Mongolici (Pu Gong Ying) and Herba cum Radice Violae (Zi Hua Di Ding), and add Rhizoma Paridis (Zao Xiu) 10g; for predominant dampness with skin ulceration, add Radix Sophorae Flavescentis (Ku Shen) 9g and Rhizoma Smilacis Glabrae (Tu Fu Ling) 20g; for predominant wind with pruritus, add Cortex Dictamni Radicis (Bai Xian Pi) 9g, Fructus Kochiae Scopariae (Di Fu Zi) 12g and Periostracum Cicadae (Chan Tui) 9g; for blood heat with red and swollen skin, add Cortex Moutan Radicis (Mu Dan Pi) 10g and Radix Paeoniae Rubra (Chi Shao) 10g; for constipation, add Radix et Rhizoma Rhei (Da Huang) 6g and Natrii Sulfas (Mang Xiao) 10g.

3) Retention of Water and Dampness

Symptoms: Pitted edema of the whole body, oliguria, general heavy sensation, sensation of stuffiness in the chest, anorexia, nausea, abdominal distention, white and greasy tongue coating, deep and slow pulse.

Therapeutic Principle: To invigorate the spleen, eliminate dampness, activate yang and promote diuresis.

Prescription: Modified Wu Pi Decoction and Wei Ling Decoction.

Modifications: For severe edema and dyspnea, add Herba Ephedrae (Ma Huang) 6g, Semen Armeniacae Amarum (Xing Ren) 9g, Fructus Perillae (Su Zi) 9g and Semen Descurainiae seu Lepidii (Ting Li Zi) 9g; for retention of dampness in the Middle Warmer with abdominal distention and fullness, add Semen Zanthoxyli (Jiao Mu) 3g, Pericarpium Areca Catechu (Da Fu Pi) 9g and Rhizoma Zingiberis Officinalis (Gan Jiang) 9g.

4) Excess of Damp-Heat

Symptoms: Anasarca, shiny and taut skin, distention and stuffiness in the chest and epigastric area, dysphoria with feverish sensation, thirst, oliguria with dark urine, or constipation, red tongue with yellow and greasy coating, deep and rapid or soft and rapid pulse.

Therapeutic Principle: To clear away heat, promote diuresis and regulate qi circulation.

Prescription: Modified Shu Zao Decoction.

Modifications: For abdominal distention and fullness, and constipation, add Radix et Rhizoma Rhei (Da Huang) 6g and Semen Descurainiae seu Lepidii (Ting Li Zi) 10g; for hematuria and dysuria, add Herba seu Radix Cirsii Japonici (Da Ji) 12g, Herba Cephalanoploris (Xiao Ji) 15g and Rhizoma Imperatae Cylindricae (Bai Mao Gen) 20g; for severe edema, stuffiness in the chest, asthmatic breathing, inability to lie flat, taut and forceful pulse, use Ting Li Da Zao Xie Fei Decoction and Wu Ling Powder; for chronic retention of damp-heat transforming into dryness that further damages yin, with dry mouth and throat, and constipation, use Zhu Ling Decoction.

5) Deficiency of Spleen Yang

Symptoms: Chronic and general pitted edema that is more pronounced below the waist, abdominal distention and stuffiness, anorexia, loose stools, sallow complexion, listlessness, fatigue, lassitude, cold limbs, oliguria, pale tongue with white and greasy or white and slippery coating, deep and slow or deep and weak pulse.

Therapeutic Principle: To warm and invigorate spleen yang to promote diuresis.

Prescription: Modified Shi Pi Decoction.

Modifications: For severe edema and loose stools, add Ramulus Cinnamomi Cassiae (Gui Zhi) 9g and Radix Astragali (Huang Qi) 12g, or Fructus Psoraleae Corylifoliae (Bu Gu Zhi) 9g and Radix Aconiti Lateralis Praeparatae (Fu Zi) 10g; for oliguria, add Ramulus Cinnamomi Cassiae (Gui Zhi) 9g and Rhizoma Alismatis Orientalis (Ze Xie) 10g; for deficiency of spleen qi with slight general edema, sallow complexion, severe edema of the eyelids and face in the early morning, edema of lower limbs on exertion, good appetite with fatigue and lassitude, normal stools or loose stools, polyuria, thin and greasy tongue coating, soft and weak pulse, use Shen Ling Bai Zhu Powder.

6) <u>Deficiency of Kidney Yang</u>

Symptoms: Recurrent and general pitted edema that is more pronounced below the waist, soreness, coldness and heaviness in the lumbar region, oliguria, extremely cold limbs, cold intolerance, listlessness, grayish dim or pale complexion, palpitation, sensation of stuffiness in the chest, dyspnea, inability to lie flat, abdominal enlargement, distention and fullness; pale and chubby tongue with white coating, deep and thready or deep, slow and forceless pulse.

Therapeutic Principle: To warm the kidney, assist yang, activate qi to promote water circulation.

Prescription: Modified Ji Sheng Shen Qi Pill and Zhen Wu Decoction.

Modifications: For edema of the eyelids and face, dull facial expression, slowness in movement, cold body and limbs, use modified You Gui Pill; for deficiency of kidney yin with recurrent edema, spiritlessness, lumbar soreness, seminal emission, dry mouth and throat, dysphoria with feverish sensation in the chest, palms and soles, red tongue, thready and weak pulse, use Zuo Gui Pill supplemented with Rhizoma Alismatis Orientalis (Ze Xie) 9g, Sclerotium Poriae Cocos (Fu Ling) 12g and Semen Malvae (Dong Kui Zi) 12g; for deficiency of liver yin and kidney yin accompanied by hyperactivity of liver yang with flushed face, dizziness, headache, palpitation, insomnia, sore and weak loins and knees, or tremors of the limbs, use Zuo Gui Pill supplemented with Concha Margaritiferae (Zhen Zhu Mu) 20g, Mastodi Ossis Fossilia (Long Gu) 20g, Concha Ostreae (Mu Li) 20g, Carapax Trionycis (Bie Jia) 15g, Herba Taxilli or Ramulus Loranthi Seu Visci (Sang Ji Sheng) 12g, Spica Prunellae Vulgaris (Xia Ku Cao) 12g and Flos Chrysanthemi Morifolii (Ju Hua) 12g.

7) Retention of Water and Blood Stasis

Symptoms: Chronic and persistent edema of the limbs or the whole body (more pronounced in the lower limbs), ecchymosis of the skin, stabbing pain in the lumbar region, or hematuria, dark purple tongue with ecchymosis and white coating, deep, thready and rough pulse.

Therapeutic Principle: To promote circulation of blood, qi and water, and remove blood stasis.

Prescription: Modified Tao Hong Si Wu Decoction and Wu Ling Powder.

Modifications: For severe anasarca, dyspnea, dysphoria with sensation of stuffiness in the chest, difficult urination, add Semen Descurainiae seu Lepidii (Ting Li Zi) 9g, Semen Zanthoxyli (Jiao Mu) 3g and Herba Lycopi Lucidi (Ze Lan) 12g; for lumbar soreness, weak knees, listlessness and fatigue, add Ji Sheng Shen Qi Pill; for deficiency of qi and yang, add Radix Astragali (Huang Qi) 12g and Radix Aconiti Lateralis Praeparatae (Fu Zi) 10g.

10. Jaundice

A. Etiology and Pathogenesis

1) Affection by Exogenous Pathogenic Factors
2) Improper Diet
3) Internal Injury due to Overstrain
4) Obstruction of Biliary Ducts by Calculi and Ascaris
5) Protracted Abdominal Mass

B. Syndrome Differentiation and Treatment

1) Damp-Heat Exterior Syndrome

Symptoms: Early stage of jaundice, mild or not remarkable yellow eyes, cold intolerance, fever, pruritus and sore of the skin, general heavy sensation, lassitude, swollen and sore throat, abdominal distention, nausea, thin and greasy tongue coating, soft and rapid pulse.

Therapeutic Principle: To clear away heat, eliminate dampness and relieve exterior syndrome.

Prescription: Modified Gan Lu Xiao Du Powder and Ma Huang Lian Qiao Chi Xiao Dou Decoction.

Modifications: For mild exterior syndrome, decrease the dosage of Herba Ephedrae (Ma Huang) and Herba Menthae Haplocalycis (Bo He); for severe yellow eyes, increase the dosage of Herba Artemisiae Scopariae (Yin Chen Hao); for severe heat, add Fructus Gardeniae Jasminoidis (Zhi Zi) 9g and Flos Lonicerae (Jin Yin Hua) 12g.

2) More Dampness than Heat

Symptoms: Yellow body and eyes (not bright yellow color), absence of fever, or low-grade fever, heavy sensation in the head, malaise, distention and fullness in the chest and abdomen, anorexia, nausea, vomiting, aversion to fatty and greasy food, loose stools, oliguria with yellow urine, thick, greasy and slight yellow tongue coating, taut and slippery r soft and slow pulse.

Therapeutic Principle: To eliminate dampness and remove turbidity.

Prescription: Modified Yin Chen Si Ling Powder.

Modifications: For distention and fullness in the chest and epigastrium, add Radix Aucklandiae Lappae (Mu Xiang) 9g, Fructus Citri Aurantii Immaturus (Zhi Shi) 9g and Cortex Magnoliae Officinalis (Hou Po) 9g; for nausea and vomiting, add Rhizoma Zingiberis Recens (Sheng Jiang) 9g, Rhizoma Pinelliae Ternatae (Ban Xia) 9g and Fructus Amomi Villosi (Sha Ren) 5g; for fever and thirst, add Radix Scutellariae Baicalensis (Huang Qin) 9g, Radix Puerariae (Ge Gen) 12g and Fructus Forsythiae Suspensae (Lian Qiao) 10g.

3) More Heat than Dampness

Symptoms: Bright yellow body and eyes, fever, thirst, or vexation, abdominal distention and fullness, dry mouth with bitter taste, nausea, vomiting, hypochondriac distending pain and tenderness, oliguria with dark yellow urine, constipation, red tongue with yellow and greasy coating, taut and rapid or slippery and rapid pulse.

Therapeutic Principle: To clear away heat and eliminate dampness.

Prescription: Modified Yin Chen Hao Decoction.

Modifications: For yellow body and eyes, add Herba Hyperici Japonici (Tian Ji Huang) 20g; for high fever and thirst, add Folium Isatidis (Da Qing Ye) 12g, Rhizoma Coptidis (Huang Lian) 9g and Cortex Phellodendri (Huang Bai) 9g; for abdominal distention and constipation, add Fructus Citri Aurantii Immaturus (Zhi Shi) 9g and Cortex Magnoliae Officinalis (Hou Po) 9g.

4) Heat Stagnation in Gallbladder Channel

Symptoms: Yellow body and eyes, right hypochondriac pain radiating to the shoulder and back, fever, or alternate fever and cold, bitter taste in the mouth, thirst, nausea, vomiting, constipation, oliguria with dark yellow urine, red tongue with yellow and greasy coating, taut and rapid pulse.

Therapeutic Principle: To clear away and purge gallbladder heat.

Prescription: Qing Dan Decoction supplemented with Radix Bupleuri (Chai Hu) 9g and Radix Scutellariae Baicalensis (Huang Qin) 9g.

Modifications: For severe hypochondriac pain, add Radix Curcumae (Yu Jin) 10g, Fructus Citri Aurantii (Zhi Ke) 9g and Radix Aucklandiae Lappae (Mu Xiang) 9g; for marked jaundice, add Herba

Artemisiae Scopariae (Yin Chen Hao) 15g, Herba Lysimachiae (Jin Qian Cao) 20g and Herba Hyperici Japonici (Tian Ji Huang) 20g; for vomiting and belching, add Semen Raphani Sativi (Lai Fu Zi) 9g and Rhizoma Pinelliae Ternatae (Ban Xia) 9g; for constipation, add Radix et Rhizoma Rhei (Da Huang) 6g and Natrii Sulfas (Mang Xiao) 10g.

5) Hyperactivity of Toxic Heat

Symptoms: Abrupt onset of bright golden colored jaundice that rapidly becomes darker, high fever, polydipsia, frequent vomiting, hypochondriac pain, abdominal fullness, unconsciousness, delirium, or epistaxis, hematochezia, ecchymosis in the skin and muscles, oliguria, constipation, crimson tongue with dry and yellow coating, taut and rapid or thready and rapid pulse.

Therapeutic Principle: To clear away heat, remove toxic substance and induce resuscitation.

Prescription: Modified Yin Chen Hao Decoction and Qing Wen Bai Du Decoction.

Modifications: For unconsciousness, add Zi Xue Pill or An Gong Niu Huang Pill; for epistaxis and hematochezia, add Cacumen Biotae Orientalis (Ce Bai Ye) 10g, Rhizoma Imperatae Cylindricae (Bai Mao Gen) 15g and Radix Lithospermi seu Macrotomiae (Zi Cao) 9g.

6) Retention of Cold-Damp in the Spleen

Symptoms: Dark yellow body and eyes, heavy sensation in the head, malaise, nausea, anorexia, abdominal distention, loose stools, spiritlessness, cold intolerance, pale tongue with white and greasy coating, soft and slow pulse.

Therapeutic Principle: To warm the Middle Warmer, dispel cold, strengthen the spleen and remove dampness.

Prescription: Modified Yin Chen Zhu Fu Decoction.

Modifications: For hypochondriac pain, add Herba Lycopi Lucidi (Ze Lan) 12g, Radix Curcumae (Yu Jin) 10g and Radix Paeoniae Rubra (Chi Shao) 10g; for loose stools, add Semen Plantaginis (Chen Qian Zi) 9g, Sclerotium Poriae Cocos (Fu Ling) 12g and Rhizoma Alismatis Orientalis (Ze Xie) 9g; for nausea, anorexia and abdominal distention, add Fructus Citri Aurantii Immaturus (Zhi Shi) 9g, Rhizoma Pinelliae Ternatae (Ban Xia) 9g and Pericarpium Citri Reticulatae (Ju Pi) 6g.

7) Retention of Blood Stasis in the Liver and Spleen

Symptoms: Chronic jaundice, dark yellow body and eyes, localized distending or pricking pain and lump in the hypochondrium, dark red tongue with petechiae, taut, thready and rough pulse.

Therapeutic Principle: To remove blood stasis and soothe the liver.

Prescription: Modified Ge Xia Zhu Yu Decoction.

Modifications: For hypochondriac pain, add Radix Curcumae (Yu Jin) 10g, Fructus Meliae Toosendan (Chuan Lian Zi) 9g and Radix Bupleuri (Chai Hu) 9g; for marked jaundice, add Herba Artemisiae Scopariae (Yin Chen Hao) 15g, Herba Hyperici Japonici (Tian Ji Huang) 20g and Herba Lysimachiae (Jin Qian Cao) 15g.

8) Deficiency of the Spleen and Blood

Symptoms: sallow complexion, pale, yellow and lusterless skin, weakness, dark urine that is more remarkable at night, spiritlessness, lassitude of the limbs, palpitation, shortness of breath, anorexia, loose stools, indolence of speaking, insomnia, pale tongue with thin and white coating, thready and weak pulse.

Therapeutic Principle: To strengthen the spleen, warm the Middle Warmer, replenish qi and nourish blood.

Prescription: Modified Xiao Jian Zhong Decoction.

Modifications: For marked deficiency of qi, add Radix Astragali (Huang Qi) 12g and Radix Codonopsitis Pilosulae (Dan Shen) 9g; for marked deficiency of blood, add Radix Angelicae Sinensis (Dang Gui) 10g, Radix Rehmanniae (Di Huang) 12g, Gelatinum Corii Asini (E Jiao) 9g and Herba Ecliptae Prostratae (Han Lian Cao) 15g; for marked yang deficiency, replace Ramulus Cinnamomi Cassiae (Gui Zhi) with Cortex Cinnamomi Cassiae (Rou Gui) 3g, and add Rhizoma Zingiberis Officinalis (Gan Jiang) 9g.

11. Spermatorrhea (Nocturnal Emission and Spontaneous Emission)

A. Etiology and Pathogenesis

1) Indulgence in Sexual Activities
2) Congenital Insufficiency
3) Emotional Disturbance
4) Improper Diet

B. Syndrome Differentiation and Treatment

1) Hyperactivity of Heart Fire and Kidney Fire

Symptoms: Insomnia with dreamful sleep, seminal emission during sleep (nocturnal emission), dysphoria with feverish sensation in the heart, vertigo, listlessness, lassitude, palpitation, restlessness, fright, amnesia, dry mouth, oliguria with dark urine, red tongue, thready and rapid pulse.

Therapeutic Principle: To remove heart fire, tranquilize the mind, nourish yin and clear away heat.

Prescription: Modified Huang Lian Qing Xin Decoction.

Modifications For hyperactive liver fire with flushed face, conjunctival congestion, restlessness, irritability, taut and rapid pulse, add Spica Prunellae Vulgaris (Xia Ku Cao) 12g and Radix Gentianae (Long Dan Cao) 5g; for yin deficiency with dizziness, tinnitus and red tongue, add Tuber Asparagi Cochinchinensis (Tian Dong) 10g and Radix Scrophulariae Ningpoensis (Xuan Shen) 10g.

2) Downward Movement of Damp-Heat

Symptoms: Frequent seminal emission, hot, dark and cloudy urine with small amount of seminal fluid, or difficult urination, bitter taste in the mouth, or thirst, restlessness, insomnia, aphthous stomatitis, foul and loose stools, or abdominal distention and stuffiness, nausea, yellow and greasy tongue coating, soft and rapid pulse.

Therapeutic Principle: To clear away heat and induce diuresis.

Prescription: Modified Bi Xie Fen Qing Decoction.

Modifications: For retention of damp-heat in the liver collaterals with dark yellow urine, itching and pain in the penis, add Radix Gentianae (Long Dan Cao) 5g, Radix Sophorae Flavescentis (Ku Shen) 9g and Caulis Akebiae (Mu Tong) 5g; for chronic illness with stagnant heat with difficult urination, distention in the lower abdomen and genitals, Patriniae Herba cum Radice (Bai Jiang Cao) 10g and Radix Paeoniae Rubra (Chi Shao) 10g.

3) Inability of Qi to Arrest Semen

Symptoms: Seminal emission on exertion and overstrain, palpitation, restlessness, insomnia, amnesia, sallow complexion, lassitude of the limbs, anorexia, loose stools, pale tongue with thin coating, thready and weak pulse.

Therapeutic Principle: To regulate and nourish the heart and spleen, replenish qi, and arrest semen.

Prescription: Modified Miao Xiang Powder.

Modifications: For failure of Middle Warmer qi to ascend, add Rhizoma Cimicifugae (Sheng Ma) 6g and Radix Bupleuri (Chai Hu) 6g.

4) Inability to Store Essence due to Kidney Deficiency

Symptoms: Frequent nocturnal emission, even spontaneous emission, lumbar soreness and weak knees, dry throat, vexation, vertigo, tinnitus, amnesia, insomnia, low-grade fever, flushed cheeks, emaciation, night sweats, loss of hair, loose teeth, red tongue with little coating, thready and rapid pulse; or persistent seminal emission, cold intolerance, cold body and limbs, impotence, premature ejaculation, cold sperm, nocturnal polyuria or oliguria, edema, clear urine, or dribbling urination, pale or lusterless complexion, tender tongue with teeth marks and white and slippery coating, deep and thready pulse.

Therapeutic Principle: To nourish kidney essence, induce astringency and stop emission.

Prescription: Modified Zuo Gui Decoction, Jin Suo Gu Jing Pill and Shui Lu Er Xian Pill.

Modifications: For yin deficiency affecting yang, leading to deficiency of both yin and yang, add Fructus Psoraleae Corylifoliae (Bu Gu Zhi) 9g, Herba Cynomorii Songarici (Suo Yang) 12g, Semen Allii Tuberosi (Jiu Cai Zi) 10g and Cornu Cervi Degelatinatum (Lu Jiao Shuang) 12g.

12. Perspiration (Hidrosis)

A. Etiology and Pathogenesis

1) Insufficiency of Lung Qi
2) Impaired Coordination between Nutritive Division/Level (ying fen) and Defensive Division/Level (wei fen)
3) Insufficiency of Heart Blood
4) Hyperactivity of Fire due to Deficiency of Yin
5) Accumulation of Pathogenic Heat

B. Syndrome Differentiation and Treatment

1) <u>Weakness of the Lung and Defensive Division/Level (Wei Fen)</u>

Symptoms: Sweating aggravated by exertion, aversion to wind, susceptibility to common cold, lassitude, lusterless complexion, thin and white tongue coating, thready and weak pulse.

Therapeutic Principle: To replenish qi and consolidate body surface.

Prescription: Modified Yu Ping Feng Powder.

Modifications: For excessive sweating, add Radix Ephedrae (Ma Huang Gen) 6g, Fructus Tritici Aestivi Levis (Fu Xiao Mai) 20g, Radix Oryzae Glutinosae (Nuo Dao Gen Xu) 20g, Mastodi Ossis Fossilia (Long Gu) 20g and Concha Ostreae (Mu Li) 20g; for severe deficiency of qi, Radix Codonopsitis Pilosulae (Dang Shen) 9g, Rhizoma Polygonati (Huang Jing) 10g and Radix Glycyrrhizae Uralensis (Gan Cao) 6g; for concurrent deficiency of yin, add Radix Ophiopogonis Japonici (Mai Dong) 10g and Fructus Schisandrae Chinensis (Wu Wei Zi) 3g.

2) <u>Incoordination between Nutritive Level (Ying) and Defensive Level (Wei)</u>

Symptoms: Sweating, aversion to wind, general aching, alternate cold and fever, or sweating in one side or part of the body, thin and white tongue coating, floating and slow pulse.

Therapeutic Principle: To regulate nutritive qi and defensive qi.

Prescription: Modified Gui Zhi Decoction.

Modifications: For excessive sweating, add Mastodi Ossis Fossilia (Long Gu) 20g and Concha Ostreae (Mu Li) 20g; for concurrent deficiency of qi, add Radix Astragali (Huang Qi) 12g; for concurrent deficiency of yang, add Radix Aconiti Lateralis Praeparatae (Fu Zi) 10g; for sweating in one side or part of the body, add Gan Mai Da Zao Decoction.

3) Insufficiency of Heart Blood

Symptoms: Spontaneous sweating or night sweating, palpitation, insomnia, listlessness, shortness of breath, lusterless complexion, pale tongue with thin coating, and thready pulse.

Therapeutic Principle: To replenish blood and nourish the heart.

Prescription: Modified Gui Pi Decoction.

Modifications: For excessive sweating, add Fructus Schisandrae Chinensis (Wu Wei Zi) 3g, Fructus Tritici Aestivi Levis (Fu Xiao Mai) 20g and Concha Ostreae (Mu Li) 20g; for severe deficiency of blood, add Radix Rehmanniae Praeparatae (Shu Di Huang) 12g, Radix Polygoni Multiflori (He Shou Wu) 12g and Fructus Lycii (Gou Qi Zi) 10g; for concurrent discomfort in the chest, dark purple tongue with ecchymosis or petechiae, add Radix Salviae Miltiorrhizae (Dan Shen) 9g, Rhizoma Ligustici Chuanxiong (Chuan Xiong) 9g, Flos Carthami Tinctorii (Hong Hua) 9g and Lignum Dalbergiae Odoriferae (Jiang Xiang) 3g.

4) Deficiency of Yin and Hyperactivity of Fire

Symptoms: Vexation, insomnia, night sweating, or spontaneous sweating, feverish sensation in palms and soles, hectic fever, flushed cheeks, emaciation, menstrual irregularities, or nocturnal seminal emission, red tongue with little coating, thready and rapid pulse.

Therapeutic Principle: To nourish yin and subdue fire.

Prescription: Modified Dang Gui Liu Huang Decoction.

Modifications: For excessive sweating, add Fructus Tritici Aestivi Levis (Fu Xiao Mai) 20g, Radix Oryzae Glutinosae (Nuo Dao Gen Xu) 20g and Concha Ostreae (Mu Li) 20g; for hectic fever and hot sensation in the bones, add Rhizoma Anemarrhenae (Zhi Mu) 10g, Cortex Lycii Radicis (Di Gu Pi) 10g, Herba Artemisiae Apiaceae seu Annuae (Qing Hao) 9g, Carapax et Plastrum Testudinis (Gui Ban) 12g and Carapax Trionycis (Bie Jia) 15g.

5) Accumulation of Pathogenic Heat

Symptoms: Continuous perspiration with sticky sweats, flushed face with a hot sensation, bitter taste in the mouth, thirst, restlessness, yellow urine, thin and yellow tongue coating, taut and rapid pulse.

Therapeutic Principle: To clear away liver heat, eliminate dampness and regulate nutritive division/level.

Prescription: Modified Long Dan Xie Gan Decoction.

Modifications: For severe interior heat and oliguria with dark urine, add Herba Artemisiae Scopariae (Yin Chen Hao) 12g; for retention of damp-heat with less predominant heat, use Si Miao Pill; for constipation, hectic fever, sweating, deep and excess pulse, use Tiao Wei Cheng Qi Decoction.

13. Acquired Immune Deficiency Syndrome (AIDS)

A. Etiology and Pathogenesis

1) Unclean Copulation
2) Perverse Behavior
3) Contact with Epidemic Pathogenic Factors
4) Insufficiency of Healthy Qi, Deficiency of Kidney Essence, and Abnormal Function of Wei (defensive), Qi, Ying (nutritive) and Xue (blood).

B. Syndrome Differentiation and Treatment

1) <u>Pathogenic Warm Factor Attacking the Lung and Impairing Yin</u>

Symptoms: Sore throat, fever, dry cough or blood-stained sputum, dyspnea, chest pain, rash, pruritus, weight loss, listlessness, night sweating, red tongue with little moisture, thin and yellow tongue coating, and thready pulse.

Therapeutic Principle: To nourish yin, clear away heat, moisten the lung and promote fluid production.

Prescription: Modified Mai Men Dong Decoction and Bai He Gu Jin Decoction.

Modifications: For persistent cough, add Fructus Aristolochiae (Ma Dou Ling) 10g and Indigo Naturalis (Qing Dai) 2g and Concha Meretricis seu Cyclinae (Hai Ge Qiao) 12g; for severe chest pain, add Herba Lycopi Lucidi (Ze Lan) 10g and Pollen Typhae (Pu Huang) 9g and Excrementum Trogopteri seu Pteromydis (Wu Ling Zhi) 9g; for persistent blood-stained sputum, add Radix Rubiae Cordifoliae (Qian Cao) 10g and Rhizoma Imperatae Cylindricae (Bai Mao Gen) 20g.

2) <u>Deficiency of the Middle Warmer with Heat Retention in the Stomach and Bowels</u>

Symptoms: Lingering fever, emaciation, shortness of breath, lassitude of the limbs, abdominal pain, diarrhea with yellow and thin stools or stools with pus and blood, tenesmus, nausea, vomiting, white and greasy tongue coating, soft and thready pulse.

Therapeutic Principle: To replenish qi, invigorate the spleen, clean the bowels and eliminate dampness.

Prescription: Modified Bu Zhong Yi Qi Decoction and Bai Tou Weng Decoction.

Modifications: For vomiting and anorexia, add Rhizoma Pinelliae Ternatae (Ban Xia) 10g, Caulis Perillae (Zi Su Geng) 9g and Rhizoma Zingiberis Recens (Sheng Jiang) 6g; for persistent abdominal pain, add Radix Aucklandiae Lappae (Mu Xiang) 9g and Radix Saposhnikoviae Divaricatae (Fang Feng) 6g; for persistent diarrhea, add Caulis Sargentodoxae Cuneatae (Hong Teng) 15g and Herba Agrimoniae Pilosae (Xian He Cao) 15g.

3) <u>Excessive Toxic Heat</u>

Symptoms: Lingering fever, sticky sweats, stuffy sensation in the chest, anorexia (poor appetite), ulcerous mouth and tongue, sticky stools and difficult defecation, yellow, sticky and powder-like tongue coating, soft and rapid pulse.

Therapeutic Principle: To clear away heat and remove turbidity.

Prescription: Modified Gan Lu Xiao Du Powder, Bai Hu Jia Ren Shen Decoction.

Example Prescription: Herba Agastache seu Pogostemonis (Huo Xiang), Herba Artemisiae Scopariae (Yin Chen Hao), Rhizoma Acori Graminei (Shi Chang Pu), Rhizoma Coptidis (Huang Lian), Fructus Amomi Cardamomi (Bai Kou Ren), Talcum (Hua Shi Fen), Rhizoma Belamcandae Chinensis (She Gan), Folium Isatidis (Da Qing Ye), and Cortex Phellodendri (Huang Bai).

4) <u>Excessive Pathogenic Heat and Phlegm Blocking the Orifice</u>

Symptoms: Fever, headache, nausea, vomiting, cloudy consciousness, or restlessness, delirium, stiff neck, convulsion, spasm of the limbs, or dementia, or epileptoid seizure, yellow and greasy tongue coating, thready and rapid or slippery and rapid pulse.

Therapeutic Principle: To clear away heart heat, induce resuscitation, cool the liver and stop wind.

Prescription: Modified Xi Huang Xuan Qiao Decoction.

Modifications: For impaired peripheral nerves with pain of the limbs and difficulty in movement, add Rhizoma Polygoni Cuspidati (Hu Zhang) 15g, Buthus Martensi (Quan Xie) 3g, Bombyx Batryticatus (Bai Jiang Can) 10g and Bombycis Mori Excrementum (Can Sha) 12g.

5) <u>Deficiency of Qi and Yin</u>

Symptoms: Low-grade fever, night sweating, dry mouth and throat, non-productive cough, spiritlessness, shortness of breath, red tongue with white coating, thready and weak pulse.

Therapeutic Principle: To replenish qi and nourish yin.

Prescription: Modified Huang Qi Sheng Mai Decoction.

Example Prescription: Radix Astragali Membranacei (Huang Qi), Radix Codonopsitis Pilosulae (Dang Shen), Radix Ophiopogonis Japonici (Mai Dong), Fructus Schisandrae Chinensis (Wu Wei Zi),

Rhizoma Anemarrhenae (Zhi Mu), stir-fried Radix Paeoniae Alba (Bai Shao Yao), Cortex Lycii Radicis (Di Gu Pi), and Fructus Ligustri Lucidi (Nu Zhen Zi).

6) <u>Deficiency of the Heart and Spleen</u>

Symptoms: Shortness of breath, spontaneous sweating, lassitude, weakness, palpitation, insomnia, irritability, cold hands and feet, diarrhea or loose stools, sallow complexion, pale tongue with white coating, thready and slow pulse.

Therapeutic Principle: To strengthen the spleen, nourish the heart, and replenish qi and blood.

Prescription: Modified Gui Pi Decoction, Bu Zhong Yi Qi Decoction.

Example Prescription: Radix Astragali Membranacei (Huang Qi), Rhizoma Atractylodis Macrocephalae (Bai Zhu), Radix Codonopsitis Pilosulae (Dang Shen), Radix Angelicae Sinensis (Dang Gui), Sclerotium Poriae Cocos (Fu Ling), Semen Ziziphi Spinosae (Suan Zao Ren), Radix Rehmanniae Praeparatae (Shi Di Huang), Radix Salviae Miltiorrhizae (Dan Shen), Radix Glycyrrhizae Uralensis (Gan Cao), Fructus Psoraleae Corylifoliae (Bu Gu Zhi) and Mastodi Ossis Fossilia (Long Gu).

Modifications: For diarrhea, add Rhizoma Dioscoreae (Shan Yao), Semen Dolichoris Lablab (Bai Bian Dou) and Semen Euryales Ferocis (Qian Shi); for nausea and vomiting, add Rhizoma Pinelliae Ternatae (Ban Xia) and Rhizoma Zingiberis Officinalis (Gan Jiang); for shortness of breath, add Fructus Schisandrae Chinensis (Wu Wei Zi) and Rhizoma Dioscoreae (Shan Yao); for yellow tongue coating, add Rhizoma Coptidis (Huang Lian) and Radix Scutellariae Baicalensis (Huang Qin).

7) <u>Deficiency of Spleen Yang and Kidney Yang</u>

Symptoms: Fever or lingering low-grade fever, emaciation, spiritlessness, palpitation, shortness of breath, dizziness, feeling of heaviness in the head, soreness of loins and knees, anorexia, nausea, or frequent hiccup and diarrhea, or diarrhea before dawn, lingering abdominal pain, cold body and limbs, spontaneous sweating, night sweating, lusterless hair and complexion, pale nails, pruritus, or thrush, pale and chubby tongue with ecchymosis or white patches, thin and white tongue coating, and deep, thready and forceless or thready and rapid pulse.

Therapeutic Principle: To invigorate the spleen, lift lucid yang, warm the kidney and astringe the bowels.

Prescription: Modified Da Tao Hua Decoction and Qi Jun Decoction, or modified Jin Gui Shen Qi Pill and Gui Pi Decoction, or modified Shi Quan Da Bu Decoction.

Example Prescription: Radix Astragali Membranacei (Huang Qi), Rhizoma Atractylodis Macrocephalae (Bai Zhu), Sclerotium Poriae Cocos (Fu Ling), Radix Aconiti Lateralis Praeparatae (Fu Zi), Cortex Cinnamomi Cassiae (Rou Gui), Radix Morindae Officinalis (Ba Ji Tian), Fructus Lycii (Gou

Qi Zi), Radix Rehmanniae Praeparatae (Shu Di Huang), Rhizoma Dioscoreae (Shan Yao), Rhizoma Alismatis Orientalis (Ze Xie), Cortex Moutan Radicis (Mu Dan Pi), Fructus Zizyphi Jujubae (Da Zao) and Radix Glycyrrhizae Uralensis (Gan Cao).

Modifications: For lingering fever, remove Cortex Cinnamomi Cassiae (Rou Gui) and add Ramulus Cinnamomi Cassiae (Gui Zhi) 10g; for persistent vomiting, add Rhizoma Pinelliae Ternatae (Ban Xia) 10g and Rhizoma Zingiberis Recens (Sheng Jiang) 3g; for persistent hiccup, add Flos Caryophylli (Ding Xiang) 5g and Calyx Diospyri Kaki (Shi Di) 6g; for persistent diarrhea, add Fructus Terminaliae Chebulae (He Zi) 6g and Pericarpium Punicae Granati (Shi Liu Pi) 10g.

8) <u>Deficiency of Liver Yin and Kidney Yin</u>

Symptoms: Dizziness, vertigo, tinnitus, deafness, afternoon low-grade fever, dry mouth and throat, soreness and weakness in the lumbar region and knees, dull pain in the hypochondriac region, dysphoria with feverish sensation in the chest, palms and soles, hectic fever, night sweats, weigh loss, weakness, alopecia (baldness), depression, red tongue with little coating, thready and rapid pulse.

Therapeutic Principle: To nourish the kidney and liver.

Prescription: Modified Liu Wei Di Huang Pill, Er Zhi Pill, San Jia Fu Mai Decoction, or Yi Guan Decoction.

Example Prescription: Radix Rehmanniae Recens (Sheng Di Huang), Fructus Corni Officinalis (Shan Zhu Yu), Rhizoma Alismatis Orientalis (Ze Xie), Rhizoma Anemarrhenae (Zhi Mu), Carapax Trionycis (Bie Jia), Fructus Ligustri Lucidi (Nu Zhen Zi), Fructus Lycii (Gou Qi Zi), Radix Ophiopogonis Japonici (Mai Dong), Herba Ecliptae Prostratae (Han Lian Cao), Cortex Moutan Radicis (Mu Dan Pi) and Flos Chrysanthemi Morifolii (Ju Hua).

9) <u>Deficiency of Lung Yin and Kidney Yin</u>

Symptoms: Low-grade fever, non-productive cough, dry mouth and throat, sore throat, hectic fever, warm sensation in the bones, weak limbs, tinnitus, dizziness, soreness and weakness in the lumbar region and knees, progressive weight loss, red tongue with little moisture, thready and rapid pulse.

Therapeutic Principle: To nourish yin and promote fluid production.

Prescription: Modified He Che Da Zao Pill.

Example Prescription: Radix Rehmanniae Recens (Sheng Di Huang), Radix Rehmanniae Praeparatae (Shu Di Huang), Placenta Hominis (Zi He Che), Tuber Asparagi Cochinchinensis (Tian Dong), Radix Ophiopogonis Japonici (Mai Dong), Carapax et Plastrum Testudinis (Gui Ban), Cortex Phellodendri (Huang Bai), Radix Achyranthis Bidentatae (Niu Xi), Fructus Schisandrae Chinensis (Wu Wei Zi) and Radix Scrophulariae Ningpoensis (Xuan Shen).

Modifications: For cough with yellow or blood-tinged sputum, and chest pain (hyperactivity of pathogenic heat in the lung), add Flos Lonicerae (Jin Yin Hua), Herba Taraxaci Mongolici (Pu Gong Ying), Semen Coicis Lacryma-jobi (Yi Yi Ren), Semen Benincasae Hispidae (Dong Gua Zi) and Herba cum Radice Houttuyniae Cordatae (Yu Xing Cao).

10) <u>Insufficiency of Kidney Essence</u>

Symptoms: Alopecia (baldness), odontoseisis (loose teeth), sparse teeth, tinnitus, deafness, absent-mindedness, forgetfulness, spiritlessness, slowness of movement, or dementia, weak lower extremities, blurred vision, sluggish responses, pale tongue, and weak pulse.

Therapeutic Principle: To nourish kidney essence.

Prescription: Modified He Che Zai Zao Pill.

Example Prescription: Radix Achyranthis Bidentatae (Niu Xi), Herba Cistanches (Rou Cong Rong), Tuber Asparagi Cochinchinensis (Tian Dong), Radix Morindae Officinalis (Ba Ji Tian), Gelatinum Corii Asini (E Jiao), Carapax et Plastrum Testudinis (Gui Ban), Carapax Trionycis (Bie Jia), Radix Paeoniae Alba (Bai Shao Yao), Cortex Eucommiae Ulmoidis (Du Zhong), and Radix Glycyrrhizae Uralensis (Gan Cao).

Modifications: For depletion of kidney essence and emaciation, add Cornu Cervi Pantotrichum (Lu Rong) and Placenta Hominis (Zi He Che); for frequent dry cough, add Radix Ophiopogonis Japonici (Mai Dong), Rhizoma Anemarrhenae (Zhi Mu) and Carapax Trionycis (Bie Jia).

11) <u>Deficiency of Kidney Yin and Kidney Yang</u>

Symptoms: Dizziness, tinnitus, soreness and weakness in the lumbar region and knees, feverish sensation in the chest, palms and soles, night sweats, or cold body and limbs, frequent urination, dry helix (ear), impotence, pale tongue with white coating, and deep, thready and forceless pulse.

Therapeutic Principle: To nourish kidney yin and kidney yang.

Prescription: Modified Jin Gui Shen Qi Pill.

Example Prescription: Radix Aconiti Lateralis Praeparatae (Fu Zi), Cortex Cinnamomi Cassiae (Rou Gui), Radix Rehmanniae Praeparatae (Shu Di Huang), Rhizoma Dioscoreae (Shan Yao), Fructus Corni Officinalis (Shan Zhu Yu), Sclerotium Poriae Cocos (Fu Ling), Rhizoma Alismatis Orientalis (Ze Xie), and Cortex Moutan Radicis (Mu Dan Pi).

12) <u>Pathogenic Heat Invading Ying (nutritive level) and Xue (blood level)</u>

Symptoms: Fever, mucocutaneous bleeding, or hematemesis, or epistaxis, or hematochezia, vexation, irritability, delirious speech, crimson tongue, taut and rapid pulse.

Therapeutic Principle: To clear away ying heat and cool blood.

Prescription: Modified Xi Jiao Di Huang Decoction, Qing Wen Bai Du Decoction, Qing Ying Decoction, or Ling Jiao Gou Teng Decoction.

Example Prescription: Radix Rehmanniae Recens (Sheng Di Huang), Radix Paeoniae Rubra (Chi Shao), Cortex Moutan Radicis (Mu Dan Pi), Fructus Gardeniae Jasminoidis (Zhi Zi), Fructus Forsythiae Suspensae (Lian Qiao), Flos Lonicerae (Jin Yin Hua), Radix Scrophulariae Ningpoensis (Xuan Shen), Rhizoma Coptidis (Huang Lian), Radix Scutellariae Baicalensis (Huang Qin), Rhizoma Acori Tatarinowii (Shi Chang Pu), Cornu Rhinocerotis (Xi Jiao), and Cornu Saigae Tataricae (Ling Yang Jiao).

13) Phlegm Stagnation and Blood Stasis

Symptoms: Lump in the hypochondriac region, enlarged lymph nodes, tumor, emaciation, sallow or black complexion, fever, bleeding, pain, dark purple tongue, and thready and rough pulse.

Therapeutic Principle: To remove blood stasis and resolve phlegm.

Prescription: Modified Tao Hong Si Wu Decoction and Xiao Luo Pill.

Example Prescription: Radix Rehmanniae Praeparatae (Shu Di Huang), Rhizoma Ligustici Chuanxiong (Chuan Xiong), Lumbricus (Di Long), Radix Paeoniae Rubra (Chi Shao), Rhizoma Arisaematis (Tian Nan Xing), Rhizoma Pinelliae Ternatae (Ban Xia), Pseudobulbus Cremastrae seu Pleiones (Shan Ci Gu), Rhizoma Curcumae Ezhu (E Zhu), Concha Ostreae (Mu Li), Bulbus Fritillariae (Bei Mu), Radix Scrophulariae Ningpoensis (Xuan Shen), and Scolopendra Subspinipes (Wu Gong).

Modifications: For excessive internal toxic heat, add Radix Semiaquilegiae (Tian Kui Zi), Herba Hedyotis Diffusae (Bai Hua She She Cao), Folium Isatidis (Da Qing Ye) and Radix Lithospermi seu Macrotomiae (Zi Cao); for qi deficiency, add Radix Astragali (Huang Qi) and Radix Codonopsitis Pilosulae (Dang Shen); for yin deficiency, add Radix Ophiopogonis Japonici (Mai Dong), Tuber Asparagi Cochinchinensis (Tian Dong), Radix Trichosanthis (Tian Hua Fen) and Fructus Ligustri Lucidi (Nu Zhen Zi).

14. Epistaxis

A. Etiology and Pathogenesis

1) Attack by Exogenous Pathogenic Factors
2) Improper Diet
3) Internal Injury due to Emotional Disturbance
4) Overstrain
5) Chronic Illness or Febrile Disease

B. Syndrome Differentiation and Treatment

1) <u>Wind-Heat Attacking the Lung</u>

Symptoms: Dry nose, nasal bleeding with bright red blood, cold intolerance, fever, dry mouth and throat, cough with yellow sputum, red tongue with thin and yellow coating, and rapid pulse.

Therapeutic Principle: To clear away lung heat and cool blood to stop bleeding.

Prescription: Modified Sang Ju Decoction.

Modifications: For sore throat, add Radix Scrophulariae Ningpoensis (Xuan Shen) 12g and Fructificatio Lasiosphaerae seu Calvatiae (Ma Bo) 3g; for thirst and dry throat, add Radix Ophiopogonis Japonici (Mai Dong) 12g, Radix Adenophorae (Sha Shen) 10g and Radix Trichosanthis (Tian Hua Fen) 10g; for severe cough, add Bulbus Fritillariae Cirrhosae (Bei Mu) 9g and Exocarpium Citri Rubrum (Ju Hong) 9g.

2) <u>Flaming-Up of Liver Fire</u>

Symptoms: Nasal bleeding, conjunctival congestion, restlessness, irritability, headache, vertigo, bitter taste in the mouth, tinnitus, red tongue with yellow coating, taut and rapid pulse.

Therapeutic Principle: To purge liver fire and cool blood to stop bleeding.

Prescription: Modified Zhi Zi Qing Gan Decoction.

Modifications: For deficiency of yin fluid, add Radix Ophiopogonis Japonici (Mai Dong) 12g, Radix Scrophulariae Ningpoensis (Xuan Shen) 10g and Radix Rehmanniae (Di Huang) 12g.

3) <u>Excessive Stomach Heat</u>

Symptoms: Nasal bleeding with bright red blood, dry nose and mouth, foul breath, epigastric discomfort, thirst with a desire to drink, restlessness, constipation, red tongue with yellow coating, and rapid pulse.

Therapeutic Principle: To purge stomach fire and cool blood to stop bleeding.

Prescription: Modified Yu Nu Decoction.

Modifications: For constipation, add Radix et Rhizoma Rhei (Da Huang) 6g; for thirst, add Radix Adenophorae (Sha Shen) 10g, Radix Trichosanthis (Tian Hua Fen) 10g and Herba Dendrobii (Shi Hu) 9g.

4) <u>Deficiency of Blood and Qi</u>

Symptoms: Nasal bleeding or bleeding in the nose, muscles and gum with light red blood, listlessness, lassitude, palpitation, shortness of breath, insomnia, pale complexion, dizziness, pale tongue with white coating, and thready or weak pulse.

Therapeutic Principle: To replenish qi and arrest blood.

Prescription: Modified Gui Pi Decoction.

Modifications: For severe bleeding, add Cacumen Biotae Orientalis (Ce Bai Ye) 12g and Pollen Typhae (Pu Huang) 9g; for severe deficiency of blood, add Fructus Mori Alba (Sang Shen) 12g and Gelatinum Corii Asini (E Jiao) 9g.

15. Gingival Hemorrhage

A. Etiology and Pathogenesis

Refer to epistaxis.

B. Syndrome Differentiation and Treatment

1) <u>Hyperactivity of Stomach Fire</u>

Symptoms: Bleeding from the gums with bright red blood, gingival redness, swelling and pain, thirst with a desire to drink, headache, foul breath, constipation, red tongue with yellow coating, full and rapid pulse.

Therapeutic Principle: To purge stomach fire and cool blood to stop bleeding.

Prescription: Modified Qing Wei Powder and Xie Xin Decoction.

Modifications: For restlessness and thirst, add Rhizoma Anemarrhenae (Zhi Mu) 10g, Radix Trichosanthis (Tian Hua Fen) 10g and Herba Dendrobii (Shi Hu) 10g; for constipation, add Natrii Sulfas (Mang Xiao) 10g and Radix et Rhizoma Rhei (Da Huang) 6g.

2) <u>Hyperactivity of Fire due to Deficiency of Yin</u>

Symptoms: Gradual onset of bleeding from gums with light red blood, which is frequently induced by attack of heat and overstrain; loose teeth, swollen gums, vertigo, red tongue with little coating, thready and rapid pulse.

Therapeutic Principle: To nourish yin, subdue fire, cool blood and stop bleeding.

Prescription: Modified Zhi Bai Di Huang Pill and Qian Gen Powder.

Modifications: For deficiency of yin with hectic fever, add Rhizoma Picrorrhizae (Hu Huang Lian) 9g and Cortex Lycii Radicis (Di Gu Pi) 10g.

16. Hemoptysis

A. Etiology and Pathogenesis

Refer to epistaxis.

B. Syndrome Differentiation and Treatment

1) <u>Heat-Dryness Attacking the Lung</u>

Symptoms: Throat itching, cough with blood-stained sputum, dry mouth and nose, or fever, difficult expectoration, red tongue with thin and yellow coating, and rapid pulse.

Therapeutic Principle: To clear away heat, moisten the lung and calm the vessels to stop bleeding.

Prescription: Modified Sang Xing Decoction.

Modifications: For fever, headache, cough and sore throat due to wind-heat attacking the lung, add Flos Lonicerae (Jin Yin Hua) 12g, Fructus Forsythiae Suspensae (Lian Qiao) 10g and Fructus Arctii Lappae (Niu Bang Zi) 9g; for dry mouth and nose and difficult expectoration due to consumption of body fluid, add Radix Ophiopogonis Japonici (Mai Dong) 12g, Tuber Asparagi Cochinchinensis (Tian Dong) 12g and Herba Dendrobii (Shi Hu) 10g.

2) Lung Heat due to Yin Deficiency

Symptoms: Cough with little blood-tinged sputum, or recurrent hemoptysis with bright red blood, dry mouth and throat, flushed cheeks, hectic fever, night sweating, red tongue with little coating, thready and rapid pulse.

Therapeutic Principle: To nourish yin, moisten the lung, cool blood and stop bleeding.

Prescription: Modified Bai He Gu Jin Decoction.

Modifications: For recurrent hemoptysis with profuse blood, add Gelatinum Corii Asini (E Jiao) 10g and Radix Notoginseng (San Qi) 9g; for hectic fever and flushed cheeks, add Herba Artemisiae Apiaceae seu Annuae (Qing Hao) 9g, Cortex Lycii Radicis (Di Gu Pi) 10g and Radix Cynanchi Atrati (Bai Wei) 9g; for night sweating, add Radix Oryzae Glutinosae (Nuo Dao Gen Xu) 15g, Fructus Schisandrae Chinensis (Wu Wei Zi) 3g, Fructus Tritici Aestivi Levis (Fu Xiao Mai) 15g and Concha Ostreae (Mu Li) 15g.

3) Liver Fire Attacking the Lung

Symptoms: Paroxysmal cough with blood-tinged sputum or bright red blood, distending pain in the chest and hypochondrium, restlessness, irritability, bitter taste in the mouth, conjunctival congestion, red tongue with thin and yellow coating, taut and rapid pulse.

Therapeutic Principle: To clear away liver fire, purge lung heat, cool blood and stop bleeding.

Prescription: Modified Xie Bai Powder and Dai Ge Powder.

Modifications: For restlessness, irritability, bitter taste in the mouth and conjunctival congestion, add Cortex Moutan Radicis (Mu Dan Pi) 10g, Fructus Gardeniae Jasminoidis (Zhi Zi) 9g and Radix Scutellariae Baicalensis (Huang Qin) 9g; for hemoptysis with profuse bright red blood, add Xi Jiao Di Huang Decoction and Yun Dan Bai Yao.

17. Hematemesis

A. Etiology and Pathogenesis

Refer to epistaxis.

B. Syndrome Differentiation and Treatment

1) <u>Excessive Stomach Heat</u>

Symptoms: Burning pain in the epigastrium, spitting of bright red or dark purple blood often with food residue, constipation with tarry stools, foul breath, red tongue with dry and yellow coating, and rapid pulse.

Therapeutic Principle: To clear away stomach heat, purge fire and cool blood to stop bleeding.

Prescription: Modified Xie Xin Decoction and Shi Hui Powder.

Modifications: For nausea and vomiting, add Ochra Haematitum (Dai Zhe Shi) 15g, Caulis Bambusae in Taeniam (Zhu Ru) 9g and Flos Inulae (Xuan Fu Hua) 9g; for marked burning sensation in the stomach, add Fructus Gardeniae Jasminoidis (Zhi Zi) 9g and Gypsum Fibrosum (Shi Gao) 30g; for dry mouth and thirst, add Radix Adenophorae (Sha Shen) 10g, Radix Ophiopogonis Japonici (Mai Dong) 12g, Rhizoma Polygonati Odorati (Yu Zhu) 12g and Herba Dendrobii (Shi Hu) 10g.

2) <u>Extravasation due to Deficiency of Qi</u>

Symptoms: Lingering and intermittent hematemesis with dark pink blood, lassitude, listlessness, pale complexion, palpitation, shortness of breath, pale tongue with white coating, thready and weak pulse.

Therapeutic Principle: To replenish qi and keep the blood circulating within the vessels.

Prescription: Modified Gui Pi Decoction.

Modifications: For aversion to cold, cold limbs, spontaneous sweating and loose stools due to deficiency of qi impairing yang, and deficiency cold in both the spleen and stomach, use Huang Tu Decoction; for profuse bleeding with extremely cold limbs, sweating and tinny pulse, emergency use Du Shen Decoction.

3) <u>Liver Fire Attacking the Stomach</u>

Symptoms: Hematemesis with bright red or dark purple blood, distending pain in the epigastrium and hypochondrium, conjunctival congestion, dry mouth, restlessness, irritability, insomnia, dreamfulness, red tongue with yellow coating, taut and rapid pulse.

Therapeutic Principle: To pure liver fire, clear away stomach heat, cool blood and stop bleeding.

Prescription: Modified Long Dan Xie Gan Decoction.

Modifications: For marked hypochondriac pain, add Rhizoma Cyperi Rotundi (Xiang Fu) 10g and Rhizoma Corydalis (Yan Hu Suo) 9g; for persistent hematemesis and stabbing pain in the epigastrium, add Radix Notoginseng (San Qi) 9g and Shi Hui Powder.

18. Hematochezia

A. Etiology and Pathogenesis

Refer to epistaxis.

B. Syndrome Differentiation and Treatment

1) <u>Damp-Heat in the Bowels</u>

Symptoms: Hematochezia with bright red blood in the stools, difficult defecation, abdominal pain, bitter taste in the mouth, poor appetite, red tongue with yellow and greasy coating, slippery and rapid pulse.

Therapeutic Principle: To clear away damp-heat, cool blood and stop bleeding.

Prescription: Modified Di Yu Powder and Huai Jiao Pill

Modifications: For anorexia, add Pericarpium Citri Reticulatae (Chen Pi) 6g and Fructus Amomi Villosi (Sha Ren) 5g; for abdominal pain, add Semen Raphani Sativi (Lai Fu Zi) 9g and Radix Curcumae (Yu Jin) 10g.

2) <u>Deficiency Cold in the Spleen and Stomach</u>

Symptoms: Hematochezia with dark purple or black blood in the stools, dull abdominal pain that is alleviated by pressure and warmth, loose stools, anorexia, cold intolerance, cold limbs, lusterless complexion, listlessness, indolence of speaking, pale tongue with white coating, and thready pulse.

Therapeutic Principle: To warm yang, invigorate the spleen, nourish blood and stop bleeding.

Prescription: Modified Huang Tu Decoction.

Modifications: For persistent hematochezia, add Ophicalcitum (Hua Rui Shi) 10g and Radix Notoginseng (San Qi) 9g; for aversion to cold and cold limbs, add Rhizoma Zingiberis Praeparatae (Pao Jiang) 6g, Cornu Cervi Degelatinatum (Lu Jiao Shuang) 10g and Folium Artemisiae Argyi (Ai Ye) 9g.

19. Hematuria

A. Etiology and Pathogenesis

Refer to epistaxis.

B. Syndrome Differentiation and Treatment

1) <u>Excessive Heat in the Lower Warmer</u>

Symptoms: A burning sensation in the urethra during urination, dark yellow urine, or hematuria with bright red blood, vexation, thirst, flushed face, aphthous stomatitis, insomnia, red tongue with thin and yellow coating, and rapid pulse.

Therapeutic Principle: To clear away heat, purge fire, cool blood and stop bleeding.

Prescription: Modified Xiao Ji Decoction.

Modifications: For thirst, add Herba Dendrobii (Shi Hu) 10g, Rhizoma Anemarrhenae (Zhi Mu) 10g and Radix Scutellariae Baicalensis (Huang Qin) 9g; for vexation and insomnia, add Rhizoma Coptidis (Huang Lian) 6g, Caulis Polygoni Multiflori (Ye Jiao Teng) 15g and Semen Ziziphi Spinosae (Suan Zao Ren) 12g.

2) Failure of the Spleen to Control Blood

Symptoms: Chronic hematuria, lusterless complexion, lassitude, poor appetite, shortness of breath, weak voice, or ecchymosis, or gingival bleeding, pale tongue, thready and weak pulse.

Therapeutic Principle: To invigorate the spleen, and replenish qi and blood.

Prescription: Modified Gui Pi Decoction.

Modifications: For collapse of qi with bearing down sensation and distention in the lower abdomen, add Rhizoma Cimicifugae (Sheng Ma) 9g and Radix Bupleuri (Chai Hu) 9g, or add Bu Zhong Yi Qi Decoction.

3) Kidney Deficiency with Hyperactivity of Fire

Symptoms: Oliguria with dark urine and blood, dizziness, tinnitus, flushed cheeks, hectic fever, listlessness, lumbar soreness, weak knees, red tongue with little coating, thready and rapid pulse.

Therapeutic Principle: To nourish yin, purge fire, cool blood and stop bleeding.

Prescription: Modified Zhi Bai Di Huang Pill.

Modifications: For vexation and insomnia, add Rhizoma Coptidis (Huang Lian) 6g and Cinnabaris (Zhu Sha) 0.5g; for vertigo, add Concha Haliotidis (Shi Jue Ming) 20g and Flos Chrysanthemi Morifolii (Ju Hua) 10g.

4) Unconsolidation of Kidney Qi

Symptoms: Chronic hematuria with pale red blood, dizziness, tinnitus, lumbar soreness, listlessness, lassitude, pale tongue, and weak pulse.

Therapeutic Principle: To replenish and restore kidney qi to stop bleeding.

Prescription: Modified Wu Bi Shan Yao Pill.

Modifications: For lumbar soreness, cold intolerance and listlessness, add sliced Cornu Cervi (Lu Jiao) 10g and Rhizoma Cibotii Barometz (Gou Ji) 12g; for excessive hematuria, add Ophicalcitum (Hua Rui Shi) 10g, Pollen Typhae (Pu Huang) 9g and Radix Notoginseng (San Qi) 9g.

Appendix I: Preparation of Decoction and Prescriptions

A prescription is a combination of proper herbs that are selected on the basis of the syndrome differentiation and treatment principle. The comprehensive actions of all herbs strengthen the effect of main drugs, eliminate the side effect of drugs, and achieve the appropriate effect of treatment.

1. Principles of Composing Prescriptions

The principles of composing prescriptions divide herbs into four groups: sovereign drug (Jun Yao, also known as monarch or principal drug), minister drug (Chen Yao), adjuvant drug (Zuo Yao, also known as assistant drug) and guiding drug (Shi Yao).

1) Sovereign Drug: A drug that has the major and leading effects in treating the cause or main symptom of a disease. Generally, sovereign drug possesses the greatest potency and the largest dosage in the herbal combination.

2) Minister Drug: A drug that helps sovereign drug to strengthen its effects on treating the main symptoms. Minister drug is also commonly used to treat the accompanying symptoms. Its potency is weaker than that of sovereign drug.

3) Adjuvant Drug: A drug that can play three roles in herbal combination. First, it can be a "supplementary drug" to strengthen medical treatment along with sovereign drug and minister drug, and it can also be used directly for secondary accompanying symptoms. Second, adjuvant drug can be a "restraining drug" to reduce or eliminate the potency, toxicity and disadvantageous factors of sovereign and minister drugs. Third, it can be a "corrigent drug", which provides paradoxical assistance, i.e., its property and flavor is opposite to sovereign drug, but it plays supplementing role in treatment. An adjuvant drug is milder than minister drug, and it is used in relatively smaller dosage.

4) Guiding Drug: A drug that has two functions. First, it can be a "meridian ushering drug" to guide other herbs in a herbal formula to reach the target channels, i.e., the affected site. Second, it can be a "mediating drug" to harmonize the effects of other drugs in the herbal combination. Its potency is relatively weaker, and it should be used in small dosage.

A herbal combination usually has one sovereign drug. Two or three sovereign drugs may be included in the combination if pathogenetic condition changes and is more complex. Minister drug can outnumber sovereign drug in the herbal combination, and adjuvant drug usually outnumbers minister drug. One or two guiding drugs are enough to be included in a formula.

Although the principles of composition of prescription is strict, the practical application is quite flexible. The prescription, including the preparation forms, dosage and herbs, can be modified according to patient's age, sex, physical condition, lifestyle; it can also be modified according to seasons, climate, environment, etc.

2. Preparations of Prescriptions

The following is the commonly used methods of preparing prescriptions and the main features of these methods.

1) Decoction

Decoction refers to the medicinal solution obtained by removing the residue after soaking and decocting the prepared herbal pieces in water for a period of time. Decoction can be easily absorbed and it generates quick healing effects. It is one of the most widely used forms in clinical practice.

2) Powder

The herbs are ground into fine powder and then well mixed for oral application and external use. The powder for oral application is usually fine powder. It is taken orally with warm boiled water. Fine powder for oral application can be taken directly without water if small amount is needed. Sometimes, the herbs are ground into coarse powder to be boiled with water, and then the residue is removed and the liquid is collected for oral application. The powder for external application should be ground into fine powder, and it is generally applied to a sore or an affected area of the body. Powder can be made easily and it can be absorbed quickly by the body. The property of powder is stable, and it is convenient to carry powder around. The quantity of herbs used to make powder is relatively small.

3) Pill

Pill refers to the round solid preparation that is made by mixing ground fine powder or extraction medicinal materials of herbs with excipient. Four types of pills are mentioned here. Other pills or boluses, such as waxed pills, water-honeyed pills, tiny pellet and drop pills, will not be listed.

(1) Honeyed Pills: They are made by mixing fine powder of herbs with refined honey. There're two kinds of honey pills, large honey pills and small honey pills. Since honey pills or boluses are soft

and moist in property, moderate, lasting and nourishing in action, they are often used in the treatment of chronic diseases or patients with weak constitution.

(2) Watered Pills: They are made by mixing fine powder of herbs with cold boiled water, distilled water, wine, vinegar, or herbal juice. Water pills are easier to be dissolved, absorbed and swallowed compared to honey pills; it is applicable to various diseases.

(3) Pasted Pills: They are made by mixing fine powder of herbs with rice paste, flour paste or yeast paste. Paste pills are characterized by strong adhesiveness, solid quality, slow decomposition and dissolution. They can prolong therapeutic effect and reduce toxicity and side effects of drugs.

(4) Condensed Pills: There are several steps to make condensed pills. First, decoct drugs or part of the drugs of a herbal formula until the decoction is concentrated to extract. Second, mix the extract with fine powder of other drugs, then dry the mixture and grind it into powder. Third, mix the powder from step 2 with water, honey or herbal juice to make pills. Condensed pills have high content of active constituents; only small amount is needed in each application.

4) Paste

Paste refers to medicinal preparations that are made by decocting drugs in water or vegetable oil and then discarding the residue. They're two types of paste, paste for oral application and paste for external application. Paste for oral application includes liquid extract, extract and decoction plaster. Paste for external application includes ointment and plaster.

(1) Decoction Plaster: It is a semi-liquid form of preparation made by decocting drugs in water repeatedly, then discarding the residue and concentrating the decoction, and finally mixing the concentrated decoction with honey or sugar. It is tasty, nourishing, small in size and high in content. It is applicable to patients with chronic diseases and weak constitution, and it can be applied for a long period of time.

(2) Ointment: It is a semi-solid form of preparation with certain viscosity, which is made by mixing the fine powder of drugs with appropriate matrix. Ointment softens and melts gradually after it is applied externally to sores, furuncles, ulcer and masses, and burns; under the circumstances, the drugs in the ointment are slowly absorbed to produce lasting therapeutic effects.

(3) Plaster: There're several steps to make plaster. First, boil drugs in vegetable oil to certain extent and remove the residue. Second, boil it again till it becomes so solid that the dripping water turns into beads. Third, mix it with yellow lead evenly and cool it down. Before it is applied to affected

area of the boy, it should be heated and spread over a piece of cloth or paper till it softens. Plaster is applicable to both local diseases and systemic diseases.

5) Alcoholic Preparation

It is an alcoholic solution obtained by soaking drugs in liquor or rice millet wine. Alcoholic preparation can also be made by stewing drugs in water (with a separation between water and drugs), and then discarding the residue and obtain the solution. It is taken orally or applied externally. Liquor is often used in tonifying and replenishing formula, and in formula for dispelling wind and dredging the collaterals.

6) Vermilion Pill

There are two types of vermilion pills, one for oral application and another for external application. Vermilion pill for oral application does not have a fixed form; it can be pellet or powder. It is made of expensive drugs and it has remarkable therapeutic effect. Vermilion pill for external application is the crystal-like product of various shapes made by heating some medicinal minerals under high temperature. It is often smashed into powder and sprinkled over the affected body part. It can also be made into medicinal paper strip or thread for external application.

7) Suppository

Suppository is a solid preparation of certain shape, made by mixing fine powder of drugs with matrix. It is inserted either into the rectum, vagina or urethra where it dissolves. Functions of suppository include killing parasites, relieving itches, moistening and astringency.

8) Granule

Granule refers to dried particles or tiny blocks made by mixing drug extracts with excipient or with fine powder of some drugs. It is taken orally after it is infused with boiled water. It is tasty, small in size, quick in action and convenient in carrying.

9) Tablet

Tablet is a flat preparation made by mixing fine powder of drugs or drug extract with excipient, and by pressing the mixture. There are many types of tablets, such as sugarcoated tablets, enteric coating tablets, buccal tablets, and effervescent tablets.

10) Syrup

Syrup is a saturated solution of sugar made by boiling drugs in water, removing the residue, concentrating the decoction and dissolving sugar in it. Syrup is sweet and can be absorbed easily. It is widely used in children.

11) Oral Liquid

Oral liquid is a refined liquid preparation made by extracting drugs by means of water of other solvent. It has agreeable taste, and it can be absorbed easily.

12) Injection

Injection is aseptic solution, suspension or powder (for preparing liquid), which has gone through the procedures of drug extraction, refining and preparing. There are several methods of applying injection, including intradermal, subcutaneous, intramuscular, intravenous, intraosseous, and intraperitoneal. It is especially suitable for patients who have difficulty in taking medicine.

3. Methods of Making a Decoction

1) Utensil for decocting drugs

An earthen jug or pot is preferable; an enamelware or aluminum ware is probably OK. Iron or copper wares are forbidden because some drugs may generate chemical reaction and side effects or may lower their solubility and generate sediment when they are heated together with iron or copper. It is advisable to use a pot with large capacity and a lid.

2) Water for decocting drugs

Tap water, well water, distilled water, spring water, clean cabbage-washing water or clean rice-washing water can by used to decoct drugs. Sometimes liquor or mixed water and wine are used. The amount of water used depends on the amount and quality of drugs and on the time needed to decoct. Drugs are usually decocted twice, or even three times. For the first decocting, water is added till it covers the drugs and is 2-3cm above them. Less water may be added for the second and third decocting. 150-200ml decoction is collected from each decocting.

3) Fire for decocting drugs

It includes "strong fire" (quick decocting) and "slow fire" (slow decocting). Strong fire is usually used first till the water boils, followed by slow fire. In addition, the choice of fire should be based on drugs' property and the time needed to decoct. Strong fire is preferable for drugs releasing exterior and promoting diuresis. These drugs are decocted for short time with relatively small amount of water. Slow fire is preferable for drugs with nourishing function; these drugs should be decocted for longer time with relatively larger amount of water. Burned drugs should be discarded.

4) Methods for decocting drugs

The drugs are usually decocted after they have been thoroughly soaked for 20-30 minutes. Moreover, the herb residue should be well pressed to get the remaining juice.

(1) Decoct first: Shells and minerals should be broken up and decocted first for about 20 minutes before adding other drugs. Some drugs that are light but in large dosage, or drugs with sand and mud, should be decocted first to obtain juice; other drugs are then decocted in the collected juice/decoction rather than in water.

(2) Decoct later: Aromatic drugs should be decocted only for about 5 minutes. When Da Huang is chiefly used for purgation, it should be decocted for 10-15 minutes. All decoct-later drugs also need to be soaked first.

(3) Wrap-decoct: Some drugs can make decoction turbid, irritate throat or stick to the pot bottom. These drugs should be wrapped first in a piece of gauze or cloth before they are decocted with other drugs.

(4) Decoct alone: Some valuable drugs should be cut into small pieces and decoct alone to obtain juice in order to preserve their ingredients. Then it is taken along with the decoction of other drugs or is taken by itself.

(5) Dissolve (Melt): Some glutinous, sticky and easily dissolved drugs should be dissolved by heat separately, and then they should be mixed with the decoction of other drugs when they are still hot.

(6) Infuse: Some aromatic or valuable drugs and drugs that are not suitable for heating or boiling, should be ground into fine powder and infused with warm boiled water or medicinal solution for oral application.

4. Methods of Taking Drugs

Methods of taking drugs also affect their therapeutic effects

1) Time for taking drugs

It is preferable to take drugs after meals if a disease is located in Upper Warmer; otherwise it is preferable to take drugs before meals if a disease is located in Lower Warmer. Drugs with tonic or purgative action should be taken before meals; those with sedatives should be taken before sleeping; and those that irritate the gastrointestinal tract should be taken after meals. Drugs for acute and serious diseases should be taken at any time, while those for chronic diseases should be taken regularly.

2) Method of taking drugs

The dosage of a decoction is one dose a day. The decoction is usually divided into two or three equal portions and they should be taken when they are warm. Under circumstances, decoction can also be taken once a day, many times a day, or be taken as tea, or even two doses can be taken in a day. The cold-natured drugs indicated for heat syndromes should be taken when they are cool; the heat-natured drugs for cold syndromes should be taken when they are warm. In serious illness, cold-natured herbs can be taken when they are hot, and hot-natured herbs can be taken when they are cool. For unconscious patients or those who have difficulty in swallowing, the decoction should be given by nasal feeding. In order to avoid toxicity and prevent them from damaging healthy qi, the drastic and toxic herbs should be started with a small dose first, increased gradually, and suspended immediately when the therapeutic effects have been achieved.

3) Nursing after taking drugs

Drugs for releasing exterior should only induce slight sweating thoroughly, not drenching sweats. Cold, uncooked or non-digestive food should not be taken after purgative formula is applied. The interaction between drugs and food must also be considered.

Appendix II: Commonly Used Herbs and Dosage

Pin Yin Name	Chinese Name	Latin Botanical Name	Common Name	Pharmaceutical Name	Dosage (gram)
A Li Shan Wu Wei Zi	阿里山五味子	Schisandra arisanensis Hayata		Fructus schisandra arisanensis	1.5-8g
A Wei	阿魏	Ferula sinkiangensis K.M.Shen; F. fukanensis K.M.Shen	Chinese Asa-fetida	Resina ferulae	1-1.5g
Ai Di Cha	矮地茶	Ardisia japonica (Horrst.) Bl	Japanese Ardisia Stem and Leaf	Ardisiae Japonicae Caulis et Folium	10-30g
Ai Pian	艾片	Blumea balsamifera DC.	Blumea Camphor; Ngai Camphor	Blumea Camphor	0.03-0.1g
Ai Ye	艾叶	Artemisia argyi Levl.et Vant.	Mugwort Leaf	Folium Artemisiae Argyi	3-10g
An Xi Xiang	安息香	Styrax benzoin Dryand; Styrax tonkinensis (Pierre)Craib ex Hartw.[S.macrothyrsus Perk.; S.hypoglaucus Perk.]	Benzoin	Benzoinum; Benzoinum Styracis	0.3-1.5g
Ba Dou	巴豆	Croton tiglium L.	Croton Seed	Fructus Crotonis; Semen Crotonis	0.1-0.3g
Ba Jiao Hui Xiang	八角茴香	Illicium verum Hook. f.	Star Anise	Fructus Anisi Stellati	3-8g
Ba Ji Tian	巴戟天	Morinda officinalis How	Morinda Root	Radix Morindae Officinalis	10-15g
Ba Yue Zha	八月扎	Akebia quinata (Thunb.) Decne.; A. trifoliata (Thunb.) koidz.; A. trifoliata (Thunb.) Koidz. var. australis (Diels) Rehd.	Akebia Fruit	Fructus Akebia	6-12g
Bai Bian Dou	白扁豆	Dolichos lablab L	Hyacinth Bean, Dolichos	Semen Dolichoris Lablab; Semen Dolichoris Album	10-30g (decoction); 6-10g

					(pill)
Bai Bu	百部	Stemona sessilifolia (Mig.) Franch. et Sav.; S. japonica(Bl) Mig.; S. tuberosa Lour	Stemona Root	Radix Stemonae	5-10g
Bai Dou Kou	白豆蔻	Amomum Kravanh Pirre ex Gagnep.; A. compactum Soland ex Maton	Cardamom	Fructus Amomi Rotundus; Fructus Amomi Kravanh	3-6g
Bai Dou Kou Ke	白豆蔻壳	Amomum Kravanh Pirre ex Gagnep.; A. compactum Soland ex Maton	Cardamom	Pericarpium Amomi Kravanh	3-6g
Bai Fan	白矾	Aluminum potassium sulfate(Chemical Name)	Alumen	Alumen	1-3g
Bai Fu Zi	白附子	Typhonium giganteum Engl.; Aconitum coreanum (Levl.) Raipaics.	Giant Typhonium Tuber	Rhizoma Typhonii	3-5g
Bai Guo	白果	Ginkgo biloba L.	Ginkgo Nut	Semen Ginkgo; Semen Ginkgo Bilobae	6-10g
Bai Guo Ye	白果叶	Ginkgo biloba L.	Ginkgo Leaf	Folium Ginkgo Bilobae	3-6g
Bai He	百合	Lilium brownii F. E. Brown.; L. alancifolium Thunb.; Lilium pumilum DC.	Lily Bulb	Bulbus Lilii	10-30g
Bai Hu Jiao	白胡椒	Piper nigrum L.	White Pepper	Fructus Piperis Albicatus	2-3g
Bai Hua She	白花蛇	Bungarus multicinctus Blyth; Agkistrodon acutus (Gunther)	Agkistrodon	Agkistrodon seu Bungarus	3-10g
Bai Hua She She Cao	白花蛇舌草	Hedyotis Diffusa Willd.; Oldenlandia Diffusa (Willd.) Roxb.	Hedyotis	Herba Hedyotis Diffusae	15-60g
Bai Ji	白及	Bletilla striata (Thunb.) Reichb. f.	Bletilla	Rhizoma Bletillae Striatae	3-10g
Bai Ji Li	白蒺藜	Tribulus Terrestris L.	Tribulus	Fructus Tribuli Alba; Frucuts Tribuli Terrestris	6-10g
Bai Jiang Can	白僵蚕	Bombyx mori L.	Silkworm	Bombyx Batryticatus	3-10g
Bai Jiang Cao	败酱草	Patrinia scabiosaefolia Fisch. Ex Link.; P. villosa Juss.	Patrinia	Patriniae Herba cum Radice	6-15g
Bai Jie Zi	白芥子	Brassica alba (L.) Boiss.; B. juncea (L.) Czern. et Coss.	White Mustard Seed	Semen Sinapis Albae	3-10g

APPENDIX II

Bai Ju Hua	白菊花	Chrysanthemum morifolium Ramat.	Chrysanthemum Flower	Chrysanthemi Flos Albus	10-15g
Bai Kou Ren	白蔻仁	Amomum Kravanh Pirre ex Gagnep.; A. compactum Soland ex Maton	Cardamom	Fructus Amomi Cardamomi	3-6g
Bai Lian	白蔹	Ampelopsis japonica (Thunb.) Makino	Ampelopis Root	Radix Ampelopsis	5-10g
Bai Mao Gen	白茅根	Imperata cylindrical (L.) Beauv. var. major (Nees.) C. E. Hubb.	Imperata Root	Rhizoma Imperatae Cylindricae; Rhizoma Imperatae	15-30g
Bai Qian	白前	Cynanchum stauntonii (Decne.) Schltr.ex Levl.; C. glaucescens (Decne.) Hand. Mazz	Cynanchum Root	Rhizoma Cynanchi Stauntonii	3-10g
Bai Shao Yao	白芍药	Paeonia lactiflora Pall.	White Peony Root	Radix Paeoniae Alba	5-10g
Bai Tou Weng	白头翁	Pulsatilla Chinensis (Bge.) Regel	Pulsatilla; Anemone	Radix Pulsatillae Chinensis; Radix Pulsatillae	6-15g
Bai Wei	白薇	Cynanchum atratum Bge.; C. versicolor Bge.	Swallowwort Root	Radix Cynanchi Atrati	3-12g
Bai Xian Pi	白鲜皮	Dictamnus dasycarpus Turcz.	Dictamnus Root Bark	Cortex Dictamni Radicis	5-10g
Bai Ying	白英	Solanum lyratum Thunb.	Climbbing Nighshade	Herba Solani Lyrati	10-25g
Bai Zhi	白芷	Angelica dahurica (Fisch ex Hoffm.) Benth. Et Hook. F.; A. dahurica (Fisch. Ex Hoffm.) Benth. Et Hook. var. formosana (Boiss.) Shan et Yuan	Angelica Root	Radix Angelicae Dahuricae	3-10g
Bai Zhu	白术	Atractylodes macrocephala Koidz.	Ovate Atractylodes Root	Rhizoma Atractylodis Macrocephalae	5-15g
Bai Zi Ren	柏子仁	Platycladus orientalis (L.) Franco; Biota orientalis (L.) Endl.	Biota Seed	Semen Platycladi; Semen Biotae Orientalis	10-20g
Ban Bian Lian	半边莲	Lobelia chinensis Lour.	Chinese Lobelia	Lobeliae Chinensis Herba cum Radice	10-20g
Ban Lan Gen	板兰根	Isatis tinctoria L.; I. indigotica Fort.; Baphicacanthus cusia Bremek.	Isatis or Baphicacanthus Root	Radix Isatidis seu Baphicacanthi; Radix Isatidis	10-15g
Ban Mao	斑蝥	Mylabris phalerata Pall.; M.	Mylabris,	Mylabris	0.03-

		eichorii L.	Cantharides		0.06g
Ban Xia	半夏	Pinellia ternata (Thunb.) Breit	Pinellia Rhizome	Rhizoma Pinelliae Ternatae; Rhizoma Pinelliae	5-10g
Ban Xia Qu	半夏曲	Pinellia ternata (Thunb.) Breit		Rhizoma Pinelliae Fermentata	5-10g
Ban Zhi Lian	半枝莲	Scutellaria barbata D. Don.	Scute Barbata	Herba Scutellaria Barbatae	10-30g
Bei Dou Gen	北豆根	Menispermum dahuricum DC.	Northern Asarum	Radix Menispermi Daurici	3-10g
Bei Mu	贝母	Fritillaria cirrhosa D. Don; F. unibracteata Hsiao et K. C. Hsiao; F. prezwalskii Maxim.; F. delavayi Franch.; F. Verticillata Willd. Var. thunbergii Bak.	Fritillaria Bulb	Bulbus Fritillariae	3-10g
Bei Mu (Chuan)	贝母(川)	Fritillaria cirrhosa D. Don; F. unibracteata Hsiao et K. C. Hsiao; F. prezwalskii Maxim.; F. delavayi Franch.	Fritillaria Bulb	Bulbus Fritillariae Cirrhosae	3-10g
Bei Mu (Zhe)	贝母(浙)	Fritillaria Verticillata Willd. Var. thunbergii Bak.	Fritillaria Bulb	Bulbus Fritillariae Thunbergii	3-10g
Bei Sha Shen	北沙参	Glehnia littoralis F. Schmidt ex Miq.	Glehnia Root	Radix Glehniae	10-15g
Bei Wu Wei Zi	北五味子	Schisandra chinensis (Turcx.) Baill.	Northern Schisandra Berry	Fructus Schisandrae Chinensis	2-6g
Bei Xi Xin	北细辛	Asarum heterotropoides Fr. Schmidt var. mandshuricum (Maxim.) Kitag.	Northern asarum	Herba cum Radice Asari	2-5g
Bi Ba	荜茇	Piper longum L.	Long Pepper	Fructus Piperis Longi	2-5g
Bi Cheng Qie	荜澄茄	Piper cubeba L.; Litsea cubeba (Lour.) Pers.	Cubeb Fruit	Fructus Cubebae	2-5g
Bi Ji	荸荠	Eleocharis dulcis (Burm. f.) Trin. ex Henschel	Water Chestnut	Rhizoma Eleocharitis	30-90g
Bi Xie	萆薢	Dioscorea hypoglauca palibin; D. septemloba Thunb.; D. futschauensis Uline	Fish Poison Yam or Tokoro	Rhizoma Dioscoreae Hypoglaucae; Rhizoma Dioscoreae Septemlobae	10-15g
Bi Ma Zi	蓖麻子	Ricinus communis, L.	Castor Bean	Semen Ricini	1-5g
Bian Dou	扁豆	Dolichos lablab L.	White Hya-	Semen Dolichoris	10-30g

			cinth Bean	Lablab; Semen Dolichoris Album	
Bian Dou Hua	扁豆花	Dolichos lablab L.	White Hyacinth Flower	Flos Dolichoris Lablab	5-10g
Bian Dou Yi	扁豆衣	Dolichos lablab L.	White Hyacinth Bean Coat	Dolichoris Lablab Testa	5-10g
Bian Xu	萹蓄	Polygonum aviculare L.	Knotgrass	Herba Polygoni Avicularis	10-15g
Bie Jia	鳖甲	Trionyx sinensis Wiegmann (=Amyda sinensis Wiegmann)	Tortoise Shell	Carapax Amydae Sinensis; Carapax Trionycis	10-30g
Bing Lang	槟榔	Areca catechu L.	Areca Seed	Semen Arecae; Semen Areca Catechu	6-15g
Bing Pian	冰片	Dryobalanops aromatica Gaertn. f.	Borneol	Borneolum Syntheticum	0.03-0.1g
Bing Tang	冰糖	Saccharum sinensis Roxb.	Rock Candy, Crystal Sugar	Crystal Sugar	10-15g
Bo He	薄荷	Mentha haplocalyx Briq.	Mint	Herba Menthae Haplocalycis; Herba Menthae	2-10g
Bu Gu Zhi	补骨脂	Psoralea corylifolia L.	Psoralea Fruit	Fructus Psoraleae Corylifoliae; Fructus Psoraleae	5-10g
Can Sha	蚕沙	Bombyx mori L. (Jia Can)	Silkworm Droppings	Bombycis Mori Excrementum	5-10g
Cang Er Cao	苍耳草	Xanthium sibiricum Patr. et Widd.	Xanthium	Herba Xanthii Sibirici	6-15g
Cang Er Zi	苍耳子	Xanthium sibiricum Patr. et Widd.	Xanthium Fruit	Fructus Xanthii Sibirici	3-10g
Cang Zhu	苍术	Atractylodes lancea (Thunb.) DC, A. chinensis (DC.) Koidz.	Atractylodes Root	Rhizoma Atractylodis	5-10g
Cao Dou Kou	草豆蔻	Alpinia katsumadai Hayata	Katsumadai	Semen Alpiniae Katsumadai	3-6g
Cao Guo	草果	Amomum tsao-ko Crevost et Lemaire	Tsaoko Fruit	Fructus Tsaoko; Fructus Amomi Tsao-Ko	3-6g
Cao Guo Ren	草果仁	Amomum tsao-ko Crevost et Lemaire	Tsaoko Fruit	Fructus Tsaoko; Fructus Amomi Tsao-Ko	3-6g
Cao He Che	草河车(蚤休)	Paris polyphylla Smith	Paris Root	Rhizoma Paridis	5-10g

Cao Jue Ming	草决明	Cassia obtusifolia L.; C. tora L.	Cassia Seed	Semen Cassiae Torae	10-15g
Cao Wu	草乌	Aconitum carmichaeli Debx.; A. kusnezoffii Reichb.	Prepared Wild Aconite	Radix Aconiti Kusnezoffii	1.5-4.5g
Ce Bai Ye	侧柏叶	Biota orientalis (L.) Endl.; Platycladus orientalis (L.) Franco	Biota Leaf	Cacumen Biotae Orientalis; Cacumen Platycladi	10-15g
Chai Hu	柴胡	Bupleurum chinense DC.; B. scorzoneraefolium Willd.	Thorowax Root	Radix Bupleuri	3-10g
Chan Pi	蟾皮	Bufo bufo gargarizans Cantor; Bufo melanostictus Schneider	Toad Skin	Cutis Bufonis	3-9g
Chan Su	蟾酥	Bufo bufo gargarizans Cantor; B. melanostictus Schneider	Toad Venom	Bufonis Venenum	0.02-0.03g
Chan Tui	蝉蜕	Cryptotympana atrata Fabr.	Cicada Molting	Periostracum Cicadae	3-10g
Chang Shan	常山	Dichroa febrifuga Lour.	Dichroa Root	Radix Dichroae Febrifugae	5-10g
Che Qian Cao	车前草	Plantago asiatica L.; P. depressa Willd	Plantago	Herba Plantaginis	10-15g
Che Qian Zi	车前子	Plantago asiatica L.; P. depressa Willd	Plantago Seed	Semen Plantaginis	5-10g
Chen Pi	陈皮	Citrus reticulata Blanco	Tangerine Peel	Pericarpium Citri Reticulatae	3-9g
Chen Sha	辰砂(朱砂)		Cinnabar	Cinnabaris	0.3-1.0g
Chen Xiang	沉香	Aquilaria agallocha Roxb.; A. sinensis (Lour.) Gilg.	Aquilaria	Lignum Aquilariae; Lignum Aquilariae Resinatum	1-1.5g
Cheng Liu	柽柳	Tamarix chinensis Lour.	Tamarisk Twig and Leaf	Cacumen Tamaricis	3-10g
Chi Fu Ling	赤茯苓	Poria cocos (Schw.) Wolf	Red Poria	Sclerotium Poriae Cocos Rubra; Poriae Rubra	10-15g
Chi Shao	赤芍	Paeonia veitchii Lynch; P. abovata Maxim.; P. lactiflora Pall.	Red Peony Root	Radix Paeoniae Rubra	6-15g
Chi Shi Zhi	赤石脂		Red Halloysite	Halloysitum Rubrum	10-20g
Chi Xiao	赤小豆	Phaseolus calcaratus Roxb.; P.	Rice Bean	Semen Phaseoli	10-30g

Dou		angularis Wight			
Chong Wei Zi	茺蔚子	Leonurus heterophyllus Sweet	Leonurus Fruit	Fructus Leonuri	6-15g
Chu Shi Zi	楮实子	Broussonetia papyrifera (L.)Vent.	Paper Mulberry Fruit	Fructus Broussonetiae	6-9g
Chu Tou Kang (Mi Pi Kang)	杵头糠（米皮糠）	Oryza sativa L.	Rice Bran	Testa Oryzae Sativae	9-30g
Chuan Jin Pi	川槿皮（木槿皮）	Hibiscus syriacus L.	Rose-of-Sharon Root Bark	Hibisci Syriaci Radicis Cortex	3-10g
Chuan Lian Zi	川楝子	Melia toosendan Sieb. et. Zucc.	Toosendan Fruit	Fructus Meliae Toosendan	3-10g
Chuan Mu Tong	川木通	Clematis armandii Franch.; C. montana Buch.-Ham	Anemone Clematis Stem; Armand Clematis Stem	Caulis Clematidis	3-6g
Chuan Mu Xiang	川木香	Vladimiria souliei (Franch.) Ling.	Common Vladimiria Root	Radix Vladiniriae Souliei	3-10g
Chuan Niu Xi	川牛膝	Cyathula officinalis Kuan	Cyathula Root	Radix Cyathulae Officinalis	10-15g
Chuan Shan Jia	穿山甲	Manis pentadactyia L.	Pangolin Scales	Squama Manitis Pentadactylae; Squama Manis	3-10g
Chuan Shan Long	穿山龙	Discorea nipponica Makino.	Japanese dioscorea	Rhizoma Dioscroea	10-15g
Chuan Wu	川乌	Aconitum carmichaeli Debx.	Prepared Aconite	Radix Aconiti Carmichaeli; Radix Aconiti	1.5-4.5g
Chuan Xin Lian	穿心莲	Andrographis paniculata (Burm. f.) Nees.	Andrographis	Herba Andrographitis Paniculatae	6-15g
Chuan Xiong	川芎	Ligusticum chuanxiong Hort.	Ligusticum, Sichuan Lovage root	Rhizoma Ligustici Chuanxiong	3-10g
Chui Pen Cao	垂盆草	Sedum sarmentosum Bunge.	Hanging Stonecrop	Herba Sedi Sarmentosi	10-30g
Chun Pi	椿皮	Ailanthus altissima (Mill.) Swingle	Ailanthus Bark	Cortex Ailanthi Altissimae; Cortex Ailanthi	3-5g
Ci Ji Li	刺蒺藜	Tribulus terrestris L.	Tribulus Fruit	Fructus Tribuli	6-10g

Ci Shi	磁石		Loadstone	Magnetitum	10-30g
Ci Wei Pi	刺猬皮	Erinaceus europaeus L.	Hedgehog's Pelt	Erinacei Pellis	3-10g
Ci Wu Jia	刺五加	Acanthopanax senticosus (Ruper. Et Maxim.) Harms.	Spiny Acanthopanax	Radix et Caulis Acanthopanacis Senticosi	5-10g
Cong Bai	葱白	Allium fistulosum L.	Scallion	Bulbus Allii Fistulosi	3-10g
Da Dou Huang Juan	大豆黄卷	Glycine max (L.) Merr.	Dried Soybean Sprout	Sojae Semen Germinatum Siccus	10-15g
Da Feng Zi	大风子	Hydnocarpus anthelmintica Pier.; H. hainanensis (Merr.) Sleum	Hydnocarpus Seed	Semen Hydnocarpi	0.3-1g
Da Fu Pi	大腹皮	Areca catechu L.	Areca Husk	Pericarpium Areca Catechu; Pericarpium Arecae	3-10g
Da Huang	大黄	Rheum palmatum L.; R. tanguticum Maxim ex Balf.; R. officinale Baill.	Rhubarb	Radix et Rhizoma Rhei	5-10g
Da Huang (Zhi)	制大黄	Rheum palmatum L.; R. tanguticum Maxim ex Balf.; R. officinale Baill.	Rhubarb	Radix et Rhizoma Rhei Praeparatae	5-10g
Da Hui Xiang	大茴香	Illicium verum Hook. F.	Star Anise	Fructus Anisi Stellati	3-8g
Da Ji	大蓟	Cirsium japonicum DC.	Cirsium	Herba seu Radix Cirsii Japonici	10-15g
Da Ji	大戟	Euphorbia pekinensis Rupr.; Knoxia valerianoides Thorel et Pitard.		Radix Euphorbiae Pekinensis; Radix Knoxiae/Euphorbiae;	1.5-3g
Da Qing Ye	大青叶	Isatis tinctoria L.; I. indigotica Fort.	Isatis Leaf	Folium Isatidis	10-20g
Da Suan	大蒜	Allium sativum L.	Garlic Bulb	Bulbus Allii Sativi	6 to 15 g
Da Zao	大枣	Ziziphus jujuba Mill. var. inermis (Bge.) Rehd.	Jujube, Chinese Date	Fructus Zizyphi Jujubae	10-30g
Dai Mao	玳瑁	Erelmochelys imbricate (L.)	Hawksbill Turtle Shell	Carapax Eretmochelydis	3-6g
Dai Zhe Shi	代赭石		Hematite	Haematitum; Ochra Haematitum	10-30g
Dan Dou Chi	淡豆豉	Glycine max (L.) Merr.	Fermented Soybean	Fermented Soybean; Semen Sojae Praeparatum	10-15g

Dan Fan	胆矾		Chalcanthite	Chalcantitum	0.1-0.3g
Dan Nan Xing	胆南星	Arisaema consanguineum Schott.; A. heterophyllum Bl.; A. amurense Maxim.	Bile-prepared Arisaema	Rhizoma Arisaematis cum Bile; Rhizoma Arisaematis cum Felle Bovis	2-5g
Dan Shen	丹参	Salvia miltiorrhiza Bge.	Salvia Root	Radix Salviae Miltiorrhizae	5-15g
Dan Zhu Ye	淡竹叶	Lophatherum gracile Brongn.	Lophatherum	Herba Lophatheri Gracilis; Herba Lophatheri	6-15g
Dang Gui	当归	Angelica sinensis (Oliv.) Diels.	Chinese angelica Root	Radix Angelicae Sinensis	5-15g
Dang Gui Wei	当归尾	Angelica sinensis (Oliv.) Diels.	Tangkuei Tails	Tail of Radix Angelicae Sinensis; Extremitas Radicis Angelicae Sinensis	5-15g
Dang Shen	党参	Codonopsis pilosula (Franch.) Nannf.	Codonopsis Root	Radix Codonopsitis Pilosulae	6-10g
Dao Dou	刀豆	Canavalia gladiata (Jacq.) DC.	Sword Bean	Semen Canavaliae	10-15g
Deng Xin Cao	灯心草	Juncus Effusus L. var. decipiens Buchen.	Juncus Pith	Medulla Junci Effusi	1.5-2.5g
Di Bie Chong	地鳖虫	Eupolyphaga sinensis Walk.; Steleophaga plancyi (Bol.)	Eupolyphaga	Eupolyphagae seu Opisthoplatia	3-10g
Di Ding	地丁	Viola yedoensis Makino.	Violet	Herba cum Radice Violae	10-20g
Di Er Cao	地耳草	Hypericum japonicum Thunb.	Lesser Hypericum	Herba Hyperici Japonici	15-30g
Di Fu Zi	地肤子	Kochia scoparia (L.) schrad.	Kochia Fruit	Fructus Kochiae Scopariae	10-15g
Di Gu Pi	地骨皮	Lycium barbarum L.; L. chinense Mill	Lycium Root Bark	Cortex Lycii Radicis; Cortex Lycii	6-15g
Di Huang	地黄	Rehmannia glutinosa Libosch. f. hueichingensis (Chao et Schih) Hsiao; Rehmannia glutinosa Libosch.	Rehmannia Root	Radix Rehmanniae	10-30g
Di Long	地龙	Pheretima aspergillum (Eperrier); Allalobophora caliginosa (Savigny) trapezoides (Ant. Duges)	Earthworm	Lumbricus	5-15g

Di Yu	地榆	Sanguisorba officinalis L.; S. officinalis var. longifolia (Bert.) Yu et Li	Sanguisorba Root	Radix Sanguisorbae Officinalis	10-15g
Di Yu Tan	地榆炭	Sanguisorba officinalis L.; S. officinalis var. longifolia (Bert.) Yu et Li	Charred Sanguisorba	Charred Radix Sanguisorbae Officinalis	10-15g
Ding Xiang	丁香	Syzygium aromaticum (L.) Merr. et Perry.	Clove	Flos Caryophylli	2-5g
Dong Chong Xia Cao	冬虫夏草	Cordyceps sinensis (Berk.) Sacc.	Cordyceps	Cordyceps Sinensis	5-10g
Dong Gua Pi	冬瓜皮	Benincasa hispida (Thunb.) Cogn.	Winter Melon Rind	Exocarpium Benincasae Hispidae	10-30g
Dong Gua Zi	冬瓜子	Benincasa hispida (Thunb.) Cogn.	Winter Melon Seed	Semen Benincasae Hispidae; Semen Benincasae	10-15g
Dong Kui Zi	冬葵子	Malva verticillata L.	Mallow Fruit	Semen Malvae	10-15g
Dou Juan	豆卷	Glycine max (L.) Merr.	Dried Soybean Sprout	Semen Sojae Germinatum Siccus	10-15g
Du Huo	独活	Angelica pubescens Maxim. F. biserrata Shan et Yuan.	Angelica Root	Radix Angelicae Pubescentis	3-10g
Du Zhong	杜仲	Eucommia ulmoides Oliv.	Eucommia Bark	Cortex Eucommiae; Cortex Eucommiae Ulmoidis	10-15g
E Bu Shi Cao	鹅不食草	Centipeda minima (L.) A.	Centipeda Herb	Herba cum Radice Centipedae	5-9g
E Guan Shi	鹅管石		Tip of Tubular Stalactites	Stalactitum	9-15g
E Jiao	阿胶	Equus Asinus L.	Donkey Hide Glue	Colla Corii Asini; Gelatinum Corii Asini	5-10g
E Zhu	莪术	Curcuma zedoraria (Berg.) Rosc.; C. aromatica Salisb.; C. Kwangsiensis S. Lee et. C.F. Liang.	Zedoaria	Rhizoma Curcumae Ezhu	3-10g
Er Cha	儿茶	Acacia catechu (L.) Willd.; Uncaria gambier Roxb.	Catechu	Acaciae seu Uncariae Pasta; Catechu	1-3g
Fan Hong Hua	番红花	Crocus sativus L.	Saffron	Stigma Croci; Stigma Croci Sativi	1.5-3g

Fan Xie Ye	番泻叶	Cassia angustifolia Vahl.; C. acutifolia Del.	Senna Leave	Folium Sennae	1.5-10g
Fang Feng	防风	Saposhnikovia divaricata (Turcz.) Schischk.	Divaricate Saposhniovia	Radix Saposhnikoviae Divaricatae; Radix Saposhnikoviae	3-10g
Fang Ji	防己	Stephania tetrandra S. Moore; Aristolochia fangchi Y.C.Wu et L.D.Chou et S.M. Hwang	Stephania	Radix Stephaniae Tetrandrae	5-10g
Fei Zi	榧子	Torreya grandis Fort.	Torreya Seeds	Semen Torreyae	30-50g
Feng Fang	蜂房	Polistes olivaceous (DeGeer).; P. japonicus Saussure; Parapolybia varia Fabricius	Wasp Nest	Vespae Nidus	2.5-4.5g
Feng Mi	蜂蜜	Apis cerana Fabricius; A. mellifera L.	Honey	Honey	15-30g
Feng Wei Cao	凤尾草	Pteris multifida Poir.	Pteris	Herba Pteridis Multifidae	10-20g
Fo Shou	佛手	Citrus medica L. var. sarcodactylis Swingle	Buddha's Hand	Fructus Citri Sarcodactyli	3-10g
Fo Shou Hua	佛手花	Citrus medica L. var. sarcodactylis Swingle	Finger Citron Flower	Flos Citri Sarcodactylidis	3-6g
Fu Hai Shi	浮海石	Costazia aculeata Canu et. Bassler	Pumice	Pumex	6-10g
Fu Ling	茯苓	Poria cocos (Schw.) Wolf	Poria	Sclerotium Poriae Cocos; Poria	10-15g
Fu Ling Pi	茯苓皮	Poria cocos (Schw.) Wolf	Poria Skin	Cortex Poriae Cocos; Cortex Poria	10-15g
Fu Long Gan	伏龙肝		Ignited Yellow Earth	Terra Flava Usta	15-30g
Fu Pen Zi	覆盆子	Rubus chingii Hu.	Rubus Berry	Fructus Rubi Chingii	3-10g
Fu Pian	附片	Aconitum carmichaeli Debx.	Aconite	Radix Aconiti Lateralis Praeparatae	3-15g
Fu Ping	浮萍	Spirodela polyrrhiza (L.) Schleid.	Duckweed or Spirodela	Herba Spirodelae	3-10g
Fu Shen	茯神	Poria cocos (Schw.) Wolf	Root Poria	Sclerotium Poriae Circum Radicem Pini; Sclerotium Poriae Cocos Pararadicis	10-15g
Fu Xiao Mai	浮小麦	Triticum aestivum L.	Light Wheat Grain	Fructus Tritici Aestivi Levis	15-30g

Pinyin	Chinese	Botanical Name	Common Name	Pharmaceutical Name	Dosage
Fu Zi	附子	Aconitum carmichaeli Debx.	Aconite	Radix Aconiti Lateralis Praeparatae	3-15g
Fu Zi (Sheng)	生附子	Aconitum carmichaeli Debx.	Aconite	Radix Aconiti Lateralis	3-15g
Gan Cao	甘草	Glycyrrhiza uralensis Fisch.; G. inflata Bat.; G. glabra L.	Licorice Root	Radix Glycyrrhizae; Radix Glycyrrhizae Uralensis	3-10g
Gan Jiang	干姜	Zingiber officinale Rosc.	Dried Ginger	Rhizoma Zingiberis Officinalis; Rhizoma Zingiberis	3-10g
Gan Lan	橄榄（青果）	Canarium album (Lour.) Raeusch.	Chinese White Olive	Fructus Canarii Albi	6-15g
Gan Qi	干漆	Rhus verniciflua Stokes	Lacquer	Resina Toxicodendri	0.06-0.1g (pill or powder)
Gan Song	甘松	Nardostachys chinensis Batal.; N. jatamanse DC.	Nardostachys Root	Rhizoma et Radix Nardostachydis	3-6g
Gan Sui	甘遂	Euphorbia kansui T.N. Liou et T.P.Wang.	Kansui Root	Radix Euphorbia Kansui; Radix Kansui	0.5-1g
Gao Ben	藁本	Ligusticum sinense Oliv.; Ligusticum jeholense Nakai et Kitag.	Chinese Luvage Root	Rhizoma et Radix Ligustici; Rhizoma Ligustici	3-10g
Gao Li Shen	高丽参	Panax ginseng C.A.Mey	Korean Ginseng Root	Radix Ginseng Coreenis	5-10g
Gao Liang Jiang	高良姜	Alpinia officinarum Hance.	Galanga	Rhizoma Alpiniae Officinarum	3-10g
Ge Fen	蛤粉	Meretrix meretrix L.; Cyclina sinensis Gmelin	Clamshell Powder	Concha Meretricis seu Cyclinae Powder	10-15g
Ge Gen	葛根	Pueraria lobata (Willd.) Ohwi.; Pueraria thomsonii Benth.	Kudzu Root	Radix Puerariae	10-20
Ge Hua	葛花	Pueraria lobata (Willd.) Ohwi.	Pueraria Flower or Kudzu Flower	Flos Puerariae	3-12
Ge Jie	蛤蚧	Gekko gecko L.	Gecko	Gecko	3-7g
Gou Ji	狗脊	Cibotium barometz (L.) J. Sm.	Cibotium Root	Rhizoma Cibotii Barometz	10-15g
Gou Qi Zi	枸杞子	Lycium barbarum L.; L. chinense Mill.	Lycium Fruit	Fructus Lycii	5-15g

Gou Teng	钩藤	Uncaria rhynchophylla (Miq.) Jacks.; U. macrophylla Wall.; U. hirsuta Havil.; U. sinensis (Oliv.) Havil.; U. sessifructus Roxb.	Uncaria Stem and Thorn	Ramulus Uncariae cum Uncis	10-15g
Gu Jing Cao	谷精草	Eriocaulon buergerianum Koern.; .E. sieboldtianum Seib. Et Zucc.	Eriocaulon Scape and Flower	Scapus et Flos Eriocaulonis	6-10g
Gu Jing Zhu	谷精珠	Eriocaulon buergerianum Koern.; .E. sieboldtianum Seib. Et Zucc.	Eriocaulon Flower	Flos Eriocauli	6-10g
Gu Sui Bu	骨碎补	Drynaria fortunei (Kunze) J. Sm.	Drynaria Root	Rhizoma Drynariae	10-20g
Gu Ya	谷芽	Oryza sativa L.	Rice Sprout	Fructus Germinatus Oryzae Sativae	10-15g
Gua Di	瓜蒂	Cucumis melo L.	Melon Stalk	Pedicellus Melo; Cucum meloc L.	2.5-5g
Gua Lou	瓜蒌	Trichosanthes Ririlowii Maxim.; T. rosthornii Harms	Trichosanthes Fruit	Fructus Trichosanthis	10-20g
Gua Lou Pi	瓜蒌皮	Trichosanthes Ririlowii Maxim.; T. rosthornii Harms	Trichosanthes Rind	Pericarpium Trichosanthis	6-10g
Gua Lou Shi	瓜蒌实	Trichosanthes Ririlowii Maxim.; T. rosthornii Harms	Trichosanthes Fruit	Fructus Trichosanthis	10-20g
Gua Lou Zi	瓜蒌子	Trichosanthes Ririlowii Maxim.; T. rosthornii Harms	Trichosanthes Seed	Semen Trichosanthis	10-15g
Guan Mu Tong	关木通	Aristolochia manshuriensis Kom	Manshurian Dutchmanspipe Stem	Caulis Aristolochiae Manshuriensis	3-6g
Guan Zhong	贯众	Dryopteris crassirhizoma Nakai.; Lunathyrium acrostichoides (Sw.) Ching ; Woodwardia unigemmata (Makino) Nakai.; Osmunda Japonica Thunb.	Dryopteris Root	Rhizoma Guanzhong; Rhizoma Dryopteris Crassirhizomae	10-15g
Gui Ban	龟板	Chinemys reevesii (Gray)	Tortoise Plastron	Plastrum Testudinis; Carapax et Plastrum Testudinis	10-30g
Gui Ban Jiao	龟板胶	Chinemys reevesii (Gray)	Tortoise Plastron Glue	Colla Testudinis Plastri; Carapax et Plastrum Testudinis	3-10g
Gui Jian Yu	鬼箭羽	Euonynus alatus (Thunb.) Sieb.	Winged Euonymus	Ramulus Euonymi	3-10g

			Twig		
Gui Zhi	桂枝	Cinnamomum cassia Presl.	Cinnamom Twig	Ramulus Cinnamomi Cassiae; Ramulus Cinnamomi	5-10g
Hai Dai (Kun Bu)	海带(昆布)	Laminaria japonica Aresch.; Ecklonia kurome Okam.	Laminaria	Thallus Laminariae	10-15g
Hai Feng Teng	海风藤	Piper futokadsura Sieb. et Zucc.	Kadsura Pepper Stem	Caulis Piperis Kadsurae	5-10g
Hai Ge Fen	海蛤粉	Meretrix meretrix L.; Cyclina sinensis Gmelin	Clamshell Powder	Concha Meretricis seu Cyclinae Powder	10-15g
Hai Ge Qiao	海蛤壳	Meretrix meretrix L.; Cyclina sinensis Gmelin	Clamshell	Concha Meretricis seu Cyclinae	10-15g
Hai Gou Shen	海狗肾	Callorhinus ursinus Linnaeus; Phoca largha Pallas; Phoca vitulina Linnaeus	Seal's Genitals	Callorhini seu Phocae Testis et Penis	3-9g
Hai Jin Sha	海金沙	Lygodium japonicum (Thunb.) Sw.	Lygodium Spores	Spora Lygodii Japonici	6-15g
Hai Ma	海马	Hippocampus kelloggi Jordanet Snvder; H. histrix Kaup; H. kudaBleeker; H. trimaculatus Leach; H. japonicus Kaup	Sea Horse	Hippocampus	3-9g
Hai Piao Xiao (Wu Zei Gu)	海螵蛸(乌贼骨)	Sepiella maindroni de Rochebrune.; Sepia esculenta Hoyle.	Cuttlefish Bone	Os Sepiae seu Sepiellae	6-12g
Hai Tong Pi	海桐皮	Erythrina variegata L. var. orientalis (L.) Merr.	Erythrina Bark	Cortex Erythrinae	6-12g
Hai Zao	海藻	Sargassum pallidum (Turn.) C Ag. ; S. fusiforme (Harv.) Setch.	Sargassum	Herba Sargassi	10-15g
Han Lian Cao (Mo Han Lian)	旱莲草(墨旱莲)	Eclipta prostrata L.	Eclipta	Herba Ecliptae Prostratae	10-30g
Han Shui Shi	寒水石	Mirabilite (Chemical Name)	Calcitum	Calcitum; Gypsum seu Calcitum	10-15g
He Huan Hua	合欢花	Albizzia julibrissin Durazz;A. kalkora (Roxb) Prain	Silk Tree Flower or Albizzia Flower	Flos Albizziae Julibrissin; Flos Albizziae	5-10g
He Huan Pi	合欢皮	Albizzia julibrissin Durazz;A. kalkora (Roxb) Prain	Silk Tree Bark	Cortex Albizziae Julibrissin; Cortex Albizziae	10-15g

He Shou Wu	何首乌	Polygonum multiflorum Thunb.	Flowery Knotweed Root or Polygonum	Radix Polygoni Multiflori	10-30g
He Shi	鹤虱	Carpesium abrotanoides L.; Daucus carota L.	Carpesium Fruit	Fructus Carpesii Abrotanoidis; Fructus Carpesii	5-15g
He Tao Ren	核桃仁	Juglans regia L.	Walnut	Semen Juglandis	10-30g
He Ye	荷叶	Nelumbo nuciflera Gaertn.	Lotus Leaf	Folium Nelumbinis Nuciferae; Folium Nelumbinis	3-10g
He Geng	荷梗	Nelumbo nuciflera Gaertn.	Lotus Stem	Petiolus Nelumbinis	9-15g
He Zi	诃子	Terminalia chebula Retz.; T. chebula Retz. var. tomentella Kurt.	Chebule	Fructus Terminaliae Chebulae; Fructus Chebulae	3-10g
Hei Dou	黑豆	Glycine max (L.) merr.	Black Soybean	Glycine Max	6-10g
Hei Zhi Ma	黑脂麻 (黑芝麻, 胡麻)	Sesamum indicum L.	Black Sesame Seed	Semen Sesami Nigrum; Semen Sesami Indici	10-30g
Hong Hua	红花	Carthamus tinctorius L.	Carthamus	Flos Carthami Tinctorii; Flos Carthami	3-10g
Hong Niang Zi	红娘子	Huechys sanguinea De Geer; H. philaemata Fabricius	Huechys	Huechys	0.15-0.5g
Hong Teng	红藤	Sargentodoxa cuneata Rehd. et Wils.	Sargentodoxa Vine	Caulis Sargentodoxae Cuneatae	10-15g
Hong Shen	红参	Panax ginseng C.A.Mey.	Red Ginseng	Radix Ginseng Rubra	5-10g
Hou Po	厚朴	Magnolia officinalis Rehd. Et Wils., Magnolia officinalis Rehd. Et Wils.var blioba Rehd.	Magnolia Bark	Cortex Magnoliae Officinalis	3-10g
Hou Po Hua	厚朴花	Magnolia officinalis Rehd. Et Wils., Magnolia officinalis Rehd. Et Wils.var blioba Rehd.	Magnolia Flower	Flos Magnoliae Officinalis	3-6g
Hu Gu	虎骨	Panthera tigris L.	Tiger Bone	Os Tigris	3-6g
Hu Huang Lian	胡黄连	Picrorrhiza Kurrooa Royle ex Benth.; P. scrophulariaeflora Pennell	Picrorhiza Root	Rhizoma Picrorrhizae	3-10g
Hu Ji Sheng	槲寄生	Viscum coloratum (Komar.)	Colored Mis-	Herba Visci	10-20g

		Nakai	tletoe		
Hu Jiao	胡椒	Piper nigrum L.	Pepper	Fructus Piperis	2-3g
Hu Lu Ba	胡芦巴	Trigonella foenum-graecum L.	Fenugreek Seed	Semen Trigonellae Foeni-graeci	3-10g
Hu Ma	胡麻 (黑脂麻, 黑芝麻)	Sesamum indicum L.	Black Sesame Seed	Semen Sesami Nigrum; Semen Sesami Indici	10-30g
Hu Po	琥珀		Amber	Succinum	1.5-3g
Hu Sui	胡荽 (香菜)	Coriandrum sativum L.	Coriander	Herba Coriandri	3-6g
Hu Tao Ren	胡桃仁	Juglans regia L.	Walnut	Semen Juglandis	10-30g
Hu Zhang	虎杖	Polygonum cuspidatum Sieb. et Zucc.	Bushy Knotweed Root	Rhizoma Polygoni Cuspidati	10-30g
Hua Jiao	花椒	Zanthoxylum bungeanum Maxim.; Z. schinifolium Sieb. et Zucc.	Zanthoxylum	Pericarpium Zanthoxyli	2-5g
Hua Ju Hong	化橘红	Citrus qrandis 'Tomentosa'; C. qrandis (L.) Osbeck	Huazhou Pomelo Rind	Exocarpium Citri Grandis Rubrum	3-10g
Hua Qi Shen	花旗参（西洋参）	Panax quinquefolium L.	American Ginseng	Radix Panacis Quinquefolii	3-6g
Hua Rui Shi	花蕊石		Ophicalcite	Ophicalcitum	10-15g
Hua Shi Fen	滑石粉		Talcum	Talcum	10-15g
Huai Hua	槐花	Sophora japonica L.	Sophora Flower	Flos Sophorae Japonicae; Flos Sophorae	10-15g
Huai Jiao	槐角	Sophora japonica L.	Sophora Fruit	Fructus Sophorae	10-15g
Huai Mi	槐米	Sophora japonica L.	Sophora Flower Bud	Flos Immaturus Sophorae Japonicae	10-15g
Huang Bai	黄柏	Phellodendron amurense Rupr.; P. chinensis Schneid.	Phellodendron Bark	Cortex Phellodendri	3-10g
Huang Dan	黄丹（铅丹）		Minjum	Minium	0.3-0.6g
Huang Jing	黄精	Polygonatum kingianum Coll et hemsl.; P. sibiricum Red.; P. cyrtonema Hua.	Polygonatum Root	Rhizoma Polygonati	10-15g
Huang Lian	黄连	Coptis chinensis Franch.; C. deltoidea C. Y. Cheng et Hsiao; C. teetoides C. Y.	Coptis Root	Rhizoma Coptidis	2-10g

		Cheng.; C. omeiensis (Chen) C. Y. Cheng			
Huang Qi	黄芪	Astragalus menbranaceus Bge. Var. mongholicus (Bge.) Hsiao; A. membranaceus (Fisch.) Bge.	Astragalus Root	Radix Astragali; Radix Astragali Membranacei	10-15g
Huang Qin	黄芩	Scutellaria baicalensis Georgi; S. amoena C.H. Wright; S. viscidula Bge. S. rehderiana Diels.	Scutellaria Root	Radix Scutellariae Baicalensis; Radix Scutellariae	3-10g
Huang Yao Zi	黄药子	Dioscorea bulbifera L.	Tuber Dioscoreae	Rhizoma Dioscoreae Bulbiferae	10-15g
Huo Ma Ren	火麻仁	Cannabis sativa L.	Hemp Seed	Semen Cannabis Sativae; Semen Cannabis	10-15g
Huo Xiang	藿香	Pogostemon cablin (Blanco) Benth.; Agastache rugosus (Fisch.et Mey.) O. Ktze	Agastache or Patchouli	Herba Agastache seu Pogostemonis; Herba Pogostemonis; Herba Agastaches	5-10g
Huo Xiao (Xiao Shi)	火硝(硝石)		Nitre	Nitrium	1.5-3g
Ji Gu Cao	鸡骨草	Arbus fruticulosus Wall. Ex Wight et Arn.	Prayer-beads	Herba cum Radice Abri	6-15g
Ji Nei Jin	鸡内金	Gallus gallus domesticus Brisson.	Gizzard Lining	Endothelium Corneum Gigeriae Galli	3-10g
Ji Xue Teng	鸡血藤	Spatholobus suberectus Dunn.; Milletia dielsiana Harms.; Millettia reticulata Benth.	Spatholobus Vine or Millettia	Radix et Caulis Jixueteng	10-15g
Jiang Can	僵蚕	Bombyx mori L.	Silkworm	Bombyx Batryticatus	3-10g
Jiang Huang	姜黄	Curcuma longa L.	Turmeric	Rhizoma Curcumae Longae	3-10g
Jiang Xiang	降香	Dalbergia odorifera T. Chen	Dalbergia	Lignum Dalbergiae Odoriferae	3-6g
Jiao Mu	椒目	Zanthoxylum bungeanum Maxim.; Z. schinifolium Sieb. et Zucc.	Zanthoxylum Seed	Semen Zanthoxyli; Pericarpium Zanthoxyli	2-5g
Jie Geng	桔梗	Platycodon grandiflorum (Jacq.) A. DC.	Balloon-flower Root	Radix Platycodonis; Radix Platycodi Grandiflori	3-9g

Jin Fei Cao	金沸草(金佛花)	Inula japonica Thunb.; I. britannica L.	Inula Flowers	Flos Inulae	3-10g
Jin Guo Lan	金果榄	Tinospora capillipes Gagn.; T. sagittata Gagn.	Tinospora Tuber	Tuber Tinosporae	3-9g
Jin Meng Shi	金礞石		Mica Schist	Lapis Micae Aureus	6-10g
Jin Qian Bai Hua She	金钱白花蛇	Bungarus multicinctus Blyth	Multibanded Krati	Bungarus Multicinctus	3-10g
Jin Qian Cao	金钱草	Lysimachia christinae Hance; Glechoma longituba (Nakai) Kupr.; Desmodium styracifolium (Osb.) Merr.; Hydrocotyle sibthorpioides Lam. Var. batrachium (Hance) Hand. – Mazz.; Dichondra repens Forst.	Moneywort	Herba Jinqiancao; Herba Lysimachiae	15-30g
Jin Yin Hua	金银花	Lonicera japonica Thunb.; L. hypoglauca Miq.; L. ☐ud an☐ DC.; L. dasystyla Rehd.	Lonicera Flower	Flos Lonicerae	10-20g
Jin Ying Zi	金樱子	Rosa laevigata Michx.	Rosa Laevigata	Fructus Rosae Laevigatae	6-18g
Jing Da Ji	京大戟	Euphorbia pekinensis Rupr.	Euphorbia Root	Radix Euphorbiae Pekinensis; Radix Euphorbiae	1.5-3g
Jing Jie	荆芥	Schizonepeta tenuifolia Brig.	Schizonepeta	Herba Schizonepetae	5-10g
Jing Jie Sui	荆芥穗	Schizonepeta tenuifolia Brig.	Herba Schizonepetae	Spica Schizonepetae	5-10g
Jing Mi	粳米	Oryza sativa L.	Stalk Rice, Nonglutinous Rice	Semen Oryzae Sativae; Fructus Oryzae Sativae	9-10g
Jiu Cai Zi	韭菜子	Allium tuberosum Rottler	Allium Seed	Semen Allii Tuberosi	5-15g
Jiu Jie Chang Pu	九节菖蒲	Anemone altaica Fisch.	Altai Anemone Root	Rhizoma Anemones Altaicae	5-10g
Jiu Xiang Chong	九香虫	Aspongopus chinensis Dallas.	Stinkbug	Aspongopus	3-5g
Ju He	橘核	Citrus reticulata Blanco.	Tangerine	Semen Citri Reticu-	3-10g

				Pip	latae	
Ju Hong	橘红	Citrus reticulata Blanco.		Red Tangerine Peel	Exocarpium Citri Rubrum; Exocarpium Citri Reticulatae Rubrum	3-10g
Ju Hua	菊花	Chrysanthemum morifolium Ramat.		Chrysanthemum	Flos Chrysanthemi Morifolii; Flos Chrysanthemi	10-15g
Ju Luo	橘络	Citrus reticulata Blanco.		Tangerine Pith	Vascular Citri Reticulatae	3-5g
Ju Pi	橘皮	Citrus reticulata Blanco		Tangerine Peel	Pericarpium Citri Reticulatae	3-9g
Ju Ye	橘叶	Citrus reticulata Blanco.		Tangerine Leaf	Folium Citri Reticulatae	6-10g
Juan Bai	卷柏	Selaginella tamariscina (Beauv.) Spr.		Selaginella	Herba Selaginellae	3-10g
Jue Ming Zi	决明子	Cassia obtusifolia L.; Cassia tora L.		Cassia Seed	Semen Cassiae	10-15g
Ku Fan	枯矾	Aluminum potassium sulfate(Chemical Name)		Alumen	Alumen	1-3g
Ku Lian Pi	苦楝皮	Melia azedarach L.; M. toosendan S. et Z.		Chinaberry Root Bark	Cortex Meliae	6-15g
Ku Shen	苦参	Sophora flavescens Ait		Sophora Flavescens	Radix Sophorae Flavescentis	3-10g
Ku Shen Zi	苦参子（鸦胆子）	Brucea javanica (L.) Merr.		Brucea Fruit	Frcutus Bruceae	1.5-2g
Ku Xing Ren	苦杏仁	Prunus armeniaca L. var. ansu Maxim. ; P. sibirica L.; P. mandschurica Koehne		Bitter Apricot Kernel	Semen Armeniacae Amarum	3-10g
Kuan Dong Hua	款冬化	Tussilago farfara L.		Tussilago Flower	Flos Farfarac	5 10g
Kun Bu	昆布	Laminaria japonica Aresch.; Ecklonia kurome Okam.		Laminaria	Thallus Laminariae; Thallus Eckloniae; Thallus Laminariae seu Eckloniae	10-15g
Lai Fu Zi	莱菔子	Raphanus sativus L.		Radish Seed	Semen Raphani Sativi; Semen Raphani	6-10g
Lao Guan Cao	老鹳草	Erodium stephanianum Willd.; Geranium wilfordii Maxim.		Cranesbill; Common Heron'sbill	Herba Erodii seu Geranii; Herba Erodii; Herba Geranii	10-30g

Lei Gong Teng	雷公藤	Tripterygium Wilfordii Hook. f.	Tripterygium Root	Radix Tripterygii Wilfordii	5-12g
Lei Wan	雷丸	Polyporus mylittae Cook. et Mass.	Omphalia	Omphalia	6-15g
Li Zhi He	荔枝核	Litchi chinensis Sonn.	Litchi Seed	Semen Litchi Chinensis	10-15g
Li Lu	藜芦	Veratrum nigrum L.	Veratrum Root and Rhizome	Radix et Rhizoma Veratri Nigri	0.3-0.9g
Li Pi	梨皮	Pyrus bretschneideri Rehd.; Pyrus pyrifolia (Burm.f.) Nakai[Ficus pyrifolia Burm.f.]; Pyrus ussuriensis Maxim.	Pericarp of Pear	Cortex Exocarpium Pyrus; Pericarpium Pyri Bretschneideri	9-15g
Lian Fang	莲房	Nelumbo nuciflera Gaertn. (Lian)	Lotus Receptacle	Receptaculum Nelumbinis	5-10g
Lian Qian Cao	连钱草	Glechoma longituba (Nakai) Kupr.	Glechoma	Herba Glechomae	15-30g
Lian Qiao	连翘	Forsythia suspensa (Thunb.) Vahl.	Forsythia Fruit	Fructus Forsythiae Suspensae; Fructus Forsythiae	6-15g
Lian Xu	莲须	Nelumbo nuciflera Gaertn. (Lian)	Lotus Stamen	Stamen Nelumbinis Nuciferae; Stamen Nelumbinis	1.5-5g
Lian Zi	莲子	Nelumbo nuciflera Gaertn. (Lian)	Lotus Seed	Semen Nelumbinis Nuciferae; Semen Nelumbinis	6-15g
Lian Zi Xin	莲子心	Nelumbo nuciflera Gaertn. (Lian)	Lotus Embryo	Plumula Nelumbinis Nuciferae	1.5-3g
Liang Mian Zhen	两面针	Zanthoxylum nitidum (Roxb.) DC.	Shiny Bramble	Radix Zanthoxyli	5-10
Ling Xiao Hua	凌霄花	Campsis grandiflora (Thunb.) K. Schum.; C. radicans (L.) Seem.	Campsis Flower	Flos Campsis	3-10g
Ling Yang Jiao	羚羊角	Saiga tatarica L.	Antelope Horn	Cornu Saigae Tataricae	1-3g
Ling Zhi	灵芝	Ganoderma lucidum (Leyss. ex. Fr.) Karst.; G. japonicum (Fr.) Lloyd.	Ganoderma	Ganoderma	3-15g
Liu Ji Nu	刘寄奴	Artemisia anomala S. Moore	Artemisiae Anomalae	Herba Artemisiae Anomalae	3-10g
Liu Yue	六月雪	Serissa foetida Comm.; S. ser-	Snow of June	Herba Serissae	10-15g

Pinyin	Chinese	Latin Name	English	Pharmaceutical	Dosage
Xue		issoides (DC) Druce	Herb, White House Bone		
Long Chi	龙齿		Dragon Tooth	Mastodi Dentis Fossilia	15-30g
Long Dan Cao	龙胆草	Gentiana scabra Bunge.; G. triflora Pall.; G. manshurica Kitag.; G. rigescens Franch.	Gentiana Root	Radix Gentianae	3-8g
Long Gu	龙骨		Dragon Bone	Fossilia Mastodi Ossis; Os Draconis; Os Draconis Fossilia	15-30g
Long Kui	龙葵	Solanum nigrum L.	Black Nightshade	Herba Solani Nigri	15-30g
Long Yan Rou	龙眼肉	Euphoria Longan (Lour.) Steud.	Longan Flesh	Arillus Longanae Euphoriae; Arillus Longan	10-15g
Lou Lu	漏芦	Rhaponticum uniflorum (L.) DC.; Echinops latifolius Tausch	Rhaponticum/Echinops Root	Radix Rhapontici seu Echinops	5-12g
Lu Dou	绿豆	Phaseolus radiatus L.	Phaseolus	Semen Phaseoli Radiati	15-30g
Lu Dou Yi	稆豆衣	Glycine max (L.) Merr.	Soybean Skin	Glycinis Testa	6-10g
Lu Feng Fang	露蜂房	Polistes olivaceous (DeGeer).; P. japonicus Saussure; Parapolybia varia Fabricius	Wasp Nest	Vespae Nidus	2.5-4.5g
Lu Gan Shi	炉甘石	□	Smithsonite	Smithsonitum	External use
Lu Gen	芦根	Phragmites communis Trin.	Phragmites Root, Reed Rhizome	Rhizoma Phragmitis Communis; Rhizoma Phragmitis	10-30g
Lu Hui	芦荟	Aloe vera L.; Aloe ferox Mill	Aloe	Herba Aloes	0.6-1.5g
Lu Jiao	鹿角	Cervus Nippon Temminck; C. elaphus L.	Deer Antler	Cornu Cervi	5-10g
Lu Jiao Jiao	鹿角胶	Cervus Nippon Temminck; C. elaphus L.	Deerhorn Glue	Colla Corni Cervi; Gelatinum Cornu Cervi	5-10g
Lu Jiao Shuang	鹿角霜	Cervus Nippon Temminck; C. elaphus L.	Degelatinated Deer Antler Powder	Cervi Cornu Degelatinatum	10-15g
Lu Lu Tong	路路通	Liquidambar taiwaniana Hance.	Sweetgum Fruit	Fructus Liquidambaris Taiwanianae	9-12g

Lu Rong	鹿茸	Cervus Nippon Temminck; C. elaphus L	Deer Velvet	Cornu Cervi Pantotrichum; Cornu Cervi Parvum	1-2g
Lu Xian Cao	鹿衔草	Pyrola rotundifolia L.; P. calliantha; P. decorata	Pyrolae	Herba Pyrolae	10-30g
Luo Bu Ma	罗布麻	Apocynum venelum L.	Doghane	Herba Apocyni Veneti	3-10g
Luo De Da	落得打（积雪草）	Centella asiatica (L.) Urban	Centella	Herba Centellae	10-30g
Luo Han Guo	罗汉果	Momordica grosvenori Swingle	Grosvenor's Momordica Fruit	Fructus Momordicae Grosvenori	15-30g
Luo Shi Teng	络石藤	Trachelospermum jasminoides (Lindl.) Lem.	Star Jasmine Stem	Caulis Trachelospermi Jasminoidis	6-15g
Ma Bian Cao	马鞭草	Verbena Officinalis L.	Verbena	Herba Verbenae	15-30g
Ma Bo	马勃	Calvatia gigantea (Batsch ex Pers.) Lloyd.; C. lilacina (Mont. Et Ber.) Lloyd; Lasiosphaera fenzlii Reich.	Puffball	Fructificatio Lasiosphaerae seu Calvatiae; Lasiosphaerae seu Calvatiae	3-6g
Ma Chi Xian	马齿苋	Portulaca oleracea L.	Portulaca	Herba Portulacae	9-15g
Ma Dou Ling	马兜铃	Aristolochia contorta Bge.; A. debilis S. et. Z.	Aristolochia Fruit	Fructus Aristolochiae	3-10g
Ma Huang	麻黄	Ephedra sinica Stapf.; E.equisetina Bunge	Ephedra	Herba Ephedrae	1.5-10g
Ma Huang Gen	麻黄根	Ephedra sinica Stapf.; E.equisetina Bge.; E. intermedia Schrenk et Mey.	Ephedra Root	Radix Ephedrae	3-10g
Ma Huang Rong	麻黄绒	Ephedra sinica Stapf.; E.equisetina Bunge	Ephedra	Herba Ephedrae	1.5-10g
Ma Qian Zi	马钱子	Strychnos pierriana A.W.Hill; S. mux-vomica L.	Nux Vomica	Semen Strychni	0.3-0.6g
Mai Dong	麦冬	Ophiopogon japonicus Ker-Gawl	Ophiopogon Tuber, Dwarf Lilyturf Tuber	Radix Ophiopogonis Japonici; Radix Ophiopogonis	10-15g
Mai Ya	麦芽	Hordeum vulgare L.	Barley Sprouts	Fructus Hordei Germinatus; Fructus Hordei Vulgaris Germinantus	10-15g

Man Jing Zi	蔓荆子	Vitex rotundifolia L.; Vitex trifolia L.	Vitex Fruit	Fructus Viticis	6-12g
Mang Xiao	芒硝	Mirabilitum	Mirbailite	Natrii Sulfas	10-15g
Mao Dong Qing	毛冬青	Ilex pubescens Hook. et Arn.	Hairy Holly Root	Radix Ilicis Pubescentis	30-60g
Mei Gui Hua	玫瑰花	Rosa rugosa Thunb.	Rosebud	Flos Rosae Rugosae	3-6g
Meng Chong	虻虫	Tabanus bivittatus Mats.	Tabanus	Tabanus; Tabanus Bivittatus	1-1.5g
Meng Shi	礞石		Chlorite/Mica Schist	Lapis Chloriti Seu Micae; Lapis Chloriti	6-10g
Mi Meng Hua	蜜蒙花	Buddleia officinalis Maxim.	Buddleia; Pale Butterflybush Flower	Flos Buddleiae	10g
Mi Pi Kang (Chu Tou Kang)	米皮糠 (杵头糠)	Oryza sativa L.	Rice Bran	Testa Oryzae Sativae	9-30g
Mi Tuo Seng	密陀僧		Litharge	Lithargyrum	0.3-1g
Ming Dang Shen	明党参	Changium smyrnioides Wolfb.	Changium Root	Radix Changii	5-10g
Mo Han Lian	墨旱莲	Eclipta prostrata L.	Eclipta	Herba Ecliptae Prostratae	10-30g
Mo Yao	没药	Commiphora myrrha Engl.; Balsamodendron ehrenbergianum Berg.	Myrrh	Myrrha	3-10g
Mu Bie Zi	木鳖子	Momordica cochinchinensis (Lour.) Spreng.	Momordica Seed	Semen Momordicae	0.5-1g
Mu Dan Pi	牡丹皮	Paeonia suffruticosa Andr.	Moutan Root Bark	Cortex Moutan; Cortex Moutan Radicis	6-12g
Mu Gua	木瓜	Chaenomeles lagenaria (Loisel.) Koidz.; C. sinensis (Thouin) Koehne	Chaenomeles Fruit	Fructus Chaenomelis	6-12g
Mu Hu Die	木蝴蝶	Oroxylum indicum (L.) Vent.	Oroxylum Seed	Semen Oroxyli	5g
Mu Jin Pi	木槿皮	Hibiscus syriacus L.	Rose-of-Sharon Root Bark	Hibisci Syriaci Radicis Cortex	3-10g

Mu Li	牡蛎	Ostrea gigas Thunb.; O. talienwhanensis Crosse.; O. rivularis Gould.	Oyster Shell	Concha Ostreae	15-30g
Mu Tong	木通	Aristolochia manshuriensis Kom.; Clematis armandii Franch.; C. montana Buch.-Ham; Akebia quinata (Thunb.) Decue.; A. trifoliata (Thunb.) Koidz., etc.	Mutong Stem; Akebia Stem	Caulis Akebiae; Caulis Aristolochiae Manshuriensis (Guan Mu Tong); Caulis Clematidis (Chuan Mu Tong)	3-6g
Mu Xiang	木香	Aucklandiae Lappa Decne. (Saussurea lappa Clarke); Vladimiria souliei (Franch.) Ling.	Saussurea	Radix Aucklandiae Lappae; Radix Aucklandiae	3-10g
Mu Zei	木贼	Equisetum hiemale L.	Equisetum	Herba Equiseti Hiemalis	3-10g
Nan Gua Zi	南瓜子	Cucurbita moschata Duch.	Pumpkin Seeds	Semen Cucurbitae Moschatae	60-120g
Nan Sha Shen	南沙参	Adenophora tetraphylla (Thunb.)Fisch.; A. stricta Miq.; A. hunanensis Nannf.	Adenophora Root	Radix Adenophorae	10-15g
Nan Wu Wei Zi	南五味子	Schisandra sphenanthera Rehd.	Southern Schisandra Berry	Fructus Schisandrae Sphenantherae	2-6g
Niu Bang Zi	牛蒡子	Arctium lappa L.	Arctium Seed	Fructus Arctii Lappae; Fructus Arctii	3-10g
Niu Huang	牛黄	Bos Taurus domesticus Gmelin	Cow Bezoar	Calculus Bovis	0.2-0.5g
Niu Xi (Huai)	牛膝（怀）	Achyranthes bidentata Blume	Achyranthes Root	Radix Achyranthis Bidentatae	10-15g
Niu Xi (Chuan)	牛膝（川）	Cyathula capitata (Wall.) Moq.; Cyathula officinalis Kuan.	Cyathula	Radix Cyathulae Officinalis	10-15g
Nu Zhen Zi	女贞子	Ligustrum lucidum Ait.	Ligustrum Fruit	Fructus Ligustri Lucidi	10-15g
Nuo Dao Gen Xu	糯稻根须	Oryza sativa L.	Glutinous Rice Root	Radix Oryzae Glutinosae	15-30g
Nuo Mi	糯米	Oryza sativa L.	Glutinous Rice	Semen Oryzae Glutinosae	9-10g
Ou Jie	藕节	Nelumbo nucifera Gaertn.	Lotus Root Node	Nodus Nelumbinis Nuciferae Rhizomatis; Nodus Nelumbinis Rhizomatis	10-15g

Pang Da Hai	胖大海	Sterculia scaphigera Wall.	Sterculia	Semen Sterculiae Scaphigerae	3-5 pieces
Pao Jiang	炮姜	Zingiber officinale Rosc.	Quick-fried Ginger	Rhizoma Zingiberis Praeparatae	3-10g
Pei Lan	佩兰	Eupatorium fortunei Turcz.	Lindley eupatorium herb	Herba Eupatorii	5-10g
Peng Sha	硼砂		Borax	Borax	1.5-3g
Pi Pa Ye	枇杷叶	Eriobotrya japonica (Thunb.) Lindl.	Loquat Leaf	Folium Eriobotryae Japonicae; Folium Eriobotryae	10-15g
Pu Gong Ying	蒲公英	Taraxacum mongolicum Hand. –Mazz.	Dandelion	Herba Taraxaci; Herba Taraxaci Mongolici	10-30g
Pu Huang	蒲黄	Typha angustifolia L.; Typha orientalis Presl.	Cattail Pollen	Pollen Typhae	3-10g
Qi Cao	蛴螬	Holotrichia diomphalia Bates; Anomala carpulenta Motsch; Mimela lucidula Hope	Northeast Giant Black Chafer	Larva of Holotrichia Diomphalia Bates; Larva Holotrichiae	2-5g
Qi Dai	脐带	Funiculus Umbilicalis	Umbilical Cord	Funiculus Umbilicalis; Taenia Umbilici Hominis	1.5-3g
Qi She	蕲蛇	Agkstrodon acutus (Gunther)	Agkistrodon	Agkistrodon	3-10g
Qian Cao (Qian Gen)	茜草(茜根)	Rubia cordifolia L.	Madder Root	Radix Rubiae Cordifoliae; Radix Rubiae	10-15g
Qian Dan	铅丹		Minium	Minium; Plumbum Rubrum	0.3-0.6g
Qian Fen	铅粉		Lead Powder, Lead Carbonate	Plumbi Carbonas et Hydrox; Hydrocerussitum	0.9-1.5g
Qian Hu	前胡	Peucedanum praeruptorum Dunn.; P. decursivum Maxim.	Peucedanum Root	Radix Peucedani	6-10g
Qian Nian Jian	千年健	Homalomena occulta (Lour.) Schott	Homalomena	Rhizoma Homalomenae Occultae	5-10g
Qian Jin Zi	千金子	Euphordia lathyris L.	Caper Euphordia Seed	Semen Euphorbiae Lathyridis	0.5-1g
Qian Li Guang	千里光	Senecio scandens Buch.-Ham.	Climbing Groundsel	Herba Sencionis Scandntis	10-30g
Qian Niu Zi	牵牛子	Pharbitisnil (L.) Choisy; Pharbitis purpurea (L.) Voigt	Morning Glory Seed	Semen Pharbitidis	3-10g
Qian Shi	芡实	Euryale ferox Salisb.	Euryale	Semen Euryales Fero-	10-15g

				cis; Semen Euryales	
Qiang Huo	羌活	Notopterygium incisum Ting.; N. forbesii Boiss.; N. franchetii Boiss.	Notopterygium Root	Rhizoma et Radix Notopterygii	3-10g
Qiang Lang	蜣螂	Catharsius molossus L.		Catharsius molossus	1.5-3g
Qin Jiao	秦艽	Gentiana macrophylla Pall.;G. straminea Maxim.; G. crassicaulis Duthie ex Burk.; G. dahurica Fisch.	Large Gentian Root	Radix Gentianae Qinjiao; Radix Gentianae Macrophyllae	5-10g
Qin Pi	秦皮	Fraxinus rhynchophylla Hance.; F. chinensis Roxb.; F. bungeana DC.; F. acuminate Ling.	Fraxinus	Cortex Fraxini	6-12g
Qing Dai	青黛	Isatis tinctoria L.; Isatis indigotica Fort.; Baphicacanthus cusia Bremek.; Polygonum tinctorium Ait.; Clerodendron cyrtophyllum Turcz.	Natural Indigo	Indigo Naturalis	1.5-3g
Qing Feng Teng	青风藤	Sinomenium acutum (Thunb.) Rehd. et Wils.; S.acutum (Thunb.) Rehd. et Wils.Var. cinoreum Rehd. et Wils.	Orient Vine	Caulis Sinomenii	6-12g
Qing Guo	青果（橄榄）	Canarium album (Lour.) Raeusch.	Chinese White Olive	Fructus Canarii Albi	6-15g
Qing Hao	青蒿	Artemisia apiacea Hance; A. annua L.	Sweet Wormwood	Herba Artemisiae Apiaceae seu Annuae; Herba Artemisiae Annuae; Herba Artemisiae	3-10g
Qing Ma Zi	苘麻子	Abutilou theophrastiMedic.	Indian Mallow Seed	Semen Abutili	10-15g
Qing Meng Shi	青礞石		Chlorite	Chloriti Lapis	6-10g
Qing Mu Xiang	青木香	Aristolochia debilis Sieb.et Zucc.; A. contorta Bge.	Birthwort Root	Radix Aristolochiae	3-10g
Qing Pi	青皮	Citrus reticulate Blanco.	Unripe Tangerine Peel	Pericarpium Citri Reticulatae Viride; Exocarpium Citri Immaturum	3-10g
Qing Xiang	青箱子	Celosia argentea L.	Celosia Seed	Semen Celosiae Ar-	6-15

Zi				genteae	
Qu Mai	瞿麦	Dianthus superbus L.; D. chinensis L.	Dianthus	Herba Dianthi	5-10g
Quan Shen	拳参	Polygonum bistorta L.	Bistort Rhizome	Rhizoma Bistortae	3-10g
Quan Xie	全蝎	Buthus martensi Karsch.	Scorpion	Scorpio; Buthus Martensi	2-5g
Ren Dong Teng	忍冬藤	Lonicera japonica Thunb.; L. hypoglauca Miq.; L. confusa DC.; L. dasystyla Rehd.	Lonicera Vine	Lonicerae Caulis et Folium; Caulis Lonicerae	10-30g
Ren Shen	人参	Panax ginseng C. A. Mey.	Ginseng	Radix Ginseng	5-10g
Ren Shen Ye	人参叶	Panax ginseng C. A. Mey	Ginseng Leaf	Folium Ginseng	5-10g
Rou Cong Rong	肉苁蓉	Cistanche salsa (C.A. Mey.) G. Beck	Cistanche	Herba Cistanches	10-20g
Rou Dou Kou	肉豆蔻	Myristica fragrans Houtt.	Nutmeg Seeds	Semen Myristicae Fragrantis; Semen Myristicae	3-10g
Rou Gui	肉桂	Cinnamomum cassia Presl	Cinamon Bark	Cortex Cinnamomi; Cortex Cinnamomi Cassiae	2-5g
Ru Xiang	乳香	Boswellia carterii Birdw.	Frankincense; Mastic	Gummi Olibanum; Olibanum	3-10g
San Leng	三棱	Sparganium stoloniferum Buch.-Ham.; Scirpus flaviatilis (Torr.) A. Gary	Sparganium; Scirpus	Rhizoma Sparganii Stoloniferi; Rhizoma Sparganii	3-10g
San Qi	三七	Panax notoginseng (Burk.) F. H. Chen.	Notoginseng Root	Radix Notoginseng	3-10g
Sang Bai Pi	桑白皮	Morus alba L.	Mulberry Root Bark	Cortex Mori Alba Radicis; Cortex Mori Radicis	10-15g
Sang Ji Sheng	桑寄生	Loranthus parasiticus (L.) Merr.; Viscum coloratum (Komar.) Nakai; Taxillus chinensis (DC.) Danser.	Mulberry Mistletoes; Loranthus	Herba Taxilli; Ramulus Loranthi Seu Visci	10-20g
Sang Piao Xiao	桑螵蛸	Paratenodera sinensis Saussure; Statilia maculata Thunb.; Mantis religiosa L.; Hierodula patellifera Serville	Mantis Cocoon Egg-case	Ootheca Mantidis	3-10g
Sang Shen	桑椹	Morus alba L.	Mulberry Fruit	Fructus Mori Alba	10-15g

Sang Ye	桑叶	Morus alba L.	Mulberry Leaf	Folium Mori; Folium Mori Alba	5-10g
Sang Zhi	桑枝	Morus alba L.	Mulberry Twig	Ramulus Mori	10-30g
Sha Ji	沙棘	Hippophae rhamnoides L.	Sea Buckthorn	Frutus Hippophae	3-9g
Sha Ren	砂仁	Amomum villosum Lour.; A. xanthioides Wall.	Amomum Fruit	Fructus Amomi; Fructus Amomi Villosi	3-6g
Sha Ren Ke	砂仁壳	Amomum villosum Lour.; A. xanthioides Wall.	Amomum Husk	Pericarpium Amomi	3-5g
Sha Shen	沙参	Adenophora tetraphylla (Thunb.)Fisch.; A. stricta Miq.; A. hunanensis Nannf.	Adenophora Root	Radix Adenophorae	10-15g
Sha Yuan Zi	沙苑子	Astragalus complanatus R. Br.	Complanate Astragalus Seed	Semen Astragali Complanati	10-20g
Shan Ci Gu	山慈姑（山茨菇）	Cremastra variabilis (BL.) Nakai; Pleione bulbocodioides (Franch.) Rolfe	Cremastra; Pleione	Pseudobulbus Cremastrae seu Pleiones	3-6g
Shan Dou Gen	山豆根	Sophora subprostrata Chun et. T. Chen; S. tonkinensis Gagnep.	Bushy Sphora Root	Radix Sophorae Subprostratae	6-10g
Shan Nai	山奈	Kaempferia galanga Linn	Kaempferia Root	Kaempferiae Rhizoma	10-20g
Shan Yang Jiao	山羊角	Naemorkedus goral Hardwicke.	Goral Horn	Cornu Naemorhedi	10-15g
Shan Yao	山药	Dioscorea opposita Thunb.	Dioscorea Root	Rhizoma Dioscoreae	10-30g
Shan Zha	山楂	Crataegus cuneata Sieb. et Zucc.; C. pinnatifida Bge. var. major N. E. Br.	Hawthorn Fruit	Fructus Crataegi	10-15g
Shan Zha Tan	山楂炭	Crataegus cuneata Sieb. et Zucc.; C. pinnatifida Bge. var. major N. E. Br.	Charred Hawthorn Fruit	Charred Fructus Crataegi	10-15g
Shan Zhu Yu	山茱萸	Cornus officinalis Sieb. Et Zucc.	Cornus Fruit	Fructus Corni Officinalis; Fructus Corni	6-12g
Shang Lu	商陆	Phytolacca acinosa Roxb.	Phytolacca	Radix Phytolaccae	5-10g
Shao Yao	芍药	Paeonia veitchii Lynch.; P. abovata Maxim.; P. lactiflora Pall.	Peony Root	Radix Paeoniae	6-15g

She Chuang Zi	蛇床子	Cnidium monnieri (L.) Cusson	Cnidium Fruit	Fructus Cnidii Monnieri	3-10g
She Gan	射干	Belancanda chinensis (L.) DC.	Belamcanda	Rhizoma Belamcandae Chinensis; Rhizoma Belamcandae	6-10g
She Han	蛇含	Potentilla kleiniana Wight et Arn.	Potentilla Reptans (A. Gray.); Herb of Klein Cinquefoil	Herba Potentillae Kleinianae	5-10g
She Tui	蛇蜕	Elaphe taeniurus Cope.; E. carinata (Guenther).	Snake Slough	Periostracum Serpentis	2-3g
She Xiang	麝香	Moschus berezovskii Flerov.; M. sifanicus Przewalski; M. moschiferus L.	Musk	Moschus	0.06-0.1g
Shen Jin Cao	伸筋草	Lycopodium clavatum L.; L. cernnum L.; Smilax nipponica Miq.	Ground Pine	Herba Lycopodii	6-15g
Shen Qu	神曲	Massa Medicata Fermentata	Medicated Leaven	Massa Medicata Fermentata	6-15g
Sheng Di Huang	生地黄	Rehmannia glutinosa Libosch. f. hueichingensis (Chao et Schih) Hsiao; Rehmannia glutinosa Libosch.	Rehmannia Root	Radix Rehmanniae Recens	10-30g
Sheng Jiang	生姜	Zingiber officinale Rosc.	Fresh Ginger	Rhizoma Zingiberis Recens	3-10g
Sheng Ma	升麻	Cimicifuga heracleifolia Kom.; C. dahurica (Turcz.) Maxim.; C. foetida L.	Cimicifuga Root	Rhizoma Cimicifugae	3-10g
Sheng Tie Luo	生铁落		Oxidized Iron Filings	Ferri Frusta	30-60g
Shi Da Gong Lao	十大功劳	Mahonia bealei (Fort.) Carr.; M. fortunei (Lindl.) Fedde.; M. japonica (Thunb.) DC.	Mahonia Leaf	Folium Mahoniae	10-15g
Shi Chang Pu	石菖蒲	Acorus gramineus Soland; Acorus tatarinowii Schott	Acorus	Rhizoma Acori Graminei; Rhizoma Acori Tatarinowii	5-10g
Shi Di	柿蒂	Diospyros kaki L. f.	Persimmon Calyx	Calyx Diospyri Kaki; Calyx Kaki	3-12g
Shi Gao	石膏	hydrous calcium sulphate (chemical name)	Gypsum	Gypsum Fibrosum	15-60g
Shi Hu	石斛	Dendrobium loddigesii Rolfe;	Dendrobium	Herba Dendrobii	6-15g

		D. fimbriatum Hook. var. oculatum Hook.; D. chrysanthum Wall.; D. candidum Wall. ex Lindl.; D. nobile Lindl	Stem		
Shi Jian Chuan	石见穿	Salvia chinensis Benth.	Chinese Sage	Herba Salviae Chinensis	10-15g
Shi Jue Ming	石决明	Haliotis diversicolor Reeve.; H. gigantea discus Reeve; H. discus hannai Ino; H. ovina Gmelin; H. Ruler (Leach); H. asinina L.; H. laevigata (Donovan)	Abalone Shell	Concha Haliotidis	15-30g
Shi Jun Zi	使君子	Quisqualis indica L.	Quisqualis	Fructus Quisqualis Indicae	6-10g
Shi Liu Pi	石榴皮	Punica granatum L.	Pomegranate Rind	Pericarpium Punicae Granati	3-10g
Shi Wei	石韦	Pyrrosia sheareri (Bak.) Ching; P. petiolosa (Christ) Ching; P. lingua (Thunb.) Farw.	Pyrrosia Leaf	Folium Pyrrosiae	5-10g
Shou Gong (Bi Hu)	守宫 (壁虎)	Gekko suinhouna Gunther	House Lizard	Gekko Swinhoana	2-5g
Shu Di Huang	熟地黄	Rehmannia glutinosa Libosch.	Cooked Rehmannia Root	Radix Rehmanniae Praeparatae	10-30g
Shu Qi	蜀漆	Dichroa febrifuga Lour.	Dichroa Leaf	Folium Dichroae	3-6g
Shui Chang Pu	水菖蒲	Acorus calamus L.	Sweetflag Rhizome	Rhizoma Acori Calami	5-10g
Shui Niu Jiao	水牛角	Bubalus bubalis L.	Water Buffalo Horn	Cornu Bubali	3-15g
Shui Zhi	水蛭	Hirudo nipponica Whitman; Whitmania pigra Whitman; W. acranulata Whitman.	Leech	Hirudo seu Whitmania; Hirudo	3-6g
Si Gua Luo	丝瓜络	Luffa cylindrica (L.) Roem.	Luffa Fiber	Fasciculus Vascularis Luffae	10-15g
Song Jie	松节	Pinus tabulae formis Carr.; P. massoniana Lamb.	Knotty Pine Wood	Lignum Pini Nodi	10-15g
Su Geng (Zi Su Geng)	苏梗	Perilla frutescens (L.) Britt.	Perilla Stem	Caulis Perillae	5-10g
Su He Xiang	苏合香	Liquidambar orientalis Mill.	Styrax	Styrax	0.3-1g

Su Mu	苏木	Caesalpinia sappan L.	Sappan Wood	Lignum Sappan	3-10g
Su Ye (Zi Su Ye)	苏叶(紫苏叶)	Perilla frutescens (L.) Britt. Var. crispa (Thunb.) Hand.-Mazz	Perilla Leaf	Folium Perillae Frutescentis; Folium Perillae	5-10g
Su Zi	苏子	Perilla frutescens (L.) Britt. Var. acuta (Thunb.) Kudo.	Perilla Fruit	Fructus Perillae	5-10g
Suan Zao Ren	酸枣仁	Ziziphus jujuba Mill.	Zizyphus	Semen Ziziphi Spinosae	10-18g
Suo Luo Zi	娑罗子	Aesculus chinensis Bge.	Horse Chestnut	Semen Aesculi	3-10g
Suo Yang	锁阳	Cynomorium songaricum Rupr.	Cynomorium Stem	Herba Cynomorii Songarici	10-15g
Ta Gan	獭肝(水獭肝)	Lutra lutra Linnaeus; Lutra perspicillata Geoffroy; Aonyx cinerea Illiger	Otter Liver	Jecur Lutrae	3-6g
Tai Zi Shen	太子参	Pseudostellaria heterophylla (Miq.) Pax ex Pax et Hoffm.	Pseudostellaria	Radix Pseudostellariae Heterophyllae; Radix Pseudostellariae	10-30g
Tan Xiang	檀香	Santalum album L.	Sandalwood	Lignum Santali Albi	1-3g
Tao Ren	桃仁	Prunus persica (Linn) Batsch.; P. davidana (Carr.) Franch.	Peach Kernel	Semen Persicae; Semen Pruni Persicae	6-10g
Tian Dong (Tian Men Dong)	天冬（天门冬）	Asparagus cochinchinensis (Lour.) Merr.	Asparagus Tuber	Radix Asparagi; Tuber Asparagi ;Tuber Asparagi Cochinchinensis	6-15g
Tian Hua Fen	天花粉	Trichosanthes kirilowii Maxim.; T. japonica Regel.	Trichosanthes Root	Radix Trichosanthis	10-15g
Tian Ji Huang (Di Er Cao)	田基黄(地耳草)	Hypericum japonicum Thunb.	Lesser Hypericum	Herba Hyperici Japonici	15-30g
Tian Kui Zi	天葵子	Semiaquilegia adoxoides (DC.) Mak.	Siemiaquilegia Tuber	Radix Semiaquilegiae	3-10g
Tian Ma	天麻	Gastrodia elata Bl.	Gastrodia	Rhizoma Gastrodiae Elatae; Rhizoma Gastrodiae	3-10g
Tian Nan Xing	天南星	Arisaema consanguineum Schott.; A. heterophyllum Bl.; A. amurense Maxim.	Arisaema	Rhizoma Arisaematis	5-15g
Tian Zhu Huang	天竺黄	Bambusa textilis Mc-Clure; Schizostachyum chinense	Bamboo Sugar	Concretio Silicea Bambusae Textillis;	3-6g

			Rendle		Concretio Silicea Bambusae	
Ting Li Zi	葶苈子		Lepidium apetalum Willd.; Descurainia sophia (L.) Schur.	Tingli Seed	Semen Descurainiae seu Lepidii	3-10g
Tong Cao	通草		Tetrapanax papyriferus (Hook.) K. Koch	Tetrapanax	Medulla Tetrapanacis Papyriferi; Medulla Tetrapanacis	2-5g
Tou Gu Cao	透骨草		Speranskia tuberculatae; Impatiens balsamina Line	Speranskia/Balsam	Herba Speranskiae seu Impatientis	6-15g
Tu Bie	土鳖		Eupolyphaga sinensis Walk.; Steleophaga plancyi (Bol.)	Eupolyphaga	Eupolyphagae seu Opisthoplatia	3-10g
Tu Bei Mu	土贝母		Bolbostemma paniculatum (Maxim.) Franquet.	Bolbostemma Tuber	Tuber Bolbostemmatis	3-10g
Tu Fu Ling	土茯苓		Smilax glabra Roxb.	Smilax	Rhizoma Smilacis Glabrae	15-60g
Tu Jing Pi	土槿皮		Pseudolarix kaempferi Gord.	Golden Larch Bark	Cortex Pseudolaricis	External use
Tu Si Zi	菟丝子		Cuscuta chinensis Lam.; C. japonica Choisy	Cuscuta	Semen Cuscutae; Semen Cuscutae Chinensis	10-15g
Wa Leng Zi	瓦楞子		Arca subcrenata Lischke; A. granosa Linnaeus; A. inflata Reeve	Ark Shell	Concha Arcae	10-30g
Wan Nian Qing	万年青（卷柏）		Selaginella tamariscina (Beauv.) Spr.	Selaginella	Herba Selaginellae	3-10g
Wang Bu Liu Xing	王不留行		Vaccaria segetalis (neck.) Garcke	Vaccaria Seed	Semen Vaccariae Segetalis	6-10g
Wei Jing	苇茎 (芦茎)		Phragmites communis Trin.	Phragmites Stalk	Caulis Phragmitis Communis; Caulis Phragmitis	10-30g
Wei Ling Cai	委陵菜		Potentilla chinensis Ser.	Chinese Sliverweed	Herba Potentillae Chinensis	8-15g
Wei Ling Xian	威灵仙		Clematis chinensis Osbeck; C. hexapetala Pall.; C. manshurica Rupr.	Clematis Root	Radix Clematidis	5-10g
Wu Bei Zi	五倍子		Rhus chinensis Mill.; R. potaninii Maxim.; R. punjabensis Stew. var. Sinica (Diels) Rehd. Et Wils.; Melaphis chinensis (Bell) Baker	Gallnut	Galla Rhois Chinensis; Galla Chinensis	1.5-6g
Wu Gong	蜈蚣 (天		Scolopendra subspinipes muti-	Centipede	Scolopendra Sub-	1-3g

(Tian Long)	龙)	lans L. Koch.		spinipes	
Wu Jia Pi	五加皮	Acanthopanax gracilistylus W.W. Smith; A. senticosus (Rupr. Et Maxim.) Harm.	Acantho-panax	Cortex Acantho-panacis Radicis	5-10g
Wu Ling Zhi	五灵脂	Trogopterus xanthipes Milne-Edwards	Squirrel Droppings,	Excrementum Trogopteri; Excrementum Trogopteri seu Pteromydis; Faeces Trogopteri	3-10g
Wu Mei	乌梅	Prunus mume (Sieb.) Sieb. Et Zucc.	Mume	Fructus Pruni Mume; Fructus Mume	10-30g
Wu Shao She	乌梢蛇	Zaocys dhumnades (Cantor)	Zaocys	Zaocys Dhumnades	5-10g
Wu Tou	乌头	Aconitum carmichaeli Debx.; A. kusnezoffii Reichb.	Prepared Wild Aconite	Radix Aconiti	1.5-4.5g
Wu Wei Zi	五味子	Schisandra chinensis (Turcx.) Baill.; Schisandra sphenanthera Rehd.	Schisandra Fruit	Fructus Schisandrae; Fructus Schisandrae Chinensis	2-6g
Wu Yao	乌药	Lindera strychnifolia (Sieb. et Zucc.) Villar	Lindera Root	Radix Linderae Strychnifoliae; Radix Linderae	3-10g
Wu Yi	芜荑	Ulmus macrocarpa Hance.	Elm Cake	Fructus Ulmi Macrocarpae Preparatus	3-10g
Wu Zei Gu (Hai Piao Xiao)	乌贼骨 (海螵蛸)	Sepiella maindroni de Rochebrune.; Sepia esculenta Hoyle.	Cuttlefish Bone	Os Sepiae seu Sepiellae	6-12g
Wu Zhu Yu	吴茱萸	Evodia rutaecarpa (Juss.) Benth.; E. rutaecarpa (Juss.) Benth. var. officinalis (Dode) Huang; E. rutaecarpa (Juss.) Benth. var. bodinieri (Dode) Huang	Evodia Fruit	Fructus Evodiae Rutaecarpae; Fructus Evodiae	1.5-5g
Xi Gua	西瓜	Citrullus vulgaris Schrad.	Watermelon	Fructus Citrulli; Pulp Citrulli	No
Xi Gua Pi	西瓜皮	Citrullus vulgaris Schrad.	Watermelon Rind	Exocarpium Citrulli	5-10g
Xi Gua Cui Yi	西瓜翠衣	Citrullus vulgaris Schrad.	The external layer of watermelon rind	Exocarpium Citrulli	5-10g
Xi He Liu	西河柳 (柽柳)	Tamarix chinensis Lour.	Tamarisk Twig and	Cacumen Tamaricis	3-10g

			Leaf		
Xi Jiao	犀角	Rhinoceros unicornis L.; R. sondaicus Desmarest.; R. sumatrensis (Fischer); R. bicornis L.; R. simus Burchell	Rhinoceros Horn	Cornu Rhinocerotis	0.5-1.5g
Xi Xian Cao	稀莶草	Siegesbeckia orientalis L.; S. pubescens Mak.; S. glabrescens Mak.	Siegesbeckia	Herba Siegesbeckiae	10-15g
Xi Xin	细辛	Asarum heteropoides Fr. Var. mandshuricum (Maxim.) Kitag.; A. sieboldii Mig.	Asarum	Herba Asari; Herba cum Radice Asari	2-5g
Xi Yang Shen	西洋参	Panax quinquefolium	American Ginseng	Radix Panacis Quinquefolii	3-6g
Xia Ku Cao	夏枯草	Prunella vulgaris L.	Prunella	Spica Prunellae Vulgaris	10-15g
Xian He Cao	仙鹤草	Agrimonia pilosa Ledeb.	Agrimony	Herba Agrimoniae Pilosae	10-15g
Xian Ling Pi	仙灵脾(淫羊藿)	Epimedium grandiflorum Morr.; E. sagittatum (Sieb. Et Zucc.) Maxim.; E. pubescens Maxim.; E. brevicornum Maxim.; E. koreanum Nakai	Epimedium	Herba Epimedii	10-15g
Xian Mao	仙茅	Curculigo orchioides Gaertz.	Curculigo	Rhizoma Curculiginis Orchioidis	3-10g
Xiang Fu	香附	Cyperus rotundus L.	Nutgrass Root	Rhizoma Cyperi; Rhizoma Cyperi Rotundi	6-12g
Xiang Jia Pi	香加皮	Periploca sepium Bge.	Chinese Silkvine Root Bark	Cortex Periplocae	5-10g
Xiang Ru	香薷	Elsholtzia splendens Nakai ex F. Maekawa; Mosla chinensis Maxim.	Elsholtzia	Herba Elsholtziae seu Moslae; Herba Moslae	3-10g
Xiang Yuan	香橼	Citrus medica L.; C. wilsonii Tanaka.	Citron	Fructus Citri Medicae seu Wilsonii	3-10g
Xiao Hui Xiang	小茴香	Foeniculum vulgare Mill.	Fennel Fruit	Fructus Foeniculi; Fructus Foeniculi Vulgaris	3-8g
Xiao Ji	小蓟	Cephalanoplos segetum (Bge.) Kitam.;C. setosum (Willd.) Kitam.	Cephalanoplos	Herba Cephalanoploris; Herba Cirsii	10-30g
Xiao Shi (Huo Xiao)	硝石(火硝)		Nitre	Nitrium	1.5-3g

Xiao Mai	小麦	Triticum aestivum L.	Wheat	Fructus Tritici; Fructus Tritici Aestivi	15-30g
Xie Bai	薤白	Allium macrostemon Bge.; A. chinense G. Don.	Chinese Garlic,	Bulbus Allii Macrostemonis; Bulbus Allii	5-10g
Xin Yi	辛夷	Magnolia biondii Pamp.; M. sprengeri Pamp.; M. denudata Desr.	Magnolia Flower	Flos Magnoliae	3-10g
Xin Yi Hua	辛夷花	Magnolia biondii Pamp.; M. sprengeri Pamp.; M. denudata Desr.	Magnolia Flower	Flos Magnoliae	3-10g
Xing Ren	杏仁	Prunus armeniaca L. var. ansu Maxim.; P. sibirica L.; P. mandschurica Koehne	Apricot Kernel	Semen Armeniacae Amarum; Semen Pruni Armeniacae	3-10g
Xiong Dan	熊胆	Ursus arctos L.; Selenarctos thibetanus G. Cuvier	Bear Gallbladder	Vesica Fellea Ursi	1.5-2.5g
Xiong Huang	雄黄		Realgar	Realgar	0.15-0.30g
Xu Chang Qing	徐长卿	Cynanchum paniculatum (Bge.) Kitag.	Paniculate Cynanchum	Radix Cynanchi Paniculati	3-10g
Xu Duan	续断	Dipsacus asper Wall.	Dipsacus	Radix Dipsaci Asperi; Radix Dipsaci	10-20g
Xu Sui Zi	续随子	Euphordia lathyris L.	Caper Euphordia Seed	Semen Euphorbiae Lathyridis	0.5-1g
Xuan Fu Hua	旋复花	Inula japonica Thunb.; I. ☐apillarie L.	Inula Flowers	Flos Inulae	3-10g
Xuan Hu Suo	玄胡索(延胡索)	Corydalis turtschaninovii Bess. F. yanhusuo Y. H. Chou et C. C. Hsu.	Corydalis	Rhizoma Corydalis	3-10g
Xuan Shen	玄参	Scrophularia ningpeonsis Hemsl.	Scrophularia Root	Radix Scrophulariae; Radix Scrophulariae Ningpoensis	10-15g
Xue Jie	血竭	Daemonorops draco Bl.	Dragon's Blood	Daemonoropis Draconis Resina; Sanguis Draconis	1-1.5g
Xue Yu Tan	血余炭	Hominis Crinis Carbonisatus	Charred Human Hair	Hominis Crinis Carbonisatus; Crinis Carbonisatus	6-10g
Xun Gu Feng	寻骨风	Aristolochia mollissima Hance	Mollissima	Rhizoma seu Herba Aristolochiae Mollissimae	10-15g

Ya Dan Zi	鸦胆子	Brucea javanica (L.) Merr.	Brucea Fruit	Frcutus Bruceae; Fructus Bruceae Javanicae	1.5-2g
Ya Zhi Cao	鸭跖草	Commelina communis L.	Common Dayflower Herb	Herba Commelinae	15-30g
Yan Hu Suo	延胡索	Corydalis turtschaninovii Bess. F. yanhusuo Y. H. Chou et C. C. Hsu.	Corydalis	Rhizoma Corydalis	3-10g
Yan Sui	芫荽 (胡荽)	Coriandrum sativum L.	Coriander	Herba Coriandri	3-6g
Yang Qi Shi	阳起石		Actinolite; Actinolite Asbestus	Actinolitum	3-6g
Ye Jiao Teng	夜交藤	Polygonum multiflorum Thunb.	Flowery Knotweed Stem	Caulis Polygoni Multiflori	15-30g
Ye Ju Hua	野菊花	Chrysanthemum indicum L.	Wild Chrysanthemum Flower	Flos Chrysanthemi Indici	10-15g
Ye Ming Sha	夜明砂	Vesperlitis superans Thomas	Bat's Droppings	Excrementum Vespertilionis Murini	3-10g
Yi Mu Cao	益母草	Leonurus heterophyllus Sweet	Leonurus	Herba Leonuri Heterophylii; Herba Leonuri	10-15g
Yi Tang	饴糖	Saccharum Granorum	Malt Sugar	Saccharum Granorum	30-60g
Yi Yi Gen	薏苡根	Coix lacryma-jobi L. var. mayuen (Roman) Stapf	Coix Root	Radix Coicis Lacryma-jobi	10-15g
Yi Yi Ren	薏苡仁	Coix lacryma-jobi L. var. mayuen (Roman) Stapf	Coix Seed	Semen Coicis Lacryma-jobi; Semen Coicis	10-30g
Yi Zhi Ren	益智仁	Alpinia oxyphylla Miq.	Alpinia Fruit	Fructus Alpiniae Oxyphyllae	3-10g
Yin Chai Hu	银柴胡	Stellaria dichotoma L. var. lanceolata Bge.	Stellaria Root	Radix Stellariae Dichotomae; Radix Stellariae	3-10g
Yin Chen Hao	茵陈蒿	Artemisia scoparia Waldst. et Kit.; A. capillaris Thunb.	Capillaris	Herba Artemisiae Scopariae	10-30g
Yin Xing	银杏	Ginkgo biloba L.	Ginkgo Nut	Semen Ginkgo Bilobae	6-10g
Yin Xing Ye	银杏叶	Ginkgo biloba L.	Ginkgo Leaf	Folium Ginkgo Bilobae	3-6g

Yin Yang Huo	淫羊藿	Epimedium grandiflorum Morr.; E. sagittatum (Sieb. Et Zucc.) Maxim.; E. pubescens Maxim.; E. brevicornum Maxim.; E. koreanum Nakai	Epimedium	Herba Epimedii	10-15g
Ying Su Ke	罂粟壳	Papaver somniferum L.	Opium Poppy Husk	Pericarpium Papaveris; Pericarpium Papaveris Somniferi	3-10g
Yu Jin	郁金	Curcuma aromatica Salisb.; C. kwangsiensis S. Lee et C. F. Liang.; C. longa L.; C. zedoaria (Berg.) Rosc.	Curcuma Tuber	Radix Curcumae	6-12g
Yu Li Ren	郁李仁	Prunus humilis Bge.; P. japonica Thunb.; P. tomentosa Thunb.	Bush Cherry Kernel	Semen Pruni	5-10g
Yu Mi Xu	玉米须	Zea mays L.	Corn Silk	Stylus Zeae Mays	15-30g
Yu Xing Cao	鱼腥草	Houttuynia cordata Thunb.	Houttuynia	Herba cum Radice Houttuyniae Cordatae	15-30g
Yu Yu Liang	禹余粮		Limonite	Limonitum	10-20g
Yu Zhu (Wei Rui)	玉竹 (葳蕤)	Polygonatum Odoratum (Mill.) Druce	Fragrant Solomonseal Rhizome	Rhizoma Polygonati Odorati	10-15g
Yuan Hu (Yan Hu Suo)	元胡(延胡索)	Corydalis turtschaninovii Bess. F. yanhusuo Y. H. Chou et C. C. Hsu.	Corydalis	Rhizoma Corydalis	3-10g
Yuan Hua	芫花	Daphne genkwa Sieb. et Zucc.	Genkwa Flower	Flos Genkwa; Flos Daphnis Genkwae	1.5-3g
Yuan Zhi	远志	Polygala tenuifolia Willd.; P. sibirica L.	Polygala Root	Radix Polygalae; Radix Polygalae Tenuifoliae	3-10g
Yue Ji Hua	月季花	Rosa chinensis Jacq.	China Tea Rose	Flos et Fructus Rosae Chinensis	3-6g
Yun Mu Xiang	云木香	Saussurea lappa Clarke	Yunnan Saussurea Root	Radix Saussureae Lappae	3-10g
Zang Qing Guo	藏青果 (西青果)	Terminalia chebula Retz.	West Olive	Fructus Immaturus Terminaliae	2-6g
Zao Jia	皂荚（皂角）	Gleditsia sinensis Lam.	Gleditsia Fruit	Fructus Gleditsiae Sinensis; Fructus	1.5-5g

				Gleditsiae	
Zao Jiao Ci	皂角刺	Gleditsia sinensis Lam.	Gleditsia Spine	Spina Gleditsiae Sinensis; Spina Gleditsiae	3-10g
Zao Xin Tu	灶心土		Ignited Yellow Earth, Oven Earth	Terra Flava Usta	15-30g
Zao Xiu (Cao He Che)	蚤休 (草河车)	Paris polyphylla Smith	Paris Root	Rhizoma Paridis	5-10g
Ze Lan	泽兰	Lycopus lucidus Turcz.; L. lucidus Turcz. var. hirtus Regel.	Lycopus	Herba Lycopi Lucidi	10-15g
Ze Qi	泽漆	Euphorbia helioscopia L.	Euphorbia	Herba Euphorbiae Helioscopiae	5-10g
Ze Xie	泽泻	Alisma orientalis (Sam.) Juzep.	Alisma Tuber	Rhizoma Alismatis Orientalis; Rhizoma Alismatis	5-10g
Zhang Nao	樟脑	Cinnamomum camphora (L.) Presl	Camphor	Camphora	0.1-0.2g
Zhe Bei Mu	浙贝母	Fritillaria Verticillata Willd. Var. thunbergii Bak.	Fritillaria Bulb	Bulbus Fritillariae Thunbergii	3-10g
Zhe Chong	蟅虫	Eupolyphaga sinensis Walk.; Steleophaga plancyi (Bol.)	Eupolyphaga	Eupolyphagae seu Steleophagae	3-10g
Zhe Shi	赭石		Hematite	Haematitum	10-30g
Zhen Zhu	珍珠	Pteria martensii (Dunker); Hyriopsis cumingii (Lea); Cristaria plicata (Leach); Anodonta woodiana (Lea)	Pearl	Margarita	0.3-1g
Zhen Zhu Mu	珍珠母	Hyriopsis cumingii (Lea); Cristaria plicata (Leach); Pteria martensii (Dunker)	Mother-of-pearl	Concha Margaritiferae	15-30g
Zhi Gan Cao	炙甘草	Glycyrrhiza uralensis Fisch.; G. ☐ud an☐ Bat.; G. glabra L.	Licorice Root	Radix Glycyrrhizae Praeparatae	3-10g
Zhi Ju Zi	枳具子	Hovenia bulcis Thunb	Japanese Raisin Tree Seed	Semen Hoveniae	4.5-9g
Zhi Ke	枳壳	Citrus aurantium L.; C. wilsonii Tanaka; Poncirus trifoliata (L.) Raf.	Mature Bitter Orange	Fructus Citri Aurantii; Fructus Aurantii	3-10g
Zhi Ma Huang	炙麻黄	Ephedra sinica Stapf.; E.equisetina Bunge	Honey-fried Ephedra	Herba Ephedrae	1.5-10g

Zhi Mu	知母	Anemarrhena asphodeloides Bge.	Anemarrhena Root	Rhizoma Anemarrhenae	6-12g
Zhi Shi	枳实	Citrus aurantium L.; C. wilsonii Tanaka; Poncirus trifoliata (L.) Raf.	Immature Bitter Orange	Fructus Citri Aurantii Immaturus	3-10g
Zhi Zi	栀子	Gardenia jasminoides Ellis.	Cape Jasmine; Gardenia Fruit	Fructus Gardeniae; Fructus Gardeniae Jasminoidis	3-10g
Zhi Zi Pi	栀子皮	Gardenia jasminoides Ellis.	Peel of Gardenia Fruit	Cortex Fructus Gardeniae	3-10g
Zhong Ru Shi	钟乳石		Tip of Tubular Stalactites	Stalactitum	9-15g
Zhu Dan Zhi	猪胆汁	Sus scrofa domestica Brisson.	Pig Gall Bladder	Vesica Fellea	6-10g
Zhu Li	竹沥	Bambusa breviflora Munro; Phyllostachys nigra (Lodd.) Munro var. henonis (Mitf.) Stapf ex Rendl	Bamboo Fluids	Succus Bambusae	30-50g
Zhu Ling	猪苓	Polyporus umbellatus (Pers.) Fries	Polyporus	Sclerotium Polypori Umbellati	5-10g
Zhu Ma Gen	苎麻根	Boehmeria nivea (L.) Gaud.	Ramie Root	Radix Boehmeriae	10-30g
Zhu Ru	竹茹	Bambusa breviflora Munro; Phyllostachys nigra (Lodd.) Munro var. henonis (Mitf.) Stapf ex Rendl	Bamboo Shavings	Caulis Bambusae in Taeniam	6-10g
Zhu Sha	朱砂		Cinnabar	Cinnabaris	0.3-1.0g
Zhu Ye	竹叶	Phyllostachys nigra (Lodd.) Munro var. henonis (Mitf.) Stapf ex Rendl	Bamboo Leaf	Folium Phyllostachydis Henonis	6-15g
Zi Bai Pi	梓白皮	Catalpa ovata G. Don	Chinese Catalpa	Cortex Catalpae Ovatae	9-15g
Zi Bei Chi	紫贝齿	Mauritia (Arabica) arabica (L.); Cypraea iynx (L.)	Cowry Shell	Concha Mauritiae; Concha Mauritiae Arabicae	10-15g
Zi Bei Tian Kui	紫背天葵	Semiaquilegia adoxoides (DC.) Mak.; Senecio nudicaulis Buch.-Ham.		Herba Senecionis Nudicaulis; Herba Semiaquilegiae	3-10g
Zi Cao	紫草	Lithospermum erythrorhizon Sieb et Zucc.; Macrotomia euchroma (Royle) pauls.	Lithospermum	Radix Lithospermi seu Macrotomiae	3-10g

Zi He Che	紫河车	Placenta Hominis		Human Placenta	Placenta Hominis	1.5-3g
Zi Hua Di Ding	紫花地丁	Viola yedoensis Makino.		Violet	Herba Violae; Herba cum Radice Violae	10-20g
Zi Ran Tong	自然铜			Pyrite	Pyritum	10-15g
Zi Shi Ying	紫石英			Fluorite	Fluoritum	9-15g
Zi Su Geng (Su Geng)	紫苏梗	Perilla frutescens (L.) Britt.		Perilla Stem	Caulis Perillae	5-10g
Zi Su Ye (Su Ye)	紫苏叶(苏叶)	Perilla frutescens (L.) Britt. var. crispa (Thunb.) Hand.-Mazz.		Perilla Leaf	Folium Perillae Frutescentis; Folium Perillae	5-10g
Zi Su Zi	紫苏子	Perilla frutescens (L.) Britt. Var. acuta (Thunb.) Kudo.		Perilla Fruit	Fructus Perillae	5-10g
Zi Wan	紫菀	Aster tataricus L. f.		Aster Root	Radix Asteris Tatarici	5-10g
Zi Zhu	紫珠(紫荆草)	Callicarpa pedunculata R. Br.; C. macrophylla Vahl.; C. nudiflora Hook. et Arn.		Callicarpa Leaf	Folium Callicarpae Formosanae; Folium Callicarpae	10-15g
Zong Lu Pi	棕榈皮	Trachycarpus fortunei H. Wendl.		Tachycarpus Stiple Fiber	Trachycarpi Petiolus Radicis; Trachycarpi Petiolus	3-10g
Zong Lu Tan	棕榈炭	Trachycarpus fortunei H. Wendl.			Trachycarpi Carbonisatus	3-10g

Appendix III: Commonly Used Herbal Prescriptions/Formula

Pin Yin Names	Chinese Names	Source Book	Ingredients	Administration
An Gong Niu huang Pill (An Gong Niu Huang Wan)	安宫牛黄丸	Analysis of Warm Diseases (Wen Bing Tiao Bian)	Calculus Bovis (Niu Huang) 30g Radix Curcumae (Yu Jin) 30g Rhizoma Coptidis (Huang Lian) 30g Cinnabaris (Zhu Sha) 30g Fructus Gardeniae (Zhi Zi) 30g Realgar (Xiong Huang) 30g Radix Scutellariae (Huang Qin) 30g Cornu Bubali (Shui Niu Jiao) 60g (It was 30g Xi Jiao in original ingredients) Borneolum Syntheticum (Bing Pian) 7.5g Moschus (She Xiang) 7.5g Margarita (Zhen Zhu) 15g (Coated by Jin Bo)	Zhen Zhu, Zhu Sha and Xiong Huang are respectively refined with water or ground into extremely fine powder. Huang Lian, Huang Qin, Zhi Zi and Yu Jin are ground into fine powder. Niu Huang, Shui Niu Jiao and Bing Pian are ground into powder, combined with above powder, sift out the mixture, and make the mixture into pills with appropriate amount of honey. Take one pill each time, once or twice daily. For infants less than three years old, take one quarter of a pill each time, once daily. For children from 4-6 years old, take half pill each time, once daily.
An Shen Ding Zhi Pill (An Shen Ding Zhi Wan)	安神定志丸	Medicine Comprehended (Yi Xue Xin Wu)	Radix Ginseng (Ren Shen) 30g Sclerotium Poriac Cocos (Fu Ling) 30g Sclerotium Poriae Circum Radicem Pini (Fu Shen) 30g Rhizoma Acori Tatarinowii (Shi Chang Pu) 15g Radix Polygalae (Yuan Zhi) 30g Mastodi Dentis Fossilia (Long Chi) 15g	Prepare the drugs into pills with honey, takes 6-9g each time with warm boiled water, twice daily.
Ba Zhen Decoction (Ba Zhen Tang). Ba Zhen Powder (Ba Zhen San, original name)	八珍汤 (原名八珍散)	Prescriptions of Auspicious Bamboo Hall (Rui Zhu Tang Fang)	Radix Angelicae Sinensis (Dang Gui) 6g Rhizoma Ligustici Chuanxiong (Chuan Xiong) 6g Radix Paeoniae Lactiflorae (Bai	Decoct the drugs in water for oral application.

| | | | Shao Yao) 6g
Radix Rehmanniae Praeparatae (Shu Di Huang) 6g
Radix Ginseng (Ren Shen) 6g
Rhizoma Atractylodis macrocephalae (Bai Zhu) 6g
Sclerotium Poriae Cocos (Fu Ling) 6g
Radix Glycyrrhizae Praeparatae (Zhi Gan Cao) 6g
Rhizoma Zingiberis Recens (Sheng Jiang) 5 slices
Fructus Zizyphi Jujubae (Da Zao) 1 piece | |
|---|---|---|---|---|
| Ba Zheng Powder (Ba Zheng San) | 八正散 | Formularies of the Bureau of People's Welfare Pharmacy (Tai Ping Hui Min He Ji Ju Fang) | Herba Dianthi (Qu Mai) 9g
Herba Polygoni Avicularis (Bian Xu) 9g
Semen Plantaginis (Che Qian Zi) 9g
Radix Glycyrrhizae Praeparatae (Zhi Gan Zao) 9g
Fructus Gardeniae Jasminoidis (Zhi Zi) 9g
Caulis Aristolochiae Manshuriensis (Mu Tong) 9g
Radix et Rhizoma Rhei (Da Huang) 9g
Medulla Junci Effusi (Deng Xin Cao)
Talcum (Hua Shi Fen) 9g | Grind the drugs except Deng Xin Cao into powder. Take 9g of the powder each time with 6g of Deng Xin Cao decocted in warm boiled water for oral application. Or decoct all drugs in water for oral application. |
| Bai He Gu Jin Decoction (Bai He Gu Jin Tang) | 百合固金汤 | Posthumous Writings of Cautious Studio (Shen Zhai Yi Shu) | Radix Rehmanniae Praeparatae (Shu Di Huang) 9g
Radix Rehmanniae Recens (Sheng Di Huang) 9g
Radix Ophiopogonis (Mai Dong) 6g
Bulbus Lilii (Bai He) 6g
Radix Paeoniae Lactiflorae (Bai Shao) 3g
Radix Angelicae Sinensis (Dang Gui) 9g
Bulbus Fritillariae (Bai Mu) 6g
Radix Glycyrrhizae (Gan Cao) 3g
Radix Scrophulariae (Xuan Shen) 3g
Radix Platycodonis (Jie Geng) 3g | Decoct the drugs in water for oral application. |
| Bai Hu Decoction (Bai Hu Tang) | 白虎汤 | Treatise on Cold Induced Diseases (Shang Han Lun) | Gypsum Fibrosum (Shi Gao) 50g
Semen Oryzae (Jing Mi) 9g
Rhizoma Anemarrhenae (Zhi Mu) 18g
Radix Glycyrrhizae Praeparatae (Gan Cao) 6g | Decoct the drugs in water for oral application. |
| Bai Hu Jia Cang | 白虎加苍 | Shang Han | Bai Hu Decoction supplemented | Decoct the drugs in |

Zhu Decoction (Bai Hu Jia Cang Zhu Tang)	术汤	Lei Zheng Huo Ren Shu	with Rhizoma Atractylodis (Cang Zhu)	water for oral application.
Bai Hu Jia Gui Zhi Decoction (Bai Hu Jia Gui Zhi Tang)	白虎加桂枝汤	Synopsis of the Golden Chamber (Jin Gui Yao Lue)	Bai Hu Decoction supplemented with Ramulus Cinnamomi Cassiae (Gui Zhi)	Decoct the drugs in water for oral application.
Bai Hu Jia Ren Shen Decoction (Bai Hu Jia Ren Shen Tang)	白虎加人参汤	Treatise on Cold Induced Diseases (Shang Han Lun)	Bai Hu Decoction supplemented with Radix Ginseng (Ren Shen)	Decoct the drugs in water for oral application.
Bai Tou Weng Decoction (Bai Tou Weng Tang)	白头翁汤	Treatise on Cold Induced Diseases (Shang Han Lun)	Cortex Fraxini (Qin Pi) 9g Rhizoma Coptidis (Huang Lian) 9g Cortex Phellodendri (Huang Bai) 9g Radix Pulsatillae (Bai Tou Weng) 6g	Decoct the drugs in water for oral application.
Bai Tou Weng Jia Gan Cao E Jiao Decoction (Bai Tou Weng Jia Gan Cao E Jiao Tang)	白头翁加干草阿胶汤		Bai Tou Weng Decoction supplemented with E Jiao and Gan Cao.	Decoct the drugs in water for oral application.
Ban Xia Bai Zhu Tian Ma Decoction (Ban Xia Bai Zhu Tian Ma Tang)	半夏白术天麻汤	Medicine Comprehended (Yi Xue Xin Wu)	Rhizoma Pinelliae (Ban Xia) 9g Rhizoma Atractylodis macrocephalae (Bai Zhu) 18g Rhizoma Gastrodiae (Tian Ma) 6g Sclerotium Poriae Cocos (Fu Ling) 6g Exocarpium Citri Rubrum (Ju Hong) 6g Radix Glycyrrhizae (Gan Cao) 3g Rhizoma Zingiberis Officinalis (Sheng Jiang) 1 slice Fructus Zizyphi Jujubae (Da Zao) 2 pcs	Decoct the drugs except Sheng Jiang and Da Zao in water for oral application, and add 1 slice of Sheng Jiang and 2 pcs of Da Zao.
Ban Xia Hou Po Decoction (Ban Xia Hou Po Tang)	半夏厚朴汤	Synopsis of the Golden Chamber (Jin Gui Yao Lue)	Rhizoma Pinelliae (Ban Xia) 12g Rhizoma Zingiberis Recens (Sheng Jiang) 15g Sclerotium Poriae Cocos (Fu Ling) 12g Cortex Magnoliae Officinalis (Hou Po) 9g Folium Perillae (Su Ye) 6g	Decoct the drugs in water for oral application.
Ban Xia Xie Xin Decoction (Ban Xia Xie Xin Tang)	半夏泻心汤	Treatise on Cold Induced Diseases (Shang Han Lun)	Rhizoma Pinelliae (Ban Xia) 12g Radix Scutellariae (Huang Qin) 9g Rhizoma Zingiberis (Gan Jiang) 9g Radix Ginseng (Ren Shen) 9g Fructus Zizyphi Jujubae (Da Zao) 4 pcs Radix Glycyrrhizae Praeparatae	Decoct the drugs in water for oral application.

			(Zhi Gan Cao) 9g Rhizoma Coptidis (Huang Lian) 3g	
Bao He Pill (Bao He Wan)	保和丸	Danxi's Experiential Therapy (Dan Xi Xin Fa)	Fructus Crataegi (Shan Zha) 18g Rhizoma Pinelliae (Ban Xia) 9g Massa Medicata Fermentata (Shen Qu) 6g Sclerotium Poriae Cocos (Fu Ling) 9g Fructus Forsythiae (Lian Qiao) 3g Semen Raphani (Lai Fu Zi) 3g Pericarpium Citri Reticulatae (Chen Pi) 3g	Decoct the drugs in water for oral application; or prepare into pills, takes 6-9g each time with warm boiled water, twice daily.
Bao Yuan Decoction (Bao Yuan Tang)	保元汤	Bo Ai Xin Jian	Radix Ginseng (Ren Shen) 3g Radix Astragali (Huang Qi) 9g Cortex Cinnamomi (Rou Gui) 1.5-2g Radix Glycyrrhizae Praeparatae (Zhi Gan Cao) 3g Rhizoma Zingiberis Recens (Sheng Jiang) 6g	Decoct the drugs in water for oral application.
Bao Zhen Decoction (Bao Zhen Tang)	保真汤	Miraculous Book of Ten Herbs (Shi Yao Shen Shu)	Radix Ginseng (Ren Shen) 9g Radix Astragali (Huang Qi) 9g Rhizoma Atractylodis Macrocephalae (Bai Zhu) 9g Sclerotium Poriae Cocos (Fu Ling) 9g Fructus Zizyphi Jujubae (Da Zao) 5 pcs Radix Asparagi (Tian Dong) 6g Radix Ophiopogonis (Mai Dong) 6g Radix Rehmanniae Recens (Sheng Di Huang) 9g Radix Rehmanniae Praeparatae (Shu Di Huang) 9g Fructus Schisandrae (Wu Wei Zi) 6g Radix Angelicae Sinensis (Dang Gui) 9g Radix Paeoniae (Shao Yao) 12g Stamen Nelumbinis (Lian Xu) 3g Cortex Lycii (Di Gu Pi) 6g Radix Bupleuri (Chai Hu) 6g Pericarpium Citri Reticulatae (Chen Pi) 4.5g Rhizoma Zingiberis Recens (Sheng Jiang) 3 slices Cortex Phellodendri (Huang Bai) 6g Rhizoma Anemarrhenae (Zhi Mu) 6g Radix Glycyrrhizae (Gan Cao) 4.5g	Decoct the drugs in water for oral application, thrice daily.
Bei Mu Gua Lou	贝母瓜篓	Medicine	Bulbus Fritillariae (Bei Mu) 15g	Decoct the drugs in

Powder (Bei Mu Gua Lou San)	散	Comprehended (Yi Xue Xin Wu)	Fructus Trichosanthis (Gua Lou) 10g Radix Trichosanthis (Tian Hua Fen) 8g Sclerotium Poriae Cocos (Fu Ling) 8g Exocarpium Citri Rubrum (Ju Hong) 8g Radix Platycodonis (Jie Geng) 8g	water for oral application.
Bi Xie Fen Qing Decoction (Bi Xie Fen Qing Yin)	萆薢分清饮	Yang Family's Formulae (Yang Shi Jia Cang Fang)	Rhizoma Dioscoreae Septemlobae (Bi Xie) 9g Rhizoma Acori Graminei (Shi Chan Pu) 9g Radix Linderae (Wu Yao) 9g Fructus Alpiniae Oxyphyllae (Yi Zhi Ren) 9g	Decoct the drugs in water for oral application.
Bie Jia Jian Pill (Bie Jia Jian Wan)	鳖甲煎丸	Synopsis of the Golden Chamber (Jin Gui Yao Lue)	Carapax Trionycis (Bie Jia) 90g Rhizoma Belamcandae (She Gan) 22.5g Radix Scutellariae (Huang Qin) 22.5g Fructus Arctii (Shu Fu) 22.5g Rhizoma Zingiberis (Gan Jiang) 22.5g Radix et Rhizoma Rhei (Da Huang) 22.5g Ramulus Cinnamomi (Gui Zhi) 22.5g Folium Pyrrosiae (Shi Wei) 22.5g Cortex Magnoliae Officinalis (Hou Po) 22.5g Radix Campsis (Zi Wei) 22.5g Colla Corii Asini (E Jiao) 22.5g Radix Bupleuri (Chai Hu) 45g Catharsius molossus (Qiang Lang) 45g Radix Paeoniae (Shao Yao) 37g Cortex Moutan (Mu Dan Pi) 37g Eupolyphagae seu Steleophagae (Zhe Chong) 37g Vespae Nidus (Feng Fang) 30g Natrii Sulfas Rubra (Chi Xiao) 90g Semen Persicae (Tao Ren) 15g Herba Dianthi (Qu Mai) 15g Radix Ginseng (Ren Shen) 7.5g Rhizoma Pinelliae (Ban Xia) 7.5g Semen Descurainiae (Ban Xia) 7.5g	Mix the drugs with wine and honey, and make them into pills, weighing 3g each. Take 1-2 pills each time, 2-3 times daily with warm water.
Bu Fei Decoction (Bu Fei Tang)	补肺汤	Yong Lei Qian Fang	Radix Astragali (Huang Qi) 9g Radix Rehmanniae Praeparatae (Shu Di Huang) 9g Cortex Mori Alba Radicis (Sang Bai Pi) 9g	Decoct the drugs in water for oral application.

			Radix Ginseng (Ren Shen) 5g Radix Asteris Tatarici (Zi Wan) 5g Fructus Schisandrae (Wu Wei Zi) 3g	
Bu Qi Yun Pi Decoction (Bu Qi Yun Pi Tang)	补气运脾汤	Standards of Diagnosis and Treatment (Zheng Zhi Zhun Sheng)	Radix Ginseng (Ren Shen) 6g Honey roasted Radix Astragali (Huang Qi) 3g Rhizoma Atractylodis Macrocephalae (Bai Zhu) 9g Sclerotium Poriae Cocos (Fu Ling) 4.5g Radix Glycyrrhizae Praeparatae (Zhi Gan Cao) 1.5g Fructus Amomi (Sha Ren) 2.4g Pericarpium Citri Reticulatae (Chen Pi) 4.5g Rhizoma Pinelliae (Ban Xia) 3g Rhizoma Zingiberis Recens (Sheng Jiang) 1 slice Fructus Ziziphi Jujubae (Da Zao) 1 pcs	Decoct the drugs in water for oral application.
Bu Tian Da Zao Pill (Bu Tian Da Zao Wan)	补天大造丸	Medicine Comprehended (Yi Xue Xin Wu)	Radix Ginseng (Ren Shen) 100g Radix Astragali Praeparatae (Zhi Huang Qi) 150g Rhizoma Atractylodis macrocephalae (Zheng Bai Zhu) 150g Radix Angelicae Sinensis (Jiu Dang Gui) 75g Semen Ziziphi Spinosae (Chao Suan Zao Ren) 75g Radix Polygalae (Chao Yuan Zhi) 75g Radix Paeoniae Alba (Jiu Bai Shao) 75g Rhizoma Dioscoreae (Shan Yao) 75g Sclerotium Poriae Cocos (Fu Ling) 75g Fructus Lycii (Jiu Gou Qi Zi) 200g Radix Rehmanniae Praeparatae (Shu Di Huang) 200g Placenta Hominis (Zi He Che) 1 whole piece Colla Corni Cervi (Lu Jiao Jiao) 500g Carapax et Plastrum Testudinis (Gui Ban Jiao) 400g	Make pills with Honey (Feng Mi), and take 12g each time with warm boiled water befoe meals.
Bu Yang Huan Wu Decoction (Bu Yang Huan Wu Tang)	补阳还五汤	Correction on the Errors of Medical Works (Yi	Radix Astragali (Huang Qi) 120g Tail of Radix Angelicae Sinensis (Dang Gui Wei) 6g Radix Paeoniae Rubra (Chi Shao)	Decoct the drugs in water for oral application.

			Lin Gai Cuo)	5g Rhizoma Ligustici Chuanxiong (Chuan Xiong) 3g Semen Persicae (Tao Ren) 3g Flos Carthami (Hong Hua) 3g Lumbricus (Di Long) 3g	
Bu Zhong Yi Qi Decoction (Bu Zhong Yi Qi Tang)	补中益气汤	Differentiation on Endogenous and Exogenous Diseases (Nei Wai Shang Bian Huo Lun)	Radix Astragali (Huang Qi) 9g Radix Glycyrrhizae Praeparatae (Zhi Gan Cao) 9g Rhizoma Atractylodis Macrocephalae (Bai Zhu) 9g Radix Ginseng (Ren Shen) 9g Radix Angelicae Sinensis (Dang Gui) 9g Pericarpium Citri Reticulatae (Chen Pi) 9g Rhizoma Cimicifugae (Sheng Ma) 9g Radix Bupleuri (Chai Hu) 9g Rhizoma Zingiberis Recens (Sheng Jiang) Fructus Zizyphi Jujubae (Da Zao)	Decoct the drugs in water for oral application.
Cang Er Powder (Cang Er San)	苍耳散	Prescriptions for Saving Lives (Ji Sheng Fang)	Radix Angelicae Dahuricae (Bai Zhi) 30g Herba Menthae (Bo He) 1.5g Flos Magnoliae (Xin Yi) 15g Fructus Xanthii Sibirici (Cang Er Zi) 7.5g	Grind the drugs into fine powder; take 6g each time with green onion and tea.
Chai Ge Jie Ji Decoction (Chai Ge Jie Ji Tang)	柴葛解肌汤	Six Books on Cold Induced Diseases (Shang Han Liu Shu)	Radix Bupleuri (Chai Hu) 6g Radix Puerariae (Ge Gen) 9g Gypsum Fibrosum (Shi Gao) 12g Rhizoma et Radix Notopterygii (Qiang Huo) 3g Radix Angelicae Dahuricae (Bai Zhi) 3g Radix Scutellariae (Huang Qin) 6g Radix Paeoniae Alba (Bai Shao) 6g Radix Platycodonis (Jie Geng) 3g Rhizoma Zingiberis Recens (Sheng Jiang) 3 slices Fructus Zizyphi Jujubae (Da Zao) 2 pcs Radix Glycyrrhizae (Gan Cao) 3g	Decoct the drugs in water for oral application.
Chai Hu Shu Gan Powder (Chai Hu Shu Gan San)	柴胡疏肝散	The Wholly Purpose of Medicine (Yi Xue Tong Zhi)	Radix Bupleuri (Chai Hu) 6g Vinegar Roasted Pericarpium Citri Reticulatae (Chen Pi) 6g Rhizoma Ligustici Chuanxiong (Chuan Xiong) 5g Radix Paeoniae (Shao Yao) 5g Fructus Citri Aurantii (Zhi Ke) 5 Rhizoma Cyperi (Xiang Fu) 5g Radix Glycyrrhizae Praeparatae	Decoct the drugs in water for oral application.

			(Zhi Gan Cao) 3g	
Chai Hu Si Wu Decoction (Chai Hu Si Wu Tang)	柴胡四物汤	Collection on Pathogenesis for Protecting Life Based on Plain Questions (Su Wen Bing Ji Qi Yi Bao Ming Ji)	Rhizoma Ligustici Chuanxiong (Chuan Xiong) 4.5g Radix Rehmanniae Praeparatae (Shu Di Huang) 4.5g Radix Angelicae Sinensis (Dang Gui) 4.5g Radix Paeoniae (Shao Yao) 4.5g Radix Bupleuri (Chai Hu) 2.4g Radix Ginseng (Ren Shen) 9g Radix Scutellariae (Huang Qin) 9g Radix Glycyrrhizae (Gan Cao) 9g Rhizoma Pinelliae Fermentata (Ban Xia Qu) 9g	Decoct the drugs in water for oral application.
Chai Shao Liu Jun Zi Decoction (Chai Shao Liu Jun Zi Tang)	柴芍六君子汤	Golden Mirror of Medicine (Yi Zong Jin Jian)	Radix Ginseng (Ren Shen) 6g Rhizoma Atractylodis Macrocephalae (Bai Zhu) 6g Sclerotium Poriae Cocos (Fu Ling) 6g Rhizoma Pineliae (Ban Xia) 6g Radix Glycyrrhizae Praeparatae (Zhi Gan Cao) 6g Pericarium Citri Reticulatae (Chen Pi) 6g Radix Bupleuri (Chai Hu) 6g Radix Paeoniae Alba (Bai Shao Yao) 6g	Decoct the drugs in water for oral application.
Chai Zhi Ban Xia Decoction (Chai Zhi Ban Xia Tang)	柴枳半夏汤	Yi Xue Ru Men	Radix Bupleuri (Chai Hu) 12g Radix Scutellariae (Huang Qin) 10g Rhizoma Pinelliae (Ban Xia) 12g Semen Trichosanthis (Gua Lou Zi) 10g Fructus Citri Aurantii (Zhi Ke) 12g Radix Platycodonis (Jie Geng) 12g Semen Pruni Armeniacae (Xing Ren) 10g Pericarpium Citri Reticulatae Viride (Qing Pi) 10g Radix Glycyrrhizae (Gan Cao) 6g	Decoct the drugs in water for oral application.
Chang Pu Yu Jin Decoction (Chang Pu Yu Jin Tang)	菖蒲郁金汤	Analysis of Warm Diseases (Wen Bing Tiao Bian)	Rhizoma Acori Tatarinowii (Shi Chang Pu) 9g Radix Curcumae (Yu Jin) 6g Stir-fried Fructus Gardeniae (Zhi Zi) 9g **Folium Phyllostachydis Henonis (Zhu Ye) 9g** Cortex Moutan Radicis (Mu Dan Pi) 9g Fructus Forsythiae (Lian Qiao) 9g Medulla Junci Effusi (Deng Xin Cao) 6g Caulis Akebiae (Mu Tong) 4.5g	Decoct the drugs except Zhu Li and Zi Jin Pian in water, and then add Zhu Li and Zi Jin PIan in the decoction for oral application.

			Succus Bambusae (Zhu Li) 15g **Zi Jin Pian** (紫金片) 1.5g	
Chen Xiang Powder (Chen Xiang San)	沉香散	Jin Gui Yi	Lignum Aquilariae Resinatum (Chen Xiang) 15g Folium Pyrrosiae (Shi Wei) 15g Talcum (Hua Shi Fen) 15g Radix Angelicae Sinensis (Dang Gui) 15g Pericarpium Citri Reticulatae (Ju Pi) 7.5g Radix Paeoniae Alba (Bai Shao Yao) 23g Semen Malvae (Dong Kui Zi) 23g Radix Glycyrrhizae Praeparatae (Zhi Gan Cao) 7.5g Semen Vaccariae Segetalis (Wang Bu Liu Xing) 15g	Grind the drugs into fine powder; take 6g each time.
Chou Xin Decoction (Chou Xin Yin)	抽薪饮	Jingyue's Complete Works (Jing Yue Quan Shu)	Radix Scutellariae (Huang Qin) 3-6g Fructus Gardeniae (Zhi Zi) 3-6g Cortex Phellodendri (Huang Bai) 3-6g Caulis Akebiae (Mu Tong) 3-6g Herba Dendrobii (Shi Hu) 3-6g Fructus Citri Aurantii (Zhi Ke) 4.5g Rhizoma Alismatis (Ze Xie) 4.5g Radix Glycyrrhizae (Gan Cao) 0.9g	Decoct the drugs in water for oral application.
Chuan Xiong Cha Tiao Powder (Chuan Xiong Cha Tiao San)	川芎茶调散	Formularies of the Bureau of People's Welfare Pharmacy (Tai Ping Hui Min He Ji Ju Fang)	Herba Menthae Haplocalycis (Bo He) 24g Rhizoma Ligustici Chuanxiong (Chuan Xiong) 12g Herba Schizonepetae (Jing Jie) 12g Herba Asari (Xi Xin) 3g Radix Saposhnikoviae (Fang Feng) 4.5g Rhizoma et Radix Notopterygii (Qiang Huo) 6g Radix Angelicae Dahuricae (Bai Zhi) 6g Radix Glycyrrhizae (Gan Cao) 6g Tea (Cha)	Add appropriate dose of tea, decoct the drugs in water for oral application; or as powder, take 6g each time, twice daily with tea after meals.
Chun Yang Zhen Ren Yang Zang Decoction (Chun Yang Zhen Ren Yang Zang Tang). Also named Zhen Ren Yang Zang Decoction (Zhen Ren Yang Zang Tang)	纯阳真人养脏汤（真人养脏汤）	Formularies of the Bureau of People's Welfare Pharmacy (Tai Ping Hui Min He Ji Ju Fang)	Radix Ginseng (Ren Shen) 9g Radix Angelicae Sinensis (Dang Gui) 9g Rhizoma Atractylodis Macrocephalae (Bai Zhu) 9g Semen Myristicae (Rou Dou Kou) 6g Cortex Cinnamomi (Rou Gui) 6g Radix Glycyrrhizae Praeparatae (Zhi Gan Cao) 6g Radix Paeoniae Alba (Bai Shao	Decoct the drugs in water for oral application before meals.

			Yao) 6g Radix Aucklandiae (Mu Xiang) 3g Fructus Chebulae (He Zi) 9g Pericarpium Papaveris (Ying Su Ke) 6g (remove pedicle, prepared with honey)	
Ci Zhu Pill (Ci Zhu Wan)	磁朱丸	Invaluable Prescriptions (Qian Jin Yao Fang)	Calcined Magnetitum (Duan Ci Shi) 200g Cinnabaris (Zhu Sha) 100g Massa Medicata Fermentata (Shen Qu) 400g	Zhu Sha is refined with water into extremely fine powder; Ci Shi and Shen Qu are ground into fine powder respectively; mix the above powder evenly and sift; and finally make pills with water and dry. Take 3g each time, twice daily.
Cong Bai Qi Wei Decoction (Cong Bai Qi Wei Yin)	葱白七味饮	Arcane Essentials from the Imperial Library (Wai Tai Mi Yao)	Bulbus Allii Fistulosi (Cong Bai) 9g Radix Puerariae (Ge Gen) 9g Radix Ophiopogonis (Mai Dong) 9g Radix Rehmanniae (Gan Di Huang) 9g Fermented Soybean (Dou Chi) 6g Rhizoma Zingiberis Recens (Sheng Jiang) 6g	Decoct the drugs in water for oral application.
Cong Chi Decoction (Cong Chi Tang)	葱豉汤	Zhou Hou Bei Ji Fang	Bulbus Allii Fistulosi (Cong Bai) 3 pcs Fermented Soybean (Dou Chi) 6g	Decoct the drugs in water for oral application. If there are no sweats after drinking the decoction, add Radix Puerariae (Ge Gen) 6g and Rhizoma Cimicifugae (Sheng Ma) 9g; if still no sweats, add Herba Ephedrae (Ma Huang) 6g.
Cong Chi Jie Geng Decoction (Cong Chi Jie Geng Tang)	葱豉桔梗汤	Edition of Popular Cold Induced Diseases (Tong Su Shang Han Lun)	Bulbus Allii Fistulosi (Cong Bai) 10g Semen Sojae Preparatum (Dan Dou Chi) 15g Herba Menthae Haplocalycis (Bo He) 5g Fructus Forsythiae Suspensae (Lian Qiao) 6g Fructus Gardeniae Jasminoidis (Zhi Zi) 9g Folium Phyllostachydis Henonis (Zhu Ye) 12g Radix Platycodi Grandiflori (Jie	Decoct the drugs in water for oral application.

			Geng) 5g Radix Glycyrrhizae (Gan Cao) 3g	
Da Bu Yin Pill (Da Bu Yin Wan). Or Da Bu Pill (original name)	大补阴丸	Danxi's Experiential Therapy (Dan Xi Xin Fa)	Radix Rehmanniae Praeparatae (Shu Di Huang) 18g Pastrum Testudinis Praeparatae (Zhi Gui Ban) 18g Cortex Phellodendri Praeparatae (Chao Huang Bai) 12g Rhizoma Anemarrhenae (Zhi Mu) 12g	Decoct the drugs in water for oral application. Or make boluses with pork spinal cord and honey; take 6-9g each time with light salty water before meals.
Da Bu Yuan Decoction (Da Bu Yuan Jian)	大补元煎	Jingyue's Complete Works (Jing Yue Quan Shu)	Radix Ginseng (Ren Shen) 3-6g Stir-fried Rhizoma Dioscoreae (Chao Shan Yao) 6g Radix Rehmanniae Praeparatae (Shu Di Huang) 6-9g Cortex Eucommiae (Du Zhong) 6g Fructus Lycii (Gou Qi Zi) 6-9g Radix Angelicae Sinensis (Dang Gui) 6-9g Fructus Corni Officinalis (Shan Zhu Yu) 3g Radix Glycyrrhizae Praeparatae (Zhi Gan Cao) 3-6g	Decoct the drugs in water for oral application.
Da Chai Hu Decoction (Da Chai Hu Tang)	大柴胡汤	Synopsis of Golden Chamber (Jin Gui Yao Lue)	Radix Bupleuri (Chai Hu) 24g Radix Scutellariae (Huang Qin) 9g Radix Paeoniae Alba (Bai Shao Yao) 9g Rhizoma Pinelliae (Ban Xia) 9g Rhizoma Zingiberis Recens (Sheng Jiang) 15g Fructus Citri Aurantii Immaturus (Zhi Shi) 9g Fructus Zizyphi Jujubae (Da Zao) 4 pcs Radix et Rhizoma Rhei (Da Huang) 6g	Decoct the drugs in water for oral application.
Da Cheng Qi Decoction (Da Cheng Qi Tang)	大承气汤	Treatise on Cold Induced Diseases (Shang Han Lun)	Cortex Magnoliae Officinalis (Hou Po) 24g Radix et Rhizoma Rhei (Da Huang) 12g Natrii Sulfas (Mang Xiao) 9g Fructus Immaturus Citri Aurantii (Zhi Shi) 12g	Decoct Hou Po and Zhi Shi prior to adding and decocting Da Huang; then remove the residue and add Mang Xiao to the decoction until it is melted. Take half warm decoction each time, twice daily. Stop taking the decoction if patients egest.
Da Ding Feng Pill (Da Ding Feng Zhu)	大定风珠	Analysis of Warm Diseases (Wen	Radix Paeoniae Alba (Bai Shao) 18g Colla Corii Asini (E Jiao) 9g Plastrum Testudinis (Gui Ban) 12g	Decoct the drugs except E Jiao and Fresh Yolk in water,

				Radix Rehmanniae Recens (Sheng Di Huang) 18g Semen Cannabis (Huo Ma Ren) 6g Fructus Schisandrae (Wu Wei Zi) 6g Concha Ostreae (Mu Li) 12g Radix Ophiopogonis (Mai Dong) 18g Radix Glycyrrhizae Praeparatae (Zhi Gan Cao) 12g Fresh Yolk (Sheng Ji Zi Huang) 2 pcs Carapax Trionycis (Bie Jia) 12g	then remove the residue and add E Jiao to the decoction until it is melted. Add Fresh Yolk and stir evenly. Take the decoction while it is still warm.
		Bing Tiao Bian)			
Da Huang Fu Zi Decoction (Da Huang Fu Zi Tang)	大黄附子汤	Synopsis of the Golden Chamber (Jin Gui Yao Lue)	Radix et Rhizoma Rhei (Da Huang) 9g Radix Aconiti Lateralis Praeparatae (Fu Zi) 12g Herba cum Radice Asari (Xi Xin) 3g	Decoct the drugs in water for oral application.
Da Huang Mu Dan Decoction (Da Huang Mu Dan Tang)	大黄牡丹汤	Synopsis of the Golden Chamber (Jin Gui Yao Lue)	Semen Benincasae (Dong Gua Zi) 15g Radix et Rhizoma Rhei (Da Huang) 12g Semen Persicae (Tao Ren) 12g Natrii Sulfas (Mang Xiao) 9g Cortex Moutan Radicis (Mu Dan Pi) 3g	Decoct the drugs except Mang Xiao in water, and then dissolve Mang Xiao in the decoction.
Da Huang Zhe Chong Pill (Da Huang Zhe Chong Wan)	大黄䗪虫丸	Synopsis of the Golden Chamber (Jin Gui Yao Lue)	Radix et Rhizoma Rhei (Da Huang) 75 Radix Scutellariae (Huang Qin) 60g Radix Glycyrrhizae (Gan Cao) 90g Semen Persicae (Tao Ren) 180g Semen Armeniacae Amarum (Xing Ren) 180g Radix Paeoniae (Shao Yao) 120g Radix Rehmanniae (Gan Di Huang) 300g Resina Toxicodendri (Gan Qi) 30g Tabanus Bivittatus (Meng Chong) 60g Hirudo seu Whitmania (Shui Zhi) 60g Larva Holotrichiae (Qi Cao) 60g Eupolyphagae seu Steleophagae (Zhe Chong) 30g	Add honey and make the drugs into pills, 3g each. Take one pill with warm boiled water each time, three times daily.
Da Jian Zhong Decoction (Da Jian Zhong Tang)	大建中汤	Synopsis of the Golden Chamber (Jin Gui Yao Lue)	Rhizoma Zingiberis (Gan Jiang) 12g Pericarpium Zanthoxyli (Hua Jiao) 6g Radix Ginseng (Ren Shen) 6g Saccharum Granonum (Yi Tang) 30g	Decoct the drugs except Yi Tang in water, and then add Yi Tang to the decoction until it is melted. Take half warm decoction each

				time, twice daily.
Da Qin Jiao Decoction (Da Qin Jiao Tang)	大秦艽汤	Collection on Pathogenesis for Protecting Life Based on Plain Questions (Su Wen Bing Ji Qi Yi Bao Ming Ji)	Radix Gentianae Macrophyllae (Qin Jiao) 9g Rhizoma Ligustici Chuanxiong (Quan Xiong) 6g Radix Angelicae Pubescentis (Du Huo) 6g Radix Angelicae Sinensis (Dang Gui) 6g Radix Paeoniae Alba (Bai Shao Yao) 6g Gypsum Fibrosum (Shi Gao) 6g Radix Glycyrrhizae (Gan Cao) 6g Rhizoma et Radix Notopterygii (Qiang Huo) 3g Radix Saposhnikoviae (Fang Feng) 3g Radix Angelicae Dahuricae (Bai Zhi) 3g Radix Scutellariae (Huang Qin) 3g Rhizoma Atractylodis Macrocephalae (Bai Zhu) 3g Sclerotium Poriae Cocos (Fu Ling) 3g Radix Rehmanniae Recens (Sheng Di Huang) 3g Radix Rehmanniae Praeparatae (Shu Di Huang) 3g Herba Asari (Xi Xin) 3g	Decoct the drugs in water for oral application.
Da Tao Hua Decoction (Da Tao Hua Tang)	大桃花汤	Invaluable Prescriptions for Emergencies (Bei Ji Qian Jin Yao Fang)	Halloysitum Rubrum (Chi Shi Zhi) 9g Rhizoma Zingiberis Officinalis (Gan Jiang) 9g Radix Angelicae Sinensis (Dang Gui) 9g Os Draconis (Long Gu) 9g Concha Ostreae (Mu Li) 9g Radix Aconiti Lateralis Praeparatae (Fu Zi) 6g Rhizoma Atractylodis Macrocephalae (Bai Zhu) 10g Radix Glycyrrhizae (Gan Cao) 3g Radix Paeoniae (Shao Yao) 3g Radix Ginseng (Ren Shen) 4.5g	Decoct the drugs in water for oral application.
Dai Ge Powder (Dai Ge San)	黛蛤散	Zhong Yao Cheng Fang Pei Ben	Indigo Naturalis (Qing Dai) 30g Concha Meretricis seu Cyclinae (Hai Ge Qiao) 300g	Grind the drugs into fine powder, mix evenly and sift. Take 6g each time, once daily.
Dan Shen Decoction (Dan Shen Yin)	丹参饮	Current Formulae in Verse (Shi	Radix Salviae Miltiorrhizae (Dan Shen) 30g Lignum Santali Albi (Tan Xiang) 3g	Decoct the drugs in water for oral application.

			Fang Ge Kuo)	Fructus Amomi Villosi (Sha Ren) 3g	
Dan Zhi Xiao Yao Powder (Dan Zhi Xiao Yao San)	丹栀逍遥散	Formularies of the Bureau of People's Pharmacy (Tai Ping Hui Min He Ji Ju Fang)	Radix Paeoniae Alba (Bai Shao) 9g Sclerotium Poriae Cocos (Fu Ling) 9g Radix Angelicae Sinensis (Dang Gui) 9g Rhizoma Atractylodis Macrocephalae (Bai Zhu) 9g Rhizoma Zinigiberis Recens (Sheng Jiang) 3g Radix Glycyrrhizae Praeparatae (Zhi Gan Cao) 4.5g Radix Bulpeuri (Chai Hu) 9g Herba Menthae (Bo He) 3g Cortex Moutan Radicis (Mu Dan Pi) 6g Fructus Gardeniae (Zhi Zi) 9g	Decoct the drugs in water for oral application. Or prepare the drugs into pills or powder, and take 6g each time, twice daily.	
Dang Gui Bu Xue Decoction (Dang Gui Bu Xue Tang)	当归补血汤	Differentiation on Endogenous and Exogenous Diseases (Nei Wai Shang Bian Huo Lun)	Radix Astragali (Huang Qi) 30g Radix Angelicae Sinensis (Dan Gui) 6g	Decoct the drugs in water for oral application.	
Dang Gui Liu Huang Decoction (Dang Gui Liu Huang Tang)	当归六黄汤	Secret Book of Orchid Chamber (Lan Shi Mi Cang)	Radix Astragali (Huang Qi) 12g Radix Angelicae Sinensis (Dang Gui) 6g Radix Rehmanniae Recens (Sheng Di Huang) 6g Radix Rehmanniae Praeparatae (Shu Di Huang) 6g Radix Scutellariae (Huang Qin) 6g Cortex Phellodendri (Huang Bai) 6g Rhizoma Coptidis (Huang Lian) 6g	Decoct the drugs in water for oral application.	
Dang Gui Si Ni Decoction (Dang Gui Si Ni Tang)	当归四逆汤	Treatise on Cold Induced Diseases (Shang Han Lun)	Radix Angelicae Sinensis (Dang Gui) 12g Ramulus Cinnamomi (Gui Zhi) 9g Radix Paeoniae Alba (Bai Shao Yao) 9g Herba Asari (Xi Xin) 3g Radix Glycyrrhizae Praeparatae (Zhi Gan Cao) 6g Medulla Tetrapanacis (Tong Cao) 6g Fructus Zizyphi Jujubae (Da Zao) 8 pcs	Decoct the drugs in water for oral application.	
Dang Gui Decoction (Dang Gui Yin Zi)	当归饮子	Prescriptions for Saving Lives (Ji	Radicis Angelicae Sinensis (Dang Gui) 9g Radix Rehmanniae Recens (Sheng	Decoct the drugs with 5 pieces of Sheng Jiang in water	

		Sheng Fang)	Di Huang) 9g Radix Paeoniae Alba (Bai Shao) 9g Rhizoma Ligustici Chuanxiong (Chuang Xiong) 9g Radix Polygoni Multiflori (He Shou Wu) 5g Herba Schizonepetae (Jing Jie Sui) 9g Radix Saposhnikoviae (Fang Feng) 9g Fructus Tribuli Alba (Bai Ji Li) 9g Radix Astragali (Huang Qi) 5g Radix Glycyrrhizae Praeparatae (Zhi Gan Zao) 5g	for oral application.
Dao Chi Powder (Dao Chi San)	导赤散	Key to Therapeutics of Children's Diseases (Xiao Er Yao Zheng Zhi Jue)	Radix Rehmanniae Recens (Sheng Di Huang) 6g Caulis Aristolochiae Manshuriensis (Mu Tong) 6g **Folium Phyllostachydis Henonis (Zhu Ye) 6g** Radix Glycyrrhizae (Gan Cao Shao) 6g	Decoct the drugs in water for oral application.
Dao Tan Decoction (Dao Tan Tang)	导痰汤	Check and Annotate Effective Prescriptions for Women (Jiao Zhu Fu Ren Liang Fang)	Rhizoma Pinelliae (Ban Xia) 9g Pericarpium Citri Reticulatae (Chen Pi) 9g Fructus Citri Aurantii Immaturus (Zhi Shi) 6g Sclerotium Poriae Cocos (Fu Ling) 12g Radix Glycyrrhizae (Gan Cao) 6g Rhizoma Arisaematis (Tian Nan Xing) 6g Rhizoma Zingiberis Recens (Sheng Jiang) 9g	Decoct the drugs in water for oral application.
Di Dang Decoction (Di Dang Tang)	抵当汤	Treatise on Cold Induced Disease (Shang Han Lun)	Hirudo seu Whitmania (Shui Zhi) 30 pcs Tabanus Bivittatus (Meng Chong) 30 pcs Semen Pruni Persicae (Tao Ren) 20 pcs Radix et Rhizoma Rhei Praeparatae (Zhi Da Huang) 48g	Decoct the drugs in water, and take 1/3 of the decoction each time for oral application.
Di Huang Decoction (Di Huang Yin Zi)	地黄饮子	Clear Synopsis on Recipes Based on Plain Quesitions of Huangdi (Huang Di Su Wen Xuan Ming Lun Fang)	Radix Rehmanniae Praeparatae (Shu Di Huang) 10g Radix Morindae Officinalis (Ba Ji Tian) 10g Fructus Corni (Shan Zhu Yu) 10g Herba Cistanches (Rou Cong Rong) 10g Radix Aconiti Lateralis Praeparatae (Pao Fu Zi) 10g Herba Dendrobii (Shi Hu) 10g	Decoct the drugs in water for oral application.

			Fructus Schisandrae Chinensis (Wu Wei Zi) 10g Cortex Cinnamomi (Rou Gui) 10g Sclerotium Poriae Cocos (Fu Ling) 10g Radix Ophiopogonis (Mai Dong) 5g Radix Polygalae (Yuan Zhi) 5g Rhizoma Acori Tatarinowii (Shi Chang Pu) 5g Rhizoma Zingiberis Recens (Sheng Jiang) 3 slices Fructus Zizyphi Jujubae (Da Zao) 2 pcs	
Di Tan Decoction (Di Tan Tang)	涤痰汤	Prescriptions for Saving Lives (Ji Sheng Fang)	Rhizoma Pinelliae (Ban Xia) 7.5g Rhizoma Arisaematis (Tian Nan Xing) 7.5g Pericarpium Citri Reticulatae (Chen Pi) 6g Fructus Citri Aurantii Immaturus (Zhi Shi) 6g Sclerotium Poriae Cocos (Fu Ling) 6g Radix Ginseng (Ren Shen) 3g Rhizoma Acori Tatarinowii (Shi Chang Pu) 3g Caulis Bambusae in Taeniam (Zhu Ru) 2.1g Rhizoma Zingiberis Recens (Sheng Jiang) 5 slices Radix Glycyrrhizae (Gan Cao) 1.5g	Decoct the drugs in water for oral application.
Di Yu Powder (Di Yu San)	地榆散	Effective Recipes (Yan Fang)	Radix Sanguisorbae Officinalis (Di Yu) 12g Radix Rubiae Cordifoliae (Qian Cao) 12g Radix Scutellariae (Huang Qin) 10g Rhizoma Coptidis (Huang Lian) 10g Fructus Gardeniae (Zhi Zi) 10g Sclerotium Poriae Cocos (Fu Ling) 12g	Decoct the drugs in water for oral application. Or grind the drug into fine powder, and take 3g each time, twice or thrice daily.
Dian Kuang Meng Xing Decoction (Dian Kuang Meng Xing Tang)	癫狂梦醒汤	Correction on the Errors of Medical Works (Yi Lin Gai Cuo)	Semen Pruni Persicae (Tao Ren) 24g Radix Bupleuri (Chai Hu) 9g Rhizoma Cyperi Rotundi (Xiang Fu) 6g Caulis Akebiae (Mu Tong) 9g Radix Paeoniae Rubra (Chi Shao) 9g Rhizoma Pinelliae (Ban Xia) 6g Pericarpium Arecae (Da Fu Pi) 9g Pericarpium Citri Reticulatae Viride	Decoct the drugs in water for oral application.

			(Qing Pi) 6g Pericarpium Citri Reticulatae (Chen Pi) 9g Cortex Mori Alba Radicis (Sang Bai Pi) 9g Fructus Perillae (Su Zi) 12g Radix Glycyrrhizae (Gan Cao) 15g	
Ding Chuan Decoction (Ding Chuan Tang)	定喘汤	Effective Prescriptions for Health Conservation (She Sheng Zhong Miao Fang)	Semen Ginkgo (Bai Guo) 9g Herba Ephedrae (Ma Huang) 9g Fructus Perillae (Su Zi) 6g Radix Glycyrrhizae (Gan Cao) 3g Flos Farfarae (Kuan Dong Hua) 9g Semen Armeniacae Amarum (Xing Ren) 6g Cortex Mori Alba Radicis (Sang Bai Pi) 9g Radix Scutellariae (Huang Qin) 6g Rhizoma Pinelliae (Ban Xia) 9g	Decoct the drugs in water for oral application.
Ding Shi Qing Luo Decoction (Ding Shi Qing Luo Yin)	丁氏清络饮	Ding Gan Ren Yi An	Radix Cynanchi Atrati (Bai Wei) Herba Dendrobii (Shi Hu) Radix Paeoniae Rubra (Chi Shao) Caulis Lonicerae (Ren Dong Teng) Radix Rehmanniae Recens (Sheng Di Huang) Cortex Lycii Radicis (Di Gu Pi) Cortex Moutan Radicis (Mu Dan Pi) Herba Artemisiae (Qing Hao) Ramulus Mori (Sang Zhi) Lumbricus (Di Long) Radix Clematidis (Wei Ling Xian) Fasciculus Vascularis Luffae (Si Gua Luo) Cornu Saigae Tataricae (Ling Yang Jiao)	Decoct Ling Yang Jiao in water first for 30 minutes, then add rest of the drugs and decoct them for oral application.
Ding Xian Pill (Ding Xian Wan)	定痫丸	Medicine Comprehended (Yi Xue Xin Wu)	Rhizoma Gastrodiae (Tian Ma) 6g Bulbus Fritillariae Cirrhosae (Chuan Bei Mu) 6g Rhizoma Pinelliae (Ban Xia) 6g Poria (Fu Ling) 6g Sclerotium Poriae Circum Radicem Pini (Fu Shen) 6g Rhizoma Arisaematis cum Bile (Dan Nan Xing) 3g Rhizoma Acori Tatarinowii (Shi Chang Pu) 3g Scorpio (Quan Xie) 3g Bombyx Batryticatus (Jiang Can) 3g Succinum (Hu Po) 3g Pericarpium Citri Reticulatae (Chen Pi) 4.5g Radix Polygalae (Yuan Zhi) 4.5g	Grind the drugs into fine powder, make Radix Glycyrrhizae (Gan Cao) 120g into ointment, add Succus Bambusae (Zhu Li) 100ml and Succus Rhizoma Zingiberis Recens (Jiang Zhi) 50ml. Stir evenly and make pills. Take 6g each time with warm boiled water, twice daily. Or add Radix Glycyrrhizae (Gan Cao) 12g to the drugs without Hu Po

				Radix Salviae Miltiorrhizae (Dan Shen) 12g Radix Ophiopogonis (Mai Dong) 12g Cinnabaris (Chen Sha) 2g	and Chen Sha, and decoct them in water; then remove the residue and add Zhu Li, Jiang Zhi, Hu Po 1g, and Chen Sha 0.5g for oral application.
Ding Xiang Shi Di Decoction (Ding Xiang Shi Di Tang)	丁香柿蒂汤	Cause of Sign and Pulse Treatment (Zheng Yin Mai Zhi)		Flos Caryophylli (Ding Xiang) 6g Calyx Diospyri Kaki (Shi Di) 6g Radix Ginseng (Ren Shen) 3g Rhizoma Zingiberis Recens (Sheng Jiang) 6g	Decoct the drugs in water for oral application.
Ding Zhi Pill (Ding Zhi Wan)	定志丸	Invaluable Prescriptions for Emergencies (Bei Ji Qian Jin Yao Fang)		Radix Codonopsitis Pilosulae (Dang Shen) 30g Sclerotium Poriae Circum Radicem Pini (Fu Shen) 30g Rhizoma Acori Tatarinowii (Shi Chang Pu) 15g Radix Polygalae (Yuan Zhi) 30g Radix Glycyrrhizae Praeparatae (Zhi Gan Cao) 15g Sclerotium Poriae Cocos (Fu Ling) 30g Rhizoma Atractylodis Macrocephalae (Bai Zhu) 15g Radix Ophiopogonis (Mai Dong) 15g	Grind the drugs into fine powder, add honey and make it into pills. Take 9g each time.
Du Huo Ji Sheng Decoction (Du Huo Ji Sheng Tang)	独活寄生汤	Invaluable Prescriptions for Emergencies (Bei Ji Qian Jin Yao Fang)		Radix Angelicae Pubescentis (Du Huo) 9g Herba Taxilli (Sang Ji Sheng) 6g Cortex Eucommiae (Du Zhong) 6g Radix Achyranthis Bidentatae (Huai Niu Xi) 6g Herba Asari (Xi Xin) 6g Radix Ginseng (Ren Shen) 6g Radix Gentianae Qinjiao (Qin Jiao) 6g Sclerotium Poriae Cocos (Fu Ling) 6g Cortex Cinnamomi Cassiae (Rou Gui) 6g Radix Saposhnikoviae (Fang Feng) 6g Rhizoma Ligustici Chuanxiong (Chuan Xiong) 6g Radix Rehmanniae Recens (Shu Di Huang) 6g Radix Glycyrrhizae (Gan Cao) 6g Radix Angelicae Sinensis (Dang Gui) 6g Radix Paeoniae Alba (Bai Shao) 6g	Decoct the drugs in water for oral application.

Du Shen Decoction (Du Shen Tang)	独参汤	Jingyue's Complete Works (Jing Yue Quan Shu)	Radix Ginseng (Ren Shen) 60g Fructus Zizyphi Jujubae (Da Zao) 5 pcs	Decoct the drugs in water for oral application.
Er Chen Decoction (Er Chen Tang)	二陈汤	Formularies of the Bureau of People's Pharmacy (Tai Ping Hui Min He Ji Ju Fang)	Rhizoma Pinelliae (Ban Xia) 15G Exocarpium Citri Rubrum (Ju Hong) 15g Sclerotium Poriae Cocos (Bai Fu Ling) 9g Radix Glycyrrhizae Praeparatae (Zhi Gan Cao) 4.5g Rhizoma Zingiberis Recens (Sheng Jiang) 7 slices Fructus Pruni Mume (Wu Mei) 1 pcs	Decoct the drugs except Sheng Jiang and Wu Mei in water, and then add 7 slices of Sheng Jiang and 1 pcs of Wu Mei for oral application.
Er Miao Powder (Er Miao San)	二妙散	Danxi's Experiential Therapy (Dan Xi Xin Fa)	Cortex Phellodendri (Huang Bai) 9g Rhizoma Atractylodis (Cang Zhu) 9g	Prepare the drugs into powder. Take 6g each time and add 3g Succus Rhizoma Zingiberis Recens (Sheng Jiang Zhi) for oral application. Or decoct the drugs for oral application.
Er Xian Decoction (Er Xian Tang)	二仙汤	Zhong Yi Fang Ji Lin Chuang Shou Ce	Rhizoma Curculiginis Orchioidis (Xian Mao) 9g Herba Epimedii (Xian Ling Pi) 9g Radix Morindae Officinalis (Ba Ji Tian) 9g Cortex Phellodendri (Huang Bai) 4.5g Rhizoma Anemarrhenae (Zhi Mu) 4.5g Radix Angelicae Sinensis (Dang Gui) 9g	Decoct the drugs in water for oral application. Twice daily.
Er Yin Decoction (Er Yin Jian)	二阴煎	Jingyue's Complete Works (Jing Yue Quan Shu)	Radix Rehmanniae Recens (Sheng Di Huang) 6-9g Radix Ophiopogonis (Mai Dong) 6-9g Fructus Zizyphi Jujubae (Da Zao) 6g Radix Glycyrrhizae Uralensis (Sheng Gan Cao) 3g Radix Scrophulariae (Xuan Shen) 4.5g Sclerotium Poriae Cocos (Fu Ling) 4.5g Rhizoma Coptidis (Huang Lian) 3-6g Caulis Akebiae (Mu Tong) 4.5g	Decoct the drugs in water for oral application before meals.

			Medulla Junci Effusi (Deng Xin Cao) 20 pcs Folium Phyllostachydis Henonis (Zhu Ye) 6g	
Er Zhi Pill (Er Zhi Wan)	二至丸	Collected Exegesis of Recipes (Yi Fang Ji Jie)	Fructus Ligustri Lucidi (Nu Zhen Zi) 500g Herba Ecliptae Prostratae (Han Lian Cao) 500g	Grind Nu Zhen Zi into fine powder and sift. Decoct Han Lian Cao twice, 1hour each time, mix the decoctions, sift and concentrate, and then add honey and Nu Zhen Zi powder to make pills. Let pills dry. Take 9g each time, twice daily.
Fang Feng Tong Sheng Powder (Fang Feng Tong Sheng San)	防风通圣散	Clear Synopsis on Recipes Based on Plain Questions of Huangdi (Huang Di Su Wen Xuan Ming Lun Fang)	Radix Saposhnikoviae (Fang Feng) 6g Rhizoma Ligustici Chuanxiong (Chuang Xiong) 6g Radix Angelicae Sinensis (Dang Gui) 6g Radix Paeoniae Alba (Bai Shao Yao) 6g Radix et Rhizoma Rhei (Da Huang) 6g Herba Menthae Haplocalycis (Bo He) 6g Herba Ephedrae (Ma Huang) 6g Fructus Forsythiae (Lian Qiao) 6g Natrii Sulfas (Mang Xiao) 6g Gypsum Fibrosum (Shi Gao) 12g Radix Scutellariae (Huang Qin) 12g Radix Platycodonis (Jie Geng) 12g Talcum (Hua Shi Fen) 20g Radix Glycyrrhizae (Gan Cao) 9g Herba Schizonepetae (Jing Jie) 3g Rhizoma Atractylodis Macrocephalae (Bai Zhu) 3g Fructus Gardeniae Jasminoidis (Zhi Zi) 3g	Prepare the drugs into pills or powder, and take 6g each time, twice daily. Or decoct the drugs with 3 slices of Sheng Jiang in water for oral application.
Fang Ji Huang Qi Decoction (Fang J Huang Qi Tang)	防己黄芪汤	Synopsis of Golden Chamber (Jin Gui Yao Lue)	Radix Stephaniae Tetrandrae (Fang Ji) 12g Radix Astragali (Huang Qi) 15g Radix Glycyrrhizae (Gan Cao) 6g Rhizoma Atractylodis Macrocephalae (Chao Bai Zhu) 9g Rhizoma Zingiberis Recens (Sheng Jiang) 4 slices Fructus Zizyphi Jujubae (Da Zao) 1 pcs	Decoct the drugs in water for oral application.

Fu Ling Pi Decoction (Fu Ling Pi Tang)	茯苓皮汤	Analysis of Warm Diseases (Wen Bing Tiao Bian)	Cortex Poriae Cocos (Fu Ling Pi) 15g Semen Coicis (Yi Yi Ren) 15g Sclerotium Polypori Umbellati (Zhu Ling) 9g Pericarpium Arecae (Da Fu Pi) 9g Medulla Tetrapanacis (Tong Cao) 9g Herba Lophatheri (Dan Zhu Ye) 6g	Decoct the drugs in water for oral application. Take 1/3 of the decoction each time.
Fu Mai Decoction (Fu Mai Tang). Also named Zhi Gan Cao Decoction.	复脉汤 (炙甘草汤)	Treatise on Cold Induced Disease (Shang Han Lun)	Radix Glycyrrhizae Praeparatae (Zhi Gan Cao) 12g Rhizoma Zingiberis Recens (Sheng Jiang) 9g Radix Ginseng (Ren Shen) 6g Radix Rehmanniae Recens (Sheng Di Huang) 50g Ramulus Cinnamomi (Gui Zhi) 9g Colla Corii Asini (E Jiao) 6g Radix Ophiopogonis (Mai Dong) 10g Semen Cannabis (Huo Ma Ren) 9g Fructus Zizyphi Jujubae (Da Zao) 30 pcs	Decoct the drugs except E Jiao in water for oral application, and stew E Jiao separately till it is melted.
Fu Yuan Huo Xue Decoction (Fu Yuan Huo Xue Tang)	复元活血汤	Medical Inventions (Yi Xue Fa Ming)	Radix Bupleuri (Chai Hu) 15g Semen Persicae (Tao Ren) 15g Radix Trichosanthis (Tian Hua Fen) 9g Radix Angelicae Sinensis (Dang Gui) 9g Radix et Rhizoma Rhei (Da Huang) 30g Flos Carthami (Hong Hua) 6g Radix Glycyrrhizae (Gan Cao) 6g Manitis Pentadactylae Squama (Chuan Shan Jia) 6g	Prepare the drugs into powder. Decoct 30g of the powder and 30ml yellow rice wine (Huang Jiu) in water each time for oral application. Or decoct all drugs in water for oral application.
Fu Zi Li Zhong Pill (Fu Zi Li Zhong Wan). Also name Fu Zi Li Zhong Decoction (Fu Zi Li Zhong Tang)	附子理中丸 (又名附子理中汤)	Treatise on Cold Induceed Diseases (Shang Han Lun)	Radix Aconiti Lateralis Praeparatae (Fu Zi) 9g Radix Ginseng (Ren Shen) 9g Radix Glycyrrhizae Praeparatae (Zhi Gan Cao) 9g Rhizoma Atractylodis Macrocephalae (Bai Zhu) 9g Rhizoma Zingiberis (Gan Jiang) 9g	Grind the drugs into coarse powder, mix it with honey, and make into pills with 9g each. Take one pill with warm boiled water each time, three times a day. Or decoct the drugs in water for oral application.
Gan Jiang Ling Zhu Decoction (Gan Jiang Ling Zhu Tang)	甘姜苓术汤	Synopsis of the Golden Chamber (Jin Gui Yao Lue)	Radix Glycyrrhizae (Gan Cao) 12g Rhizoma Zingiberis (Gan Jiang) 12g Sclerotium Poriae Cocos (Fu Ling) 12g Rhizoma Atractylodis Macrocepha-	Decoct the drugs in water for oral application.

Formula	Chinese	Source	Ingredients	Administration
			lae (Bai Zhu) 12g	
Gan Lu Xiao Du Powder (Gan Lu Xiao Du Dan)	甘露消毒丹	Experience of Medicine Secretly Pass on (Yi Xiao Mi Chuang)	Talcum (Hua Shi Fen) 15g Herba Artemisiae Scopariae (Yin Chen Hao) 11g Radix Scutellariae (Huang Qin) 10g Rhizoma Acori Graminei (Shi Chang Pu) 6g Bulbus Fritillariae Cirrhosae (Chuan Bei Mu) 5g Caulis Akebiae (Mu Tong) 5g Herba Agastache seu Pogostemonis (Huo Xiang) 4g Rhizoma Belamcandae (She Gan) 4g Fructus Forsythiae Suspensae (Lian Qiao) 4g Herba Menthae (Bo He) 4g Fructus Amomi Rotundus (Bai Dou Kou) 4g	Prepare the drugs into powder, and take 6-9g each time with warm boiled water. Or decoct the drugs for oral application.
Gan Mai Da Zao Decoction (Gan Mai Da Zao Tang)	甘麦大枣汤	Synopsis of the Golden Chamber (Jin Gui Yao Lue)	Fructus Tritici Aestivi (Xiao Mai) 30g Fructus Zizyphi Jujubae (Da Zao) 10 pcs Radix Glycyrrhizae (Gan Cao) 15g	Decoct the drugs in water for oral application.
Ge Gen Huang Qin Huang Lian Decoction (Ge Gen Huang Qin Huang Lian Tang)	葛根黄芩黄连汤	Treatise on Cold Induced Diseases (Shang Han Lun)	Radix Puerariae (Ge Gen) 24g Radix Scutellariae (Huang Qin) 9g Rhizoma Coptidis (Huang Lian) 9g Radix Glycyrrhizae Praeparatae (Zhi Gan Cao) 6g	Decoct the drugs in water for oral application.
Ge Gen Qin Lian Decoction (Ge Gen Qin Lian Tang)	葛根芩连汤	Treatise on Cold Induced Diseases (Shang Han Lun)	Radix Puerariae (Ge Gen) 24g Radix Scutellariae (Huang Qin) 9g Rhizoma Coptidis (Huang Lian) 9g Radix Glycyrrhizae Praeparatae (Zhi Gan Cao) 6g	Decoct the drugs in water for oral application.
Ge Gen Decoction (Ge Gen Tang)	葛根汤	Treatise on Cold Induced Diseases (Shang Han Lun)	Radix Puerariae (Ge Gen) Herba Ephedrae (Ma Huang) Rhizoma Zingiberis Recens (Sheng Jiang) Ramulus Cinnamomi (Gui Zhi) Radix Paeoniae (Shao Yao) Radix Glycyrrhizae Praeparatae (Zhi Gan Cao) Fructus Zizyphi Jujubae (Da Zao)	Decoct the drugs in water for oral application.
Ge Hua Jie Cheng Decoction (Ge Hua Jie Cheng San)	葛花解醒汤	Treatise on the Spleen and Stomach (Pi Wei Lun)	Flos Puerariae (Ge Hua) 15g Fructus Amomi Kravanh (Bai Dou Kou) 15g Fructus Amomi (Sha Ren) 15g Pericarpium Citri Reticulatae Viride (Qing Pi) 0.9g Pericarpium Citri Reticulatae (Ju Pi) 4.5g Radix Ginseng (Ren Shen) 4.5g	Grind the drugs into extremely fine powder, mix evenly. Take 10g each time with warm boiled water.

			Rhizoma Atractylodis Macrocephalae (Bai Zhu) 6g Sclerotium Poriae Cocos (Fu Ling) 4.5g Massa Medicata Fermentata (Shen Qu) 6g Rhizoma Zingiberis (Gan Jiang) 6g Sclerotium Polypori Umbellati (Zhu Ling) 4.5g Rhizoma Alismatis (Ze Xie) 6g Radix Aucklandiae (Mu Xiang) 1.5g	
Ge Xia Zhu Yu Decoction (Ge Xia Zhu Yu Tang)	膈下逐瘀汤	Correction on the Errors of Medical Works (Yi Lin Gai Cuo)	Excrementum Trogopteri (Wu Ling Zhi) 6g Radix Angelicae Sinensis (Dang Gui) 9g Semen Pruni Persicae (Tao Ren) 9g Radix Linderae (Wu Yao) 6g Radix Glycyrrhizae (Gan Cao) 9g Flos Carthami Tinctorii (Hong Hua) 9g Rhizoma Ligustici Chuanxiong (Chuan Xiong) 6g Cortex Moutan Radicis (Mu Dan Pi) 6g Radix Paeoniae Rubra (Chi Shao) 6g Rhizoma Cyperi Rotundi (Xiang Fu) 4.5g Fructus Citri Aurantii (Zhi Ke) 4.5g Rhizoma Corydalis (Yan Hu Suo) 3g	Decoct the drugs in water for oral application.
Gu Chong Decoction (Gu Chong Tang)	固冲汤	Discourse on Medical Problems by Integrated Traditional Chinese and Western Medicine (Yi Xue Zhong Zhong Can Xi Lu)	Rhizoma Atractylodis Macrocephalae (Bai Zhu) 30g Radix Astragali (Sheng Huang Qi) 18g Os Draconis (Long Gu) 24g Concha Ostreae (Mu Li) 24g Fructus Corni (Shan Zhu Yu) 24g Radix Paeoniae Alba (Sheng Bai Shao) 12g Os Sepiae seu Sepiellae (Hai Piao Xiao) 12g Radix Rubiae (Qian Cao) 9g Trachycarpi Carbonisa tus (Zong Bian Tan) 6g Galla Chinensis (Wu Bei Zi) 1.5g	Decoct the drugs in water for oral application. Grind Galla Chinensis into powder and take half with water each time, twice daily.
Gu Jing Pill (Gu Jing Wan)	固经丸	Danxi's Experiential Therapy (Dan Xi Xin Fa)	Cortex Phellodendri (Huang Bai) 6g Radix Scutellariae (Huang Qin) 9g Cortex Ailanthi (Chun Pi) 9g Radix Paeoniae Alba (Bai Shao Yao) 9g Plastrum Testudinis (Gui Ban) 9g	Decoct the drugs in water for oral application. Or prepare into pills, take 6-9g each time, twice daily.

			Rhizoma Cyperi (Xiang Fu) 5g	
Gua Di Powder (Gua Di San)	瓜蒂散	Treatise on Cold Induced Diseases (Shang Han Lun)	Pedicellus Melo (Gua Di) 3g Semen Phaseoli (Chi Xiao Dou) 3g Fermented Soybean (Dan Dou Chi) 9g	Decoct the drugs in water for oral application. Or prepare Gua Di and Chi Xiao Dou into powder, and take 1-3g each time with Dou Chi decoction.
Gua Lou Gui Zhi Decoction (Gua Lou Gui Zhi Tang)	瓜蒌桂枝汤	Synopsis of the Golden Chamber (Jin Gui Yao Lue)	Fructus Trichosanthis (Gua Lou Shi) 6g Ramulus Cinnamomi (Gui Zhi) 9g Radix Paeoniae (Shao Yao) 9g Radix Glycyrrhizae (Gan Cao) 6g Rhizoma Zingiberis Recens (Sheng Jiang) 9g Fructus Zizyphi Jujubae (Da Zao) 12 pcs	Decoct the drugs for oral application.
Gua Lou Xie Bai Bai Jiu Decoction (Gua Lou Xie Bai Bai Jiu Tang)	瓜蒌薤白白酒汤	Synopsis of the Golden Chamber (Jin Gui Yao Lue)	Fructus Trichosanthis (Gua Lou Shi) 15g Bulbus Allii Macrostemonis (Xie Bai) 12g White Spirit (Bai Jiu) 100ml	Decoct the drugs for oral application.
Gua Lou Xie Bai Ban Xia Decoction (Gua Lou Xie Bai Ban Xia Tang)	瓜蒌薤白半夏汤	Synopsis of the Golden Chamber (Jin Gui Yao Lue)	Fructus Trichosanthis (Gua Lou Shi) 15g Bulbus Allii Macrostemonis (Xie Bai) 12g Rhizoma Pinelliae (Ban Xia) 12g White Spirit (Bai Jiu) 100ml	Decoct the drugs for oral application.
Gui Lu Er Xian Glue (Gui Lu Er Xian Jiao)	龟鹿二仙胶	Convenience for Treatment (Yi Bian)	Cornu Cervi (Lu Jiao) 5000g Plastrum Testudinis (Gui Ban) 2500g Fructus Lycii (Gou Qi Zi) 900g Radix Ginseng (Ren Shen) 450g	Boil the drugs into glue on top of a lead jar. Take 4.5g with wine (Jiu) at the first time before meal and increase the dosage gradually to 9g each time.
Gui Pi Decoction (Gui Pi Tang)	归脾汤	Classification and Treatment of Traumatic Diseases (Zheng Ti Lei Yao)	Radix Ginseng (Ren Shen) 9g Rhizoma Atractylodis Macrocephalae (Bai Zhu) 9g Sclerotium Poriae Circum Radicem Pini (Fu Shen) 9g Semen Zizyphi Spinosae (Suan Zao Ren) 9g Arillus Longan (Long Yan Rou) 9g Radix Astragali (Huang Qi) 9g Radix Angelicae Sinensis (Dang Gui) 9g Radix Polygalae (Yuan Zhi) 9g Radix Aucklandiae Lappae (Mu Xiang) 5g Radix Glycyrrhizae Praeparatae	Decoct the drugs in water for oral application.

			(Zhi Gan Cao) 3g Rhizoma Zingiberis Recens (Sheng Jiang) 2 slices Fructus Zizyphi Jujubae (Da Zao) 3 pcs	
Gui Shao Di Huang Decoction (Gui Shao Di Huang Tang)	归芍地黄汤	Bing Yin Mai Zhi	Radix Angelicae Sinensis (Dang Gui) Radix Paeoniae Alba (Bai Shao Yao) Radix Rehmanniae Recens (Sheng Di Huang) Fructus Corni Officinalis (Shan Zhu Yu) Rhizoma Dioscoreae (Shan Yao) Cortex Moutan Radicis (Mu Dan Pi) Sclerotium Poriae Cocos (Fu Ling) Rhizoma Alismatis (Ze Xie)	Decoct the drugs in water for oral application.
Gui Shao Liu Jun Zi Decoction (Gui Shao Liu Jun Zi Tang)	归芍六君子汤	Bi Hua Yi Jing	Radix Angelicae Sinensis (Dang Gui) 6g Radix Paeoniae Alba (Bai Shao Yao) 6g Radix Ginseng (Ren Shen) 4.5g Rhizoma Atractylodis Macrocephalae (Bai Zhu) 4.5g Sclerotium Poriae Cocos (Fu Ling) 4.5g Pericarpium Citri Reticulatae (Chen Pi) 3g Rhizoma Pinelliae (Ban Xia) 3g Radix Glycyrrhizae Praeparatae (Zhi Gan Cao) 1.5g	Decoct the drugs in water for oral application.
Gui Zhi Decoction (Gui Zhi Tang)	桂枝汤	Treatise on Cold Induced Diseases (Shang Han Lun)	Ramulus Cinnamomi (Gui Zhi) 9g Radix Paeoniae Alba (Bai Shao Yao) 9g Rhizoma Zingiberis Recens (Sheng Jiang) 9g Fructus Zizyphi Jujubae (Da Zao) 3 pcs Radix Glycyrrhizae Praeparatae (Gan Cao) 6g	Decoct the drugs in water for oral application, and then take some hot gruel and lie in warm bed to induce slight perspiration.
Gui Zhi Fu Ling Pill (Gui Zhi Fu Ling Wan)	桂枝茯苓丸	Synopsis of the Golden Chamber (Jin Gui Yao Lue)	Ramulus Cinnamomi (Gui Zhi) 6g Sclerotium Poriae Cocos (Fu Ling) 6g Cortex Moutan Radicis (Mu Dan Pi) 6g Semen Persicae (Tao Ren) 6g Radix Paeoniae (Shao Yao) 6g	Make the drugs into pills with honey (Feng Mi), and take 3-5g daily. Or decoct the drugs in water for oral application.
Gui Zhi Gan Cao Long Gu Mu Li Decoction (Gui Zhi Gan Cao Long	桂枝甘草龙骨牡蛎汤	Treatise on Cold Induceed Diseases (Shang Han	Ramulus Cinnamomi (Gui Zhi) 3g Radix Glycyrrhizae Praeparatae (Zhi Gan Cao) 6g Calcined Os Draconis (Long Gu)	Decoct the drugs in water for oral application.

Gu Mu Li Tang)		Lun)	6g Calcined Concha Ostreae (Mu Li) 6g	
Gui Zhi Shao Yao Zhi Mu Decoction (Gui Zhi Shao Yao Zhi Mu)	桂枝芍药知母汤	Synopsis of the Golden Chamber (Jin Gui Yao Lue)	Ramulus Cinnamomi (Gui Zhi) 12g Radix Paeoniae (Shao Yao) 9g Radix Glycyrrhizae Praeparatae (Zhi Gan Cao) 6g Herba Ephedrae (Ma Huang) 6g Rhizoma Atractylodis Macrocephalae (Bai Zhu) 15g Rhizoma Anemarrhenae (Zhi Mu) 12g Radix Saposhnikoviae (Fang Feng) 12g Radix Aconiti Lateralis Praeparatae (Fu Zi) 10g Rhizoma Zingiberis Recens (Sheng Jiang) 15g	Decoct the drugs in water for oral application.
Gun Tan Pill (Gun Tan Wan). Also named Meng Shi Gun Tan Pill (Meng Shi Gun Tan Wan)	滚痰丸 (又名礞石滚痰丸)	Main Discussions on Health Cultivation of Taiding (Tai Ding Yang Sheng Zhu Lun)	Radix et Rhizoma Rhei (Da Huang) 240g Radix Scutellariae (Huang Qin) 240g Lapis Chloriti (Meng Shi) 30g Lignum Aquilariae Resinatum (Chen Xiang) 15g	Make the drugs into pills with water. Take 6-9g each time with warm biled water, once or twice daily.
Guo Min Decoction (Guo Min Jian)	过敏煎	Effective Recipes (Yan Fang)	Radix Bupleuri (Chai Hu) 15g Radix Paeoniae Alba (Bai Shao Yao) 12g Radix Saposhnikoviae (Fang Feng) 12g Fructus Schisandrae Chinensis (Wu Wei Zi) 6g Fructus Pruni Mume (Wu Mei) 6g	Decoct the drugs in water for oral application.
Hai Zao Yu Hu Decoction (Hai Zao Yu Hu Tang)	海藻玉壶汤	Golden Mirror of Medicine (Yi Zong Jin Jian)	Herba Sargassi (Hai Zao) 3g Thallus Laminariae (Hai Dai) 1.5g Thallus Eckloniae (Kun Bu) 3g Rhizoma Pinelliae (Ban Xia) 3g Pericarpium Citri Reticulatae (Chen Pi) 3g Pericarpium Citri Reticulatae Viride (Qing Pi) 3g Fructus Forsythiae (Lian Qiao) 3g Bulbus Fritillariae (Bei Mu) 3g Radix Angelicae Sinensis (Dang Gui) 3g Rhizoma Ligustici Chuanxiong (Chuan Xiong) 3g Radix Angelicae Pubescentis (Du Huo) 3g Radix Glycyrrhizae (Gan Cao) 3g	Decoct the drugs in water for oral application.

Hao Qin Qing Dan Decoction (Hao Qin Qing Dan Tang)	蒿芩清胆汤	Revised Edition of Popular Cold Induced Diseases (Chong Ding Tong Su Shang Han Lun)	Herba Artemisiae Annuae (Qing Hao) 4.5-6g Caulis Bambusae in Taenia (Zhu Ru) 9g Rhizoma Pinelliae (Ban Xia) 4.5g Poriae Rubra (Chi Fu Ling) 9g Radix Scutellariae (Huang Qin) 4.5-9g Fructus Citri Aurantii (Zhi Ke) 4.5g Pericarpium Citri Reticulatae (Chen Pi) 4.5g Bi Yu Powder (Bi Yu San) 9g composed of Talcum (Hua Shi Fen), Radix Glycyrrhizae (Gan Cao) and Indigo Naturalis (Qing Dai)	Decoct the drugs in water for oral application.
He Che Da Zao Pill (He Che Da Zao)	河车大造丸	Fu Shou Jing Fang	Placenta Hominis (Zi He Che) 100g Radix Rehmanniae Praeparatae (Shu Di Huang) 200g Cortex Eucommiae (Du Zhong) 150g Radix Asparagi (Tian Dong) 100g Radix Ophiopogonis (Mai Dong) 100g Carapax et Plastrum Testudinis (Gui Ban) 200g Cortex Phellodendri (Huang Bai) 150g Radix Achyranthis Bidentatae (Niu Xi) 100g	Grind the drugs into fine powder, sift and mix evenly. Add 80-100g of honey, and make the powder into pills. Take 9g each time.
Hou Po Wen Zhong Decoction (Hou Po Wen Zhong Tang)	厚朴温中汤	Differentiation on Endogenous and Exogenous Diseases (Nei Wai Shang Bian Huo Lun)	Cortex Magnoliae Officinalis (Hou Po) 10g Pericarpium Citri Reticulatae (Chen Pi) 10g Rhizoma Zingiberis (Gan Jiang) 3g Semen Alpiniae Katsumadai (Cao Dou Kou) 5g Sclerotium Poriae Cocos (Fu Ling) 5g Radix Aucklandiae (Mu Xiang) 5g Radix Glycyrrhizae Praeparatae (Zhi Gan Cao) 5g	Decoct the drugs in water for oral application. Or grind the drugs into powder, decoct powder 10g with fresh ginger 3 slices, and remove residue.
Hua Ban Decoction (Hua Ban Tang)	化斑汤	Analysis of Warm Diseases (Wen Bing Tiao Bian)	Gypsum Fibrosum (Shi Gao) 30g Rhizoma Anemarrhenae (Zhi Mu) 12g Radix Glycyrrhizae (Gan Cao) 9g Radix Scrophulariae (Xuan Shen) 9g Cornu Bubali (Shui Niu Jiao) 60g [to replace Cornu Rhinocerotis (Xi Jiao) 6g] Semen Oryzae Sativae (Jing Mi) 9g	Decoct the drugs in water for oral application. Take 1/3 each time, thrice daily. Decoct the residue for bedtime oral application.
Hua Chong Pill	化虫丸	Formularies	Plumbi Carbonas et Hydrox (Qian	Grind the drugs into

(Hua Chong Wan)		of the Bureau of People's Pharmacy (Tai Ping Hui Min He Ji Ju Fang)	Fen) 1500g Fructus Carpesii (He Shi) 1500g Semen Arecae (Bing Lang) 1500g Cortex Meliae (Ku Lian Pi) 1500g Alumen (Ku Fan) 375g	fine powder and make into pillets with flour. Take 6g each time with thin gruel before mails, once daily. 1g for one year old children.
Hua Gan Decoction (Hua Gan Jian)	化肝煎	Jingyue's Complete Works (Jing Yue Quan Shu)	Cortex Moutan Radicis (Mu Dan Pi) 4.5g Fructus Gardeniae (Zhi Zi) 4.5g Radix Paeoniae Alba (Bai Shao Yao) 6g Pericarpium Citri Reticulatae Viride (Qing Pi) 6g Pericarpium Citri Reticulatae (Chen Pi) 6g Rhizoma Alismatis (Ze Xie) 4.5g Tuber Bolbostemmatis (Tu Bei Mu) 6-9g	Decoct the drugs in water for oral application before meals.
Huai Hua Powder (Huai Hua San)	槐花散	Prescriptions for Universal Relief and ability (Pu Ji Ben Shi Fang)	Flos Sophorae (Huai Hua) 9g Cacumen Biotae (Ce Bai Ye) 9g Herba Schizonepetae (Jing Jie Sui) 9g Fructus Citri Aurantii (Zhi Ke) 9g	Decoct the drugs in water for oral application.
Huan Shao Pill (Huan Shao Dan)	还少丹	Collected Exegesis of Recipes (Yi Fang Ji Jie)	Radix Rehmanniae Praeparatae (Shu Di Huang) Fructus Lycii (Gou Qi Zi) Fructus Corni Officinalis (Shan Zhu Yu) Herba Cistanches (Rou Cong Rong) Radix Morindae Officinalis (Ba Ji Tian) Fructus Foeniculi Vulgaris (Xiao Hui Xiang) Cortex Eucommiae (Du Zhong) Radix Achyranthis Bidentatae (Huai Niu Xi) Fructus Broussonetiae (Chu Shi Zi) Sclerotium Poriae Cocos (Fu Ling) Rhizoma Dioscoreae (Shan Yao) Fructus Zizyphi Jujubae (Da Zao) Rhizoma Acori Tatarinowii (Shi Chang Pu) Radix Polygalae Tenuifoliae (Yuan Zhi) Fructus Schisandrae Chinensis (Wu Wei Zi) (Equal in dosage)	Grind the drugs into powder, and make pills with honey. Take 6-9g each time, twice daily.
Huang Lian E Jiao Decoction (Huang	黄连阿胶	Treatise on Cold Indu-	Rhizoma Coptidis (Huang Lian) 12g	Decoct the drugs except E Jiao and

Formula	Chinese	Source	Ingredients	Preparation
(Huang Lian E Jiao)	汤	ceed Diseases (Shang Han Lun)	Radix Scutellariae (Huang Qin) 6g Colla Corii Asini (E Jiao) 9g Radix Paeoniae Alba (Bai Shao Yao) 6g Egg Yolk (Ji Zi Huang) 2 pcs	Egg Yolk in water, remove residue, and add E Jiao to the decoction until it is melted. Then add yolk and mix evenly.
Huang Lian Jie Du Decoction (Huang Lian Jie Du Tang)	黄连解毒汤	A Handbook of Prescriptions for Emergencies (Zhou Hou Bei Zi Fang)	Radix Scutellariae (Huang Qin) 9g Rhizoma Coptidis (Huang Lian) 9g Cortex Phellodendri (Huang Bai) 6g Fructus Gardeniae (Zhi Zi) 9g	Decoct the drugs in water for oral application.
Huang Lian Shang Qing Pill (Huang Lian Shang Qing Wan)	黄连上清丸	Zhong Guo Yao Dian	Radix et Rhizoma Rhei Praeparatae (Jiu Da Huang) 320g Rhizoma Coptidis (Huang Lian) 10g Radix Scutellariae (Huang Qin) 80g Cortex Phellodendri (Jiu Huang Bai) 40g Fructus Gardeniae Jasminoidis (Zhi Zi) 80g Fructus Forsythiae (Lian Qiao) 80g Flos Chrysanthemi (Ju Hua) 160g Radix Platycodonis (Jie Geng) 80g Herba Menthae (Bo He) 40g Rhizoma Ligustici Chuanxiong (Chuan Xiong) 40g Fructus Viticis (Man Jing Zi) 80g Radix Saposhnikoviae (Fang Feng) 40g Spica Schizonepetae (Jing Jie Sui) 80g Radix Angelicae Dahuricae (Bai Zhi) 80g Gypsum Fibrosum (Shi Gao) 40g Flos Inulae (Xuan Fu Hua) 20g Radix Glycyrrhizae (Gan Cao) 40g	Grind the drugs into fine powder, sift and mix evenly. For every 100g of powder, add 150-170g of honey and make it into pills (6g per pill). Take 6-12g each time, twice daily.
Huang Lian Shang Qing Pill (Huang Lian Shang Qing Wan)	黄连上清丸	Ci He Ting Ji Fang	Radix et Rhizoma Rhei (Da Huang) 36g Rhizoma Coptidis (Huang Lian) 24g Radix Scutellariae (Huang Qin) 24g Cortex Phellodendri (Huang Bai) 24g Fructus Gardeniae Jasminoidis (Zhi Zi) 24g Rhizoma Curcumae Longae (Jiang Huang) 18g Fructus Forsythiae (Lian Qiao) 18g Flos Chrysanthemi (Ju Hua) 12g Tail of Radix Angelicae Sinensis (Dang Gui Wei) 12g	Grind the drugs into fine powder, and make into pills with honey. Take 9g each time.

			Radix Platycodonis (Jie Geng) 6g Radix Puerariae (Ge Gen) 6g Herba Menthae (Bo He) 12g Radix Scrophulariae (Xuan Shen) 12g Radix Trichosanthis (Tian Hua Fen) 6g Rhizoma Ligustici Chuanxiong (Chuan Xiong) 6g	
Huang Lian Qing Xin Decoction (Huang Lian Qing Xin Yin)	黄连清心饮	Shen Shi Zun Sheng Shu	Rhizoma Coptidis (Huang Lian) Radix Rehmanniae Recens (Sheng Di Huang) Radix Angelicae Sinensis (Dang Gui) Radix Glycyrrhizae (Gan Cao) Sclerotium Poriae Circum Radicem Pini (Fu Shen) Radix Polygalae (Yuan Zhi) Semen Ziziphi Spinosae (Suan Zao Ren) Radix Ginseng (Ren Shen) Semen Nelumbinis (Lian Zi) 10g	Decoct the drugs in water for oral application after meals.
Huang Lian Wen Dan Decoction (Huang Lian Wen Dan Tang)	黄连温胆汤	Invaluable Prescriptions for Emergencies (Bei Ji Qian Jin Yao Fang)	Rhizoma Coptidis (Huang Lian) 6-9g Pericarpium Citri Reticulatae (Chen Pi) 9g Rhizoma Pinelliae (Ban Xia) 6g Fructus Citri Aurantii Immaturus (Zhi Shi) 6g Caulis Bambusae in Taeniam (Zhu Ru) 6g Sclerotium Poriae Cocos (Fu Ling) 4.5g Radix Glycyrrhizae Praeparatae (Zhi Gan Cao) 3g Rhizoma Zingiberis Recens (Sheng Jiang) 5 slices Fructus Zizyphi Jujubae (Da Zao) 1 piece	Decoct the drugs in water for oral application.
Huang Lian Xiang Ru Decoction (Huang Lian Xiang Ru Yin)	黄连香薷饮	Collected Exegesis of Recipes (Yi Fang Ji Jie)	Herba Elsholtziae seu Moslae (Xiang Ru) 4.5g Cortex Magnoliae Officinalis (Hou Po) 4.5g Semen Dolichoris Lablab (Bian Dou) 9g Rhizoma Coptidis (Huang Lian) 6g	Decoct the drugs in water for oral application.
Huang Long Decoction (Huang Long Tang)	黄龙汤	Six Books on Cold Induced Diseases (Shang Han Liu Lun)	Radix et Rhizoma Rhei (Da Huang) 9g Natrii Sulfas (Mang Xiao) 6g Fructus Citri Aurantii Immaturus (Zhi Shi) 6g Cortex Magnoliae Officinalis (Hou	Decoct the drugs except Mang Xiao in water, and then dissolve Mang Xiao in the decoction for oral application.

			Po) 6g Radix Angelicae Sinensis (Dang Gui) 9g Radix Ginseng (Ren Shen) 6g Radix Glycyrrhizae (Gan Cao) 3g Radix Platycodonis (Jie Geng) 3g Rhizoma Zingiberis Recens (Sheng Jiang) 3 slices Fructus Zizyphi Jujubae (Da Zao) 2 pcs	
Huang Qi Decoction (Huang Qi Tang)	黄芪汤	Jin Gui Yi	Radix Astragali (Huang Qi) Pericarpium Citri Reticulatae (Chen Pi) Semen Cannabis (Huo Ma Ren) White Honey	Decoct the drugs in water for oral application.
Huang Qi Jian Zhong Decoction (Huang Qi Jian Zhong Tang)	黄芪建中汤	Synopsis of the Golden Chamber (JinGui Yao Lue)	Radix Astragali (Huang Qi) 5g Radix Paeoniae (Shao Yao) 18g Ramulus Cinnamomi (Gui Zhi) 9g Radix Glycyrrhizae Praeparatae (Zhi Gan Cao) 6g Rhizoma Zingiberis Recens (Sheng Jiang) 9g Fructus Zizyphi Jujubae (Da Zao) 4 pcs Saccharum Granorum (Yi Tang) 30g	Decoct the drugs in water for oral application.
Huang Qi Gui Zhi Wu Wu Decoction (Huang Qi Gui ZhiWu Wu Tang)	黄芪桂枝五物汤	Synopsis of the Golden Chamber (JinGui Yao Lue)	Radix Astragali (Huang Qi) 9g Radix Paeoniae Alba (Bai Shao Yao) 9g Ramulus Cinnamomi (Gui Zhi) 9g Rhizoma Zingiberis Recens (Sheng Jiang) 18g Fructus Zizyphi Jujubae (Da Zao) 4 pcs	Decoct the drugs in water for oral application.
Huang Qi Liu Yi Powder (Huang Qi Liu Yi San)	黄芪六一散	Formularies of the Bureau of People's Welfare Pharmacy (Tai Ping Hui Min He Ji Ju Fang)	Radix Astragali (Huang Qi) Radix Glycyrrhizae (Gan Cao)	Decoct the drugs in water for oral application.
Huang Qi Sheng Mai Decoction (Huang Qi Sheng Mai Yin)	黄芪生脉饮	The Origin of Medicine (Yi Xue Qi Yuan)	Modified Sheng Mai Powder (Sheng Mai San) supplemented with Radix Astragali (Huang Qi) Note: replace Radix Ginseng (Ren Shen) with Radix Codonopsitis Pilosulae (Dang Shen)	Decoct the drugs in water for oral application.
Huang Tu Decoction (Huang Tu Tang)	黄土汤	Synopsis of the Golden Chamber (JinGui Yao	Radix Glycyrrhizae (Gan Cao) 9g Radix Rehmanniae Recens (Gan Di Huang) 9g Rhizoma Atractylodis Macrocepha-	Decoct Zao Xin Tu first in water and collect the decoction; then add other drugs

		Lue)	lae (Bai Zhu) 9g Radix Aconiti Lateralis Praeparatae (Fu Zi) 9g Colla Corii Asini (E Jiao) 9g Radix Scutellariae (Huang Qin) 9g Terra Flava Usta (Zao Xin Tu) 30g	except E Jiao in the decoction and decoct again. Finally melt E Jiao in the decoction for oral application.
Huai Jiao Pill (Huai Jiao Wan)	槐角丸	Danxi's Experiential Therapy (Dan Xi Xin Fa)	Fructus Sophorae (Huai Jiao) 60g Radix Sanguisorbae Officinalis (Di Yu) 30g Radix Scutellariae (Huang Qin) 30g Radix Angelicae Sinensis (Dang Gui) 30g Stir-fried Fructus Citri Aurantii (Chao Zhi Ke) 30g Radix Saposhnikoviae (Fang Feng) 30g	Grind the drugs into fine powder, sift and mix evenly. Then add honey to make pills (for every 100g of powder, add 130-150g of honey). Take 9g each time, twice daily.
Hui Yang Jiu Ji Decoction (Hui Yang Jiu Ji Tang)	回阳救急汤	Six Books on Cold Induced Diseases (Shang Han Liu Shu)	Radix Aconiti Lateralis Praeparatae (Fu Zi) 9g Rhizoma Zingiberis (Gan Jiang) 6g Cortex Cinnamomi (Rou Gui) 3g Radix Ginseng (Ren Shen) 6g Rhizoma Atractylodis Macrocephalae Praeparatae (Chao Mai Zhu) 9g Sclerotium Poriae Cocos (Fu Ling) 9g Pericarpium Citri Reticulatae (Chen Pi) 6g Radix Glycyrrhizae Praeparatae (Zhi Gan Cao) 6g Fructus Schisandrae Chinensis (Wu Wei Zi) 3g Rhizoma Pinelliae (Ban Xia) 9g Rhizoma Zingiberis Recens (Sheng Jiang) 2 slices	Decoct the drugs in water for oral application. Before taking, add 0.1g Moschus (She Xiang).
Huo Luo Pill (Huo Luo Dan). Also named Xiao Huo Luo Pill (Xiao Huo Luo Dan)	活络丹	Formularies of the Bureau of People's Welfare Pharmacy (Tai Ping Hui Min He Ji Ju Fang)	Rhizoma Arisaematis (Tian Nan Xing) 180g Radix Aconiti Carmichaeli (Chuan Wu) 180g Radix Aconiti Kusnezoffii (Cao Wu) 180g Lumbricus (Di Long) 180g Olibanum (Ru Xiang) 66g Myrrha (Mo Yao) 66g	Prepare the drugs into boluses with honey (3g per bolus). Take one bolus each time with old wine or warm boiled water.
Huo Luo Xiao Ling Pill (Huo Luo Xiao Ling Dan)	活络效灵丹	Discourse on Medical Problems by Integrated Traditional Chinese and Western Medicine (Yi Xue Zhong	Radix Angelicae Sinensis (Dang Gui) 15g Radix Salviae Miltiorrhizae (Dan Shen) 15g Gummi Olibanum (Ru Xiang) 15g Myrrha (Mo Yao) 15g	Decoct the drugs in water for oral application. Or grind the drugs into fine power, and take 1/4 each time with warm wine.

		Zhong Can Xi Lu)		
Huo Po Xia Ling Decoction (Huo Po Xia Ling Tang)	藿朴夏苓汤	Shi Wen Shi Yi Zhi Liao Fa	Herba Agastache seu Pogostemonis (Huo Xiang) 6g Cortex Magnoliae Officinalis (Hou Po) 3g Rhizoma Pinelliae (Ban Xia) 5g Semen Pruni Armeniacae (Xing Ren) 9g Fructus Amomi Cardamomi (Bai Kou Ren) 2g Semen Coicis (Yi Yi Ren) 12g Sclerotium Poriae Cocos (Fu Ling) 9g Sclerotium Polypori Umbellati (Zhu Ling) 5g Rhizoma Alismatis (Ze Xie) 5g Medulla Tetrapanacis (Tong Cao) 3g	Decoct the drugs in water for oral application.
Huo Xiang Zheng Qi Powder (Huo Xiang Zheng Qi San)	藿香正气散	Formularies of the Bureau of People's Welfare Pharmacy (Tai Ping Hui Ming He Ji Ju Fang)	Herba Agastaches (Huo Xiang) 9g Pericarpium Arecae (Da Fu Pi) 6g Folium Perillae Frutescentis (Zi Su Ye) 6g Sclerotium Poriae Cocos (Fu Ling) 6g Radix Angelicae Dahuricae (Bai Zhi) 6g Radix Platycodonis (Jie Geng) 6g Rhizoma Atractylodis Macrocephalae (Bai Zhu) 6g Rhizoma Pinelliae (Ban Xia) 6g Pericarpium Citri Reticulatae (Chen Pi) 6g Cortex Magnoliae Officinalis (Hou Po) 6g Radix Glycyrrhizae Praeparatae (Gan Cao) 7.5g Rhizoma Zingiberis Recens (Sheng Jiang) Fructus Zizyphi Jujubae (Da Zao)	Prepare the drugs into powder. Take 6g powder each time with 2 slices of Sheng Jiang and 2 pcs of Da Zao and decoct in water for oral application. Or decoct the drugs with Sheng Jiang and Da Zao in water for oral application.
Ji Chuan Decoction (Ji Chuan Jian)	济川煎	Jingyue's Complete Works (Jing Yue Quan Shu)	Radix Angelicae Sinensis (Dang Gui) 9-15g Radix Achyranthis Bidentatae (Niu Xi) 6g Herba Cistanches (Rou Cong Rong) 6-9g Rhizoma Alismatis (Ze Xie) 4.5g Rhizoma Cimicifugae (Sheng Ma) 1.5-3g Fructus Aurantii (Zhi Ke) 3g	Decoct the drugs in water for oral application.
Ji Jiao Li Huang Pill (Ji Jiao Li	己椒苈黄	Synopsis of the Golden	Radix Stephaniae Tetrandrae (Fang Ji) 30g	Grind the drugs into fine powder and

Huang Wan)	丸	Chamber (Jin Gui Yao Lue)	Semen Zanthoxyli (Jiao Mu) 30g Semen Descurainiae seu Lepidii (Ting Li Zi) 30g Radix et Rhizoma Rhei (Da Huang) 30g	make into pills with honey. Take 3g each time, thrice daily.
Ji Sheng Shen Qi Pill (Ji Sheng Shen Qi Wan)	济生肾气丸	Prescriptions for Saving Lives (Ji Sheng Fang)	Radix Aconiti Lateralis Praeparatae (Fu Zi) 30g Fructus Schisandrae Chinensis (Wu Wei Zi) 30g Fructus Corni Officinalis (Shan Zhu Yu) 30g Rhizoma Dioscoreae (Shan Yao) 30g Cortex Moutan Radicis (Mu Dan Pi) 30g Cornu Cervi Pantotrichum (Lu Rong) 30g Radix Rehmanniae Praeparatae (Shu Di Huang) 30g Cortex Cinnamomi (Rou Gui) 15g Sclerotium Poriae Cocos (Fu Ling) 30g Rhizoma Alismatis (Ze Xie) 30g	Grind the drugs into fine powder and make into pills with honey. Take 6-9g each time with light salty water or gruel.
Ji Sheng Xiao Ji Decoction (Ji Sheng Xiao Ji Yin Zi). Also named Xiao Ji Decoction (Xiao Ji Yin Zi).	济生小蓟饮子（又名小蓟饮子）	Prescriptions for Saving Lives (Ji Sheng Fang)	Radix Rehmanniae Recens (Sheng Di Huang) 9g Herba Cephalanoploris (Xiao Ji) 9g Talcum (Hua Shi Fen) 9g Medulla Tetrapanacis (Tong Cao) 9g Pollen Typhae (Pu Huang) 9g Nodus Nelumbinis Rhizomatis (Ou Jie) 9g Herba Lophatheri (Dan Zhu Ye) 9g Radix Angelicae Sinensis (Dang Gui) 9g Fructus Gardeniae (Zhi Zi) 9g Radix Glycyrrhizae (Gan Cao) 9g	Decoct the drugs in water for oral application.
Jia Jian Wei Rui Decoction (Jia Jian Wei Rui Tang)	加减葳蕤汤	Revised Edition of Popular Cold Induced Diseases (Chong Ding Tong Su Shang Han Lun)	Rhizoma Polygonati Odorati (Sheng Yu Zhu) 9g Bulbus Allii Fistulosi (Sheng Cong Bai) 6g Radix Platycodonis (Jie Geng) 4.5g Radix Cynanchi Atrati (Bai Wei) 3g Semen Sojae Preparatum (Dan Dou Chi)12g Herba Menthae (Bo He) 4.5g Radix Glycyrrhizae Praeparatae (Zhi Gan Cao) 1.5g Fructus Zizyphi Jujubae (Da Zao) 2 pcs	Decoct the drugs in water for oral application.
Jia Wei Er Miao Powder (Jia Wei Er	加味二妙散	Danxi's Experiential	Cortex Phellodendri (Huang Bai) 6g Radix Angelicae Sinensis (Dang	Prepare the drugs into powder. Take 6g

Miao San)		Therapy (Dan Xi Xin Fa)	Gui) 6g Rhizoma Atractylodis (Cang Zhu) 9g Radix Cyathulae Officinalis (Chuan Niu Xi) 6g Radix Stephaniae Tetrandrae (Fang Ji) 6g Rhizoma Dioscoreae Hypoglaucae (Bi Xie) 6g Carapax et Plastrum Testudinis (Gui Ban) 6g	each time and add 3g Succus Rhizoma Zingiberis Recens (Sheng Jiang Zhi) for oral application. Or decoct the drugs for oral application.
Jia Wei Jie Geng Decoction (Jia Wei Jie Geng Tang)	加味桔梗汤	Medicine Comprehended (Yi Xue Xin Wu)	Radix Platycodonis (Jie Geng) 2.4g Radix Glycyrrhizae (Gan Cao) 4.5g Bulbus Fritillariae (Bei Mu) 4.5g Exocarpium Citri Rubrum (Ju Hong) 2.4g Flos Lonicerae (Jin Yin Hua) 15g Semen Coicis (Yi Yi Ren) 15g Semen Descurainiae seu Lepidii (Ting Li Zi) 2.4g Rhizoma Bletillae Striatae (Bai Ji) 2.4g	Decoct the drugs in water for oral application.
Jia Wei Si Wu Decoction (Jia Wei Si Wu Tang)	加味四物汤	Jin Gui Yi	Radix Rehmanniae Recens (Sheng Di Huang) 6g Radix Angelicae Sinensis (Dang Gui) 3g Radix Paeoniae Alba (Bai Shao) 3g Rhizoma Ligustici Chuanxiong (Chuan Xiong) 1.5g Fructus Viticis (Man Jing Zi) 1.5g Flos Chrysanthemi (Ju Hua) 2.1g Radix Scutellariae (Huang Qin) 3g Radix Glycyrrhizae (Gan Cao) 0.9g	Decoct the drugs in water for oral application.
Jian Pi Pill (Jian Pi Wan)	健脾丸	Standards of Diagnosis and Treatment (Zheng Zhi Zhun Sheng)	Rhizoma Atractylodis Macrocephalae (Bai Zhu) 15g Radix Aucklandiae (Mu Xiang) 5g Wine processed Rhizoma Coptidis (Jiu Huang Lian) 5g Radix Glycyrrhizae Praeparatae (Zhi Gan Cao) 5g Sclerotium Poriae Cocos (Fu Ling) 12g Radix Ginseng (Ren Shen) 9g Massa Medicata Fermentata (Shen Qu) 6g Pericarpium Citri Reticulatae (Chen Pi) 6g Fructus Amomi (Sha Ren) 6g Stir-fried Fructus Hordei Germinatus (Chao Mai Ya) 6g Fructus Crataegi (Shan Zha) 6g Rhizoma Dioscoreae (Shan Yao) 6g	Decoct the drugs in water for oral application. Or prepare the drugs into pills; take 6-9g each time with warm boiled water, twice daily.

			Semen Myristicae (Rou Dou Kou) 6g	
Jiao Tai Pill (Jiao Tai Wan)	交泰丸	Han Shi Yi Tong	Rhizoma Coptidis (Huang Lian) 15g Cortex Cinnamomi (Rou Gui) 1.5g	Make the drugs into pills with honey. Take the pills with light salty water before meals
Jin Gui Shen Qi Pill (Jin Gui Shen Qi Wan). Also named Shen Qi Pill (Shen Qi Wan)	金匮肾气丸 (又名肾气丸)	Synopsis of the Golden Chamber (Jin Gui Yao Lue)	Radix Rehmanniae Recens (Sheng Di Huang) 24g Rhizoma Dioscoreae (Shan Yao) 12g Fructus Corni (Shan Zhu Yu) 12g Rhizoma Alismatis (Ze Xie) 9g Sclerotium Poriae Cocos (Fu Ling) 9g Cortex Moutan Radicis (Mu Dan Pi) 9g Ramulus Cinnamomi (Gui Zhi) 3g Radix Aconiti Lateralis Praeparatae (Pao Fu Zi) 3g	Decoct the drugs in water for oral application. Or make the drugs into pills; take 6-9g each time with warm boiled water or wine.
Jin Gui Xie Xin Decoction (Jin Gui Xie Xin Tang). Also named Xie Xin Decoction (Xie Xin Tang)	金匮泻心汤 (又名泻心汤)	Synopsis of the Golden Chamber (Jin Gui Yao Lue)	Radix et Rhizoma Rhei (Da Huang) 6g Rhizoma Coptidis (Huang Lian) 3g Radix Scutellariae (Huang Qin) 3g	Decoct the drugs in water for oral application.
Jin Ling Zi Powder (Jin Ling Zi San)	金铃子散	Pocket-Size Decoction (Xiu Zhen Fang)	Fructus Meliae Toosendan (Chuan Lian Zi) 9g Rhizoma Corydalis (Xuan Hu Suo) 9g	Grind the drugs into fine powder; take 9g each time with wine (Jiu) or warm boiled water. Or decoct the drugs in water for oral application.
Jin Suo Gu Jing Pill (Jin Suo Gu Jing Wan)	金锁固精丸	Collected Exegesis of Recipes (Yi Fang Ji Jie)	Semen Astragali Complanati (Sha Yuan Zi) 12g Semen Euryales Ferocis (Qian Shi) 12g Stamen Nelumbinis Nuciferae (Lian Xu) 12g Concha Ostreae (Mu Li) 9g Os Draconis (Long Gu) 9g Semen Nelumbinis Nuciferae (Lian Zi) 6g	Decoct the drugs in water for oral application. Or make the drugs into pills with the paste of Lian Zi; take 6g each time with light salty water.
Jing Fang Bai Du Powder (Jing Fang Bai Du San)	荆防败毒散	Wai Ke Li Li	Radix Saposhnikoviae (Fang Feng) 6g Herba Schizonepetae (Jing Jie) 6g Radix Ginseng (Ren Shen) 6g Rhizoma et Radix Notopterygii (Qiang Huo) 6g Radix Angelicae Pubescentis (Du Huo) 6g Radix Bupleuri (Chai Hu) 6g	Decoct the drugs in water for oral application.

			Radix Peucedani (Qian Hu) 6g Radix Platycodonis (Jie Geng) 6g Fructus Citri Aurantii (Zhi Ke) 6g Sclerotium Poriae Cocos (Fu Ling) 6g Rhizoma Ligustici Chuanxiong (Chuan Xiong) 6g Radix Glycyrrhizae (Gan Cao) 3g	
Jiu Wei Qiang Huo Decoction (Jiu Wei Qiang Huo Tang)	九味羌活汤	Difficult Medical Problem (Ci Shi Nan Zhi)	Rhizoma et Radix Notopterygii (Qiang Huo) 9g Radix Saposhnikoviae (Fang Feng) 9g Rhizoma Atractylodis (Cang Zhu) 9g Herba Asari (Xi Xin) 3g Rhizoma Ligustici Chuanxiong (Chuan Xiong) 6g Radix Angelicae Dahuricae (Bai Zhi) 6g Radix Rehmanniae Recens (Sheng Di Huang) 6g Radix Scutellariae (Huang Qin) 6g Radix Glycyrrhizae (Gan Cao) 6g	Decoct the drugs in water for oral application.
Jiu Xian Powder (Jiu Xian San)	九仙散	Precious Warning for Health (Wei Sheng Bao Jian)	Radix Ginseng (Ren Shen) 9g Flos Farfarae (Kuan Dong Hua) 9g Cortex Mori Alba Radicis (Sang Bai Pi) 9g Radix Platycodonis (Jie Geng) 9g Fructus Schisandrae Chinensis (Wu Wei Zi) 9g Colla Corii Asini (E Jiao) 9g Fructus Mume (Wu Mei) 9g Bulbus Fritillariae (Bei Mu) 6g Pericarpium Papaveris (Ying Su Ke) 6g (parched with honey until it becomes yellow)	Make the drugs into powder and take 6g each time with warm boiled water. Or decoct the drugs in water for oral application.
Ju Pi Zhu Ru Decoction (Ju Pi Zhu Ru Tang)	橘皮竹茹汤	Synopsis of the Golden Chamber (Jin Gui Yao Lue)	Pericarpium Citri Reticulatae (Ju Pi) 12g Rhizoma Zingiberis Recens (Sheng Jiang) 9g Caulis Bambusae in Taeniam (Zhu Ru) 12g Fructus Zizyphi Jujubae (Da Zao) 6 pcs Radix Glycyrrhizae (Gan Cao) 6g Radix Ginseng (Ren Shen) 3g	Decoct the drugs in water for oral application.
Juan Bi Decoction (Juan Bi Tang)	蠲痹汤	Yang's Formulae Handed Down by Family (Yang Shi Jia Cang	Radix Astragali (Huang Qi) 4.5g Radix Angelicae Sinensis (Dang Gui) 4.5g Radix Paeoniae Alba (Bai Shao Yao) 4.5g Rhizoma et Radix Notopterygii	Decoct the drugs in water for oral application.

	Fang)		(Qiang Huo) 4.5g Radix Saposhnikoviae (Fang Feng) 4.5g Rhizoma Curcumae Longae (Jiang Huang) 4.5g Radix Glycyrrizae (Gan Cao) 1.5g Rhizoma Zingiberis Recens (Sheng Jiang) 5 slices	
Kai Yu Er Chen Decoction (Kai Yu Er Chen Tang)	开郁二陈汤	Wan Shi Nu Ke	Rhizoma Pinelliae (Ban Xia) 2.1g Pericarpium Citri Reticulatae (Chen Pi) 3g Sclerotium Poriae Cocos (Fu Ling) 3g Radix Glycyrrhizae (Gan Cao) 1.5g Rhizoma Atractylodis (Cang Zhu) 3g Pericarpium Citri Reticulatae Viride (Qing Pi) 2.1g Rhizoma Cyperi (Xiang Fu) 3g Radix Aucklandiae (Mu Xiang) 1.5g Semen Areca Catechu (Bing Lang) 2.1g Rhizoma Ligustici Chuanxiong (Chuan Xiong) 3g Rhizoma Curcumae Ezhu (E Zhu) 2.1g	Decoct the drugs in water with Rhizoma Zingiberis Recens (Sheng Jiang) for oral application.
Ke Xue Formula (Ke Xue Fang)	咳血方	Danxi's Experiential Therapy (Dan Xi Xin Fa)	Indigo Naturalis (Qing Dai) 6g Semen Trichosanthis (Gua Lou Zi) 9g Pumex (Fu Hai Shi) 9g Fructus Gardeniae (Zhi Zi) 9g Fructus Chebulae (He Zi) 6g	Decoct the drugs in water for oral application.
Li Zhong Pill (Li Zhong Wan). Also name Li Zhong Decoction (Li Zhong Tang)	理中丸 (又名理中汤)	Treatise on Cold Induceed Diseases (Shang Han Lun)	Radix Ginseng (Ren Shen) 9g Radix Glycyrrhizae Praeparatae (Zhi Gan Cao) 9g Rhizoma Atractylodis Macrocephalae (Bai Zhu) 9g Rhizoma Zingiberis (Gan Jiang) 9g	Grind the drugs into coarse powder, mix it with honey, and make into pills with 9g each. Take one pill with warm boiled water each time, three times a day. Or decoct the drugs in water for oral application.
Lian Po Decoction (Lian Po Yin)	连朴饮	Treatise on Cholera Morbus (Huo Luan Lun)	Cortex Magnoliae Officinalis (Hou Po) 6g Rhizoma Coptidis (Huang Lian) 3g Rhizoma Acori Tatarinowii (Shi Chang Pu) 3g Rhizoma Pinelliae (Ban Xia) 3g Semen Sojae Preparatum (Dan Dou Chi) 9g Fructus Gardeniae (Zhi Zi) 9g	Decoct the drugs in water for oral application.

			Rhizoma Phragmitis (Lu Gen) 60g	
Liang Fu Pill (Liang Fu Wan)	良附丸	Liang Fang Ji Ye	Rhizoma Alpiniae Officinarum (Gao Liang Jiang) 4.5g Rhizoma Cyperi (Xiang Fu) 4.5g	Grind the drugs into powder separately, and make pill with gruel, succus of fresh ginger and salt.
Liang Ge Powder (Liang Ge San)	凉膈散	Formularies of the Bureau of People's Welfare Pharmacy (Tai Ping Hui Min He Ji Ju Fang)	Fructus Forsythiae (Lian Qiao) 12g Radix et Rhizoma Rhei (Da Huang) 6g Radix Glycyrrhizae (Gan Cao) 6g Fructus Gardeniae (Zhi Zi) 3g Radix Scutellariae (Huang Qin) 3g Herba Menthae (Bo He) 3g Lophatheri Gracilis Herba (Dan Zhu Ye) Natrii Sulfas (Mang Xiao) 6g	Grind the drugs into coarse powder, take 6g each time and decoct it with a little Folium Phyllostachydis (Zhu Ye) and honey (Feng Mi) in water for oral application. Or decoct the drugs in water for oral application.
Ling Gan Wu Wei Jiang Xin Decoction (Ling Gan Wu Wei Jiang Xin Tang)	苓甘五味姜辛汤	Synopsis of Golden Chamber (Jin Gui Yao Lue)	Sclerotium Poriae Cocos (Fu Ling) 12g Radix Glycyrrhizae (Gan Cao) 9g Rhizoma Zingiberis (Gan Jiang) 9g Herba Asari (Xi Xin) 5g Fructus Schisandrae Chinensis (Wu Wei Zi) 5g	Decoct the drugs in water for oral application.
Ling Gui Zhu Gan Decoction (Ling Gui Zhu Gan Tang)	苓桂术甘汤	Synopsis of Golden Chamber (Jin Gui Yao Lue	Poria (Fu Ling) 12g Ramulus Cinnamomi (Gui Zhi) 9g Rhizoma Atractylodis Macrocephalae (Bai Zhu) 6g Radix Glycyrrhizae Praeparatae (Zhi Gan Cao) 6g	Decoct the drugs in water for oral application.
Ling Jiao Gou Teng Decoction (Ling Jiao Gou Teng Tang)	羚角钩藤汤	Edition of Popular Cold Induced Diseases (Tong Su Shang Han Lun)	Cornu Saigae tataricae (Ling Yang Jiao) 4.5g Folium Mori (Sang Ye) 6g Bulbus Fritillariae Cirrhosae (Chuan Bei Mu) 12g Radix Rehmanniae Recens (Sheng Di Huang) 15g Ramulus Uncariae cum Uncis (Gou Teng) 9g Flos Chrysanthemi (Ju Hua) 9g Sclerotium Poriae Circum Radicem Pini (Fu Shen) 9g Radix Paeoniae Alba (Bai Shao Yao) 9g Radix Glycyrrhizae (Sheng Gan Cao) 3g Caulis Bambusae in Taeniam (Zhu Ru) 15g	Decoct Ling Yang Jiao and Zhu Ru in water first for 30 minutes, then add rest of the drugs and decoct them for oral application.
Ling Yang Jiao Decoction (Ling Yang Jiao Tang)	羚羊角汤	Yi Chun Sheng Yi	Cornu Saigae Tataricae (Ling Yang Jiao) 6g Carapax et Plastrum Testudinis	Smash Shi Jue Ming into pieces. Decoct the drugs in water for

			(Gui Ban) 24g Radix Rehmanniae Recens (Sheng Di Huang) 18g Cortex Moutan Radicis (Mu Dan Pi) 4.5g Radix Paeoniae Alba (Bai Shao Yao) 3g Radix Bupleuri (Chai Hu) 3g Herba Menthae (Bo He) 3g Periostracum Cicadae (Chan Tui) 3g Flos Chrysanthemi (Ju Hua) 6g Spica Prunellae Vulgaris (Xia Ku Cao) 4.5g Concha Haliotidis (Shi Jue Ming) 24g Fructus Zizyphi Jujubae (Da Zao) 10 pcs	oral application.
Liu Jun Zi Decoction (Liu Jun Zi Tang)	六君子汤	Check and Annotate Effective Prescriptions for Women (Jiao Zhu Fu Ren Liang Fang)	Radix Ginseng (Ren Shen) 6g Rhizoma Atractylodis Macrocephalae (Bai Zhu) 6g Sclerotium Poriae Cocos (Fu Ling) 6g Rhizoma Pineliae (Ban Xia) 6g Radix Glycyrrhizae Praeparatae (Gan Cao) 6g Pericarium Citri Reticulatae (Chen Pi) 6g	Decoct the drugs in water for oral application.
Liu Mo Decoction (Liu Mo Tang)	六磨汤	Standards of Diagnosis and Treatment (Zheng Zhi Zhun Sheng)	Lignum Aquilariae Resinatum (Chen Xiang) Radix Aucklandiae (Mu Xiang) Semen Areca Catechu (Bing Lang) Radix Linderae (Wu Yao) Fructus Citri Aurantii Immaturus (Zhi Shi) Radix et Rhizoma Rhei (Da Huang) (equal in dosage)	Grind each drug with 75ml of water separately; then mix the juice of all the drugs evenly and take it when it is warm.
Liu Wei Di Huang Pill (Liu Wei Di Huang Wan)	六味地黄丸	Key to Thrapeutics of Children's Diseases (Xiao Er Yao Zheng Zhi Jue)	Radix Rehmanniae Praeparatae (Shu Di Huang) 24g Fructus Corni (Shan Zhu Yu) 12g Rhizoma Dioscoreae (Shan Yao) 12g Cortex Moutan Radicis (Mu Dan Pi) 9g Sclerotium Poriae Cocos (Fu Ling) 9g Rhizoma Alismatis (Ze Xie) 9g	Decoct the drugs in water for oral application. Or make boluses, and take 6-9g each time with warm boiled water or light salty water before meals.
Liu Yi Powder (Liu Yi San). Also named Yi Yuan Powder (Yi Yuan San)	六一散	Clear Synopsis on Recipes Based on Plain Questions of	Talcum (Hua Shi Fen) 18g Radix Glycyrrhizae (Gan Cao) 3g	Decoct the drugs in water for oral application.

			Huang Di (Huang Di Su Wen Xuan Ming Lun Fang)		
Long Dan Xie Gan Decoction (Long Dan Xie Gan Tang)	龙胆泻肝汤		Collected Exegesis of Recipes (Yi Fang Ji Jie)	Radix Gentianae (Long Dan Cao) 6g Radix Bupleuri (Chai Hu) 6g Rhizoma Alismatis (Ze Xie) 12g Semen Plantaginis (Che Qian Zi) 9g Caulis Akebiae (Mu Tong) 6g Radix Rehmanniae Recens (Sheng Di Huang) 9g Radix Angelicae Sinensis (Dang Gui) 3g Fructus Gardeniae (Zhi Zi) 9g Radix Scutellariae (Huang Qin) 9g Radix Glycyrrhizae (Sheng Gan Cao) 6g	Decoct the drugs in water for oral application. Or prepare the drugs into pills; take 6g each time, twice daily.
Ma Huang Decoction (Ma Huang Tang)	麻黄汤		Treatise on Cold Induced Diseases (Shang Han Lun)	Herba Ephedrae (Ma Huang) 9g Ramulus Cinnamomi (Gui Zhi) 6g Semen Armeniacae Amarum (Xing Ren) 6g Radix Glycyrrhizae Praeparatae (Zhi Gan Cao) 3g	Decoct the drugs in water for oral application. And cover a patient's body with a quilt for mild perspiration.
Ma Huang Lian Qiao Chi Xiao Dou Decoction (Ma Huang Lian Qiao Chi Xiao Dou Tang)	麻黄连翘赤小豆汤		Treatise on Cold Induced Diseases (Shang Han Lun)	Herba Ephedrae (Ma Huang) 6g Semen Armeniacae Amarum (Xing Ren) 6g Radix Glycyrrhizae Praeparatae (Zhi Gan Cao) 6g Cortex Catalpae Ovatae (Zi Bai Pi) 18g Fructus Forsythiae (Lian Qiao) 6g Semen Phaseoli (Chi Xiao Dou) 18g Rhizoma Zingiberis Recens (Sheng Jiang) 6g Fructus Zizyphi Jujubae (Da Zao) 12 pcs	Cortex Catalpae Ovatae (Zi Bai Pi) can be replaced with Cortex Mori Alba Radicis (Sang Bai Pi). Decoct Herba Ephedrae (Ma Huang) first, then add other drugs and decoct. Take 1/2 of the decoction each time, twice daily.
Ma Huang Xing Ren Gan Cao Shi Gao Decoction (Ma Huang Xing Ren Gan Cao Shi Gao Tang). Also known as Ma Xing Gan Shi Decoction or Ma Xing Shi Gan Decoction (Ma Xing Gan Shi Tang or Ma Xing Shi Gan Tang)	麻黄杏仁甘草石膏汤 (又名麻杏甘石汤, 麻杏石甘汤)		Treatise on Cold Induced Diseases (Shang Han Lun)	Gypsum Fibrosum (Shi Gao) 18g Herba Ephedrae (Ma Huang) 9g Semen Armeniacae Amarum (Xing Ren) 9g Radix Glycyrrhizae Praeparatae (Gan Cao) 6g	Decoct the drugs in water for oral application.

Formula	Chinese	Source	Ingredients	Administration
Ma Xing Shi Gan Decoction (Ma Xing Shi Gan Tang)	麻杏石甘汤	Treatise on Cold Induced Diseases (Shang Han Lun)	Gypsum Fibrosum (Shi Gao) 18g Herba Ephedrae (Ma Huang) 9g Semen Armeniacae Amarum (Xing Ren) 9g Radix Glycyrrhizae Praeparatae (Gan Cao) 6g	Decoct the drugs in water for oral application.
Ma Zi Ren Pill (Ma Zi Ren Wan). Also named Pi Yue Pill (Pi Yue Wan)	麻子仁丸	Treatise on Cold Induced Diseases (Shang Han Lun)	Semen Cannabis (Huo Ma Ren) 21g Radix et Rhizoma Rhei (Da Huang) 12g Radix Paeoniae Alba (Bai Shao) 9g Fructus Immaturus Citri Aurantii (Zhi Shi) 9g Cortex Magnoliae Officinalis (Chuan Po) 9g Semen Armeniacae Amarum (Xing Ren) 9g	Decoct the drugs in water and then add 20-30ml honey to the decoction for oral application. Or make the drugs into pills with honey, and take 6-9g each time with warm boiled water, once or twice daily.
Mai Men Dong Decoction (Mai Men Dong Tang)	麦门冬汤	Synopsis of the Golden Chamber (Jin Gui Yao Lue)	Radix Ophiopogonis (Mai Dong) 42g Rhizoma Pinelliae (Ban Xia) 6g Semen Oryzae Sativae (Jing Mi) 3g Fructus Zizyphi Jujubae (Da Zao) 4 pcs Radix Ginseng (Ren Shen) 9g Radix Glycyrrhizae (Gan Cao) 6g	Decoct the drugs in water for oral application.
Mai Wei Di Huang Pill (Mai Wei Di Huang Wan). Also named Ba Wei Di Huang Pill (Ba Wei Di Huang Wan).	麦味地黄丸 (又名八味地黄丸)	Yi Ji	Radix Rehmanniae Praeparatae (Shu Di Huang) 24g Fructus Corni (Shan Zhu Yu) 24g Rhizoma Dioscoreae (Shan Yao) 12g Cortex Moutan Radicis (Mu Dan Pi) 6g Rhizoma Alismatis (Ze Xie) 6g Sclerotium Poriae Cocos (Fu Ling) 12g Radix Ophiopogonis (Mai Dong) 15g Fructus Schisandrae Chinensis (Wu Wei Zi) 15g	Grind the drug into fine powder and make pills with honey. Take 9g each time before meals.
Meng Shi Gun Tan Pill (Meng Shi Gun Tan Wan). Also named Gun Tan Pill (Gun Tan Wan)	礞石滚痰丸 (又名滚痰丸)	Main Discussions on Health Cultivation of Taiding (Tai Ding Yang Sheng Zhu Lun)	Radix et Rhizoma Rhei (Da Huang) 240g Radix Scutellariae (Huang Qin) 240g Lapis Chloriti (Meng Shi) 30g Lignum Aquilariae Resinatum (Chen Xiang) 15g	Make the drugs into pills with water. Take 6-9g each time with warm biled water, once or twice daily.
Miao Xiang Powder (Miao Xiang San)	妙香散	Shen Shi Zun Sheng Shu	Rhizoma Dioscoreae (Shan Yao) 30g Sclerotium Poriae Cocos (Fu Ling) 30g Sclerotium Poriae Circum Radicem Pini (Fu Shen) 30g	Grind the drugs into fine powder (grind She Xiang and Chen Sha separately). Take 6g each time with warm wine.

APPENDIX III   599

			Radix Polygalae (Yuan Zhi) 30g Radix Astragali (Huang Qi) 30g Radix Ginseng (Ren Shen) 15g Radix Platycodonis (Jie Geng) 15g Radix Glycyrrhizae Praeparatae (Zhi Gan Cao) 15g Radix Aucklandiae (Mu Xiang) 75g Cinnabaris (Chen Sha) 9g Moschus (She Xiang) 3g	
Niu Huang Qing Xin Pill (Niu Huang Qing Xin Wan). Also named Wan Shi Niu Huang Qing Xin Pill, Wan Shi Niu Huang Pill.	牛黄清心丸（又名万氏牛黄清心丸, 万氏牛黄丸）	Hereditary Physician's Mastery of Medicine for Sore and Nail-form Boil (Chuang Ding Shi Yi Xin Fa)	Cinnabaris (Chen Sha) 4g Rhizoma Coptidis (Huang Lian) 15g Radix Scutellariae (Huang Qin) 9g Fructus Gardeniae (Zhi Zi) 9g Radix Curcumae (Yu Jin) 6g Calculus Bovis (Niu Huang) 1g	Prepare the drugs into pill. Take 3g each time with decoction of Medulla Junci Effusi (Deng Xin Cao).
Niu Huang Zhi Bao Pill (Niu Huang Zhi Bao Dan)	牛黄至宝丹	Yi Lin Sheng Mo Da Quan	Radix Ginseng (Ren Shen) 30g Concretio Silicea Bambusae (Tian Zhu Huang) 30g Radix Polygoni Multiflori (He Shou Wu) 30g Rhizoma Arisaematis (Tian Nan Xing) 15g Cornu Bubali (Shui Niu Jiao) 100g [to replace the original Cornu Rhinocerotis (Xi Jiao)] Cinnabaris (Zhu Sha) 30g Realgar (Xiong Huang) 30g Carapax Eretmochelydis (Sheng Dai Mao) 30g Succinum (Hu Po) 30g Calculus Bovis (Niu Huang) 15g Moschus (She Xiang) 7.5g Borneolum Syntheticum (Bing Pian) 7.5g Benzoinum (An Xi Xiang) 45g Gold Foil (Jin Bo) 50 pcs Silver Foil (Yin Bo) 50 pcs	Shui Niu Jiao, Dai Mao, An Xi Xiong and Hu Po are respectively ground into fine powder. Zhu Sha and Xiong Huang are respectively refined with water into extremely fine powder. Grind Niu Huang, She Xiang and Bing Pian into fine powder. Grind other drugs into fine powder. Mix the above powder and grind it, then sift it evenly and make it into pills with honey. Take one pill (3g) each time, once or twice daily.
Nuan Gan Decoction (Nuan Gan Jian)	暖肝煎	Jingyue's Complete Works (Jing Yue Quan Shu)	Radix Angelicae Sinensis (Dang Gui) 6-9g Fructus Lycii (Gou Qi Zi) 9g Fructus Foeniculi (Xiao Hui Xiang) 6g Cortex Cinnamomi (Rou Gui) 3-6g Radix Linderae (Wu Yao) 6g Lignum Aquilariae Resinatum (Chen Xiang) 3g Sclerotium Poriae Cocos (Fu Ling) 6g Rhizoma Zingiberis Recens (Sheng	Decoct the drugs in water for oral application.

			Jiang) 3g	
Ping Chuan Gu Ben Decoction (Ping Chuan Gu Ben Tang)	平喘固本汤	Effective Recipes (Yan Fang)	Radix Codonopsitis Pilosulae (Dang Shen) 9g Fructus Schisandrae Chinensis (Wu Wei Zi) 3g Cordyceps Sinensis (Dong Chong Xia Cao) 9g Semen Juglandis (Hu Tao Ren) 9g Lignum Aquilariae Resinatum (Chen Xiang) 3g Magnetitum (Ci Shi) 9g Funiculus Umbilicalis (Qi Dai) 9g Fructus Perillae (Su Zi) 9g Flos Farfarae (Kuan Dong Hua) 9g Rhizoma Pinelliae (Ban Xia) 9g Exocarpium Citri Rubrum (Ju Hong) 9g	Decoct the drugs in water for oral application.
Ping Wei Powder (Ping Wei San)	平胃散	Brief Prescriptions for People's Welfare (Jian Yao Ji Zhong Fang)	Rhizoma Atractylodis (Cang Zhu) 12g Cortex Magnoliae Officinalis (Hou Po) 9g Pericarpium Citri Reticulatae (Chen Pi) 6g Radix Glycyrrhizae Praeparatae (Zhi Gan Cao) 3g Fructus Zizyphi Jujubae (Da Zao) Rhizoma Zingiberis Recens (Sheng Jiang)	Prepare the drugs except Da Zao and Sheng Jiang into powder. Take 6g powder each time and decoct with 2 slices of Sheng Jiang and 2 pcs of Da Zao for oral application. Or decoct the drugs in water for oral application.
Pu Ji Xiao Du Decoction (Pu Ji Xiao Du Yin, or Pu Ji Xiao Du Yin Zi)	普济消毒饮（子）	Effective Prescriptions Tested by Dongyuan (Dong Yuan Shi Xiao Fang)	Radix Scutellariae (Huang Qin) 15g Rhizoma Coptidis (Huang Lian) 15g Exocarpium Citri Rubrum (Ju Hong) 6g [or replace it with Pericarpium Citri Reticulatae (Chen Pi)] Radix Glycyrrhizae (Gan Cao) 6g Radix Scrophulariae (Xuan Shen) 6g Radix Bupleuri (Chai Hu) 6g Radix Platycodonis (Jie Geng) 6g Fructus Forsythiae (Lian Qiao) 3g Radix Isatidis (Ban Lan Gen) 3g Lashiosphaerae seu Calvatiae Fructificato (Ma Bo) 3g Fructus Arctii Lappae (Niu Bang Zi) 3g Herba Menthae (Bo He) 3g [or replace it with Radix Ginseng (Ren Shen)] Bombyx Batryticatus (Jiang Can) 2g Rhizoma Cimicifugae (Sheng Ma) 2g	Decoct the drugs in water for oral application.

Qi Bao Mei Ran Pill (Qi Bao Mei Ran Dan)	七宝美髯丹	Prescriptions of Benevolent Hall (Ji Shan Tang Fang)	Radix Polygoni Multiflori Bubra (Chi He Shou Wu) 500g Radix Polygoni Multiflori Alba (Bai He Shou Wu) 500g Radix Achyranthis Bidentatae (Niu Xi) 250g Poria Rubra (Chi Fu Ling) 500g Poria Alba (Bai Fu Ling) 500g Radix Angelicae Sinensis (Dang Gui) 250g Fructus Psoraleae (Bu Gu Zhi) 120g Semen Cuscutae (Tu Si Zi) 250g Fructus Lycii (Gou Qi Zi) 250g	Soak and steam He Shou Wu in water that has been used to wash rice. Soak Fu Ling in milk. Bu Gu Zhi is parched with Semen Sesami Nigrum (Hei Zhi Ma). Make the drugs into pills with honey, and take 9g each time, thrice daily (with warm wine in the morning, with decoction of fresh ginger at noon, and with salty water in the evening).
Qi Fu Decoction (Qi Fu Yin)	七福饮	Jingyue's Complete Works (Jing Yue Quan Shu)	Radix Rehmanniae Praeparatae (Shu Di Huang) 6-9g Radix Angelicae Sinensis (Dang Gui) 6-9g Radix Ginseng (Ren Shen) 6-9g Rhizoma Atractylodis Macrocephalae (Bai Zhu) 4.5g Radix Glycyrrhizae Praeparatae (Zhi Gan Cao) 3g Radix Polygalae (Yuan Zhi) 0.9-1.5g Semen Ziziphi Spinosae (Suan Zao Ren) 6g	Decoct the drugs in water for oral application before meals.
Qi Ge Powder (Qi Ge San)	启膈散	Medicine Comprehended (Yi Xue Xin Wu)	Radix Salviae Miltiorrhizae (Dan Shen) 9g Radix Adenophorae (Sha Shen) 9g Bulbus Fritillariae Cirrhosae (Chuan Bei Mu) 4.5g Sclerotium Poriae Cocos (Fu Ling) 3g Radix Curcumae (Yu Jin) 1.5g Folium Nelumbinis Basis (He Ye Di) 2 pcs Pericarpium Amomi (Sha Ren Ke) 1.2g Testa Oryzae Sativae (Chu Tou Kang) 1.5g	Decoct the drugs in water for oral application.
Qi Ju Di Huang Pill (Qi Ju Di Huang Wan)	杞菊地黄丸	Yi Ji	Fructus Lycii (Gou Qi Zi) 9g Flos Chrysanthemi (Ju Hua) 9g Radix Rehmanniae Praeparatae (Shu Di Huang) 24g Fructus Corni (Shan Zhu Yu) 12g Rhizoma Dioscoreae (Shan Yao) 12g Cortex Moutan Radicis (Mu Dan	Decoct the drugs in water for oral application. Or make boluses, and take 6-9g each time with warm boiled water or light salty water before meals.

			Pi) 9g Sclerotium Poriae Cocos (Fu Ling) 9g Rhizoma Alismatis (Ze Xie) 9g	
Qi Jun Decoction (Qi Jun Tang)	启峻汤	Zhang Shi Yi Tong	Radix Ginseng (Ren Shen) 4.5g Radix Astragali (Huang Qi) 4.5g Radix Angelicae Sinensis (Dang Gui) 4.5g Stir-fried Rhizoma Atractylodis Macrocephalae (Chao Bai Zhu) 4.5g Pericarpium Citri Reticulatae (Chen Pi) 2.4g Radix Glycyrrhizae Praeparatae (Zhi Gan Cao) 1.5g Cortex Cinnamomi (Rou Gui) 1.5g Sclerotium Poriae Cocos (Fu Ling) 4.5g Rhizoma Zingiberis (Pao Gan Jiang) 1.2g Fleshy Fruits 2.4g Lignum Aquilariae Resinatum (Chen Xiang) 2.4g Radix Aconiti Lateralis Praeparatae (Fu Zi) 4.5g	Fleshy Fruits include berry (tomato, grapes), hesperidium, pepo (cucumber, water melon), pome (pear, apple) and drupe (plum, cherry, and peach). Decoct the drugs in water for oral application.
Qi Li Powder (Qi Li San)	七厘散	Record of Co-Longevity (Tong Shou Lu)	Sanguis Draconis (Xue Jie) 30g Moschus (She Xiang) 0.4g Borneolum Syntheticum (Bing Pian) 0.36g Olibanum (Ru Xiang) 4.5g Myrrha (Mo Yao) 4.5g Flos Carthami (Hong Hua) 4.5g Cinnabaris (Zhu Sha) 3.6g Catechu (Er Cha) 7.2g	Grind the drugs into fine powder, seal it and store it. Take 0.5-1.5g each time with yellow wine or warm water. For external use, take appropriate amount of powder and paste it with wine to the wound.
Qi Wei Du Qi Pill (Qi Wei Du Qi Wan)	七味都气丸	Yi Zong Ji Ren Bian	Radix Rehmanniae Praeparatae (Shu Di Huang) 24g Fructus Corni (Shan Zhu Yu) 12g Rhizoma Dioscoreae (Shan Yao) 12g Cortex Moutan Radicis (Mu Dan Pi) 9g Sclerotium Poriae Cocos (Fu Ling) 9g Rhizoma Alismatis (Ze Xie) 9g Fructus Schisandrae Chinensis (Wu Wei Zi) 9-15g	Decoct the drugs in water for oral application. Or make boluses, and take 6-9g each time with warm boiled water or light salty water, twice daily.
Qi Wei Bai Zhu Powder (Qi Wei Bai Zhu San)	七味白术散	Key to Therapeutics of Children's Diseases	Radix Ginseng (Ren Shen) 6g Sclerotium Poriae Cocos (Fu Ling) 12g Rhizoma Atractylodis Macrocepha-	Grind into coarse powder, and take 6g each time. Or decoct the drugs in water for

Formula	Chinese	Source	Ingredients	Preparation
	(Xiao Er Yao Zheng Zhi Jue)		lae (Bai Zhu) 12g Radix Glycyrrhizae (Gan Cao) 3g Herba Agastache seu Pogostemonis (Huo Xiang Ye) 12g Radix Aucklandiae (Mu Xiang) 6g Radix Puerariae (Ge Gen) 15g	oral application.
Qian Gen Powder (Qian Gen San)	茜根散	Jingyue's Complete Works (Jing Yue Quan Shu)	Radix Rubiae Cordifoliae (Qian Cao) 30g Radix Scutellariae (Huang Qin) 30g Colla Corii Asini (E Jiao) 30g Cacumen Biotae Orientalis (Ce Bai Ye) 30g Radix Rehmanniae Recens (Sheng Di Huang) 30g Radix Glycyrrhizae (Gan Cao) 15g	Grind the drugs into powder. Decoct 12g of powder with 225ml of water and Rhizoma Zingiberis Recens (Sheng Jiang) 3 slices for oral application.
Qian Jin Wei Jing Decoction (Qian Jin Wei Jing Tang)	<千金>苇茎汤	Invaluable Prescriptions for Emergencies (Bei Ji Qian Jin Yao Fang)	Fresh Rhizoma Phragmitis (Lu Gen) 60g Semen Coicis (Yi Yi Ren) 30g Semen Benincasae (Dong Gua Zi) 30g Semen Persicae (Tao Ren) 9g	Decoct the drugs in water for oral application.
Qian Zheng Powder (Qian Zheng San)	牵正散	Yang's Formulae Handed Down by Family (Yang Shi Jia Cang Fang)	Rhizoma Typhonii (Bai Fu Zi) 5g Bombyx Batryticatus (Bai Jiang Can) 5g Scorpio (Quan Xie) 5g	Decoct the drugs in water for oral application. Or grind the drugs into fine powder, and take 3g each time with warm wine, twice or thrice daily.
Qiang Huo Sheng Shi Decoction (Qiang Huo Sheng Shi Tang)	羌活胜湿汤	Treatise on the Spleen and Stomach (Pi Wei Lun)	Rhizoma et Radix Notopterygii (Qiang Huo) 9g Radix Angelicae Pubescentis (Du Huo) 9g Ligustici Rhizoma et Radix (Gao Ben) 6g Radix Saposhnikoviae (Fang Feng) 6g Radix Glycyrrhizae Praeparatae (Zhi Gan Cao) 6g Fructus Viticis (Man Jing Zi) 5g Rhizoma Ligustici Chuanxiong (Chuan Xiong) 5g	Decoct the drugs in water for oral application.
Qin Jiao Bie Jia Powder (Qin Jiao Bie Jia San)	秦艽鳖甲散	Precious Warning for Health (Wei Sheng Bao Jian)	Radix Gentianae Qinjiao (Qin Jiao) 15g Carapax Trionycis (Bie Jia) 30g Radix Bupleuri (Chai Hu) 30g Radix Angelicae Sinensis (Dang Gui) 15g Cortex Lycii Radicis (Di Gu Pi) 30g Herba Artemisiae Apiaceae seu Annuae (Qing Hao) 5 pcs Rhizoma Anemarrhenae (Zhi Mu)	Grind the drugs except Qing Hao and Wu Mei into coarse powder. Decoct 15g of powder with 200ml of water, 5 pcs of Qing Hao and 1 piece of Wu Mei each time before meals.

| | | | 15g
Fructus Pruni Mume (Wu Mei) 1 piece | |
| --- | --- | --- | --- | --- |
| Qing Dan Decoction (Qing Dan Tang) | 清胆汤 | Effective Recipes (Yan Fang) | Radix et Rhizoma Rhei (Da Huang) 10g (decoct later)
Fructus Gardeniae (Zhi Zi) 10g
Rhizoma Coptidis (Huang Lian) 5g
Radix Bupleuri (Chai Hu) 10g
Radix Paeoniae Alba (Bai Shao Yao) 12g
Herba Taraxaci (Pu Gong Ying) 15g
Herba Lysimachiae (Jin Qian Cao) 15g
Fructus Trichosanthis (Gua Lou) 10g
Radix Curcumae (Yu Jin) 10g
Rhizoma Corydalis (Yan Hu Suo) 10g
Fructus Meliae Toosendan (Chuan Lian Zi) 10g | Decoct the drugs in water for oral application, twice daily. |
| Qing E Pill (Qing E Wan) | 青娥丸 | Formularies of the Bureau of People's Welfare Pharmacy (Tai Ping Hui Min He Ji Ju Fang) | Fructus Psoraleae (Bu Gu Zhi) 240g
Cortex Eucommiae (Du Zhong) 480g
Semen Juglandis (Hu Tao Ren) 150g
Bulbus Allii Sativi (Da Suan) 120g | Grind the drugs into fine powder. Add 50-70g of honey to 100g of powder and make pills. Take 9g each time with warm wine before meals, twice or thrice daily. |
| Qing Gong Decoction (Qing Gong Tang) | 清宫汤 | Analysis of Warm Diseases (Wen Bing Tiao Bian) | Radix Scrophulariae (Xuan Shen) 9g
Plumula Nelumbinis Nuciferae (Lian Zi Xin) 1.5g
Folium Phyllostachydis Henonis (Zhu Ye) 6g
Fructus Forsythiae (Lian Qiao) 6g
Cornu Rhinocerotis (Xi Jiao) 6g [replaced with Cornu Bubali (Shui Niu Jiao) 30g]
Radix Ophiopogonis (Mai Dong) 9g | Decoct the drugs in water for oral application. |
| Qing Gu Powder (Qing Gu San) | 清骨散 | Standards of Diagnosis and Treatment (Zheng Zhi Zhun Sheng) | Radix Stellariae (Yin Chai Hu) 5g
Rhizoma Picrorrhizae (Hu Huang Lian) 3g
Radix Gentianae Macrophyllae (Qin Jiao) 3g
Carapax Trionycis (Bie Jia) 3g
Cortex Lycii (Di Gu Pi) 3g
Herba Artemisiae Annuae (Qing Hao) 3g
Rhizoma Anemarrhenae (Zhi Mu) 3g | Decoct the drugs in water for oral application. |

				Radix Glycyrrhizae (Gan Cao) 2g	
Qing Hao Bie Jia Decoction (Qing Hao Bie Jia Tang)	青蒿鳖甲汤	Analysis of Warm Diseases (Wen Bing Tiao Bian)		Carapax Trionycis (Bie Jia) 15g Herba Artemisiae Annuae (Qing Hao) 6g Radix Rehmanniae Recens (Sheng Di Huang) 12g Rhizoma Anemarrhenae (Zhi Mu) 6g Cortex Moutan Radicis (Mu Dan Pi) 9g	Decoct the drugs in water for oral application.
Qing Jin Hua Tan Decoction (Qing Jin Hua Tan Tang)	清金化痰汤	The Wholly Purpose of Medicine (Yi Xue Tong Zhi)		Radix Scutellariae (Huang Qin) 4.5g Fructus Gardeniae (Zhi Zi) 4.5g Radix Platycodi Grandiflori (Jie Geng) 6g Radix Glycyrrhizae (Gan Cao) 1.2g Bulbus Fritillariae (Bei Mu) 3g Rhizoma Anemarrhenae (Zhi Mu) 3g Radix Ophiopogonis (Mai Dong) 3g Cortex Mori Alba Radicis (Sang Bai Pi) 3g Semen Trichosanthis (Gua Lou Zi) 3g Exocarpium Citri Rubrum (Ju Hong) 3g Sclerotium Poriae Cocos (Fu Ling) 3g	Decoct the drugs in water for oral application after meals.
Qing Qi Hua Tan Pill (Qing Qi Hua Tan Wan)	清气化痰丸	Textual Research on Prescriptions (Yi Fang Kao)		Rhizoma Arisaematis cum Bile (Dan Nan Xing) 9g Rhizoma Pinelliae Praeparatae (Zhi Ban Xia) 9g Semen Trichosanthis (Gua Lou Zi) 6g Radix Scutellariae (Huang Qin) 6g Pericarpium Citri Reticulatae (Chen Pi) 6g Semen Armeniacae Amarum (Xing Ren) 6g Fructus Citri Aurantii Immaturus (Zhi Shi) 6g Sclerotium Poriae Cocos (Fu Ling) 6g	Grind the drugs into fine powder and make the powder into pillets with succus of fresh ginger. Take 6g each time with warm boiled water. Or decoct the drugs in water with 3 slices of Rhizoma Zingiberis Recens (Sheng Jiang) for oral application.
Qing Shu Yi Qi Decoction (Qing Shu Yi Qi Tang)	清暑益气汤	Compendium on Warm Diseases (Wen Re Jing Wei)		Radix Panacis Quinquefolii (Xi Yang Shen) 5g Herba Dendrobii (Shi Hu) 15g Radix Ophiopogonis (Mai Dong) 9g Rhizoma Coptidis (Huang Lian) 3g Folium Phyllostachydis Henonis (Zhu Ye) 6g [or replace it with Herba Lophatheri (Dan Zhu Ye)]	Decoct the drugs in water for oral application.

			Petiolus Nelumbinis (He Geng) 15g Rhizoma Anemarrhenae (Zhi Mu) 6g Radix Glycyrrhizae (Gan Cao) 3g Semen Oryzae Sativae (Jing Mi) 15g Exocarpium Citrulli (Xi Gua Cui Yi) 30g	
Qing Wei Powder (Qing Wei San)	清胃散	Treatise on the Spleen and Stomach (Pi Wei Lun)	Rhizoma Cimicifugae (Sheng Ma) 9g Radix Rehmanniae Recens (Sheng Di Huang) 6g Radix Angelicae Sinensis (Dang Gui) 6g Rhizoma Coptidis (Huang Lian) 9g Cortex Moutan Radicis (Mu Dan Pi) 6g Gypsum (Shi Gao)	Decoct the drugs in water for oral application.
Qing Wen Bai Du Decoction (Qing Wen Bai Du Yin)	清瘟败毒饮	A View of Warm Diseases with Rahes (Yi Zhen Yi De)	Gypsum Fibrosum (Shi Gao) 24g Radix Rehmanniae Recens (Sheng Di Huang) 6g Cornu Bubali (Shui Niu Jiao) 6g [to replace Cornu Rhinocerotis (Xi Jiao)] Rhizoma Coptidis (Huang Lian) 3g Fructus Gardeniae (Zhi Zi) 6g Radix Platycodonis (Jie Geng) 6g Radix Scutellariae (Huang Qin) 6g Rhizoma Anemarrhenae (Zhi Mu) 6g Radix Paeoniae Rubra (Chi Shao) 6g Radix Scrophulariae (Xuan Shen) 6g Fructus Forsythiae (Lian Qiao) 6g Radix Glycyrrhizae (Gan Cao) 6g Cortex Moutan Radicis (Mu Dan Pi) 6g Folium Phyllostachydis Henonis (Zhu Ye) 6g	Decoct Shi Gao and Shui Niu Jiao in water first, then add other drugs and decoct. Oral application.
Qing Xin Lian Zi Decoction (Qing Xin Lian Zi Yin)	清心莲子饮	Formularies of the Bureau of People's Welfare Pharmacy (Tai Ping Hui Min He Ji Ju Fang)	Radix Scutellariae (Huang Qin) 15g Radix Ophiopogonis (Mai Dong) 15g Cortex Lycii Radicis (Di Gu Pi) 15g Semen Plantaginis (Che Qian Zi) 15g Radix Glycyrrhizae Praeparatae (Zhi Gan Cao) 15g Semen Nelumbinis (Lian Zi) 22.5g Sclerotium Poriae Cocos (Fu Ling) 22.5g Radix Astragali (Huang Qi) 22.5g	Grind the drugs into powder. Decoct 9g of powder each time for oral application before meals.

			Radix Ginseng (Ren Shen) 22.5g	
Qing Yi Decoction (Qing Yi Tang)	清胰汤	Effective Recipes (Yan Fang)	Radix Bupleuri (Chai Hu) 15g Radix Scutellariae (Huang Qin) 9g Rhizoma Coptidis (Huang Lian) 9g Radix Aucklandiae (Mu Xiang) 9g Radix Paeoniae Alba (Bai Shao Yao) 15g Rhizoma Corydalis (Yan Hu Suo) 9g Radix et Rhizoma Rhei (Da Huang, decoct later) 15g Natrii Sulfas (Mang Xiao) 9g	Decoct the drugs except Mang Xiao in water, remove the residue, and then dissolve Mang Xiao in the decoction.
Qing Ying Decoction (Qing Ying Tang)	清营汤	Analysis of Warm Diseases (Wen Bing Tiao Bian)	Cornu Bubali (Shui Niu Jiao) 30g [to replace Cornu Rhinocerotis (Xi Jiao)] Radix Rehmanniae Recens (Sheng Di Huang) 15g Radix Scrophulariae (Xuan Shen) 9g Folium Phyllostachydis Henonis (Zhu Ye Xin) 3g Radix Ophiopogonis (Mai Dong) 9g Radix Salviae Miltiorrhizae (Dan Shen) 6g Rhizoma Coptidis (Huang Lian) 5g Flos Lonicerae (Jin Yin Hua) 9g Fructus Forsythiae (Lian Qiao) 6g	Decoct the drugs in water for oral application.
Qing Zao Jiu Fei Decoction (Qing Zao Jiu Fei Tang)	清燥救肺汤	Principles and Prohibitions of Medical Profession (Yi Men Fa Lu)	Folium Mori (Sang Ye) 9g Gypsum Fibrosum (Shi Gao) 8g Radix Ophiopogonis (Mai Dong) 4g Radix Glycyrrhizae (Gan Cao) 3g Semen Sesami Indici (Hei Zhi Ma) 3g Colla Corii Asini (E Jiao) 3g Semen Armeniacae Amarum (Xing Ren) 2g Radix Ginseng (Ren Shen) 2g Folium Eriobotryae (Pi Pa Ye) 3g	Decoct the drugs in water for oral application.
Qing Zhong Decoction (Qing Zhong Tang)	清中汤	The Wholly Purpose of Medicine (Yi Xue Tong Zhi)	Rhizoma Coptidis (Huang Lian) 6g Fructus Gardeniae (Zhi Zi) 6g Rhizoma Pinelliae (Ban Xia) 3g Sclerotium Poriae Cocos (Fu Ling) 4.5g Pericarpium Citri Reticulatae (Chen Pi) 4.5g Semen Alpiniae Katsumadai (Cao Dou Kou) 2.1g Radix Glycyrrhizae (Gan Cao) 2.1g	Decoct the drugs in water with Rhizoma Zingiberis Recens (Sheng Jiang) 3 slices for oral application before meals.
Ren Shen Bai Du Powder (Ren Shen	人参败毒	Formularies of the Bureau	Radix Ginseng (Ren Shen) 9g Rhizoma et Radix Notopterygii	Decoct the drugs in water for oral appli-

Formula	Chinese	Source	Ingredients	Preparation
Bai Du San)	散	of People's Welfare Pharmacy (Tai Ping Hui Min He Ji Ju Fang)	(Qiang Huo) 9g Radix Angelicae Pubescentis (Du Huo) 9g Radix Bupleuri (Chai Hu) 9g Radix Peucedani (Qian Hu) 9g Rhizoma Ligustici Chuanxiong (Chuan Xiong) 9g Fructus Citri Aurantii (Zhi Ke) 9g Radix Platycodonis (Jie Geng) 9g Sclerotium Poriae Cocos (Fu Ling) 9g Radix Glycyrrhizae (Gan Cao) 9g Rhizoma Zingiberis Recens (Sheng Jiang) 3 slices Herba Menthae (Bo He) 2g	cation. Or prepare the drugs except Sheng Jiang and Bo He into powder, and take 6g of the powder each time and decoct with Sheng Jiang and Bo He for oral application.
Ren Shen Decoction (Ren Shen Tang)	人参汤	Treatise on Cold Induced Diseases (Shang Han Lun)	Radix Ginseng (Ren Shen) Rhizoma Zingiberis (Gan Jiang) Radix Glycyrrhizae Praeparatae (Zhi Gan Cao) Rhizoma Atractylodis Macrocephalae (Bai Zhu)	Decoct the drugs in water for oral application.
Ren Shen Hu Tao Decoction (Ren Shen Hu Tao Tang)	人参胡桃汤	Revised Edition of Yan's Prescriptions for Saving Lives (Chong Ding Yan Shi Ji Sheng Fang)	Radix Ginseng (Ren Shen) 6g Semen Juglandis (Hu Tao Ren) 30g Rhizoma Zingiberis Recens (Sheng Jiang) 5 slices Fructus Zizyphi Jujubae (Da Zao) 2 pcs	Decoct the drugs in water for oral application.
Ren Shen Si Ni Decoction (Ren Shen Si Ni Tang). Also named Si Ni Jia Ren Shen Decoction (Si Ni Jia Ren Shen Tang)	人参四逆汤 (又名四逆加人参汤)	Treatise on Cold Induced Diseases (Shang Han Lun)	Radix Ginseng (Ren Shen) 6g Radix Glycyrrhizae Praeparatae (Zhi Gan Cao) 6g Rhizoma Zingiberis (Gan Jiang) 9g Radix Aconiti Lateralis Praeparatae (Fu Zi) 15g	Decoct the drugs in water for oral application.
Ren Shen Yang Rong Decoction (Ren Shen Yang Rong Tang)	人参养荣汤	Formularies of the Bureau of People's Welfare Pharmacy (Tai Ping Hui Min He Ji Ju Fang)	Radix Angelicae Sinensis (Dang Gui) 6g Radix Paeoniae Lactiflorae (Bai Shao Yao) 6g Radix Rehmanniae Praeparatae (Shu Di Huang) 6g Radix Ginseng (Ren Shen) 6g Rhizoma Atractylodis macrocephalae (Bai Zhu) 6g Sclerotium Poriae Cocos (Fu Ling) 6g Radix Glycyrrhizae Praeparatae (Zhi Gan Cao) 6g Radix Astragali (Huang Qi) 6g Cortex Cinnamomi (Rou Gui) 6g Fructus Schisandrae (Wu Wei Zi)	Decoct the drugs in water for oral application.

			4g Radix Polygalae (Yuan Zhi) 6g Pericarpium Citri Reticulatae (Ju Pi) 6g Rhizoma Zingiberis Recens (Sheng Jiang) 5 slices Fructus Zizyphi Jujubae (Da Zao) 1 piece	
Run Chang Pill (Run Chang Wan)	润肠丸	Shen Shi Zun Sheng Shu	Radix Angelicae Sinensis (Dang Gui) 30g Radix Rehmanniae Recens (Sheng Di Huang) 30g Semen Cannabis (Huo Ma Ren) 30g Semen Pruni Persicae (Tao Ren) 30g Fructus Citri Aurantii (Zhi Ke) 30g	Grind the drugs into powder and make pills with honey. Take 9g each time before meals.
San Ao Decoction (San Ao Tang)	三拗汤	Formularies of the Bureau of People's Welfare Pharmacy (Tai Ping Hui Min He Ji Ju Fang)	Herba Ephedrae (Ma Huang) 30g Semen Pruni Armeniacae (Xing Ren) 30g Radix Glycyrrhizae (Gan Cao) 30g (equal in dosage)	Grind the drugs into coarse powder. Decoct 15g of powder each time with 5 slices of ginger for oral application.
San Bi Decoction (San Bi Tang)	三痹汤	Effective Prescriptions for Women (Fu Ren Liang Fang)	Radix Dipsaci Asperi (Xu Duan) 30g Cortex Eucommiae (Du Zhong) 30g Radix Saposhnikoviae (Fang Feng) 30g Cortex Cinnamomi (Rou Gui Xin) 30g Herba cum Radice Asari (Xi Xin) 30g Radix Ginseng (Ren Shen) 30g Sclerotium Poriae Cocos (Fu Ling) 30g Radix Angelicae Sinensis (Dang Gui) 30g Radix Paeoniae Alba (Bai Shao Yao) 30g Radix Astragali (Huang Qi) 30g Radix Cyathulae Officinalis (Chuan Niu Xi) 30g Radix Glycyrrhizae (Gan Cao) 30g Radix Gentianae Qinjiao (Qin Jiao) 15g Radix Rehmanniae Recens (Sheng Di Huang) 15g Rhizoma Ligustici Chuanxiong (Chuan Xiong) 15g Radix Angelicae Pubescentis (Du	Grind the drugs into powder. Decoct 15g each time with Rhizoma Zingiberis Recens (Sheng Jiang) 3 slices and Fructus Zizyphi Jujubae (Da Zao) 1 piece for oral application before meals.

			Huo) 15g	
San Jia Fu Mai Decoction (San Jia Fu Mai Tang)	三甲复脉汤	Analysis of Warm Diseases (Wen Bing Tiao Bian)	Radix Glycyrrhizae Praeparatae (Zhi Gan Cao) 18g Radix Rehmanniae Recens (Sheng Di Huang) 18g Radix Paeoniae Alba (Bai Shao Yao) 18g Radix Ophiopogonis (Mai Dong) 15g Semen Cannabis (Huo Ma Ren) 9g Colla Corii Asini (E Jiao) 9g Concha Ostreae (Mu Li) 15g Carapax Trionycis (Bie Jia) 24g Carapax et Plastrum Testudinis (Gui Ban) 30g	Decoct the drugs except E Jiao in water, then remove the residue and add E Jiao to the decoction until it is melted. Take the decoction while it is still warm
San Leng Decoction (San Leng Tang)	三棱汤	Clear Synopsis on Recipes Based on Plain Questions (Xuan Ming Lun Fang)	Rhizoma Sparganii (San Leng) 60g Rhizoma Atractylodis Macrocephalae (Bai Zhu) 30g Rhizoma Curcumae Ezhu (E Zhu) 15g Radix Angelicae Sinensis (Dang Gui) 15g Semen Areca Catechu (Bing Lang) 9g Radix Aucklandiae (Mu Xiang) 9g	Grind the drugs into powder. Take 9g each time with boiled water after meals, thrice daily. Or decoct 9g of powder each time for oral application.
San Miao Powder (San Miao San)	三妙散	Danxi's Experiential Therapy (Dan Xi Xin Fa)	Er Miao Powder supplemented with Radix Achyranthis Bidentatae (Niu Xi)	Same as Er Miao Powder (Er Miao San)
San Ren Decoction (San Ren Tang)	三仁汤	Analysis of Warm Diseases (Wen Bing Tiao Bian)	Semen Armeniacae Amarum (Xing Ren) 15g Talcum (Hua Shi Fen) 18g Medulla Tetrapanacis (Tong Cao) 6g Fructus Amomi Rotundus (Bai Dou Kou) 6g **Folium Phyllostachydis Henonis (Zhu Ye) 6g** Cortex Magnoliae Officinalis (Hou Po) 6g Semen Coicis (Sheng Yi Yi Ren) 18g Rhizoma Pinelliae (Ban Xia) 15g	Decoct the drugs in water for oral application.
San Wu Bei Ji Pill (San Wu Bei Ji Wan)	三物备急丸	Synopsis of Golden Chamber (Jin Gui Yao Lue)	Radix et Rhizoma Rhei (Da Huang) 3g Fructus Crotonis (Ba Dou) 3g Rhizoma Zingiberis (Gan Jiang) 3g	Prepare the drugs into pills or powder. Take 0.6-1.5g each time with warm water or wine. It can be administered with nasal feeding too.

Formula	Chinese	Source	Ingredients	Preparation
San Zi Yang Qin Decoction (San Zi Yang Qin Tang)	三子养亲汤	All Effectiv Prescriptions (Jie Xiao Fang)	Semen Sinapis Albae (Bai Jie Zi) 9g Fructus Perillae (Su Zi) 9g Semen Raphani Sativi (Lai Fu Zi) 9g	Smash the drugs and wrap them with a piece of cloth before decocting in water. Drink the decoction frequently.
Sang Bai Pi Decoction (Sang Bai Pi)	桑白皮汤	Jingyue's Complete Works (Jing Yue Quan Shu)	Cortex Mori Alba Radicis (Sang Bai Pi) 2.4g Rhizoma Pinelliae (Ban Xia) 2.4g Fructus Perillae (Su Zi) 2.4g Semen Pruni Armeniacae (Xing Ren) 2.4g Bulbus Fritillariae (Bei Mu) 2.4g Radix Scutellariae (Huang Qin) 2.4g Rhizoma Coptidis (Huang Lian) 2.4g Fructus Gardeniae (Zhi Zi) 2.4g	Decoct the drugs in water with 3 slices of Rhizoma Zingiberis Recens (Sheng Jiang) for oral application.
Sang Ju Decoction (Sang Ju Yin)	桑菊饮	Analysis of Warm Diseases (Wen Bing Tiao Bian)	Folium Mori (Sang Ye) 8g Semen Armeniacae Amarum (Xing Ren) 6g Radix Platycodonis (Jie Geng) 6g Rhizoma Phragmitis (Lu Gen) 6g Fructus Forsythiae Suspensae (Lian Qiao) 5g Flos Chrysanthemi Morifolii (Ju Hua) 3g Herba Menthae (Bo He) 3g Radix Glycyrrhizae (Sheng Gan Cao) 3g	Decoct the drugs in water for oral application.
Sang Piao Xiao Powder (Sang Piao Xiao San)	桑螵蛸散	Augmented Materia Medica (Ben Cao Yan Yi)	Radix Ginseng (Ren Shen) 9g Radix Polygalae (Yuan Zhi) 9g Ootheca Mantidis (Sang Piao Xiao) 9g Os Draconis (Long Gu) 9g Carapax et Plastrum Testudinis (Gui Ban) 9g Radix Angelicae Sinensis (Dang Gui) 9g Rhizoma Acori Graminei (Shi Chang Pu) 9g Sclerotium Poriae Circum Radicem Pini (Fu Shen) 9g	Decoct the drugs in water for oral application. Or prepare the drugs into powder, and take 6g each time before sleep.
Sang Xing Decoction (Sang Xing Tang)	桑杏汤	Analysis of Warm Diseases (Wen Bing Tiao Bian)	Folium Mori (Sang Ye) 3g Semen Armeniacae Amarum (Xing Ren) 4.5g Radix Adenophorae (Sha Shen) 6g Bulbus Fritillariae Thunbergii (Zhe Bei Mu) 3g Semen Sojae Preparatum (Dan Dou Chi) 3g Cortex Fructus Gardeniae (Zhi Zi Pi) 3g	Decoct the drugs in water for oral application.

			Cortex Exocarpium Pyrus (Li Pi) 3g	
Sha Shen Mai Dong Decoction (Sha Shen Mai Dong Tang)	沙参麦冬汤	Analysis of Warm Diseases (Wen Bing Tiao Bian)	Radix Adenophorae (Sha Shen) 9g Radix Ophiopogonis (Mai Dong) 9g Rhizoma Polygonati Odorati (Yu Zhu) 6g Radix Trichosanthis (Tian Hua Fen) 4.5g Semen Dolichoris Lablab (Bian Dou) 4.5g Folium Mori Alba (Sang Ye) 4.5g Radix Glycyrrhizae (Gan Cao) 3g	Decoct the drugs in water for oral application, twice daily.
Sha Shen Qing Fei Decoction (Sha Shen Qing Fei Tang)	沙参清肺汤	Effective Recipes (Yan Fang)	Radix Glehniae (Bei Sha Shen) Radix Astragali (Huang Qi) Radix Pseudostellariae (Tai Zi Shen) Cortex Albizziae (He Huan Pi) Rhizoma Bletillae Striatae (Bai Ji) Radix Glycyrrhizae (Gan Cao) Radix Platycodonis (Jie Geng) Semen Coicis (Yi Yi Ren) Semen Benincasae (Dong Gua Zi)	Decoct the drugs in water for oral application.
Shao Fu Zhu Yu Decoction (Shao Fu Zhu Yu Tang)	少腹逐瘀汤	Correction on the Errors of Medical Works (Yi Lin Gai Cuo)	Fructus Foeniculi Vulgaris (Xiao Hui Xiang) 7 grains Rhizoma Zingiberis (Gan Jiang) 0.6g Rhizoma Corydalis (Yan Hu Suo) 3g Radix Angelicae Sinensis (Dang Gui) 9g Rhizoma Ligustici Chuanxiong (Chuan Xiong) 6g Cortex Cinnamomi (Rou Gui) 3g Radix Paeoniae Rubra (Chi Shao) 6g Pollen Typhae (Pu Huang) 9g Excrementum Trogopteri (Wu Ling Zhi) 6g Myrrha (Mo Yao) 6g	Decoct the drugs in water for oral application.
Shao Yao Di Huang Decoction (Shao Yao Di Huang Tang), also named Xi Jiao Di Huang Decoction	芍药地黄汤 (又名犀角地黄汤)	Particle Prescriptions (Xiao Pin Fang)	Cornu Bubali (Shui Niu Jiao) 30g [to replace Cornu Rhinocerotis (Xi Jiao) in original recipe] Radix Rehmanniae Recens (Sheng Di Huang) 24g Radix Paeoniae (Shao Yao) 12g Cortex Moutan Radicis (Mu Dan Pi) 9g	Decoct the drugs in water for oral application.
Shao Yao Gan Cao Decoction (Shao Yao Gan Cao Tang)	芍药甘草汤	Treatise on Cold Induced Diseases (Shang Han Lun)	Radix Paeoniae (Shao Yao) 12g Radix Glycyrrhizae Praeparatae (Zhi Gan Cao) 12g	Decoct the drugs in water for oral application.

Shao Yao Decoction (Shao Yao Tang)	芍药汤	Collection on Pathogenesis for Protecting Life Based on Plain Questions (Su Wen Bing Ji Qi Yi Bao Ming Ji)	Radix Paeoniae (Shao Yao) 30g Radix Angelicae Sinensis (Dang Gui) 15g Radix Scutellariae (Huang Qin) 15g Rhizoma Coptidis (Huang Lian) 15g Radix et Rhizoma Rhei (Da Huang) 9g Radix Aucklandiae (Mu Xiang) 6g Semen Arecae (Bing Lang) 6g Radix Glycyrrhizae Praeparatae (Zhi Gan Cao) 6g Cortex Cinnamomi (Rou Gui) 5g	Decoct the drugs in water for oral application.
She Gan Ma Huang Decoction (She Gan Ma Huang Tang)	射干麻黄汤	Synopsis of the Golden Chamber (Jin Gui Yao Lue)	Rhizoma Belamcandae (She Gan) 9g Herba Ephedrae (Ma Huang) 12g Herba cum Radice Asari (Xi Xin) 9g Radix Asteris Tatarici (Zi Wan) 9g Flos Farfarae (Kuan Dong Hua) 9g Rhizoma Pinelliae (Ban Xia) 9g Fructus Schisandrae Chinensis (Wu Wei Zi) 3g Rhizoma Zingiberis Recens (Sheng Jiang) 12g Fructus Zizyphi Jujubae (Da Zao) 7 pcs	Decoct Ma Huang two times first, then add other drugs and decoct. Take 1/3 of the decoction each time, thrice daily.
Shen Fu Decoction (Shen Fu Tang)	参附汤	Effective Prescriptions for Women (Fu Ren Liang Fang)	Radix Ginseng (Ren Shen) 6g Radix Aconiti Lateralis Praeparatae (Fu Zi) 12g Rhizoma Zingiberis Recens (Sheng Jiang) 10 slices Fructus Zizyphi Jujubae (Da Zao) 5 pcs	Decoct the drugs in water for oral application before meals.
Shen Fu Long Mu Decoction (Shen Fu Long Mu Tang)	参附龙牡汤	Effective Recipes (Yan Fang)	Radix Ginseng (Ren Shen) 6g Radix Aconiti Lateralis Praeparatae (Fu Zi) 12g Os Draconis (Long Gu) 30g Concha Ostreae (Mu Li) 30g Rhizoma Zingiberis Recens (Sheng Jiang) 10 slices Fructus Zizyphi Jujubae (Da Zao) 5 pcs	Decoct Long Gu and Mu Li first, then add other drugs and decoct.
Shen Fu Yang Rong Decoction (Shen Fu Yang Rong Tang)	参附养荣汤	Wen Yi Lun	Radix Angelicae Sinensis (Dang Gui) 3g Radix Paeoniae Alba (Bai Shao Yao) 3g Radix Rehmanniae Recens (Sheng Di Huang) 9g Radix Ginseng (Ren Shen) 3g Radix Aconiti Lateralis Praeparatae (Fu Zi) 2.1g	Decoct the drugs in water for oral application.

			Rhizoma Zingiberis (Gan Jiang) 3g	
Shen Fu Zai Zao Pill (Shen Fu Zai Zao Wan)	参附再造丸	Edition of Popular Cold Induced Diseases (Tong Su Shang Han Lun)	Radix Ginseng (Ren Shen) 6g Radix Aconiti Lateralis Praeparatae (Fu Zi) 6g Ramulus Cinnamomi (Gui Zhi) 10g Rhizoma et Radix Notopterygii (Qiang Huo) 10g Radix Astragali (Huang Qi) 15g Herba cum Radice Asari (Xi Xin) 3g Radix Saposhnikoviae (Fang Feng) 18g Radix Glycyrrhizae Praeparatae (Zhi Gan Cao) 6g	Decoct the drugs in water for oral application.
Shen Ge Powder (Shen Ge San). Also named Shen Jie Powder (Shen Jie San)	参蛤散(又名参蚧散)	Prescriptions for Saving Lives (Ji Sheng Fang)	Radix Ginseng (Ren Shen) 9g Gecko (Ge Jie) 2 pcs	Grind into powder. Take 1-2g each time, twice or thrice daily.
Shen Ling Bai Zhu Powder (Shen Ling Bai Zhu San)	参苓白术散	Formularies of the Bureau of People's Welfare Pharmacy (Tai Ping Hui Min He Ji Ju Fang)	Rhizoma Atractylodis Macrocephalae (Bai Zhu) 12g Radix Ginseng (Ren Shen) 12g Rhizoma Dioscoreae (Shan Yao) 12g Semen Dolichoris Lablab (Bai Bian Dou) 6g Semen Nelumbinis (Lian Zi) 6g Sclerotium Poriae Cocos (Fu Ling) 12g Radix Glycyrrhizae Praeparatae (Zhi Gan Cao) 12g Semen Coicis (Yi Yi Ren) 6g Fructus Amomi Villosi (Sha Ren) 6g Radix Platycodonis (Jie Geng) 6g	Decoct the drugs in water for oral application. Or prepare the drugs into powder; take 6g each time with the decoction of Fructus Zizyphi Jujubae (Da Zao).
Shen Qi Di Huang Decoction (Shen Qi Di Huang Tang)	参芪地黄汤	Shen Shi Zun Sheng Shu	Radix Codonopsitis Pilosulae (Dang Shen) Radix Astragali (Huang Qi) Radix Rehmanniae Praeparatae (Shu Di Huang) Rhizoma Alismatis (Ze Xie) Rhizoma Dioscoreae (Shan Yao) Cortex Moutan Radicis (Mu Dan Pi) Fructus Corni Officinalis (Shan Zhu Yu)	Decoct the drugs in water for oral application.
Shen Qi Pill (Shen Qi Wan)	肾气丸	Synopsis of the Golden Chamber (Jin Gui Yao Lue)	Radix Rehmanniae Recens (Sheng Di Huang) 24g Rhizoma Dioscoreae (Shan Yao) 12g Fructus Corni (Shan Zhu Yu) 12g Rhizoma Alismatis (Ze Xie) 9g	Decoct the drugs in water for oral application. Or make the drugs into pills; take 6-9g each time with warm boiled water or

			Sclerotium Poriae Cocos (Fu Ling) 9g Cortex Moutan Radicis (Mu Dan Pi) 9g Ramulus Cinnamomi (Gui Zhi) 3g Radix Aconiti Lateralis Praeparatae (Pao Fu Zi) 3g	wine.
Shen Su Decoction (Shen Su Yin)	参苏饮	Formularies of the Bureau of People's Pharmacy (Tai Ping Hui Min He Ji Ju Fang)	Radix Ginseng (Ren Shen) 6g Folium Perillae (Zi Su Ye) 6g Radix Puerariae (Ge Gen) 6g Rhizoma Pinelliae (Ban Xia) 6g Radix Peucedani (Qian Hu) 6g Sclerotium Poriae Cocos (Fu Ling) 6g Fructus Aurantii (Zhi Ke) 4g Radix Platycodonis (Jie Geng) 4g Radix Aucklandiae (Mu Xiang) 4g Pericarpium Citri Reticulatae (Chen Pi) 4g Radix Glycyrrhizae Praeparatae (Zhi Gan Cao) 4g Rhizoma Zingiberis Recens (Sheng Jiang) 7 slices Fructus Zizyphi Jujubae (Da Zao) 1 pcs	Prepare the drugs except Sheng Jiang and Da Zao into powder, and then decoct the powder with Sheng Jiang and Da Zao in water of oral application. Or decoct all the drugs in water for oral application.
Shen Tong Zhu Yu Decoction (Shen Tong Zhu Yu Tang)	身痛逐瘀汤	Correction on the Errors of Medical Works (Yi Lin Gai Cuo)	Radix Gentianae Qinjiao (Qin Jiao) 3g Rhizoma Ligustici Chuanxiong (Chuan Xiong) 6g Semen Pruni Persicae (Tao Ren) 9g Flos Carthami Tinctorii (Hong Hua) 9g Radix Glycyrrhizae (Gan Cao) 6g Rhizoma et Radix Notopterygii (Qiang Huo) 3g Myrrha (Mo Yao) 6g Radix Angelicae Sinensis (Dang Gui) 9g Excrementum Trogopteri seu Pteromydis (Wu Ling Zhi) 6g Rhizoma Cyperi Rotundi (Xiang Fu) 3g Radix Cyathulae Officinalis (Chuan Niu Xi) 9g Lumbricus (Di Long) 6g	Decoct the drugs in water for oral application.
Shen Xian Huo Ming Decoction (Shen Xian Huo Ming Yin). Also named Xian Fang Huo Ming Decoction (Xian Fang	神仙活命饮	Effective Prescriptions for Women (Nu Ke Wan Jin Fang)	Radix Angelicae Dahuricae (Bai Zhi) 3g Bulbus Fritillariae (Bei Mu) 6g Radix Saposhnikoviae (Fang Feng) 6g Radix Paeoniae Rubra (Chi Shao) 6g	Add appropriate amount of wine and decoct the drugs in water for oral application.

Huo Ming Yin).			Radix Angelicae Sinensis (Dang Gui) 6g Radix Glycyrrhizae (Gan Cao) 6g Spina Gleditsiae (Zao Jiao Ci) 6g Squama Manis Praeparatae (Zhi Chuan Shan Jia) 6g Radix Trichosanthis (Tian Hua Fen) 6g Olibanum (Ru Xiang) 6g Myrrha (Mo Yao) 6g Flos Lonicerae (Jin Yin Hua) 9g Pericarpium Citri Reticulatae (Chen Pi) 9g	
Sheng Hua Decoction (Sheng Hua Tang)	生化汤	Fuqingzhu's Gynecology (Fu Qing Zhu Nu Ke)	Radix Angelicae Sinensis (Dang Gui) 24g Rhizoma Ligustici Chuanxiong (Chuan Xiong) 9g Semen Persicae (Tao Ren) 6g Rhizoma Zingiberis Praeparatae (Pao Jiang) 2g Radix Glycyrrhizae Praeparatae (Zhi Gan Cao) 2g	Decoct the drugs in water with appropriate amount of yellow rice wine and urine of boys under 12 for oral application.
Sheng Ma Ge Gen Decoction (Sheng Ma Ge Gen Tang)	升麻葛根汤	Formularies of the Bureau of People's Welfare Pharmacy (Tai Ping Hui Min He Ji Ju Fang)	Rhizoma Cimicifugae (Sheng Ma) 6g Radix Puerariae (Ge Gen) 9g Radix Paeoniae (Shao Yao) 6g Radix Glycyrrhizae Praeparatae (Zhi Gan Cao) 6g	Decoct the drugs in water for oral application.
Sheng Mai Powder (Sheng Mai San)	升脉散	The Origin of Medicine (Yi Xue Qi Yuan)	Radix Ginseng (Ren Shen) 9g Radix Ophiopogonis (Mai Dong) 9g Fructus Schisandrae Chinensis (Wu Wei Zi) 6g	Decoct the drugs in water for oral application.
Sheng Tie Luo Decoction (Sheng Tie Luo Yin)	生铁落饮	Medicine Comprehended (Yi Xue Xin Wu)	Radix Asparagi (Tian Dong) 9g Radix Ophiopogonis (Mai Dong) 9g Bulbus Fritillariae (Bei Mu) 9g Rhizoma Arisaematis cum Bile (Dan Nan Xing) 3g Exocarpium Citri Rubrum (Ju Hong) 3g Radix Polygalae (Yuan Zhi) 3g Rhizoma Acori Tatarinowii (Shi Chang Pu) 3g Fructus Forsythiae (Lian Qiao) 3g Sclerotium Poriae Cocos (Fu Ling) 3g Sclerotium Poriae Circum Radicem Pini (Fu Shen) 3g Radix Scrophulariae (Xuan Shen)	Decoct Ferri Frusta (Sheng Tie Luo) in water first, and then add other drugs to decoct for oral application.

			4.5g Ramulus Uncariae cum Uncis (Gou Teng) 4.5g Radix Salviae Miltiorrhizae (Dan Shen) 4.5g Cinnabaris (Chen Sha) 0.9g Ferri Frusta (Sheng Tie Luo) 60g	
Sheng Yu Decoction (Sheng Yu Tang)	圣愈汤	Golden Mirror of Medicine (Yi Zong Jin Jian)	Si Wu Decoction (Si Wu Tang) supplemented with Radix Ginseng (Ren Shen) and Radix Astragali (Huang Qi)	Decoct the drugs in water for oral application.
Shi Bu Pill (Shi Bu Wan)	十补丸	Prescriptions for Saving Lives (Ji Sheng Fang)	Radix Aconiti Lateralis Praeparatae (Pao Fu Zi) 10g Fructus Schisandrae Chinensis (Wu Wei Zi) 10g Fructus Corni (Shan Zhu Yu) 5g Rhizoma Dioscoreae Praeparatae (Chao Shan Yao) 5g Cortex Moutan Radicis (Mu Dan Pi) 5g Cornu Cervi Pantotrichum (Lu Rong) 5g Radix Rehmanniae Praeparatae (Shu Di Huang) 5g Cortex Cinnamomi (Rou Gui) 5g Sclerotium Poriae Cocos (Fu Ling) 5g Rhizoma Alismatis (Ze Xie) 5g	Prepare the drugs into pills, and take 9g each time with wine or salty water before meals. Or decoct the drugs in water for oral application.
Shi Hui Powder (Shi Hui San)	十灰散	Miraculous Book of Ten Herbs (Shi Yao Shen Shu)	Herba seu Radix Cirsii Japonici (Da Ji) 9g Herba Cephalanoploris (Xiao Ji) 9g Folium Nelumbinis (He Ye) 9g Cacumen Platycladi (Ce Bai Ye) 9g Rhizoma Imperatae (Bai Mao Gen) 9g Radix Rubiae (Qian Cao) 9g Fructus Gardeniae (Zhi Zi) 9g Radix et Rhizoma Rhei (Da Huang) 9g Cortex Moutan Radicis (Mu Dan Pi) 9g Trachycarpi Petiolus Radicis (Zong Lu Pi) 9g	The drugs are charred and ground into powder. Jing Mo is properly ground in an appropriate amount of lotus or carrot juice and then mix with 9-15g of the powder for oral application. Or decoct the drugs in water for oral application.
Shi Pi Powder (Shi Pi San)	实脾散	Revised Edition of Yan's Prescriptions for Saving Lives (Chong Ding Yan Shi Ji Sheng Fang)	Cortex Magnoliae Officinalis (Hou Po) 6g Rhizoma Atractylodis Macrocephalae (Bai Zhu) 6g Fructus Chaenomelis (Mu Gua) 6g Radix Aucklandiae (Mu Xiang) 6g Fructus Tsaoko (Cao Guo Ren) 6g Semen Arecae (Bing Lang) 6g Radix Aconiti Lateralis Praeparatae	Prepare the drugs into powder. Take 6g each time, and decoct it with Rhizoma Zingiberis Recens (Sheng Jiang) and Fructus Zizyphi Jujubae (Da Zao) in water for oral appli-

			(Pao Fu Zi) 6g Sclerotium Poriae Cocos (Bai Fu Ling) 6g Rhizoma Zingiberis (Gan Jiang) 6g Radix Glycyrrhizae Praeparatae (Zhi Gan Cao) 3g	cation.
Shi Pi Decoction (Shi Pi Yin)	实脾饮	Revised Edition of Yan's Prescriptions for Saving Lives (Chong Ding Yan Shi Ji Sheng Fang)	Cortex Magnoliae Officinalis (Hou Po) 6g Rhizoma Atractylodis Macrocephalae (Bai Zhu) 6g Fructus Chaenomelis (Mu Gua) 6g Radix Aucklandiae (Mu Xiang) 6g Fructus Tsaoko (Cao Guo Ren) 6g Semen Arecae (Bing Lang) 6g Radix Aconiti Lateralis Praeparatae (Pao Fu Zi) 6g Sclerotium Poriae Cocos (Bai Fu Ling) 6g Rhizoma Zingiberis (Gan Jiang) 6g Radix Glycyrrhizae Praeparatae (Zhi Gan Cao) 3g	Decoct all the drugs in water for oral application.
Shi Quan Da Bu Decoction (Shi Quan Da Bu Tang)	十全大补汤	Prescriptions of Auspicious Bamboo Hall (Rui Zhu Tang Fang)	Ba Zhen Decoction (Ba Zhen Tang) supplemented with Radix Astragali (Huang Qi) and Cortex Cinnamomi (Rou Gui)	Decoct the drugs in water for oral application.
Shi Wei Powder (Shi Wei San)	石苇散	Zheng Zhi Hui Bu	Folium Pyrrosiae (Shi Wei) Semen Malvae (Dong Kui Zi) Herba Dianthi (Qu Mai) Talcum (Hua Shi Fen) Semen Plantaginis (Che Qian Zi)	Make the drugs into pills. Take 6-9g each time.
Shi Xiao Pill (Shi Xiao Wan). Also named Zhi Shi Xiao Pi Pill (Zhi Shi Xiao Pi Wan)	失笑丸（又名枳实消痞丸）	Secret Book of Orchid Chamber (Lan Shi Mi Cang)	Rhizoma Zingiberis (Gan Jiang) 6g Radix Glycyrrhizae Praeparatae (Zhi Gan Cao) 6g Fructus Hordei Germinatus (Mai Ya) 6g Sclerotium Poriae Cocos (Bai Fu Ling) 6g Rhizoma Atractylodis Macrocephalae (Bai Zhu) 6g Rhizoma Pinelliae Fermentata (Ban Xia Qu) 9g Radix Ginseng (Ren Shen) 9g Cortex Magnoliae Officinalis (Hou Po) 12g Fructus Citri Aurantii Immaturus (Zhi Shi) 15g Rhizoma Coptidis (Huang Lian) 15g	Make the drugs into pills. Take 6-9g each time with warm boiled water, twice daily. Or decoct the drugs in water for oral application.
Shi Xiao Powder (Shi Xiao San)	失笑散	Formularies of the Bureau of People's	Excrementum Trogopteri (Wu Ling Zhi) 6g Pollen Typhae (Pu Huang) 6g	Grind the drugs into fine powder, and take 6g each time

		Welfare Pharmacy (Tai Ping Hui Min He Ji Ju Fang)		with yellow rice wine or vinegar, twice daily. Or wrap the drugs by gauze and decoct in water.
Shi Zao Decoction (Shi Zao Tang)	十枣汤	Treatise on Cold Induced Diseases (Shang Han Lun)	Radix Kansui (Gan Sui) Flos Genkwa (Yuan Hua) Radix Euphorbiae Pekinensis (Da Ji) Equal in dosage	Grind the drugs into fine powder and put into capsules (1-2g in each capsule). Decoct 10 pcs of Fructus Zizyphi Jujubae (Da Zao), and take one capsule with the decoction each time in the morning before meals, once daily.
Shu Gan Powder (Shu Gan San)	疏肝散	Bing Yin Mai Zhi	Radix Bupleuri (Chai Hu) Caulis Perillae (Su Geng) Pericarpium Citri Reticulatae Viride (Qing Pi) Ramulus Uncariae cum Uncis (Gou Teng) Fructus Gardeniae (Zhi Zi) Radix Paeoniae Alba (Bai Shao Yao) Pericarpium Citri Reticulatae (Chen Pi) Radix Glycyrrhizae (Gan Cao)	Decoct the drugs in water for oral application.
Shu Zao Decoction (Shu Zao Yin Zi)	疏凿饮子	Prescriptions for Saving Lives (Ji Sheng Fang)	Rhizoma Alismatis (Ze Xie) 6g Semen Phaseoli (Chi Xiao Dou) 6g Radix Phytolaccae (Shang Lu) 6g Rhizoma et Radix Notopterygii (Qiang Huo) 6g Pericarpium Arecae (Da Fu Pi) 6g Semen Zanthoxyli (Jiao Mu) 6g Caulis Akebiae (Mu Tong) 6g Radix Gentianae Macrophyllae (Qin Jiao) 6g Semen Arecae (Bing Lang) 6g Cortex Poria (Fu Ling Pi) 6g Rhizoma Zingiberis Recens (Sheng Jiang) 5 slices	Decoct the drugs in water for oral application. Or grind the drugs into powder, and take 9g each time with decoction of Sheng Jiang.
Shui Lu Er Xian Pill (Shui Lu Er Xian Dan)	水陆二仙丹	Standards of Diagnosis and Treatment (Zheng Zhi Zhun Sheng)	Fructus Rosae Laevigatae (Jin Ying Zi) Semen Euryales Ferocis (Qian Shi)	Make pills and take 6-9g each time with light salty water, twice daily.
Shun Qi Dao Tan Decoction (Shun Qi Dao Tan)	顺气导痰汤	Effective Recipes (Yan Fang)	Rhizoma Pinelliae (Ban Xia) 9g Pericarpium Citri Reticulatae (Chen Pi) 9g	Decoct the drugs in water for oral application.

			Sclerotium Poriae Cocos (Fu Ling) 12g Radix Glycyrrhizae (Gan Cao) 6g Rhizoma Zingiberis Recens (Sheng Jiang) 9g Rhizoma Arisaematis cum Bile (Dan Nan Xing) 6g Fructus Citri Aurantii Immaturus (Zhi Shi) 6g Radix Aucklandiae (Mu Xiang) 6g Rhizoma Cyperi Rotundi (Xiang Fu) 6g	
Shun Qi He Zhong Decoction (Shun Qi He Zhong)	顺气和中汤	Standards of Diagnosis and Treatment (Zheng Zhi Zhun Sheng)	Radix Astragali (Huang Qi) 4.5g Radix Ginseng (Ren Shen) 3g Rhizoma Atractylodis Macrocephalae (Bai Zhu) 1.5g Pericarpium Citri Reticulatae (Chen Pi) 1.5g Radix Angelicae Sinensis (Dang Gui) 1.5g Radix Paeoniae Alba (Bai Shao Yao) 1.5g Radix Glycyrrhizae Praeparatae (Zhi Gan Cao) 2.1g Rhizoma Cimicifugae (Sheng Ma) 0.9g Radix Bupleuri (Chai Hu) 0.9g Fructus Viticis (Man Jing Zi) 0.6g Rhizoma Ligustici Chuanxiong (Chuan Xiong) 0.6g Herba cum Radice Asari (Xi Xin) 0.6g	Decoct the drugs in water for oral application after meals.
Si Jun Zi Decoction (Si Jun Zi Tang)	四君子汤	Formularies of the Bureau of People's Welfare Pharmacy (Tai Ping Hui Min He Ji Ju Fang)	Radix Ginseng (Ren Shen) 6g Rhizoma Atractylodis Macrocephalae (Bai Zhu) 6g Sclerotium Poriae Cocos (Fu Ling) 6g Radix Glycyrrhizae Praeparatae (Gan Cao) 6g	Decoct the drugs in water for oral application.
Si Miao Pill (Si Miao Wan)	四妙丸	Cheng Fang Bian Du	Cortex Phellodendri (Huang Bai) 9g Rhizoma Atractylodis (Cang Zhu) 9g Radix Achyranthis Bidentatae (Niu Xi) 12g Semen Coicis (Yi Yi Ren) 12g	Decoct the drugs in water for oral application. Or make the drugs into pills, and take 6g each time.
Si Miao Yong An Decoction (Si Miao Yong An Tang)	四妙勇安汤	New Compilation of Effective Recipes (Yan Fang Xin Bian)	Flos Lonicerae (Jin Yin Hua) 45g Radix Scrophulariae (Xuan Shen) 45g Radix Angelicae Sinensis (Dang Gui) 30g Radix Glycyrrhizae (Gan Cao) 15g	Decoct the drugs in water for oral application.

Si Ni Powder (Si Ni San)	四逆散	Treatise on Cold Induced Diseases (Shang Han Lun)	Radix Glycyrrhizae Praeparatae (Zhi Gan Cao) 6g Fructus Citri Aurantii Immaturus (Zhi Shi) 6g Radix Bupleuri (Chai Hu) 6g Radix Paeoniae Alba (Bai Shao Yao) 6g	Decoct the drugs in water for oral application.
Si Ni Decoction (Si Ni Tang)	四逆汤	Treatise on Cold Induced Diseases (Shang Han Lun)	Radix Glycyrrhizae Praeparatae (Zhi Gan Cao) 6g Rhizoma Zingiberis (Gan Jiang) 9g Radix Aconiti Lateralis (Sheng Fu Zi) 15g	Decoct the drugs in water for oral application.
Si Ni Jia Ren Shen Decoction (Si Ni Jia Ren Shen Tang)	四逆加人参汤	Treatise on Cold Induced Diseases (Shang Han Lun)	Radix Ginseng (Ren Shen) 6g Radix Glycyrrhizae Praeparatae (Zhi Gan Cao) 6g Rhizoma Zingiberis (Gan Jiang) 9g Radix Aconiti Lateralis Praeparatae (Fu Zi) 15g	Decoct the drugs in water for oral application.
Si Shen Pill (Si Shen Wan)	四神丸	Standards of Diagnosis and Treatment (Zheng Zhi Zhun Sheng)	Semen Myristicae (Rou Dou Kou) 6g Fructus Psoraleae (Bu Gu Zhi) 12g Fructus Schisandrae Chinensis (Wu Wei Zi) 6g Fructus Evodiae (Wu Zhu Yu) 3g Rhizoma Zingiberis Recens (Sheng Jiang) 6g Fructus Zizyphi Jujubae (Da Zao) 5 pcs	Decoct the drugs in water for oral application. Or prepare the drugs except Sheng Jiang and Da Zao into pills, and take 6g each time with the decoction of Sheng Jiang and Da Zao before meals.
Si Wei Hui Yang Decoction (Si Wei Hui Yang Yin)	四味回阳饮	Jingyue's Complete Works (Jing Yue Quan Shu)	Radix Ginseng (Ren Shen) 30-60g Radix Aconiti Lateralis Praeparatae (Fu Zi) 6-9g Rhizoma Zingiberis (Gan Jiang) 6-9g Radix Glycyrrhizae Praeparatae (Zhi Gan Cao) 3-6g	Decoct the drugs in water for oral application.
Si Wu Decoction (Si Wu Tang)	四物汤	Clandestine Prescriptions for Wounds and Bonesetting Handed down by the Fairy (Xian Shou Li Shang Xu Duan Mi Fang)	Radix Rehmanniae Praeparatae (Shu Di Huang) 12g Radix Angelicae Sinensis (Dang Gui) 6g Radix Paeoniae Alba (Bai Shao) 6g Rhizoma Ligustici Chuanxiong (Chuan Xiong) 3g	Decoct the drugs in water for oral application.
Su He Xiang Pill (Su He Xiang Wan). Original name Chi Li Qie Pill (Chi Li Qie Wan)	苏合香丸	Prescriptions for Benefiting Health (Guang Ji Fang)	Styrax (Su He Xiang) 15g Borneolum Syntheticum (Bing Pian) 15g Olibanum (Ru Xiang) 15g Moschus (She Xiang) 30g Benzoinum (An Xi Xiang) 30g	1) Zhu Sha is refined with water into extremely fine powder; 2) She Xiang, Bing Pian and Shui Niu Jiao are ground into

			Radix Aucklandiae (Mu Xiang) 30g Rhizoma Cyperi (Xiang Fu) 30g Lignum Santali Albi (Tan Xiang) 30g Flos Caryophylli (Ding Xiang) 30g Lignum Aquilariae Resinatum (Chen Xiang) 30g Fructus Piperis Longi (Bi Ba) 30g Rhizoma Atractylodis Macrocephalae (Bai Zhu) 30g Fructus Chebulae (He Zi) 30g Cinnabaris (Zhu Sha) 30g Cornu Bubali (Shui Niu Jiao) 60g [to replace Cornu Rhinocerotis (Xi Jiao)]	fine powder; 3) the rest drugs except Su He Xiang are ground into fine powder; 4) mix powder from 1), 2) and 3) evenly and sift. 5) Finally, melt Su He Xiang and add honey to make pills, and let the pills dry in low temperature. Take one pill each time with warm boiled water, once or twice daily. Decrease the dosage accordingly for children. For coma patients, use nasal feeding.
Su Zi Jiang Qi Decoction (Su Zi Jiang Qi Tang)	苏子降气汤	Formularies of the Bureau of People's Welfare Pharmacy (Tai Ping Hui Min He Ji Ju Fang)	Fructus Perillae (Zi Su Zi) 9g Rhizoma Pinelliae (Ban Xia) 9g Radix Angelicae Sinensis (Dang Gui) 6g Radix Glycyrrhizae Praeparatae (Zhi Gan Cao) 6g Radix Peucedani (Qian Hu) 6g Cortex Magnoliae Officinalis (Hou Po) 6g Cortex Cinnamomi (Rou Gui) 6g Rhizoma Zingiberis Recens (Sheng Jiang) 2 slices Fructus Zizyphi Jujubae (Da Zao) 1 piece Folium Perillae (Zi Su Ye) 5 leaves	Decoct the drug in water for oral application.
Suan Zao Ren Decoction (Suan Zao Ren Tang)	酸枣仁汤	Synopsis of the Golden Chamber (Jin Gui Yao Lue)	Semen Zizyphi Spinosae (Suan Zao Ren) 15g Sclerotium Poriae Cocos (Fu Ling) 6g Rhizoma Ligustici Chuanxiong (Chuan Xiong) 6g Radix Glycyrrhizae (Gan Cao) 3g Rhizoma Anemarrhenae (Zhi Mu) 6g	Decoct the drug in water for oral application.
Suo Quan Pill (Suo Quan Wan)	缩泉丸	Secret Prescriptions of Wei Family (Wei Shi Jia Cang Fang)	Fructus Alpiniae Oxyphyllae (Yi Zhi Ren) 9g Radix Linderae (Wu Yao) 9g Rhizoma Dioscoreae (Shan Yao) 9g	Decoct the drug in water for oral application. Or make Wu Yao and Yi Zhi Ren into pills with the paste of Shan Yao, and take 6g each time with salty water or thin rice gruel.

Name	Chinese	Source	Ingredients	Preparation
Tai Shan Pan Shi Powder (Tai Shan Pan Shi San)	泰山磐石散	Medical Complete Book, Ancient and Modern (Gu Jin Yi Tong Da Quan)	Radix Ginseng (Ren Shen) 9g Radix Astragali (Huang Qi) 9g Rhizoma Atractylodis Macrocephalae (Bai Zhu) 4.5g Radix Glycyrrhizae Praeparatae (Zhi Gan Cao) 4.5g Radix Angelicae Sinensis (Dan Gui) 9g Rhizoma Ligustici Chuanxiong (Chuan Xiong) 7g Radix Paeoniae Alba (Bai Shao Yao) 7g Radix Rehmanniae Praeparatae (Shu Di Huang) 7g Radix Dipsaci (Xu Duan) 6g Semen Oryzae Sativae (Nuo Mi) 6g Radix Scutellariae (Huang Qin) 6g Fructus Amomi Villosi (Sha Ren) 4.5g	Decoct the drugs in water for oral application. Take two doses every week for two or three months after the second month of pregnancy.
Tao He Cheng Qi Decoction (Tao He Cheng Qi Tang)	桃核承气汤	Treatise on Cold Induced Diseases (Shang Han Lun)	Semen Persicae (Tao Ren) 12g Radix et Rhizoma Rhei (Da Huang) 12g Ramulus Cinnamomi (Gui Zhi) 6g Radix Glycyrrhizae Praeparatae (Zhi Gan Cao) 6g Natrii Sulfas (Mang Xiao) 6g	Decoct the drugs except Mang Xiao in water, and then melt Mang Xiao in the decoction.
Tao Hong Si Wu Decoction (Tao Hong Si Wu Tang)	桃红四物汤	Clandestine Prescriptions for Wounds and Bonesetting Handed down by the Fairy (Xian Shou Li Shang Xu Duan Mi Fang)	Si Wu Decoction (Si Wu Tang) supplemented with Semen Persicae (Tao Ren) and Flos Carthami (Hong Hua)	Decoct the drugs in water for oral application.
Tao Hong Decoction (Tao Hong Yin)	桃红饮	Lei Zheng Zhi Cai	Semen Persicae (Tao Ren) Flos Carthami (Hong Hua) Rhizoma Ligustici Chuanxiong (Chuan Xiong) Tail of Radix Angelicae Sinensis (Dang Gui Wei) Radix Clematidis (Wei Ling Xian)	Decoct the drugs in water and add little Moschus (She Xiang) for oral application.
Tao Ren Cheng Qi Decoction (Tao Ren Cheng Qi Tang)	桃仁承气汤	Treatise on Cold Induced Diseases (Shang Han Lun)	Tiao Wei Cheng Qi Decoction (Tiao Wei Cheng Qi Tang) supplemented with Semen Persicae (Tao Ren) and Ramulus Cinnamomi (Gui Zhi)	Decoct drugs except Natrii Sulfas (Mang Xiao) in water, remove the residue, and then dissolve Mang Xiao in the decoction.

Tao Ren Hong Hua Decoction (Tao Ren Hong Hua Jian)	桃仁红花煎	Su An Yi An	Radix Salviae Miltiorrhizae (Dan Shen) Radix Paeoniae Rubra (Chi Shao) Semen Persicae (Tao Ren) Flos Carthami (Hong Hua) Rhizoma Cyperi Rotundi (Xiang Fu) Rhizoma Corydalis (Yan Hu Suo) Pericarpium Citri Reticulatae Viride (Qing Pi) Radix Angelicae Sinensis (Dang Gui) Rhizoma Ligustici Chuanxiong (Chuan Xiong) Radix Rehmanniae Recens (Sheng Di Huang)	Decoct the drugs in water for oral application.
Tian Ma Gou Teng Decoction (Tian Ma Gou Teng Yin)	天麻钩藤饮	New Concepts for Diagnosis and Treatment of Miscellaneous Diseases (Za Bing Zheng Zhi Xin Yi)	Caulis Polygoni Multiflori (Ye Jiao Teng) 9g Concha Haliotidis (Shi Jue Ming) 18g Herba Taxilli (Sang Ji Sheng) 9g Ramulus Uncariae cum Uncis (Gou Teng) 12g Sclerotium Poriae Circum Radicem Pini (Fu Sheng) 9g Herba Leonuri (Yi Mu Cao) 9g Radix Achyranthis Bidentatae (Niu Xi) 12g Cortex Eucommiae (Du Zhong) 9g Rhizoma Gastrodiae (Tian Ma) 9g Fructus Gardeniae (Zhi Zi) 9g Radix Scutellariae (Huang Qin) 9g	Decoct the drugs in water for oral application.
Tian Tai Wu Yao Powder (Tian Tai Wu Yao San). Also named Wu Yao Powder (Wu Yao San)	天台乌药散 (又名乌药散)	Complete Record of Holy Benevolence (Sheng Ji Zong Lu)	Radix Linderae (Wu Yao) 9g Radix Aucklandiae (Mu Xiang) 9g Fructus Foeniculi (Xiao Hui Xiang) 9g Pericarpium Citri Reticulatae Viride (Qing Pi) 9g Rhizoma Alpiniae Officinarum (Gao Liang Jiang) 9g Semen Arecae (Bing Lang) 6g Fructus Meliae Toosendan (Chuan Lian Zi) 12g Fructus Crotonis (Ba Dou) 12g	Roast Ba Dou and Chuan Lian Zi until they turn black, remove Ba Dou from the mixture, and decoct all the drugs for oral application. Take appropriate amount of yellow rice wine each time. Or make the drugs into powder, and take 3g each time with warm wine.
Tian Wang Bu Xin Pill (Tian Wang Bu Xin Dan)	天王补心丹	Check and Annotate Effective Prescriptions for Women (Jiao Zhu Fu	Radix Rehmanniae Recens (Sheng Di Huang) 15g Radix Ginseng (Ren Shen) 5g Sclerotium Poriae Cocos (Bai Fu Ling) 5g Radix Polygalae (Yuan Zhi) 5g	Decoct the drugs in water for oral application. Or make pellets coated by Cinnabaris (Zhu Sha), and take 6-9g each time

		Ren Liang Fang)	Radix Scrophulariae (Xuan Shen) 5g Semen Biotae Orientalis (Bai Zi Ren) 10g Radix Platycodonis (Jie Geng) 5g Radix Asparagi (Tian Dong) 10g Radix Salviae Miltiorrhizae (Dan Shen) 5g Semen Zizyphi Spinosae (Suan Zao Ren) 10g Radix Ophiopogonis (Mai Dong) 10g Radix Angelicae Sinensis (Dang Gui) 10g Fructus Schisandrae Chinensis (Wu Wei Zi) 10g	with warm boiled water or decoction of Arillus Longan (Long Yan Rou) before sleep.
Tiao Wei Cheng Qi Decoction (Tiao Wei Cheng Qi Tang)	调胃承气汤	Treatise on Cold Induced Diseases (Shang Han Lun)	Radix Glycyrrhizae Praeparatae (Zhi Gan Cao) 6g Natrii Sulfas (Mang Xiao) 15g Radix et Rhizoma Rhei (Da Huang) 12g	Decoct Da Huang and Zhi Gan Cao, remove the residue, and then dissolve Mang Xiao in the decoction.
Tiao Ying Decoction (Tiao Ying Yin)	调营饮	Standards of Diagnosis and Treatment (Zheng Zhi Zhun Sheng)	Rhizoma Curcumae Ezhu (E Zhu) Rhizoma Ligustici Chuanxiong (Chuan Xiong) Radix Angelicae Sinensis (Dang Gui) Rhizoma Corydalis (Yan Hu Suo) Radix Paeoniae Rubra (Chi Shao) Herba Dianthi (Qu Mai) Radix et Rhizoma Rhei (Da Huang) Semen Areca Catechu (Bing Lang) Pericarpium Citri Reticulatae (Chen Pi) Pericarpium Areca Catechu (Da Fu Pi) Semen Descurainiae seu Lepidii (Ting Li Zi) Sclerotium Poriae Cocos Rubra (Chi Fu Ling) Cortex Mori Alba Radicis (Sang Bai Pi) Herba cum Radice Asari (Xi Xin) Cortex Cinnamomi (Rou Gui) Radix Glycyrrhizae Praeparatae (Zhi Gan Cao) Rhizoma Zingiberis Recens (Sheng Jiang) Fructus Zizyphi Jujubae (Da Zao) Radix Angelicae Dahuricae (Bai Zhi)	Decoct the drugs in water for oral application.
Ting Li Da Zao	葶苈大枣	Synopsis of	Semen Descurainiae seu Lepidii	Decoct Da Zao first,

Formula	Chinese	Source	Ingredients	Administration
Xie Fei Decoction (Ting Li Da Zao Xie Fei Tang)	泻肺汤	the Golden Chamber (Jin Gui Yao Lue)	(Ting Li Zi) 9g Fructus Zizyphi Jujubae (Da Zao) 12 pcs	then add Ting Li Zi and decoct for oral application.
Tong Qiao Huo Xue Decoction (Tong Qiao Huo Xue Tang)	通窍活血汤	Correction on the Errors of Medical Works (Yi Lin Gai Cuo)	Radix Paeoniae Rubra (Chi Shao) 6g Rhizoma Ligustici Chuanxiong (Chuan Xiong) 4.5g Semen Persicae (Tao Ren) 12g Flos Carthami (Hong Hua) 9g Bulbus Allii Fistulosi (Lao Cong) 9g Rhizoma Zingiberis Recens (Sheng Jiang) 9g Fructus Zizyphi Jujubae (Da Zao) 15g Moschus (She Xiang) 0.5g Yellow Rice Wine	Decoct the drugs in water for oral application.
Tong Xie Formula (Tong Xie Yao Fang)	痛泻要方	Danxi's Experiential Therapy (Dan Xi Xin Fa)	Rhizoma Atractylodis Macrocephalae Praeparatae (Chao Bai Zhu) 9g Radix Paeoniae Alba Praeparatae (Chao Bai Shao) 6g Pericarpium Citri Reticulatae (Chen Pi) 4.5g Radix Saposhnikoviae (Fang Feng) 3g	Decoct the drugs in water for oral application.
Tong You Decoction (Tong You Tang)	通幽汤	Secret Book of Orchid Chamber (Lan Shi Mi Cang)	Radix Rehmanniae Recens (Sheng Di Huang) 1.5g Radix Rehmanniae Praeparatae (Shu Di Huang) 1.5g Radix Angelicae Sinensis (Dang Gui) 3g Semen Pruni Persicae (Tao Ren) 0.3g Flos Carthami (Hong Hua) 0.3g Rhizoma Cimicifugae (Sheng Ma) 3g Radix Glycyrrhizae Praeparatae (Zhi Gan Cao) 3g	Decoct the drugs in water; then add 1.5g of Semen Areca Catechu (Bing Lang) fine powder for oral application before meals.
Wan Dai Decoction (Wan Dai Tang)	完带汤	Fu Qingzhu's Gynecology (Fu Qing Zhu Nu Ke)	Rhizoma Atractylodis Macrocephalae (Bai Zhu) 30g Rhizoma Dioscoreae (Shan Yao) 30g Radix Paeoniae Alba (Bai Shao Yao) 15g Semen Plantaginis (Che Qian Zi) 9g Rhizoma Atractylodis (Cang Zhu) 9g Radix Ginseng (Ren Shen) 6g Radix Glycyrrhizae (Gan Cao) 3g Radix Bupleuri (Chai Hu) 2g Pericarpium Citri Reticulatae (Chen Pi) 2g	Decoct the drugs in water for oral application.

			Flos Schizonepetae (Jing Jie Sui Tan) 2g	
Wan Shi Niu Huang Qing Xin Pill (Wan Shi Niu Huang Qing Xin Wan). Also named Niu Huang Qing Xin Pill (Niu Huang Qing Xin Wan).	万氏牛黄清心丸 (又名牛黄清心丸)	Hereditary Physician's Mastery of Medicine for Sore and Nail-form Boil (Chuang Ding Shi Yi Xin Fa)	Cinnabaris (Chen Sha) 4g Rhizoma Coptidis (Huang Lian) 15g Radix Scutellariae (Huang Qin) 9g Fructus Gardeniae (Zhi Zi) 9g Radix Curcumae (Yu Jin) 6g Calculus Bovis (Niu Huang) 1g	Prepare the drugs into pill. Take 3g each time with decoction of Medulla Junci Effusi (Deng Xin Cao).
Wan Shi Niu Huang Pill (Wan Shi Niu Huang Wan). Also named Niu Huang Qing Xin Pill (Niu Huang Qing Xin Wan).	万氏牛黄丸 (又名牛黄清心丸)	Hereditary Physician's Mastery of Medicine for Sore and Nail-form Boil (Chuang Ding Shi Yi Xin Fa)	Cinnabaris (Chen Sha) 4g Rhizoma Coptidis (Huang Lian) 15g Radix Scutellariae (Huang Qin) 9g Fructus Gardeniae (Zhi Zi) 9g Radix Curcumae (Yu Jin) 6g Calculus Bovis (Niu Huang) 1g	Prepare the drugs into pill. Take 3g each time with decoction of Medulla Junci Effusi (Deng Xin Cao).
Wei Jing Decoction (Wei Jing Tang)	苇茎汤	Arcane Essentials from the Imperial Library (Wai Tai Mi Yao)	Caulis Phragmitis (Wei Jing) 60g Semen Coicis (Yi Yi Ren) 30g Semen Benincasae (Dong Gua Zi) 30g Semen Persicae (Tao Ren) 9g	Decoct the drugs in water for oral application.
Wei Ling Decoction (Wei Ling Tang)	胃苓汤	Danxi's Experiential Therapy (Dan Xi Xin Fa)	Rhizoma Atractylodis (Cang Zhu) Cortex Magnoliae Officinalis (Hou Po) Pericarpium Citri Reticulatae (Chen Pi) Rhizoma Atractylodis Macrocephalae (Bai Zhu) Sclerotium Poriae Cocos (Fu Ling) Rhizoma Alismatis (Ze Xie) Sclerotium Polypori Umbellati (Zhu Ling) Radix Glycyrrhizae (Gan Cao) Cortex Cinnamomi (Rou Gui) Rhizoma Zingiberis Recens (Sheng Jiang) Fructus Zizyphi Jujubae (Da Zao)	Grind the drugs into coarse powder. Decoct 15g with 5 slices of Rhizoma Zingiberis Recens (Sheng Jiang) and 2 pcs of Fructus Zizyphi Jujubae (Da Zao) for oral application.
Wei Rui Decoction (Wei Rui Tang)	葳蕤汤	Revised Edition of Popular Cold Induced Diseases (Chong Ding Tong Su Shang Han Lun)	Rhizoma Polygonati Odorati (Sheng Yu Zhu) 9g Bulbus Allii Fistulosi (Sheng Cong Bai) 6g Radix Platycodonis (Jie Geng) 4.5g Radix Cynanchi Atrati (Bai Wei) 3g Semen Sojae Preparatum (Dan Dou Chi) 12g Herba Menthae (Bo He) 4.5g Radix Glycyrrhizae Praeparatae (Zhi Gan Cao) 1.5g	Decoct the drugs in water for oral application.

			Fructus Ziziphi Jujubae (Da Zao) 2 pcs	
Wen Dan Decoction (Wen Dan Tang)	温胆汤	Treatise on Three Categories of Pathogenic Factors and Prescriptions (San Yin Ji Yi Bing Zheng Fang Lun)	Pericarpium Citri Reticulatae (Chen Pi) 9g Rhizoma Pinelliae (Ban Xia) 6g Fructus Citri Aurantii Immaturus (Zhi Shi) 6g Caulis Bambusae in Taeniam (Zhu Ru) 6g Sclerotium Poriae Cocos (Fu Ling) 4.5g Radix Glycyrrhizae Praeparatae (Zhi Gan Cao) 3g Rhizoma Zingiberis Recens (Sheng Jiang) 5 slices Fructus Ziziphi Jujubae (Da Zao) 1 piece	Decoct the drugs in water for oral application.
Wen Jing Decoction (Wen Jing Tang)	温经汤	Synopsis of the Golden Chamber (Jin Gui Yao Lue)	Fructus Evodiae (Wu Zhu Yu) 9g Radix Ophiopogonis (Mai Dong) 9g Rhizoma Pinelliae (Ban Xia) 6g Rhizoma Zingiberis Recens (Sheng Jiang) 6g Radix Angelicae Sinensis (Dang Gui) 6g Rhizoma Ligustici Chuanxiong (Chuan Xiong) 6g Radix Paeoniae (Shao Yao) 6g Radix Ginseng (Ren Shen) 6g Ramulus Cinnamomi (Gui Zhi) 6g Cortex Moutan Radicis (Mu Dan Pi) 6g Radix Glycyrrhizae (Gan Cao) 6g Colla Corii Asini (E Jiao) 6g	Decoct the drugs except E Jiao in water, and then melt E Jiao in the decoction for oral application.
Wen Pi Decoction (Wen Pi Tang)	温脾汤	Invaluable Prescriptions for Emergencies (Bei Ji Qian Jin Yao Fang)	Radix et Rhizoma Rhei (Da Huang) 15g Radix Angelicae Sinensis (Dang Gui) 9g Rhizoma Zingiberis (Gan Jiang) 9g Radix Aconiti Lateralis Praeparatae (Fu Zi) 6g Radix Ginseng (Ren Shen) 6g Natrii Sulfas (Mang Xiao) 6g Radix Glycyrrhizae (Gan Cao) 6g	Decoct the drugs in water for oral application.
Wu Bi Shan Yao Pill (Wu Bi Shan Yao Wan)	无比山药丸	Formularies of the Bureau of People's Pharmacy (Tai Ping Hui Min He Ji Ju Fang)	Radix Rehmanniae Praeparatae (Shu Di Huang) 30g Fructus Corni (Shan Zhu Yu) 30g Rhizoma Dioscoreae (Shan Yao) 60g Sclerotium Poriae Circum Radicem Pini (Fu Shen) [or Sclerotium Poriae Cocos (Fu	Make boluses with honey, and take 6-9g each time with wine before meals, twice daily.

			Ling)]30g Rhizoma Alismatis (Ze Xie) 30g Herba Cistanches (Rou Cong Rong) 120g Semen Cuscutae Chinensis (Tu Si Zi) 90g Fructus Schisandrae Chinensis (Wu Wei Zi) 180g Halloysitum Rubrum (Chi Shi Zhi) 30g Radix Morindae Officinalis (Ba Ji Tian) 30g Cortex Eucommiae (Du Zhong) 90g Radix Achyranthis Bidentatae (Niu Xi) 30g	
Wu Ji Powder (Wu Ji San)	五积散	Formularies of the Bureau of People's Pharmacy (Tai Ping Hui Min He Ji Ju Fang)	Rhizoma Atractylodis (Cang Zhu) 12g Radix Platycodonis (Jie Geng) 9g Fructus Aurantii (Zhi Ke) 6g Pericarpium Citri Reticulatae (Chen Pi) 6g Herba Ephedrae (Ma Huang) 6g Radix Paeoniae Alba (Bai Shao Yao) 3g Radix Angelicae Dahuricae (Bai Zhi) 3g Rhizoma Ligustici Chuanxiong (Chuan Xiong) 3g Radix Angelicae Sinensis (Dang Gui) 3g Radix Glycyrrhizae Praeparatae (Zhi Gan Cao) 3g Cortex Cinnamomi (Rou Gui) 3g Sclerotium Poriae Cocos (Fu Ling) 3g Rhizoma Pinelliae (Ban Xia) 3g Cortex Magnoliae Officinalis (Hou Po) 4g Rhizoma Zingiberis (Gan Jiang) 4g	Prepare the drugs into powder, and take 9g each time, twice daily. Or Decoct the drugs in water for oral application.
Wu Ji Pill (Wu Ji Wan)	戊己丸	Danxi's Experiential Therapy (Dan Xi Xin Fa)	Rhizoma Coptidis (Huang Lian) Fructus Evodiae (Wu Zhu Yu) Radix Paeoniae Alba (Bai Shao Yao)	The three drugs are equal in dosage. Prepare the drugs into pills, and take 3g each time. Or decoct the drugs in water for oral application.
Wu Ling Powder (Wu Ling San)	五苓散	Treatise on Cold Induced Diseases (Shang Han Lun)	Sclerotium Poriae Cocos (Fu Ling) 9g Sclerotium Polypori Umbellati (Zhu Ling) 9g Rhizoma Atractylodis Macrocepha-	Prepare the drugs into powder, and take 6g each time with warm boiled water. Or decoct the

Formula	Chinese	Source	Ingredients	Preparation
			lae (Bai Zhu) 9g Rhizoma Alismatis (Ze Xie) 15g Ramulus Cinnamomi (Gui Zhi) 6g	drugs in water for oral application.
Wu Mei Pill (Wu Mei Wan)	乌梅丸	Treatise on Cold Induced Diseases (Shang Han Lun)	Fructus Mume (Wu Mei) 30g Herba Asari (Xi Xin) 3g Rhizoma Coptidis (Huang Lian) 9g Rhizoma Zingiberis (Gan Jiang) 9g Pericarpium Zanthoxyli (Hua Jiao) 6g Cortex Phellodendri (Huang Bai) 6g Radix Aconiti Lateralis Praeparatae (Fu Zi) 6g Ramulus Cinnamomi (Gui Zhi) 6g Radix Ginseng (Ren Shen) 6g Radix Angelicae Sinensis (Dang Gui) 6g	Decoct the drugs in water for oral application. Or prepare the drugs into pills with honey, and take 9g each time, twice or thrice daily.
Wu Mo Decoction (Wu Mo Yin Zi)	五磨饮子	Collected Exegesis of Recipes (Yi Fang Ji Jie)	Radix Linderae (Wu Yao) Lignum Aquilariae Resinatum (Chen Xiang) Semen Areca Catechu (Bing Lang) Fructus Citri Aurantii Immaturus (Zhi Shi) Radix Aucklandiae (Mu Xiang) (equal in dosage)	Grind the drugs with white spirit for oral application.
Wu Pi Powder (Wu Pi San). Also named Wu Pi Decoction (Wu Pi Yin	五皮散 (又名五皮饮)	Hua's Reserved Canon on Medicine (Hua Shi Zhong Zang Jing)	Cortex Poriae Cocos (Fu Ling Pi) 9g Pericarpium Areca (Da Fu Pi) 9g Cortex Rhizoma Zingiberis Recens (Sheng Jiang Pi) 9g Cortex Mori Alba Radicis (Sang Bai Pi) 9g Pericarpium Citri Reticulatae (Chen Pi) 9g	Prepare the drugs into power, and decoct 9g of the powder each time for oral application. Or decoct the five drugs in water for oral application.
Wu Tou Decoction (Wu Tou Tang)	乌头汤	Synopsis of the Golden Chamber (Jin Gui Yao Lue)	Radix Aconiti Carmichaeli (Chuan Wu) 6g Herba Ephedrae (Ma Huang) 9g Radix Paeoniae (Shao Yao) 9g Radix Astragali (Huang Qi) 9g Radix Glycyrrhizae (Gan Cao) 9g	Decoct the drugs in water, remove residue, add honey and decoct again.
Wu Wei Xiao Du Decoction (Wu Wei Xiao Du Yin)	五味消毒饮	Golden Mirror of Medicine (Yi Zong Jin Jian)	Flos Lonicerae (Jin Yin Hua) 9g Herba Taraxaci Mongolici (Pu Gong Ying) 5g Herba Violae (Zi Hua Di Ding) 5g Flos Chrysanthemi Indici (Ye Ju Hua) 5g Herba Senecionis Nudicaulis (Zi Bei Tian Kui) 5g	Add appropriate amount of wine and decoct the drugs in water for oral application. And cover the patient with quilts to induce sweating.
Wu Yao Powder (Wu Yao San). Also named Tian Tai Wu Yao Powder (Tian Tai Wu	乌药散 (又名天台乌药散)	Complete Record of Holy Benevolence (Sheng Ji	Radix Linderae (Wu Yao) 9g Radix Aucklandiae (Mu Xiang) 9g Fructus Foeniculi (Xiao Hui Xiang) 9g Pericarpium Citri Reticulatae	Roast Ba Dou and Chuan Lian Zi until they turn black, remove Ba Dou from the mixture, and

Yao San).		Zong Lu)	Viride (Qing Pi) 9g Rhizoma Alpiniae Officinarum (Gao Liang Jiang) 9g Semen Arecae (Bing Lang) 6g Fructus Meliae Toosendan (Chuan Lian Zi) 12g Fructus Crotonis (Ba Dou) 12g	decoct all the drugs for oral application. Take appropriate amount of yellow rice wine each time. Or make the drugs into powder, and take 3g each time with warm wine.
Wu Yin Decoction (Wu Yin Jian)	五阴煎	Jingyue's Complete Works (Jing Yue Quan Shu)	Radix Rehmanniae Praeparatae (Shu Di Huang) 15-30g Rhizoma Dioscoreae (Shan Yao) 6g Semen Dolichoris Lablab (Bian Dou) 6-9g Radix Glycyrrhizae Praeparatae (Zhi Gan Cao) 3-6g Sclerotium Poriae Cocos (Fu Ling) 4.5g Radix Paeoniae (Shao Yao) 6g Fructus Schisandrae Chinensis (Wu Wei Zi) 20 grains Radix Ginseng (Ren Shen) dosage at will Rhizoma Atractylodis Macrocephalae (Bai Zhu) 3-6g	Decoct the drugs in water with 20 grains of Semen Nelumbinis (Lian Zi) for oral application.
Wu Zhi An Zhong Decoction (Wu Zhi An Zhong Tang)	五汁安中饮	Effective Recipes (Yan Fang)	Chinese Chives Juice 10ml Milk 60ml Fresh Ginger Juice 10ml Pear Juice 10ml Lotus Root Juice 10ml	Mix and drink.
Wu Zhi Decoction (Wu Zhi Yin)	五汁饮	Analysis of Warm Diseases (Wen Bing Tiao Bian)	Pear Juice 30g Juice of Rhizoma Eleocharitis (Bi Ji, water chestnut juice) 20g Jouice of fresh Rhizoma Phragmitis Communis (Lu Gen, fresh reed rhizome juice) 25g Juice of Radix Ophiopogonis (Mai Dong, dwarf lilyturf tuber juice) 10g Juice of Nodus Nelumbinis Rhizomatis (Ou Jie, lotus root juice) 20g	Mix and drink. Or decoct the juices in water for oral application.
Wu Zhu Yu Decoction (Wu Zhu Yu Tang)	吴茱萸汤	Treatise on Cold Induced Diseases (Shang Han Lun)	Fructus Evodiae (Wu Zhu Yu) 15g Rhizoma Zingiberis Recens (Sheng Jiang) 18g Fructus Zizyphi Jujubae (Da Zao) 4 pcs Radix Ginseng (Ren Shen) 9g	Decoct the drugs in water for oral application.
Wu Zi Yan Zong Pill (Wu Zi Yan Zong Wan)	五子衍宗丸	Danxi's Experiential Therapy (Dan Xi Xin Fa)	Fructus Lycii (Gou Qi Zi) 240g Fructus Rubi Chingii (Fu Pen Zi) 120g Semen Cuscutae Chinensis (Tu Si Zi) 240g	Grind the drugs into fine powder and make pills with honey. Take 9g each time with warm

				Fructus Schisandrae Chinensis (Wu Wei Zi) 60g Semen Plantaginis (Che Qian Zi) 60g	boiled water, light salty water or wine, twice daily.
Xi Huang Xuan Qiao Decoction (Xi Huang Xuan Qiao Tang)	犀黄宣窍汤	Shi Bing Lun		Cornu Bubali (Shui Niu Jiao, decoct first) 30g [to replace Cornu Rhinocerotis (Xi Jiao) 2.4g] Ramulus Uncariae cum Uncis (Gou Teng) 9g Fructus Forsythiae (Lian Qiao) 9g Cornu Saigae Tataricae (Ling Yang Jiao, deoct first) 3g Bulbus Fritillariae Cirrhosae (Chuan Bei Mu) 15g Rhizoma Acori Tatarinowii (Shi Chang Pu) 3g	Decoct Shui Niu Jiao and Ling Yang Jiao first, and then add other drugs to decoct. Grind 1 bolus of Niu Huang Zhi Bao Pill (Niu Huang Zhi Bao Dan 牛黄至宝丹) into fine powder and mix with the decoction for oral application.
Xi Jiao Di Huang Decoction (Xi Jiao Di Huang Tang). Also named Shao Yao Di Huang Decoction	犀角地黄汤	Particle Prescriptions (Xiao Pin Fang)		Cornu Bubali (Shui Niu Jiao) 30g [to replace Cornu Rhinocerotis (Xi Jiao) in original recipe] Radix Rehmanniae Recens (Sheng Di Huang) 24g Radix Paeoniae (Shao Yao) 12g Cortex Moutan Radicis (Mu Dan Pi) 9g	Decoct the drugs in water for oral application.
Xi Xian Powder (Xi Xian San)	稀涎散	Standards of Diagnosis and Treatment (Zheng Zhi Zhun Sheng)		Semen Crotonis (Ba Dou) 6 grains (smash each grain into two pcs) Fructus Gleditsiae (Zao Jia) 9g Alumen (Bai Fan) 30g	Melt Alumen (Bai Fan) first, then add other two drugs, mix evenly, calcine until Alumen (Bai Fan) is dried up, light and crisp. Take 0.9g each time and blow into mouth or nose. Or take 1.5g each time with decoction of Medulla Junci Effusi (Deng Xin Cao) for oral application.
Xi Xin Decoction (Xi Xin Tang)	洗心汤	Bian Zheng Lu		Radix Ginseng (Ren Shen) 30g Radix Glycyrrhizae (Gan Cao) 3g Rhizoma Pinelliae (Ban Xia) 15g Pericarpium Citri Reticulatae (Chen Pi) 9g Radix Aconiti Lateralis Praeparatae (Fu Zi) 3g Sclerotium Poriae Circum Radicem Pini (Fu Shen) 30g Semen Ziziphi Spinosae (Suan Zao Ren) 30g Massa Medicata Fermentata (Shen Qu) 9g Rhizoma Acori Tatarinowii (Shi	Decoct the drugs in water for oral application.

			Chang Pu) 3g	
Xian Fang Huo Ming Decoction (Xian Fang Huo Ming Yin). Also named Shen Xian Huo Ming Decoction (Shen Xian Huo Ming Yin)	仙方活命饮	Effective Prescriptions for Women (Nu Ke Wan Jin Fang)	Radix Angelicae Dahuricae (Bai Zhi) 3g Bulbus Fritillariae (Bei Mu) 6g Radix Saposhnikoviae (Fang Feng) 6g Radix Paeoniae Rubra (Chi Shao) 6g Radix Angelicae Sinensis (Dang Gui) 6g Radix Glycyrrhizae (Gan Cao) 6g Spina Gleditsiae (Zao Jiao Ci) 6g Squama Manis Praeparatae (Zhi Chuan Shan Jia) 6g Radix Trichosanthis (Tian Hua Fen) 6g Olibanum (Ru Xiang) 6g Myrrha (Mo Yao) 6g Flos Lonicerae (Jin Yin Hua) 9g Pericarpium Citri Reticulatae (Chen Pi) 9g	Add appropriate amount of wine and decoct the drugs in water for oral application.
Xiang Fu Xuan Fu Hua Decoction (Xiang Fu Xuan Fu Hua Tang)	香附旋覆花汤	Analysis of Warm Diseases (Wen Bing Tiao Bian)	Rhizoma Cyperi Rotundi (Xiang Fu) Flos Inulae (Xuan Fu Hua) Fructus Perillae (Su Zi) Semen Coicis (Yi Yi Ren) Rhizoma Pinelliae (Ban Xia) Sclerotium Poriae Cocos (Fu Ling) Pericarpium Citri Reticulatae (Ju Pi)	Decoct the drugs in water for oral application.
Xiang Ru Powder (Xiang Ru San)	香薷散	Formularies of the Bureau of People's Pharmacy (Tai Ping Hui Min He Ji Ju Fang)	Herba Moslae (Xiang Ru) 12g Cortex Magnoliae Officinalis (Hou Po) 6g Semen Dolichoris Album (Bai Bian Dou) 6g	Decoct the drugs in water for oral application. Or add a little wine when decocting.
Xiang Sha Liu Jun Zi Decoction (Xiang Sha Liu Jun Zi Tang)	香砂六君子汤	Formularies of the Bureau of People's Welfare Pharmacy (Tai Ping Hui Min He Ji Ju Fang)	Si Jun Zi Decoction (Si Jun Zi Tang) supplemented with Rhizoma Pinelliae (Ban Xia), Fructus Amomi (Sha Ren), Pericarpium Citri Reticulatae (Che Pi), Radix Aucklandiae (Mu Xiang)	Decoct the drugs in water for oral application.
Xiang Su Powder (Xiang Su San)	香苏散	Formularies of the Bureau of People's Welfare Pharmacy (Tai Ping Hui Min He Ji Ju Fang)	Rhizoma Cyperi Rotundi (Xiang Fu) 120g Folium Perillae Frutescentis (Zi Su Ye) 120g Pericarpium Citri Reticulatae (Chen Pi) 60g Radix Glycyrrhizae Prep (Zhi Gan Cao) 30g	Grind into coarse powder. Decoct 9g each time for oral application, thrice daily.

Xiao Ban Xia Jia Fu Ling Decoction (Xiao Ban Xia Jia Fu Ling Tang)	小半夏加茯苓汤	Synopsis of the Golden Chamber (Jin Gui Yao Lue)	Rhizoma Pinelliae (Ban Xia) 18g Rhizoma Zingiberis Recens (Sheng Jiang) 15g Sclerotium Poriae Cocos (Fu Ling) 9g	Decoct the drugs in water for oral application. Take 1/2 of decoction each time, twice daily.
Xiao Chai Hu Decoction (Xiao Chai Hu Tang)	小柴胡汤	Treatise on Cold Induced Diseases (Shang Han Lun)	Radix Bupleuri (Chai Hu) 24g Rhizoma Pinelliae (Ban Xia) 9g Radix Scutellariae (Huang Qin) 9g Radix Ginseng (Ren Shen) 9g Radix Glycyrrhizae Praeparatae (Zhi Gan Cao) 9g Rhizoma Zingiberis Recens (Sheng Jiang) 9g Fructus Ziziphi Jujubae (Da Zao) 4 pcs	Decoct the drugs in water for oral application.
Xiao Cheng Qi Decoction (Xiao Cheng Qi Tang)	小承气汤	Treatise on Cold Induced Diseases (Shang Han Lun)	Radix et Rhizoma Rhei (Da Huang) 12g Cortex Magnoliae Officinalis (Hou Po) 6g Fructus Immaturus Citri Aurantii (Zhi Shi) 7g	Decoct the drugs simultaneously in water for oral application.
Xiao Feng Powder (Xiao Feng San)	消风散	Orthodox Manual of Surgery (Wai Ke Zheng Zong)	Herba Schizonepetae (Jing Jie) 6g Radix Saposhnikoviae (Fang Feng) 6g Radix Angelicae Sinensis (Dang Gui) 6g Radix Rehmanniae Recens (Sheng Di Huang) 6g Radix Sophorae Flavescentis (Ku Shen) 6g Rhizoma Atractylodis (Cang Zhu) 6g Periostracum Cicadae (Chan Tui) 6g Semen Sesami Indici (Hei Zhi Ma) 6g Fructus Arctii (Nui Bang Zi) 6g Rhizoma Anemarrhenae (Zhi Mu) 6g Gypsum Fibrosum (Shi Gao) 6g Caulis Akebiae (Mu Tong) 3g Radix Glycyrrhizae (Gan Cao) 3g	Decoct the drugs in water for oral application.
Xiao He Powder (Xiao He San)	消核散	Golden Mirror of Medicine (Yi Zong Jin Jian)	Herba Sargassi (Hai Zao) 90g Concha Ostreae (Mu Li) 120g Radix Scrophulariae (Xuan Shen) 120g Semen Oryzae Glutinosae (Nuo Mi) 240g Radix Glycyrrhizae (Gan Cao) 30g Huechys (Hong Niang Zi) 28 pcs	Stir-fry Semen Oryzae Glutinosae (Nuo Mi) with Huechys (Hong Niang Zi) until they turn into brown color, remove Huechys, and grind Semen Oryzae Glutinosae with other

				drugs into fine powder. Take 3-4.5g each time with wine.
Xiao Luo Pill (Xiao Luo Wan)	消瘰丸	Medicine Comprehended (Yi Xue Xin Wu)	Steamed Radix Scrophulariae (Xuan Shen) 12g Calcined Concha Ostreae (Duan Mu Li) 12g Steamed Bulbus Fritillariae (Bei Mu) 12g	Grind the drugs into powder (grind Mu Li with vinegar) and make pills with honey. Take 9g each time with warm boiled water, twice daily.
Xiao Huo Luo Pill (Xiao Huo Luo Dan). Originally named Huo Luo Pill (Huo Luo Dan)	小活络丹	Formularies of the Bureau of People's Welfare Pharmacy (Tai Ping Hui Min He Ji Ju Fang)	Rhizoma Arisaematis (Tian Nan Xing) 180g Radix Aconiti Carmichaeli (Chuan Wu) 180g Radix Aconiti Kusnezoffii (Cao Wu) 180g Lumbricus (Di Long) 180g Olibanum (Ru Xiang) 66g Myrrha (Mo Yao) 66g	Prepare the drugs into boluses with honey (3g per bolus). Take one bolus each time with old wine or warm boiled water.
Xiao Ji Decoction (Xiao Ji Yin Zi). Also named Ji Sheng Xiao Ji Decoction (Ji Sheng Xiao Ji Yin Zi)	小蓟饮子（又名济生小蓟饮子）	Prescriptions for Saving Lives (Ji Sheng Fang)	Radix Rehmanniae Recens (Sheng Di Huang) 9g Herba Cephalanoploris (Xiao Ji) 9g Talcum (Hua Shi Fen) 9g Medulla Tetrapanacis (Tong Cao) 9g Pollen Typhae (Pu Huang) 9g Nodus Nelumbinis Rhizomatis (Ou Jie) 9g Herba Lophatheri (Dan Zhu Ye) 9g Radix Angelicae Sinensis (Dang Gui) 9g Fructus Gardeniae (Zhi Zi) 9g Radix Glycyrrhizae (Gan Cao) 9g	Decoct the drugs in water for oral application.
Xiao Jian Zhong Decoction (Xiao Jian Zhong Tang)	小建中汤	Treatise on Cold Induced Diseases (Shang Han Lun)	Radix Paeoniae (Shao Yao) 18g Ramulus Cinnamomi (Gui Zhi) 9g Rhizoma Zingiberis Recens (Sheng Jiang) 9g Fructus Zizyphi Jujubae Fructus (Da Zao) 4 pcs Saccharum Granorum (Yi Tang) 30g Radix Glycyrrhizae Praeparatae (Zhi Gan Cao) 6g	Decoct the drugs except Yi Tang in water, and then melt Yi Tang in the decoction for oral application.
Xiao Ke Formula (Xiao Ke Fang)	消渴方	Danxi's Experiential Therapy (Dan Xi Xin Fa)	Rhizoma Coptidis (Huang Lian) Radix Trichosanthis (Tian Hua Fen) Radix Rehmanniae Recens (Sheng Di Huang) Nodus Nelumbinis Rhizomatis (Ou Jie) Milk	Mix Rhizoma Coptidis Powder (Huang Lian), Radix Trichosanthis Powder (Tian Hua Fen), Radix Rehmanniae Recens Juice (Sheng Di Huang), Nelumbinis

				Rhizoma Zingiberis Recens (Sheng Jiang) Honey (Feng Mi)	Rhizomatis Juice (Ou Zhi), Milk, Rhizoma Zingiberis Recens Juice (Sheng Jiang) and honey thoroughly for oral application.
Xiao Qing Long JiaShi Gao Decoction (Xiao Qing Long JiaShi Gao Tang)	小青龙加石膏汤	Treatise on Cold Induced Diseases (Shang Han Lun)		Xiao Qing Long Decoction (Xiao Qing Long Tang) supplemented with Gypsum Fibrosum (Shi Gao)	Decoct the drugs in water for oral application.
Xiao Qing Long Decoction (Xiao Qing Long Tang)	小青龙汤	Treatise on Cold Induced Diseases (Shang Han Lun)		Rhizoma Pinelliae (Ban Xia) 6g Herba Ephedrae (Ma Huang) 9g Radix Paeoniae (Shao Yao) 9g Herba Asari (Xi Xin) 3g Radix Glycyrrhizae Praeparatae (Zhi Gan Cao) 9g Ramulus Cinnamomi (Gui Zhi) 9g Fructus Schisandrae Chinensis (Wu Wei Zi) 3g Rhizoma Zingiberis (Gan Jiang) 9g	Decoct the drugs in water for oral application.
Xiao Xian Xiong Decoction (Xiao Xian Xiong Tang)	小陷胸汤	Treatise on Cold Induced Diseases (Shang Han Lun)		Rhizoma Coptidis (Huang Lian) 6g Rhizoma Pinelliae (Ban Xia) 9g Fructus Trichosanthis (Gua Lou Shi) 20g	Decoct the drugs in water for oral application.
Xiao Xu Ming Decoction (Xiao Xu Ming Tang)	小续命汤	Invaluable Prescriptions (Qian Jin Yao Fang)		Herba Ephedrae (Ma Huang) 3g Radix Stephaniae Tetrandrae (Fang Ji) 3g Radix Ginseng (Ren Shen) 3g Radix Paeoniae (Shao Yao) 3g Rhizoma Ligustici Chuanxiong (Chuan Xiong) 3g Ramulus Cinnamomi (Gui Zhi) 3g Radix Aconiti Lateralis Praeparatae (Fu Pian) 2g Radix Saposhnikoviae (Fang Feng) 4.5g Semen Pruni Armeniacae (Xing Ren) 3g Radix Scutellariae (Huang Qin) 3g Radix Glycyrrhizae (Gan Cao) 3g Rhizoma Zingiberis Recens (Sheng Jiang) 15g	Decoct Herba Ephedrae (Ma Huang) first, and then add other drugs to decoct for oral application.
Xiao Yao Powder (Xiao Yao San)	逍遥散	Formularies of the Bureau of People's Pharmacy (Tai Ping Hui Min He Ji Ju Fang)		Radix Paeoniae Alba (Bai Shao) 9g Sclerotium Poriae Cocos (Fu Ling) 9g Radix Angelicae Sinensis (Dang Gui) 9g Rhizoma Atractylodis Macrocephalae (Bai Zhu) 9g	Decoct the drugs in water for oral application. Or prepare the drugs into pills or powder, and take 6g each time, twice daily.

			Rhizoma Zinigiberis Recens (Shao Sheng Jiang) 3g Radix Glycyrrhizae Praeparatae (Zhi Gan Cao) 4.5g Radix Bulpeuri (Chai Hu) 9g Herba Menthae (Bo He) 3g	
Xie Bai Powder (Xie Bai San). Also named Xie Fei Powder (Xie Fei San)	泻白散（又名泻肺散）	Key to Therapeutics of Children's Diseases (Xiao Er Yao Zheng Zhi Jue)	Cortex Mori Alba Radicis (Sang Bai Pi) 9g Cortex Lycii (Di Gu Pi) 9g Radix Glycyrrhizae Praeparatae (Zhi Gan Cao) 3g Semen Oryzae Sativae (Geng Mi) 9g	Decoct the drugs in water for oral application.
Xie Fei Powder (Xie Fei San). Also named Xie Bai Powder (Xie Bai San).	泻肺散（又名泻白散）	Key to Therapeutics of Children's Diseases (Xiao Er Yao Zheng Zhi Jue)	Cortex Mori Alba Radicis (Sang Bai Pi) 9g Cortex Lycii (Di Gu Pi) 9g Radix Glycyrrhizae Praeparatae (Zhi Gan Cao) 3g Semen Oryzae Sativae (Geng Mi) 9g	Decoct the drugs in water for oral application.
Xie Huang Powder (Xie Huang San)	泻黄散	Key to Therapeutics of Children's Diseases (Xiao Er Yao Zheng Zhi Jue)	Herba Agastache seu Pogostemonis (Huo Xiang) 21g Fructus Gardeniae (Zhi Zi) 3g Gypsum Fibrosum (Shi Gao) 15g Radix Glycyrrhizae (Gan Cao) 90g Radix Saposhnikoviae (Fang Feng) 120g	Smash the drugs into small pieces, stir-fry with honey and wine; then grind into fine powder. Decoct 3-6g each time for oral application.
Xie Xin Decoction (Xie Xin Tang)	泻心汤	Synopsis of the Golden Chamber (Jin Gui Yao Lue)	Radix et Rhizoma Rhei (Da Huang) 6g Rhizoma Coptidis (Huang Lian) 3g Radix Scutellariae (Huang Qin) 3g	Decoct the drugs in water for oral application.
Xin Jia Huang Long Decoction (Xin Jia Huang Long Tang)	新加黄龙汤	Six Books on Cold Induced Diseases (Shang Han Liu Lun)	Substract Hou Po, Zhi Shi, Jie Geng and Da Zao from Huang Long Decoction (Huang Long Tang), and add Xuan Shen, Sheng Di Huang, Mai Dong and Hai Shen to it	Decoct the drugs except Mang Xiao in water, and then dissolve Mang Xiao in the decoction for oral application.
Xin Jia Xiang Ru Decoction (Xin Jia Xiang Ru Yin)	新加香薷饮	Analysis of Warm Diseases (Wen Bing Tiao Bian)	Herba Moslae (Xiang Ru) 6g Flos Lonicerae (Jin Yin Hua) 9g Flos Dolichoris Lablab (Xian Bian Dou Hua) 9g Cortex Magnoliae Officinalis (Hou Po) 6g Fructus Forsythiae (Lian Qiao) 6g	Decoct the drugs in water for oral application.
Xing Lou Cheng Qi Decoction (Xing Lou Cheng Qi Tang)	星蒌承气汤	Lin Chuang Zhong Yi Ni Ke Xue	Rhizoma Arisaematis cum Bile (Dan Nan Xing) 15g Fructus Trichosanthis (Gua Lou) 15g Radix et Rhizoma Rhei (Da Huang) 10g Natrii Sulfas (Mang Xiao) 10g	Decoct the drugs in water for oral application.

Xing Pi Decoction (Xing Pi Tang)	醒脾汤	Golden Mirror of Medicine (Yi Zong Jin Jian)	Radix Ginseng (Ren Shen) Rhizoma Atractylodis Macrocephalae (Bai Zhu) Sclerotium Poriae Cocos (Fu Ling) Rhizoma Gastrodiae Elatae (Tian Ma) Rhizoma Pinelliae (Ban Xia) Exocarpium Citri Rubrum (Ju Hong) Scorpio (Quan Xie) Bombyx Batryticatus (Jiang Can) Radix Glycyrrhizae (Gan Cao) Rhizoma Arisaematis cum Bile (Dan Nan Xing) Semen Oryzae Sativae (Jing Mi) Rhizoma Zingiberis Recens (Sheng Jiang)	Decoct the drugs in water for oral application.
Xing Su Powder (Xing Su San)	杏苏散	Analysis of Warm Diseases (Wen Bing Tiao Bian)	Semen Armeniacae Amarum (Xing Ren) 9g Folium Perillae (Su Ye) 9g Radix Peucedani (Qian Hu) 9g Rhizoma Pinelliae (Ban Xia) 9g Sclerotium Poriae Cocos (Fu Ling) 9g Pericarpium Citri Reticulatae (Chen Pi) 6g Radix Platycodonis (Jie Geng) 6g Fructus Aurantii (Zhi Ke) 6g Radix Glycyrrhizae (Gan Cao) 3g Rhizoma Zingiberis Recens (Sheng Jiang) 3 slices Fructus Zizyphi Jujubae (Da Zao) 3 pcs	Decoct the drugs in water for oral application.
Xiong Xin Dao Tan Decoction (Xiong Xin Dao Tan Tang)	芎辛导痰汤	Qi Xiao Liang Fang	Rhizoma Ligustici Chuanxiong (Chuan Xiong) 4.5g Herba cum Radice Asari (Xi Xin) 4.5g Rhizoma Arisaematis (Tian Nan Xing) 4.5g Pericarpium Citri Reticulatae (Chen Pi) 4.5g Sclerotium Poriae Cocos (Fu Ling) 4.5g Rhizoma Pinelliae (Ban Xia) 6g Fructus Citri Aurantii Immaturus (Zhi Shi) 3g Radix Glycyrrhizae (Gan Cao) 3g Rhizoma Zingiberis Recens (Sheng Jiang) 7 slices	Decoct the drugs in water for oral application after meals.
Xiong Zhi Shi Gao Decoction (Xiong Zhi Shi Gao Tang)	芎芷石膏汤	Golden Mirror of Medicine (Yi Zong	Rhizoma Ligustici Chuanxiong (Chuan Xiong) Radix Angelicae Dahuricae (Bai	Decoct the drugs in water for oral application.

		(Jin Jian)	Zhi) Gypsum Fibrosum (Shi Gao) Flos Chrysanthemi (Ju Hua) Rhizoma et Radix Ligustici (Gao Ben) Rhizoma et Radix Notopterygii (Qiang Huo)	
Xuan Bi Decoction (Xuan Bi Tang)	宣痹汤	Analysis of Warm Diseases (Wen Bing Tiao Bian)	Radix Stephaniae Tetrandrae (Fang Ji) 15g Semen Pruni Armeniacae (Xing Ren) 15g Fructus Forsythiae (Lian Qiao) 9g Talcum (Hua Shi Fen) 15g Semen Coicis (Yi Yi Ren) 15g Rhizoma Pinelliae (Ban Xia) 9g Bombycis Mori Excrementum (Can Sha) 9g Semen Phaseoli (Chi Xiao Dou) 9g Fructus Gardeniae (Zhi Zi) 9g	Decoct the drugs in water for oral application. Take 1/3 of the decoction each time, thrice daily.
Xuan Fu Dai Zhe Decoction (Xuan Fu Dai Zhe Tang)	旋覆代赭汤	Treatise on Cold Induced Diseases (Shang Han Lun)	Flos Inulae (Xuan Fu Hua) 9g Radix Ginseng (Ren Shen) 6g Rhizoma Zingiberis Recens (Sheng Jiang) 10g Ochra Haematitum (Dai Zhe Shi) 9g Radix Glycyrrhizae Praeparatae (Zhi Gan Cao) 6g Rhizoma Pinelliae (Ban Xia) 9g Fructus Zizyphi Jujubae (Da Zao) 4 pcs	Decoct the drugs in water for oral application.
Xue Fu Zhu Yu Decoction (Xue Fu Zhu Yu Tang)	血府逐瘀汤	Correction on the Errors of Medical Works (Yi Lin Gai Cuo)	Semen Persicae (Tao Ren) 12g Radicis Angelicae Sinensis (Dang Gui) 9g Radix Rehmanniae (Sheng Di Huang) 9g Flos Carthami (Hong Hua) 9g Radix Achyranthis Bidentatae (Niu Xi) 9g Fructus Citri Aurantii (Zhi Ke) 6g Radix Paeoniae Rubra (Chi Shao) 6g Radix Platycodonis (Jie Geng) 4.5g Rhizoma Ligustici Chuanxiong (Chuan Xiong) 4.5g Radix Bupleuri (Chai Hu) 3g Radix Glycyrrhizae (Gan Cao) 6g	Decoct the drugs in water for oral application.
Yang He Decoction (Yang He Tang)	阳和汤	Life-saving Manual of Diagnosis and Treatment of External Dis-	Radix Rehmanniae Praeparatae (Shu Di Huang) 30g Cortex Cinnamomi (Rou Gui) 3g Herba Ephedrae (Ma Huang) 2g Colla Corni Cervi (Lu Jiao Jiao) 9g Semen Sinapis Albae (Bai Jie Zi) 6g	Decoct the drugs in water for oral application.

		eases (Wai Ke Zheng Zhi Quan Sheng Ji)	Charred Rhizoma Zingiberis (Jiang Tan) 2g Radix Glycyrrhizae (Sheng Gan Cao) 3g	
Yang Gan Pill (Yang Gan Wan)	羊肝丸	Lei Yuan Fang	Excrementum Vespertilionis Murini (Ye Ming Sha) 30g Periostracum Cicadae (Chan Tui) 30g Herba Equiseti Hiemalis (Mu Zei) 30g Radix Angelicae Sinensis (Dang Gui) 30g Lamb Liver (Yang Gan) 120g	Cook lamb liver thoroughly, and mash it into paste. Grind other drugs into powder, mix the powder with mashed lamb liver and make pills.
Yang Xin Decoction (Yang Xin Tang)	养心汤	Effective Recipes from Benevolent Houses (Ren Zhai Zhi Zhi Fang)	Radix Astragali (Huang Qi) 15g Sclerotium Poriae Cocos (Fu Ling) 15g Sclerotium Poriae Circum Radicem Pini (Fu Shen) 15g Rhizoma Pinelliae Fermentata (Ban Xia Qu) 15g Radix Angelicae Sinensis (Dang Gui) 15g Rhizoma Ligustici Chuanxiong (Chuan Xiong) 15g Radix Polygalae (Yuan Zhi) 7.5g Cortex Cinnamomi (Rou Gui) 7.5g Semen Platycladi (Bai Zi Ren) 7.5g Semen Ziziphi Spinosae (Suan Zao Ren) 7.5g Fructus Schisandrae Chinensis (Wu Wei Zi) 7.5g Radix Ginseng (Ren Shen) 7.5g Radix Glycyrrhizae Praeparatae (Zhi Gan Cao) 12g	Grind the drugs into powder, decoct 15g each time with Rhizoma Zingiberis Recens (Sheng Jiang) 3g and Fructus Ziziphi Jujubae (Da Zao) 2 pcs in water for oral application. Or prepare the drugs into pills and take 9g each time. Or decoct the drugs in water for oral application.
Yang Yin Qing Fei Decoction (Yang Yin Qing Fei Tang)	养阴清肺汤	Jade Key to the Secluded Chamber (Chong Lou Yu Yao)	Radix Rehmanniae Recens (Sheng Di Huang) 12g Radix Ophiopogonis (Mai Dong) 9g Radix Glycyrrhizae (Gan Cao) 3g Radix Scrophulariae (Xuan Shen) 9g Bulbus Fritillariae (Bei Mu) 5g Cortex Moutan Radicis (Mu Dan Pi) 5g Herba Menthae (Bo He) 3g Stir-fired Radix Paeoniae Alba (Chao Bai Shao Yao) 5g	Decoct the drugs in water for oral application.
Yi Gong Powder (Yi Gong San)	异功散	Formularies of the Bureau of People's Welfare Pharmacy	Si Jun Zi Decoction (Si Jun Zi Tang) supplemented with Pericarpium Citri Reticulatae (Chen Pi)	Decoct the drugs in water for oral application.

		(Tai Ping Hui Min He Ji Ju Fang)		
Yi Guan Decoction (Yi Guan Jian)	一贯煎	Supplement to Classified Case Records of Celebrated Physicians (Xu Ming Yi Lei An)	Radix Rehmanniae Recens (Sheng Di Huang) 18g Fructus Lycii (Gou Qi Zi) 18g Radix Glehniae (Bei Sha Shen) 9g Radix Ophiopogonis (Mai Dong) 9g Radix Angelicae Sinensis (Dang Gui) 9g Fructus Meliae Toosendan (Chuan Lian Zi) 4.5g	Decoct the drugs in water for oral application.
Yi Huang Decoction (Yi Huang Tang)	易黄汤	Fu Qingzhu's Gynecology (Fu Qing Zhu Nu Ke)	Rhizoma Dioscoreae (Shan Yao) 30g Semen Euryales (Qian Shi) 30g Cortex Phellodendri (Huang Bai) 6g Semen Plantaginis (Che Qian Zi) 3g Semen Ginkgo (Bai Guo) 12g	Decoct the drugs in water for oral application.
Yi Wei Decoction (Yi Wei Tang)	益胃汤	Analysis of Warm Diseases (Wen Bing Tiao Bian)	Radix Adenophorae (Sha Shen) 9g Radix Ophiopogonis (Mai Dong) 15g Radix Rehmanniae Recens (Sheng Di Huang) 15g Rhizoma Polygonati Odorati (Yu Zhu) 4.5g Crystal Sugar (Bing Tang) 3g	Decoct the drugs in water for oral application. Take 1/2 of decoction each time.
Yi Yi Ren Decoction (Yi Yi Ren Tang)	薏苡仁汤	Lei Zheng Zhi Cai	Semen Coicis (Yi Yi Ren) Rhizoma Atractylodis (Cang Zhu) Rhizoma et Radix Notopterygii (Qiang Huo) Radix Angelicae Pubescentis (Du Huo) Herba Ephedrae (Ma Huang) Radix Saposhnikoviae (Fang Feng) Radix Aconiti Carmichaeli (Chuan Wu) Radix Angelicae Sinensis (Dang Gui) Rhizoma Ligustici Chuanxiong (Chuan Xiong) Radix Glycyrrhizae (Gan Cao) Rhizoma Zingiberis Recens (Sheng Jiang)	Decoct the drugs in water for oral application.
Yi Yuan Powder (Yi Yuan San). Also named Liu Yi Powder (Liu Yi San).	益元散（又名六一散）	Clear Synopsis on Recipes Based on Plain Questions of Huang Di (Huang Di Su Wen Xuan	Talcum (Hua Shi Fen) 18g Radix Glycyrrhizae (Gan Cao) 3g	Decoct the drugs in water for oral application.

		Ming Lun Fang)		
Yin Chen Hao Decoction (Yin Chen Hao Tang)	茵陈蒿汤	Treatise on Cold Induced Diseases (Shang Han Lun)	Herba Artemisiae Scopariae (Yin Chen Hao) 6g Fructus Gardeniae (Zhi Zi) 9g Radix et Rhizoma Rhei (Da Huang) 6g	Decoct the drugs in water for oral application.
Yin Chen Si Ling Powder (Yin Chen Si Ling San)	茵陈四苓散	Effective Recipes (Yan Fang)	Herba Artemisiae Scopariae (Yin Chen Hao) 15-30g Sclerotium Poriae Cocos (Fu Ling) 9g Rhizoma Atractylodis Macrocephalae (Bai Zhu) 9g Rhizoma Alismatis Orientalis (Ze Xie) 15g Sclerotium Polypori Umbellati (Zhu Ling) 9g	Decoct the drugs in water for oral application. Take 1/2 of the decoction each time, twice daily.
Yin Chen Wei Ling Decoction (Yin Chen Wei Ling Tang)	茵陈胃苓汤	Gan Zheng Ji Yao	Herba Artemisiae Scopariae (Yin Chen Hao) 24g Rhizoma Atractylodis (Cang Zhu) 3g Cortex Magnoliae Officinalis (Hou Po) 3g Pericarpium Citri Reticulatae (Chen Pi) 4.5g Rhizoma Atractylodis Macrocephalae (Bai Zhu) 4.5g Sclerotium Poriae Cocos (Fu Ling) 9g Rhizoma Alismatis (Ze Xie) 4.5g Sclerotium Polypori Umbellati (Zhu Ling) 4.5g Radix Glycyrrhizae (Gan Cao) 1.5g Ramulus Cinnamomi (Gui Zhi) 1.5g	Decoct the drugs in water for oral application.
Yin Chen Wu Ling Powder (Yin Chen Wu Ling San)	茵陈五苓散	Synopsis of the Golden Chamber (Jin Gui Yao Lue)	Wu Ling Powder (Wu Ling San) 15g supplemented with Herba Artemisiae Scopariae (Yin Chen Hao) 30g	Mix evenly. Take 6g each time with gruel before meals, thrice daily.
Yin Chen Zhu Fu Decoction (Yin Chen Zhu Fu Tang)	茵陈术附汤	Medicine Comprehended (Yi Xue Xin Wu)	Herba Artemisiae Scopariae (Yin Chen Hao) 3g Rhizoma Atractylodis Macrocephalae (Bai Zhu) 6g Radix Aconiti Lateralis Praeparatae (Fu Zi) 1.5g Cortex Cinnamomi (Rou Gui) 0.9g Rhizoma Zingiberis (Gan Jiang) 1.5g Radix Glycyrrhizae Praeparatae (Zhi Gan Cao) 3g	Decoct the drugs in water for oral application.
Yin Qiao Powder (Yin Qiao San)	银翘散	Analysis of Warm Dis-	Flos Lonicerae (Jin Yin Hua) 15g Fructus Forsythiae (Lian Qiao) 15g	Decoct the drugs in water for oral appli-

		eases (Wen Bing Tiao Bian)	Radix Platycodonis (Jie Geng) 9g Fructus Arctii (Niu Bang Zi) 9g Herba Menthae (Bo He) 9g Radix Glycyrrhizae (Gan Cao) 6g Semen Sojae Praeparatum (Dan Dou Chi) 6g Herba Lophatheri (Dan Zhu Ye) 6g Spica Schizonepetae (Jing Jie Sui) 6g Rhizoma Phragmitis (Lu Gen) 18g	cation. Or Prepare the drugs except Lu Gen into powder, and decoct 9g each time with the decoction of Fresh Rhizoma Phragmitis (Xian Lu Gen) for oral application.
You Gui Pill (You Gui Wan)	右归丸	Jingyue's Complete Works (Jing Yue Quan Shu)	Radix Rehmanniae Praeparatae (Shu Di Huang) 24g Colla Corni Cervi (Lu Jiao Jiao) 12g Rhizoma Dioscoreae (Shan Yao) 12g Fructus Lycii (Gou Qi Zi) 12g Semen Cuscutae (Tu Si Zi) 12g Cortex Eucommiae (Du Zhong) 12g Radix Aconiti Lateralis Praeparatae (Fu Zi) 6-18g Cortex Cinnamomi (Rou Gui) 6-12g Fructus Corni (Shan Zhu Yu) 9g Radix Angelicae Sinensis (Dang Gui) 9g	Decoct the drugs in water for oral application. Or Prepare the drugs into pills, and take 9g each time with warm boiled water or light salty water.
Yu Gong Powder (Yu Gong San)	禹功散	Confucians' Duties to Their Parents (Ru Men Shi Qin)	Semen Pharbitidis (Qian Niu Zi) 12g Fructus Foeniculi (Xiao Hui Xiang) 3g Rhizoma Zingiberis Recens (Sheng Jiang) 6g	Decoct the drugs in water for oral application. Or grind the drugs except Sheng Jiang into fine powder, and take 3-6g each time with10ml of Succus Rhizoma Zingiberis Recens (Sheng Jiang Zhi) before sleep.
Yu Nu Decoction (Yu Nu Jian)	玉女煎	Jingyue's Complete Works (Jing Yue Quan Shu)	Radix Rehmanniae Praeparatae (Shu Di Huang) 9-30g Radix Ophiopogonis (Mai Dong) 6g Rhizoma Anemarrhenae (Zhi Mu) 5g Radix Achyranthis Bidentatae (Niu Xi) 5g Gypsum Fibrosum (Shi Gao) 9-15g	Decoct the drugs in water for oral application.
Yu Ping Feng Powder (Yu Ping Feng San)	玉屏风散	Observing and Studying Primary Prescriptions (Jiu Yuan Fang)	Radix Astragali Praeparatae (Zhi Huang Qi) 12g Rhizoma Atractylodis Macrocephalae (Bai Zhu) 12g Radix Saposhnikoviae (Fang Feng) 6g	Decoct the drugs in water for oral application. Or prepare the drugs except Da Zao into powder, and take 6g each

			Fructus Zizyphi Jujubae (Da Zao) 4 pcs	time with the decoction of Da Zao after meals.
Yu Ye Decoction (Yu Ye Tang)	玉液汤	Discourse on Medical Problems by Integrated Traditional Chinese and Western Medicine (Yi Xue Zhong Zhong Can Xi Lu)	Rhizoma Dioscoreae (Shan Yao) 30g Radix Astragali (Huang Qi) 15g Rhizoma Anemarrhenae (Zhi Mu) 18g Endothelium Corneum Gigeriae Galli (Ji Nei Jin) 6g Radix Puerariae (Ge Gen) 4.5g Fructus Schisandrae Chinensis (Wu Wei Zi) 9g Radix Trichosanthis (Tian Hua Fen) 9g	Decoct the drugs in water for oral application.
Yu Zhen Powder (Yu Zhen San)	玉真散	Orthodox Manual of External Medicine (Wai Ke Zheng Zong)	Rhizoma Arisaematis (Tian Nan Xing) 6g Radix Saposhnikoviae (Fang Feng) 6g Radix Angelicae Dahuricae (Bai Zhi) 6g Rhizoma Gastrodiae (Tian Ma) 6g Rhizoma et Radix Notopterygii (Qiang Huo) 6g Rhizoma Typhonii (Bai Fu Zi) 6g	Decoct the drugs in water for oral application. Or grind the drugs into powder and take 3-6g each time with warm wine, thrice daily. Encourage perspiration and avoid wind after taking the drugs.
Yue Bi Decoction (Yue Bi Tang)	越婢汤	Synopsis of the Golden Chamber (Jin Gui Yao Lue)	Gypsum Fibrosum (Shi Gao) 25g Herba Ephedrae (Ma Huang) 18g Radix Glycyrrhizae Praeparatae (Gan Cao) 6g Rhizoma Zingiberis Recens (Sheng Jiang) 9g Fructus Zizyphi Jujubae (Da Zao) 15 pcs	Decoct Herba Ephedrae (Ma Huang) in water first, and then add other drugs to decoct for oral application. Take 1/3 of the decoction each time, thrice daily.
Yue Bi Jia Ban Xia Decoction (Yue Bi Jia Ban Xia Tang)	越婢加半夏汤	Synopsis of the Golden Chamber (Jin Gui Yao Lue)	Gypsum Fibrosum (Shi Gao) 25g Herba Ephedrae (Ma Huang) 18g Radix Glycyrrhizae Praeparatae (Gan Cao) 6g Rhizoma Zingiberis Recens (Sheng Jiang) 9g Fructus Zizyphi Jujubae (Da Zao) 15 pcs Rhizoma Pinelliae (Ban Xia) 9g	Decoct Herba Ephedrae (Ma Huang) in water first, and then add other drugs to decoct for oral application. Take 1/3 of the decoction each time, thrice daily.
Yue Bi Jia Zhu Decoction (Yue Bi Jia Zhu Tang)	越婢加术汤	Synopsis of the Golden Chamber (Jin Gui Yao Lue)	Gypsum Fibrosum (Shi Gao) 25g Herba Ephedrae (Ma Huang) 18g Radix Glycyrrhizae Praeparatae (Gan Cao) 6g Rhizoma Zingiberis Recens (Sheng Jiang) 9g	Decoct Herba Ephedrae (Ma Huang) in water first, and then add other drugs to decoct for oral application. Take

			Fructus Zizyphi Jujubae (Da Zao) 15 pcs Rhizoma Atractylodis Macrocephalae (Bai Zhu) 12g	1/3 of the decoction each time, thrice daily.
Yue Hua Pill (Yue Hua Wan)	月华丸	Medicine Comprehended (Yi Xue Xin Wu)	Radix Adenophorae (Sha Shen) 30g Radix Ophiopogonis (Mai Dong) 30g Radix Asparagi (Tian Dong) 30g Radix Rehmanniae Recens (Sheng Di Huang) 30g Radix Rehmanniae Praeparatae (Shu Di Huang) 30g Colla Corii Asini (E Jiao) 30g Rhizoma Dioscoreae (Shan Yao) 30g Sclerotium Poriae Cocos (Fu Ling) 15g Folium Mori Alba (Sang Ye) 60g Flos Chrysanthemi (Ju Hua) 60g Radix Stemonae (Bai Bu) 30g Radix Notoginseng (San Qi) 15g Bulbus Fritillariae Cirrhosae (Chuan Bei Mu) 30g Jecur Lutrae (Ta Gan) 15g	Decoct the drugs except Colla Corii Asini (E Jiao) in water until they become ointment, and then melt E Jiao in the ointment, and add honey to make pills. Take 9g each time, thrice daily.
Yue Ju Pill (Yue Ju Wan)	越鞠丸	Danxi's Experiential Therapy (Dan Xi Xin Fa)	Rhizoma Cyperi (Xiang Fu) 6g Rhizoma Atractylodis (Cang Zhu) 6g Rhizoma Ligustici Chuanxiong (Chuan Xiong) 6g Fructus Gardeniae (Zhi Zi) 6g Massa Medicata Fermentata (Shen Qu) 6g	Decoct the drugs in water for oral application. Or make the drugs into pills, and take 6-9g each time with warm boiled water.
Zai Zao Powder (Zai Zao San)	再造散	Six Books on Cold Induced Diseases (Shang Han Liu Lun)	Radix Astragali (Huang Qi) 6g Radix Ginseng (Ren Shen) 3g Ramulus Cinnamomi (Gui Zhi) 3g Radix Glycyrrhizae (Gan Cao) 3g Radix Aconiti Lateralis Praeparatae (Fu Zi) 3g Herba Asari (Xi Xin) 3g Rhizoma et Radix Notopterygii (Qiang Huo) 3g Radix Saposhnikoviae (Fang Feng) 3g Rhizoma Ligustici Chuanxiong (Chuan Xiong) 3g Rhizoma Zingiberis Recens Praeparatae (Wei Sheng Jiang) 3g Fructus Zizyphi Jujubae (Da Zao) 2 pcs Stir-fried Radix Paeoniae Alba (Chao Bai Shao Yao) 2g	Decoct the drugs in water for oral application.
Zan Yu Pill (Zan	赞育丹	Jingyue's	Radix Rehmanniae Praeparatae	Make the drugs into

Yu Dan)		Complete Works (Jing Yue Quan Shu)	(Shu Di Huang) 24g Rhizoma Atractylodis Macrocephalae (Bai Zhu) 24g Radix Angelicae Sinensis (Dang Gui) 18g Fructus Lycii (Gou Qi Zi) 18g Cortex Eucommiae (Du Zhong) 12g Rhizoma Curculiginis Orchioidis (Xian Mao) 12g Radix Morindae Officinalis (Zhi Ba Ji Tian) 12g Fructus Corni Officinalis (Shan Zhu Yu) 12g Herba Epimedii (Yin Yang Huo) 12g Herba Cistanches (Rou Cong Rong) 12g Semen Allii Tuberosi (Jiu Cao Zi) 12g Fructus Cnidii Monnieri (She Chuang Zi) 6g Radix Aconiti Lateralis Praeparatae (Fu Zi) 6g Cortex Cinnamomi (Rou Gui) 6g	pills with honey. Take 9g each time with warm boiled water. Could add Radix Ginseng (Ren Shen) and Cornu Cervi Pantotrichum (Lu Rong) to the prescription.
Zeng Ye Cheng Qi Decoction (Zeng Ye Cheng Qi Tang)	增液承气汤	Analysis of Warm Diseases (Wen Bing Tiao Bian)	Radix Scrophulariae (Xuan Shen) 30g Radix Ophiopogonis (Mai Dong) 24g Radix Rehmanniae Recens (Sheng Di Huang) 24g Radix et Rhizoma Rhei (Da Huang) 9g Natrii Sulfas (Mang Xiao) 4.5g	Decoct the drugs except Mang Xiao in water, and then dissolve Mang Xiao in the decoction for oral application.
Zeng Ye Decoction (Zeng Ye Tang)	增液汤	Analysis of Warm Diseases (Wen Bing Tiao Bian)	Radix Scrophulariae (Xuan Shen) 30g Radix Ophiopogonis (Mai Dong) 24g Radix Rehmanniae Recens (Sheng Di Huang) 24g	Decoct the drugs in water for oral application.
Zhen Fang Bai Pill (Zhen Fang Bai Wan Zi)	真方白丸子	Prescriptions of Auspicious Bamboo Hall (Rui Zhu Tang Fang)	Rhizoma Pinelliae (Ban Xia) 30g Rhizoma Typhonii (Bai Fu Zi) 30g Rhizoma Arisaematis (Tian Nan Xing) 30g Rhizoma Gastrodiae Elatae (Tian Ma) 30g Radix Aconiti Carmichaeli (Chuan Wu) 30g Scorpio (Quan Xie) 30g Radix Aucklandiae (Mu Xiang) 30g Fructus Citri Aurantii (Zhi Ke) 30g	Grind the drugs into fine powder and make pills with fresh ginger juice. Take 9g each time with tea or wine after meals, thrice daily.
Zhen Gan Xi Feng	镇肝熄风	Discourse on	Radix Glycyrrhizae (Gan Cao) 4.5g	Decoct the drugs in

Decoction (Zhen Gan Xi Feng Tang)	汤	Medical Problems by Integrated Traditional Chinese and Western Medicine (Yi Xue Zhong Zhong Can Xi Lu)	Radix Achyranthis Bidentatae (Niu Xi) 30g Ochra Haematitum (Dai Zhe Shi) 30g Os Draconis (Long Gu) 15g Concha Ostreae (Mu Li) 15g Plastrum Testudinis (Gui Ban) 15g Radix Paeoniae Alba (Bai Shao Yao) 15g Radix Scrophulariae (Xuan Shen) 15g Radix Asparagi (Tian Dong) 15g Fructus Hordei Germinatus (Mai Ya) 6g Herba Artemisiae Scopariae (Yin Chen Hao) 6g Fructus Meliae Toosendan (Chuan Lian Zi) 6g	water for oral application.
Zhen Ren Yang Zang Decoction (Zhen Ren Yang Zang Tang). Also named Chun Yang Zhen Ren Yang Zang Decoction (Chun Yang Zhen Ren Yang Zang Tang)	真人养脏汤（纯阳真人养脏汤）	Formularies of the Bureau of People's Welfare Pharmacy (Tai Ping Hui Min He Ji Ju Fang)	Radix Ginseng (Ren Shen) 9g Radix Angelicae Sinensis (Dang Gui) 9g Rhizoma Atractylodis Macrocephalae (Bai Zhu) 9g Semen Myristicae (Rou Dou Kou) 6g Cortex Cinnamomi (Rou Gui) 6g Radix Glycyrrhizae Praeparatae (Zhi Gan Cao) 6g Radix Paeoniae Alba (Bai Shao Yao) 6g Radix Aucklandiae (Mu Xiang) 3g Fructus Chebulae (He Zi) 9g Pericarpium Papaveris (Ying Su Ke) 6g (remove pedicle, prepared with honey)	Decoct the drugs in water for oral application before meals.
Zhen Wu Decoction (Zhen Wu Tang)	真武汤	Treatise on Cold Induced Diseases (Shang Han Lun)	Sclerotium Poriae Cocos (Fu Ling) 9g Radix Paeoniae Alba (9g) Rhizoma Zingiberis Recens (Sheng Jiang) 9g Rhizoma Atractylodis Macrocephalae (Bai Zhu) 6g Radix Aconiti Lateralis Praeparatae (Fu Zi) 9g	Decoct the drugs in water for oral application before meals.
Zheng Qi Tian Xiang Powder (Zheng Qi Tian Xiang San)	正气天香散	Bao Ming Ge Kuo	Radix Linderae (Wu Yao) 60g Rhizoma Cyperi Rotundi (Xiang Fu) 240g Pericarpium Citri Reticulatae (Chen Pi) 30g Folium Perillae Frutescentis (Zi Su Ye) 30g Rhizoma Zingiberis (Gan Jiang)	Grind the drugs into fine powder. Take 9g each time with warm boiled water.

			30g	
Zhi Bai Di Huang Pill (Zhi Bai Di Huang Wan)	知柏地黄丸	Key to Thrapeutics of Children's Diseases (Xiao Er Yao Zheng Zhi Jue)	Liu Wei Di Huang Pill (Liu Wei Di Huang Wan) supplemented with Radix Anemarrhenae (Zhi Mu) and Cortex Phellodendri (Huang Bai)	Decoct the drugs in water for oral application. Or make boluses, and take 6-9g each time with warm boiled water or light salty water before meals.
Zhi Bao Pill (Zhi Bao Dan)	至宝丹	Prescriptions of Magical Garden (Ling Yuan Fang)	Cornu Bubali (Shui Niu Jiao) 100g [to replace the original Cornu Rhinocerotis (Xi Jiao)] Cinnabaris (Zhu Sha) 30g Realgar (Xiong Huang) 30g Carapax Eretmochelydis (Sheng Dai Mao) 30g Succinum (Hu Po) 30g Calculus Bovis (Niu Huang) 0.3g Moschus (She Xiang) 0.3g Borneolum Syntheticum (Bing Pian) 0.3g Benzoinum (An Xi Xiang) 45g Gold Foil (Jin Bo) 50 pcs Silver Foil (Yin Bo) 50 pcs	Shui Niu Jiao, Dai Mao, An Xi Xiong and Hu Po are respectively ground into fine powder. Zhu Sha and Xiong Huang are respectively refined with water into extremely fine powder. Grind Niu Huang, She Xiang and Bing Pian into fine powder. Mix the above powder and grind it, then sift it evenly and make it into pills with honey. Take one pill (3g) each time, once or twice daily.
Zhi Gan Cao Decoction (Zhi Gan Cao Tang). Also named Fu Mai Decoction (Fu Mai Tang)	炙甘草汤 （又名复脉汤）	Treatise on Cold Induced Diseases (Shang Han Lun)	Radix Glycyrrhizae Praeparatae (Zhi Gan Cao) 12g Rhizoma Zingiberis Recens (Sheng Jiang) 9g Radix Ginseng (Ren Shen) 6g Radix Rehmanniae Recens (Sheng Di Huang) 50g Ramulus Cinnamomi (Gui Zhi) 9g Colla Corii Asini (E Jiao) 6g Radix Ophiopogonis (Mai Dong) 10g Semen Cannabis (Huo Ma Ren) 9g Fructus Zizyphi Jujubae (Da Zao) 30 pcs	Decoct the drugs except E Jiao in water for oral application, and stew E Jiao separately till it is melted.
Zhi Jing Powder (Zhi Jing San)	止痉散	Yang's Formulae Handed Down by Family (Yang Shi Jia Cang Fang)	Scorpio (Quan Xie) 5g Scolopendra Subspinipes (Wu Gong) 3g	Decoct the drugs in water for oral application. Or grind the drugs into fine powder, and take 3g each time with warm wine, twice or thrice daily.

Zhi Mi Decoction (Zhi Mi Tang)	指迷汤	Bian Zheng Lu	Radix Ginseng (Ren Shen) 15g Rhizoma Atractylodis Macrocephalae (Bai Zhu) 30g Rhizoma Pinelliae (Ban Xia) 9g Massa Medicata Fermentata (Shen Qu) 9g Rhizoma Arisaematis cum Bile (Dan Nan Xing) 3g Pericarpium Citri Reticulatae (Chen Pi) 1.5g Rhizoma Acori Tatarinowii (Shi Chang Pu) 1.5g Radix Aconiti Lateralis Praeparatae (Fu Zi) 0.9g Semen Myristicae (Rou Dou Kou) 3g Radix Glycyrrhizae (Gan Cao) 3g	Decoct the drugs in water for oral application. Radix Ginseng (Ren Shen) could be replaced with Radix Codonopsitis Pilosulae (Dang Shen).
Zhi Mi Fu Ling Pill (Zhi Mi Fu Ling Wan)	指迷茯苓丸	Quan Sheng Zhi Mi Fang	Sclerotium Poriae Cocos (Fu Ling) 30g Fructus Citri Aurantii (Zhi Ke) 15g Rhizoma Pinelliae (Ban Xia) 60g Natrii Sulfas (Mang Xiao) 7.5g Rhizoma Zingiberis Recens (Sheng Jiang)	Grind the first four drugs into powder and make pills with Rhizoma Zingiberis Recens (Sheng Jiang) juice. Take 3g each time after meals.
Zhi Shi Dao Zhi Pill (Zhi Shi Dao Zhi Wan)	枳实导滞丸	Treatise on Differentiation of Internal and External Injuries (Nei Wai Shang Bian Huo Lun)	Radix et Rhizoma Rhei (Da Huang) 9g Fructus Citri Aurantii Immaturus (Zhi Shi) 9g Massa Medicata Fermentata (Shen Qu) 9g Sclerotium Poriae Cocos (Fu Ling) 6g Radix Scutellariae (Huang Qin) 6g Rhizoma Coptidis (Huang Lian) 6g Rhizoma Atractylodis Macrocephalae (Bai Zhu) 6g Rhizoma Alismatis (Ze Xie) 6g	Decoct the drugs in water for oral application. Or prepare the drugs into pills, and take 6-9g each time with warm boiled water, twice daily.
Zhi Shi Xiao Pi Pill (Zhi Shi Xiao Pi Wan). Also named Shi Xiao Pill (Shi Xiao Wan)	枳实消痞丸（又名失笑丸）	Secret Book of Orchid Chamber (Lan Shi Mi Cang)	Rhizoma Zingiberis (Gan Jiang) 6g Radix Glycyrrhizae Praeparatae (Zhi Gan Cao) 6g Fructus Hordei Germinatus (Mai Ya) 6g Sclerotium Poriae Cocos (Bai Fu Ling) 6g Rhizoma Atractylodis Macrocephalae (Bai Zhu) 6g Rhizoma Pinelliae Fermentata (Ban Xia Qu) 9g Radix Ginseng (Ren Shen) 9g Cortex Magnoliae Officinalis (Hou Po) 12g Fructus Citri Aurantii Immaturus	Make the drugs into pills. Take 6-9g each time with warm boiled water, twice daily. Or decoct the drugs in water for oral application.

| | | | (Zhi Shi) 15g
Rhizoma Coptidis (Huang Lian) 15g | |
|---|---|---|---|---|
| Zhi Shi Xie Bai Gui Zhi Decoction (Zhi Shi Xie Bai Gui Zhi Tang) | 枳实薤白桂枝汤 | Synopsis of the Golden Chamber (Jin Gui Yao Lue) | Substract Bai Jiu from Gua Lou Xie Bai Bai Jiu Decoction (Gua Lou Xie Bai Bai Jiu Tang), and add Fructus Citri Aurantii Immaturus (Zhi Shi), Ramulus Cinnamomi (Gui Zhi) and Cortex Magnoliae Officinalis (Hou Po) to it. | Decoct the drugs in water for oral application. |
| Zhi Sou Powder (Zhi Sou San) | 止嗽散 | Medicine Comprehended (Yi Xue Xin Wu) | Radix Platycodonis (Jie Geng) 12g
Herba Schizonepetae (Jing Jie) 12g
Radix Asteris Tatarici (Zi Wan) 12g
Radix Stemonae (Bai Bu) 12g
Rhizoma Cynanchi Stauntonii (Bai Qian) 12g
Pericarpium Citri Reticulatae (Chen Pi) 6g
Radix Glycyrrhizae Praeparatae (Zhi Gan Cao) 3g | Decoct the drugs in water for oral application. |
| Zhi Zi Qing Gan Decoction (Zhi Zi Qing Gan Tang) | 栀子清肝汤 | Lei Zheng Zhi Cai | Fructus Gardeniae (Zhi Zi)
Cortex Moutan Radicis (Mu Dan Pi)
Radix Bupleuri (Chai Hu)
Radix Angelicae Sinensis (Dang Gui)
Radix Paeoniae Alba (Bai Shao Yao)
Sclerotium Poriae Cocos (Fu Ling)
Rhizoma Ligustici Chuanxiong (Chuan Xiong)
Fructus Arctii Lappae (Niu Bang Zi)
Radix Glycyrrhizae (Gan Cao) | Decoct the drugs in water for oral application. |
| Zhong Man Fen Xiao Pill (Zhong Man Fen Xiao Wan) | 中满分消丸 | Secret Book of Orchid Chamber (Lan Shi Mi Cang) | Cortex Magnoliae Officinalis (Hou Po) 30g
Fructus Citri Aurantii Immaturus (Zhi Shi) 15g
Rhizoma Coptidis (Huang Lian) 15g
Radix Scutellariae (Huang Qin) 36g
Rhizoma Anemarrhenae (Zhi Mu) 12g
Rhizoma Pinelliae (Ban Xia) 15g
Pericarpium Citri Reticulatae (Chen Pi) 9g
Sclerotium Poriae Cocos (Fu Ling) 6g
Sclerotium Polypori Umbellati (Zhu Ling) 3g
Rhizoma Alismatis Orientalis (Ze Xie) 9g | Grind the drugs into powder and make pills with water. Take 6g each time before meals. |

				Fructus Amomi Villosi (Sha Ren) 6g
Rhizoma Zingiberis (Gan Jiang) 6g
Rhizoma Curcumae Longae (Jiang Huang) 3g
Radix Ginseng (Ren Shen) 3g
Rhizoma Atractylodis Macrocephalae (Bai Zhu) 3g
Radix Glycyrrhizae Praeparatae (Zhi Gan Cao) 3g	
Zhu Che Pill (Zhu Che Wan)	驻车丸	Invaluable Prescriptions for Emergencies (Bei Ji Qian Jin Yao Fang)	Rhizoma Coptidis (Huang Lian) 18g
Colla Corii Asini (E Jiao) 9g
Radix Angelicae Sinensis (Dang Gui) 9g
Rhizoma Zingiberis (Gan Jiang) 6g	Grind the drugs into fine powder, sift and make pills with water and vinegar. Take 6-9g each time, twice or thrice daily.
Zhu Ling Decoction (Zhu Ling Tang)	猪苓汤		Sclerotium Polypori Umbellati (Zhu Ling) 9g
Sclerotium Poriae Cocos (Fu Ling) 9g
Rhizoma Alismatis (Ze Xie) 9g
Talcum (Hua Shi Fen) 9g
Colla Corii Asini (E Jiao) 9g	Decoct the drugs except E Jiao in water. E Jiao is melted separately and added in the decoction for oral application.
Zhu Sha An Shen Pill (Zhu Sha An Shen Wan)	朱砂安神丸	Differentiation on Endogenous and Exogenous Diseases (Nei Wai Shang Bian Huo Lun)	Cinnabaris (Zhu Sha) 1g
Rhizoma Coptidis (Huang Lian) 18g
Radix Glycyrrhizae (Gan Cao) 16.5g
Radix Rehmanniae Recens (Sheng Di Huang) 4.5g
Radix Angelicae Sinensis (Dang Gui) 7.5g	Grind Zhu Sha separately in water, and prepare the drugs into pills with honey. Take 6-9g each time with warm boiled water before sleep.
Zhu Ye Shi Gao Decoction (Zhu Ye Shi Gao Tang)	竹叶石膏汤	Treatise on Cold Induced Diseases (Shang Han Lun)	Folium Phyllostachydis Henonis (Zhu Ye) 6g
Gypsum Fibrosum (Shi Gao) 50g
Rhizoma Pinelliae (Ban Xia) 9g
Radix Ophiopogonis (Mai Dong) 18g
Radix Ginseng (Ren Shen) 6g
Radix Glycyrrhizae Praeparatae (Zhi Gan Cao) 6g
Semen Oryzae Sativae (Jing Mi) 9g	Decoct the drugs in water for oral application.
Zi Shui Qing Gan Decoction (Zi Shui Qing Yin)	滋水清肝饮	Yi Zong Ji Ren Bian	Radix Rehmanniae Recens (Sheng Di Huang)
Fructus Corni Officinalis (Shan Zhu Yu)
Sclerotium Poriae Cocos (Fu Ling)
Radix Angelicae Sinensis (Dang Gui)
Rhizoma Dioscoreae (Shan Yao)
Cortex Moutan Radicis (Mu Dan Pi)	Decoct the drugs in water for oral application.

			Rhizoma Alismatis (Ze Xie) Radix Bupleuri (Chai Hu) Radix Paeoniae Alba (Bai Shao Yao) Fructus Gardeniae (Zhi Zi) Semen Ziziphi Spinosae (Suan Zao Ren)	
Zi Xue. Also named Zi Xue Pellet (Zi Xue Dan)	紫雪（又名紫雪丹）	Arcane Essentials from the Imperial Library (Wai Tai Mi Yao)	Gypsum Fibrosum (Shi Gao) 1.5g Calcitum (Han Shui Shi) 1.5g Talcum (Hua Shi Fen) 1.5g Magnetitum (Ci Shi) 1.5g Cornu Bubali (Shui Niu Jiao) 30g [to preplace original Cornu Rhinocerotis (Xi Jiao)] Cornu Saigae Tataricae (Ling Yang Jiao) 150g Lignum Aquilariae Resinatum (Chen Xiang) 150g Radix Aucklandiae (Mu Xiang) 150g Radix Scrophulariae (Xuan Shen) 500g Rhizoma Cimicifugae (Sheng Ma) 500g Radix Glycyrrhizae Praeparatae (Zhi Gan Cao) 240g Flos Caryophylli (Ding Xiang) 30g Natrii Sulfas (Mang Xiao) 5kg Nitrium (Xiao Shi) 950g Moschus (She Xiang) 1.5g Cinnabaris (Zhu Sha) 90g Gold (Huang Jin) 300g	Smash Shi Gao, Han Shui Shi, Hua Shi and Ci Shi into masses, and decoct them in water for three times. Decoct Xuan Shen, Mu Xiang, Chen Xiang, Sheng Ma, Gan Cao and Diang Xiang with the above decoction for three times, then mix the decoctions, sift them, and condense the filtrate into ointment. Smash Mang Xiao and Xiao Shi, and add them into the ointment, mix evenly, make them dry, and grind them into moderate or fine powder. Make Ling Yang Jiao into fine powder, refine Zhu Sha with water into extremely fine powder, grind Shui Niu Jiao and She Xiang into fine powder, and finally mix the above powder evenly, sift them (without Huang Jin), and pack the mixture in vials (1.5g each). Take 1.5-3g each time, twice daily.
Zuo Gui Pill (Zuo Gui Wan)	左归丸	Jingyue's Complete Works (Jing Yue Quan Shu)	Radix Rehmanniae Praeparatae (Shu Di Huang) 24g Rhizoma Dioscoreae (Shan Yao) 12g Fructus Lycii (Gou Qi Zi) 12g Fructus Corni (Shan Zhu Yu) 12g	Decoct the drugs in water for oral application. Or make them into boluses with honey, and take 9g each time with

			Semen Cuscutae (Tu Si Zi) 12g Colla Corni Cervi (Lu Jiao Jiao) 12g Colla Testudinis Plastri (Gui Ban Jiao) 12g Radix Cyathulae Officinalis (Chuan Niu Xi) 12g	warm boiled water or light salty water before meals.
Zuo Gui Decoction (Zuo Gui Yin)	左归饮	Jingyue's Complete Works (Jing Yue Quan Shu)	Radix Rehmanniae Praeparatae (Shu Di Huang) 24g Rhizoma Dioscoreae (Shan Yao) 12g Fructus Lycii (Gou Qi Zi) 12g Fructus Corni (Shan Zhu Yu) 12g Sclerotium Poriae Cocos (Fu Ling) 12g Radix Glycyrrhizae (Gan Cao) 6g	Decoct the drugs in water for oral application.
Zuo Jin Pill (Zuo Jin Wan). Also named Hui Ling Pill (Hui Ling Wan), Yu Lian Pill (Yu Lian Wan)	左金丸（又名回令丸，黄连丸）	Danxi's Experiential Therapy (Dan Xi Xin Fa)	Rhizoma Coptidis (Huang Lian) 12g Fructus Evodiae (Wu Zhu Yu) 2g	Prepare the drugs into pills, and take 3g each time. Or decoct them in water for oral application.

INDEX

1

12 Regular Channels, 61, 62
15 Collaterals, 61

8

8 Extraordinary Channels, 61

A

An Gong Niu huang Pill, 558
An Shen Ding Zhi Pill, 155, 442, 558
Anger, 14, 15, 26, 38, 216, 248, 440, 446

B

Ba Zhen Decoction, 224, 231, 310, 314, 323, 329, 393, 420, 431, 461, 478, 558, 619
Ba Zhen Powder, 558
Ba Zheng Powder, 53, 60, 270, 293, 296, 559
Bai He Gu Jin Decoction, 48, 112, 129, 263, 264, 396, 498, 506, 559
Bai Hu Decoction, 69, 71, 184, 465, 559, 560
Bai Hu Jia Cang Zhu Decoction, 58, 559
Bai Hu Jia Gui Zhi Decoction, 58, 382, 386, 560
Bai Hu Jia Ren Shen Decoction, 71, 346, 499, 560
Bai Tou Weng Decoction, 49, 70, 215, 498, 560
Bai Tou Weng Jia Gan Cao E Jiao Decoction, 560
Ban Xia Bai Zhu Tian Ma Decoction, 164, 359, 458, 470, 479, 560
Ban Xia Hou Po Decoction, 444, 486, 560
Ban Xia Xie Xin Decoction, 55, 560
Bao He Pill, 46, 375, 378, 475, 481, 486, 561
Bao Yuan Decoction, 336, 352, 471, 472, 561
Bao Zhen Decoction, 129, 561
Bei Mu Gua Lou Powder, 561
Bi Xie Fen Qing Decoction, 495, 562
Bie Jia Jian Pill, 234, 235, 239, 329, 330, 562
Bu Fei Decoction, 27, 47, 98, 102, 112, 115, 118, 151, 201, 562
Bu Qi Yun Pi Decoction, 228, 563
Bu Tian Da Zao Pill, 130, 563
Bu Yang Huan Wu Decoction, 29, 168, 171, 176, 185, 342, 396, 405, 407, 412, 417, 421, 438, 459, 563
Bu Zhong Yi Qi Decoction, 27, 30, 43, 107, 206, 216, 265, 283, 287, 294, 437, 478, 482, 484, 498, 500, 509, 564

C

Cang Er Powder, 564
Chai Ge Jie Ji Decoction, 564
Chai Hu Shu Gan Powder, 39, 205, 209, 222, 237, 245, 248, 249, 324, 328, 393, 433, 443, 471, 475, 564
Chai Hu Si Wu Decoction, 147, 565
Chai Shao Liu Jun Zi Decoction, 257, 565
Chai Zhi Ban Xia Decoction, 135, 565
Chang Pu Yu Jin Decoction, 162, 241, 281, 565
Channels and Collaterals, 61, 65, 66, 67, 382, 385, 398, 399, 406
Chen Xiang Powder, 297, 566
Chou Xin Decoction, 462, 566
Chuan Xiong Cha Tiao Powder, 402, 467, 566
Chun Yang Zhen Ren Yang Zang Decoction, 566, 648
Ci Zhu Pill, 372, 567
Cong Bai Qi Wei Decoction, 147, 567
Cong Chi Decoction, 56, 144, 567
Cong Chi Jie Geng Decoction, 89, 567

D

Da Bu Pill, 568
Da Bu Yin Pill, 40, 568
Da Bu Yuan Decoction, 27, 52, 133, 287, 451, 469, 568
Da Chai Hu Decoction, 68, 106, 250, 256, 568
Da Cheng Qi Decoction, 50, 59, 69, 71, 254, 362, 474, 486, 568
Da Ding Feng Pill, 57, 421, 568
Da Huang Fu Zi Decoction, 484, 569
Da Huang Mu Dan Decoction, 569
Da Huang Zhe Chong Pill, 239, 307, 446, 569
Da Jian Zhong Decoction, 258, 474, 569
Da Qin Jiao Decoction, 417, 570
Da Tao Hua Decoction, 500, 570
Dai Ge Powder, 55, 97, 111, 141, 328, 506, 570
Dan Shen Decoction, 171, 206, 210, 473, 570
Dan Zhi Xiao Yao Powder, 293, 432, 443, 471, 571
Dang Gui Bu Xue Decoction, 29, 301, 309, 313, 571
Dang Gui Decoction, 571
Dang Gui Liu Huang Decoction, 497, 571
Dang Gui Si Ni Decoction, 70, 171, 176, 472, 571
Dao Chi Powder, 37, 59, 435, 572
Dao Tan Decoction, 36, 132, 167, 374, 379, 403, 407, 421, 572, 639
Di Dang Decoction, 29, 572

Di Huang Decoction, 232, 279, 305, 335, 366, 375, 422, 463, 572
Di Tan Decoction, 116, 158, 170, 201, 418, 425, 444, 457, 460, 471, 573
Di Yu Powder, 230, 508, 573
Dian Kuang Meng Xing Decoction, 446, 448, 573
Ding Chuan Decoction, 105, 574
Ding Shi Qing Luo Decoction, 387, 574
Ding Xian Pill, 424, 574
Ding Xiang Shi Di Decoction, 575
Ding Zhi Pill, 446, 575
Du Huo Ji Sheng Decoction, 383, 388, 476, 575
Du Shen Decoction, 112, 116, 162, 180, 213, 335, 507, 576

E

Eight Parameters, 18
Eight Principles, 18
Er Chen Decoction, 49, 55, 96, 101, 107, 114, 140, 144, 281, 348, 356, 359, 471, 486, 576
Er Miao Powder, 576, 611
Er Xian Decoction, 133, 360, 576
Er Yin Decoction, 446, 448, 576
Er Zhi Pill, 290, 321, 501, 577
Exterior Syndrome, 18, 491

F

Fang Feng Tong Sheng Powder, 577
Fang Ji Huang Qi Decoction, 261, 263, 307, 379, 488, 577
Fear, 15, 24, 424, 447
Five Elements, 23
Five Endogenous Pathogenetic Factors, 16
Five Phases, 23
Four Cycles, 24
Four Divisions, 70
Fright, 15, 424, 447, 451
Fu Ling Pi Decoction, 281, 578
Fu Mai Decoction, 57, 578, 649
Fu Viscera, 33
Fu Yuan Huo Xue Decoction, 578
Fu Zi Li Zhong Decoction, 44, 69, 231, 238, 246, 375, 474, 482, 578
Fu Zi Li Zhong Pill, 268, 578

G

Gan Jiang Ling Zhu Decoction, 475, 578
Gan Lu Xiao Du Powder, 191, 491, 499, 579
Gan Mai Da Zao Decoction, 445, 497, 579
Ge Gen Decoction, 579
Ge Gen Huang Qin Huang Lian Decoction, 579
Ge Gen Qin Lian Decoction, 191, 219, 322, 481, 579
Ge Hua Jie Cheng Decoction, 463, 579

Ge Xia Zhu Yu Decoction, 197, 217, 224, 231, 239, 245, 257, 317, 323, 487, 493, 580
Grief, 15, 447
Gu Chong Decoction, 580
Gu Jing Pill, 580
Gua Di Powder, 581
Gua Lou Gui Zhi Decoction, 581
Gua Lou Xie Bai Bai Jiu Decoction, 581, 651
Gua Lou Xie Bai Ban Xia Decoction, 170, 176, 197, 471, 581
Gui Lu Er Xian Glue, 581
Gui Pi Decoction, 30, 35, 45, 54, 155, 171, 213, 272, 310, 316, 332, 335, 338, 371, 438, 441, 445, 450, 451, 453, 455, 478, 497, 500, 505, 507, 509, 581
Gui Shao Di Huang Decoction, 287, 582
Gui Shao Liu Jun Zi Decoction, 245, 582
Gui Zhi Decoction, 67, 68, 474, 496, 582
Gui Zhi Fu Ling Pill, 106, 270, 582
Gui Zhi Gan Cao Long Gu Mu Li Decoction, 152, 157, 582
Gui Zhi Shao Yao Zhi Mu Decoction, 387, 583
Gun Tan Pill, 583, 599
Guo Min Decoction, 106, 583

H

Hai Zao Yu Hu Decoction, 222, 355, 583
Hao Qin Qing Dan Decoction, 584
He Che Da Zao Pill, 109, 317, 478, 501, 584
Hou Po Wen Zhong Decoction, 584
Hua Ban Decoction, 290, 584
Hua Chong Pill, 310, 584
Hua Gan Decoction, 210, 585
Huai Hua Powder, 30, 585
Huai Jiao Pill, 508, 589
Huan Shao Pill, 428, 585
Huang Lian E Jiao Decoction, 54, 69, 441, 450, 585
Huang Lian Jie Du Decoction, 300, 320, 586
Huang Lian Qing Xin Decoction, 494, 587
Huang Lian Shang Qing Pill, 37, 468, 586
Huang Lian Wen Dan Decoction, 36, 41, 42, 55, 156, 158, 241, 264, 270, 301, 306, 412, 424, 440, 472, 587
Huang Lian Xiang Ru Decoction, 465, 468, 587
Huang Long Decoction, 587, 638
Huang Qi Decoction, 484, 588
Huang Qi Gui Zhi Wu Wu Decoction, 588
Huang Qi Jian Zhong Decoction, 206, 209, 257, 338, 588
Huang Qi Liu Yi Powder, 372, 588
Huang Qi Sheng Mai Decoction, 499, 588
Huang Tu Decoction, 507, 508, 588
Hui Yang Jiu Ji Decoction, 342, 589
Huo Luo Pill, 400, 408, 589, 636
Huo Luo Xiao Ling Pill, 210, 589
Huo Po Xia Ling Decoction, 362, 590
Huo Xiang Zheng Qi Powder, 57, 58, 480, 485, 590

I

Interior Syndrome, 19
Internal Cold, 17
Internal Dampness, 17
Internal Dryness, 17
Internal Heat, 17
Internal Wind, 17

J

Ji Chuan Decoction, 485, 590
Ji Jiao Li Huang Pill, 266, 268, 590
Ji Sheng Shen Qi Pill, 52, 165, 202, 239, 268, 277, 279, 305, 307, 352, 392, 490, 491, 591
Ji Sheng Xiao Ji Decoction, 591, 636
Jia Jian Wei Rui Decoction, 147, 591
Jia Wei Er Miao Powder, 439, 591
Jia Wei Jie Geng Decoction, 125, 592
Jia Wei Si Wu Decoction, 469, 592
Jian Pi Pill, 592
Jiao Tai Pill, 54, 593
Jin Gui Shen Qi Pill, 27, 51, 108, 152, 168, 246, 267, 297, 306, 314, 346, 363, 370, 428, 434, 473, 500, 502, 593
Jin Gui Xie Xin Decoction, 30, 593
Jin Ling Zi Powder, 593
Jin Suo Gu Jing Pill, 366, 496, 593
Jing Fang Bai Du Powder, 56, 89, 144, 593
Jiu Wei Qiang Huo Decoction, 594
Jiu Xian Powder, 594
Joy, 1, 14, 15, 26
Ju Pi Zhu Ru Decoction, 28, 594
Juan Bi Decoction, 58, 382, 594

K

Kai Yu Er Chen Decoction, 224, 595
Ke Xue Formula, 595

L

Li Zhong Decoction, 45, 55, 69, 223, 258, 478, 480, 487, 595
Li Zhong Pill, 216, 250, 595
Lian Po Decoction, 44, 595
Liang Fu Pill, 44, 45, 49, 204, 474, 596
Liang Ge Powder, 37, 135, 596
Ling Gan Wu Wei Jiang Xin Decoction, 596
Ling Gui Zhu Gan Decoction, 32, 37, 98, 159, 196, 379, 486, 596
Ling Jiao Gou Teng Decoction, 72, 265, 503, 596
Ling Yang Jiao Decoction, 418, 466, 478, 596
Liu Jun Zi Decoction, 98, 108, 140, 304, 597
Liu Mo Decoction, 483, 597
Liu Wei Di Huang Pill, 51, 98, 168, 283, 297, 302, 314, 339, 365, 370, 410, 422, 433, 441, 445, 450, 469, 485, 501, 597, 649
Liu Yi Powder, 90, 481, 597, 642
Long Dan Xie Gan Decoction, 30, 39, 41, 42, 59, 212, 253, 348, 354, 361, 404, 425, 440, 452, 454, 478, 498, 507, 598
Lower Warmer, 33, 270, 271, 296, 306, 508, 516

M

Ma Huang Decoction, 68, 261, 268, 598
Ma Huang Lian Qiao Chi Xiao Dou Decoction, 262, 264, 268, 275, 279, 488, 491, 598
Ma Huang Xing Ren Gan Cao Shi Gao Decoction, 598
Ma Xing Shi Gan Decoction, 48, 71, 93, 96, 118, 121, 135, 138, 144, 598, 599
Ma Zi Ren Pill, 396, 483, 599
Mai Men Dong Decoction, 30, 487, 498, 599
Mai Wei Di Huang Pill, 133, 369, 599
Melancholy, 15, 444
Meng Shi Gun Tan Pill, 36, 446, 448, 583, 599
Miao Xiang Powder, 495, 599
Middle Warmer, 33, 65, 270, 297, 306, 359, 361, 443, 462, 474, 477, 482, 486, 487, 489, 493, 494, 495, 498

N

Niu Huang Qing Xin Pill, 36, 426, 600, 628
Niu Huang Zhi Bao Pill, 600, 633
Nuan Gan Decoction, 41, 474, 600

P

Pensiveness, 15, 24, 248, 271, 442
Ping Chuan Gu Ben Decoction, 102, 601
Ping Wei Powder, 55, 371, 481, 601
Pu Ji Xiao Du Decoction, 601

Q

Qi Bao Mei Ran Pill, 602
Qi Fu Decoction, 427, 431, 602
Qi Ge Powder, 226, 602
Qi Ju Di Huang Pill, 55, 165, 268, 290, 329, 357, 363, 372, 469, 602
Qi Jun Decoction, 500, 603
Qi Li Powder, 603
Qi Wei Bai Zhu Powder, 370, 603
Qi Wei Du Qi Pill, 108, 603
Qian Gen Powder, 332, 335, 505, 604
Qian Jin Wei Jing Decoction, 59, 111, 121, 125, 153, 472, 604
Qian Zheng Powder, 407, 417, 604
Qiang Huo Sheng Shi Decoction, 57, 89, 144, 468, 604

Qin Jiao Bie Jia Powder, 129, 604
Qing Dan Decoction, 249, 492, 605
Qing E Pill, 477, 605
Qing Gong Decoction, 393, 466, 605
Qing Gu Powder, 60, 354, 605
Qing Hao Bie Jia Decoction, 72, 184, 323, 606
Qing Jin Hua Tan Decoction, 32, 111, 118, 140, 153, 606
Qing Qi Hua Tan Pill, 99, 142, 606
Qing Shu Yi Qi Decoction, 465, 606
Qing Wei Powder, 45, 59, 403, 505, 607
Qing Wen Bai Du Decoction, 118, 280, 300, 314, 390, 493, 503, 607
Qing Xin Lian Zi Decoction, 284, 607
Qing Yi Decoction, 253, 254, 608
Qing Ying Decoction, 71, 122, 184, 320, 323, 331, 466, 503, 608
Qing Zao Jiu Fei Decoction, 48, 139, 395, 410, 608
Qing Zhong Decoction, 256, 608

R

Ren Shen Bai Du Powder, 608
Ren Shen Decoction, 473, 609
Ren Shen Hu Tao Decoction, 52, 609
Ren Shen Si Ni Decoction, 157, 353, 609
Ren Shen Yang Rong Decoction, 29, 152, 609
Run Chang Pill, 484, 610

S

San Ao Decoction, 48, 93, 96, 121, 138, 610
San Bi Decoction, 399, 610
San Jia Fu Mai Decoction, 72, 282, 287, 501, 611
San Jiao, 26, 33
San Leng Decoction, 329, 611
San Miao Powder, 611
San Ren Decoction, 205, 270, 611
San Wu Bei Ji Pill, 611
San Zi Yang Qin Decoction, 32, 49, 96, 101, 107, 108, 114, 140, 612
Sang Bai Pi Decoction, 48, 59, 97, 101, 612
Sang Ju Decoction, 57, 71, 93, 121, 139, 504, 612
Sang Piao Xiao Powder, 53, 612
Sang Xing Decoction, 93, 139, 145, 395, 506, 612
Seven Emotions, 14, 30
Sha Shen Mai Dong Decoction, 98, 133, 136, 141, 228, 324, 346, 613
Sha Shen Qing Fei Decoction, 126, 613
Shao Fu Zhu Yu Decoction, 475, 613
Shao Yao Decoction, 49, 614
Shao Yao Di Huang Decoction, 613, 633
Shao Yao Gan Cao Decoction, 210, 613
She Gan Ma Huang Decoction, 105, 614
Shen Fu Decoction, 35, 102, 116, 119, 122, 157, 172, 181, 301, 419, 458, 614

Shen Fu Long Mu Decoction, 178, 189, 242, 371, 466, 614
Shen Fu Yang Rong Decoction, 192, 614
Shen Fu Zai Zao Pill, 146, 615
Shen Ge Powder, 52, 115, 615
Shen Ling Bai Zhu Powder, 98, 216, 263, 379, 410, 481, 490, 615
Shen Qi Di Huang Decoction, 264, 269, 287, 291, 301, 305, 615
Shen Qi Pill, 288, 593, 615
Shen Su Decoction, 90, 146, 616
Shen Tong Zhu Yu Decoction, 272, 387, 399, 476, 616
Shen Xian Huo Ming Decoction, 616, 634
Sheng Hua Decoction, 617
Sheng Ma Ge Gen Decoction, 617
Sheng Mai Powder, 35, 56, 107, 118, 122, 133, 151, 155, 161, 171, 177, 181, 185, 192, 202, 338, 349, 366, 370, 458, 466, 473, 588, 617
Sheng Tie Luo Decoction, 448, 617
Sheng Yu Decoction, 188, 342, 371, 618
Shi Bu Pill, 618
Shi Hui Powder, 212, 507, 508, 618
Shi Pi Decoction, 197, 237, 268, 276, 290, 355, 434, 490, 619
Shi Pi Powder, 618
Shi Quan Da Bu Decoction, 29, 317, 365, 500, 619
Shi Wei Powder, 293, 619
Shi Xiao Pill, 619, 650
Shi Xiao Powder, 36, 171, 206, 249, 376, 471, 619
Shi Zao Decoction, 32, 135, 620
Shu Gan Powder, 28, 620
Shu Zao Decoction, 276, 489, 620
Shui Lu Er Xian Pill, 287, 496, 620
Shun Qi Dao Tan Decoction, 447, 620
Shun Qi He Zhong Decoction, 469, 621
Si Jun Zi Decoction, 27, 43, 56, 102, 223, 279, 324, 351, 352, 444, 621, 634, 641
Si Miao Pill, 280, 287, 290, 306, 386, 400, 410, 476, 498, 621
Si Miao Yong An Decoction, 387, 621
Si Ni Decoction, 69, 122, 189, 357, 474, 622
Si Ni Jia Ren Shen Decoction, 609, 622
Si Ni Powder, 54, 369, 486, 622
Si Shen Pill, 55, 165, 216, 231, 482, 622
Si Wei Hui Yang Decoction, 109, 162, 213, 622
Si Wu Decoction, 29, 147, 314, 365, 469, 618, 622, 624
Six Channels, 60
Six Climatic Causes, 13, 18
Six Pathogenic Factors, 13
Six Pernicious Influences, 13
Six Stages, 60
Spirit, 73, 581
Su He Xiang Pill, 36, 172, 176, 241, 342, 418, 444, 458, 459, 460, 466, 472, 622
Su Zi Jiang Qi Decoction, 28, 33, 105, 200, 623
Suan Zao Ren Decoction, 41, 55, 442, 623
Summer Heat, 13

Suo Quan Pill, 294, 623

T

Tai Shan Pan Shi Powder, 624
Tao He Cheng Qi Decoction, 68, 446, 624
Tao Hong Decoction, 383, 624
Tao Hong Si Wu Decoction, 132, 152, 176, 188, 234, 307, 314, 321, 324, 336, 356, 371, 380, 412, 433, 491, 503, 624
Tao Ren Cheng Qi Decoction, 29, 624
Tao Ren Hong Hua Decoction, 156, 180, 624
TCM, 9, 10, 33, 34, 35, 50, 73, 78, 79, 81, 83
Tian Ma Gou Teng Decoction, 39, 57, 164, 307, 359, 416, 420, 434, 468, 477, 625
Tian Tai Wu Yao Powder, 37, 625, 631
Tian Wang Bu Xin Pill, 35, 155, 188, 191, 193, 349, 445, 625
Tiao Wei Cheng Qi Decoction, 50, 69, 71, 498, 624, 626
Tiao Ying Decoction, 238, 265, 626
Ting Li Da Zao Xie Fei Decoction, 32, 49, 132, 152, 177, 181, 196, 276, 391, 489, 626
Tong Qiao Huo Xue Decoction, 405, 425, 429, 432, 461, 470, 479, 627
Tong Xie Formula, 216, 482, 627
Tong You Decoction, 227, 627
Triple Warmer, 26, 33, 61, 62, 65, 264, 267, 268, 281, 301, 322

U

Upper Warmer, 33, 270, 516

W

Wan Dai Decoction, 627
Wan Shi Niu Huang Pill, 600, 628
Wan Shi Niu Huang Qing Xin Pill, 600, 628
Wei Jing Decoction, 48, 628
Wei Ling Decoction, 44, 49, 58, 219, 237, 270, 275, 480, 489, 628
Wei Rui Decoction, 91, 628
Wen Dan Decoction, 36, 171, 266, 321, 446, 471, 473, 479, 486, 629
Wen Jing Decoction, 29, 629
Wen Pi Decoction, 629
Wu Bi Shan Yao Pill, 272, 294, 297, 310, 509, 629
Wu Ji Pill, 630
Wu Ji Powder, 630
Wu Ling Powder, 68, 115, 132, 181, 201, 238, 261, 262, 265, 268, 269, 287, 307, 357, 489, 491, 630, 643
Wu Mei Pill, 70, 631
Wu Mo Decoction, 209, 631
Wu Pi Decoction, 262, 268, 269, 275, 276, 284, 307, 489, 631

Wu Pi Powder, 631
Wu Tou Decoction, 386, 398, 631
Wu Wei Xiao Du Decoction, 133, 184, 220, 254, 262, 275, 289, 372, 488, 631
Wu Yao Powder, 625, 631
Wu Yin Decoction, 321, 632
Wu Zhi An Zhong Decoction, 227, 632
Wu Zhi Decoction, 31, 632
Wu Zhu Yu Decoction, 37, 467, 632
Wu Zi Yan Zong Pill, 287, 290, 317, 453, 632

X

Xi Huang Xuan Qiao Decoction, 499, 633
Xi Jiao Di Huang Decoction, 30, 72, 118, 184, 241, 289, 323, 331, 335, 339, 341, 392, 503, 506, 613, 633
Xi Xian Powder, 32, 633
Xi Xin Decoction, 428, 432, 469, 633
Xian Fang Huo Ming Decoction, 195, 616, 634
Xiang Fu Xuan Fu Hua Decoction, 136, 634
Xiang Ru Powder, 634
Xiang Sha Liu Jun Zi Decoction, 43, 309, 634
Xiang Su Powder, 46, 634
Xiao Ban Xia Jia Fu Ling Decoction, 37, 306, 634
Xiao Chai Hu Decoction, 68, 253, 635
Xiao Cheng Qi Decoction, 50, 69, 71, 220, 378, 635
Xiao Feng Powder, 635
Xiao He Powder, 33, 635
Xiao Huo Luo Pill, 589, 636
Xiao Ji Decoction, 30, 271, 279, 284, 332, 509, 591, 636
Xiao Jian Zhong Decoction, 44, 45, 474, 494, 636
Xiao Ke Formula, 369, 636
Xiao Luo Wan, 636
Xiao Qing Long Decoction, 32, 48, 97, 100, 105, 637
Xiao Qing Long JiaShi Gao Decoction, 637
Xiao Xian Xiong Decoction, 36, 44, 471, 472, 637
Xiao Xu Ming Decoction, 406, 637
Xiao Yao Powder, 28, 39, 55, 234, 348, 357, 374, 452, 453, 463, 471, 637
Xie Bai Powder, 55, 111, 141, 328, 391, 506, 638
Xie Fei Powder, 638
Xie Huang Powder, 59, 638
Xie Xin Decoction, 59, 212, 435, 446, 505, 507, 593, 638
Xin Jia Huang Long Decoction, 638
Xin Jia Xiang Ru Decoction, 90, 145, 481, 638
Xing Lou Cheng Qi Decoction, 416, 638
Xing Pi Decoction, 425, 638
Xing Su Powder, 32, 94, 138, 639
Xiong Zhi Shi Gao Decoction, 403, 468, 639
Xuan Bi Decoction, 195, 640
Xuan Fu Dai Zhe Decoction, 28, 640
Xue Fu Zhu Yu Decoction, 29, 36, 106, 132, 158, 165, 167, 170, 175, 188, 196, 197, 202, 220, 227, 270,

272, 297, 333, 342, 372, 376, 380, 441, 444, 446, 471, 640

Y

Yang Gan Pill (Yang Gan Wan), 641
Yang He Decoction, 328, 640
Yang Xin Decoction, 35, 151, 434, 447, 450, 641
Yang Yin Qing Fei Decoction, 48, 641
Yi Gong Powder, 267, 641
Yi Guan Decoction, 40, 210, 239, 246, 250, 359, 438, 501, 642
Yi Huang Decoction, 642
Yi Wei Decoction, 60, 205, 207, 396, 485, 642
Yi Yi Ren Decoction, 386, 642
Yi Yuan Powder, 597, 642
Yin and Yang, 18, 21, 22, 23, 62, 129, 133, 192, 241, 288, 291, 305, 360, 361, 366, 370, 395, 422, 442, 458
Yin Chen Hao Decoction, 41, 42, 234, 238, 242, 244, 250, 393, 492, 493, 643
Yin Chen Si Ling Powder, 492, 643
Yin Chen Wei Ling Decoction, 244, 643
Yin Chen Wu Ling Powder, 58, 316, 643
Yin Chen Zhu Fu Decoction, 493, 643
Yin Qiao Powder, 57, 89, 124, 145, 183, 187, 191, 194, 268, 270, 271, 407, 643
You Gui Pill, 51, 157, 168, 172, 313, 338, 346, 353, 362, 365, 388, 451, 469, 477, 479, 490, 644
Yu Gong Powder, 238, 644
Yu Nu Decoction, 223, 335, 339, 369, 391, 396, 504, 644
Yu Ping Feng Powder, 90, 98, 107, 146, 264, 267, 496, 644
Yu Ye Decoction, 645
Yu Zhen Powder, 645
Yue Bi Decoction, 645
Yue Bi Jia Ban Xia Decoction, 101, 200, 645
Yue Bi Jia Zhu Decoction, 261, 275, 488, 645
Yue Hua Pill, 128, 195, 646

Yue Ju Pill, 646

Z

Zai Zao Powder, 646
Zan Yu Pill, 451, 454, 646
Zang Viscera, 33
Zeng Ye Cheng Qi Decoction, 647
Zeng Ye Decoction, 31, 391, 485, 647
Zhen Fang Bai Pill, 416, 647
Zhen Gan Xi Feng Decoction, 40, 404, 412, 417, 647
Zhen Ren Yang Zang Decoction, 49, 482, 566, 648
Zhen Wu Decoction, 52, 56, 69, 115, 152, 157, 159, 172, 177, 181, 189, 196, 198, 201, 263, 268, 277, 284, 288, 290, 307, 379, 473, 490, 648
Zheng Qi Tian Xiang Powder, 204, 474, 648
Zhi Bai Di Huang Pill, 51, 60, 155, 271, 284, 294, 321, 332, 428, 454, 505, 509, 649
Zhi Bao Pill, 57, 60, 72, 116, 393, 418, 424, 466, 649
Zhi Gan Cao Decoction, 35, 155, 158, 171, 180, 188, 192, 473, 578, 649
Zhi Jing Powder, 649
Zhi Mi Decoction, 432, 649
Zhi Mi Fu Ling Pill, 387, 650
Zhi Shi Dao Zhi Pill, 28, 475, 481, 650
Zhi Shi Xiao Pi Pill, 619, 650
Zhi Shi Xie Bai Gui Zhi Decoction, 171, 472, 651
Zhi Sou Powder, 93, 651
Zhi Zi Qing Gan Decoction, 504, 651
Zhong Man Fen Xiao Pill, 238, 651
Zhu Che Pill, 217, 652
Zhu Ling Tang, 652
Zhu Sha An Shen Pill, 35, 155, 441, 446, 652
Zhu Ye Shi Gao Decoction, 122, 126, 465, 652
Zi Shui Qing Gan Decoction, 235, 362, 652
Zi Xue. Also named Zi Xue Pellet, 653
Zuo Gui Decoction, 177, 496, 654
Zuo Gui Pill, 51, 168, 172, 277, 313, 388, 426, 428, 433, 449, 477, 479, 490, 653
Zuo Jin Pill, 54, 205, 210, 486, 654

www.ingramcontent.com/pod-product-compliance
Ingram Content Group UK Ltd.
Pitfield, Milton Keynes, MK11 3LW, UK
UKHW051257180426
11947UKWH00020B/1763